# Noninvasive Physiological Measurement

This book explains the principles and techniques of microwave physiological sensing and introduces fundamental results of the noninvasive sensing of physiological signatures, vital signs, as well as life detection. Specifically, noninvasive microwave techniques for contact, contactless, and remote sensing of circulatory and respiratory movements and physiological volume changes are discussed.

*Noninvasive Physiological Measurement: Wireless Microwave Sensing*, is written by a pioneering researcher in microwave noninvasive physiological sensing and leading global expert in microwaves in biology and medicine. The book reviews current advances in noninvasive cardiopulmonary sensing technology and measurement. It includes measurements of the vital signs and physiological signatures from laboratory research and clinical testing. The book discusses the applicable domains and scenarios in which there is an interaction of radio frequency (RF) and microwaves with biological matter in gas, fluid, or solid form, both from inside and outside of the human or animal body. The book also provides examples for healthcare monitoring and diagnostic applications through wearables, devices, or remote contactless sensors for physiological signals and signature, vital signs, and body motion sensing. This book is an essential guide to understanding the human body's interaction with microwaves and noninvasive physiological sensing and monitoring.

This book is intended for researchers and professionals in biomedical, electrical, and computer engineering with an interest in antenna, sensors, microwaves, signal processing, and medical applications. It will also be of interest to healthcare professionals, technologists, and practitioners interested in noninvasive physiological sensing and patient monitoring.

**Dr. James C. Lin's** pioneering work inspired many researchers to follow, and many more to follow them. He is recognized as one of the world's most renowned scientists who has studied microwave and RF radiation in biology and medicine. He has served as a professor of bioengineering, electrical and computer engineering, physiology and biophysics, and physical and rehabilitation medicine.

# Noninvasive Physiological Measurement
## Wireless Microwave Sensing

James C. Lin

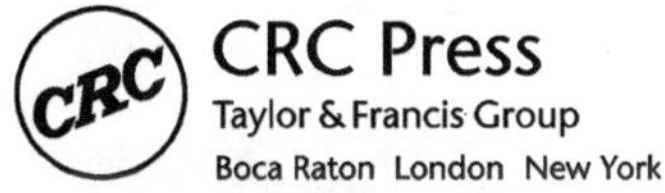


CRC Press is an imprint of the
Taylor & Francis Group, an informa business

Designed cover image: James C. Lin

First edition published 2024
by CRC Press
2385 NW Executive Center Drive, Suite 320, Boca Raton FL 33431

and by CRC Press
4 Park Square, Milton Park, Abingdon, Oxon, OX14 4RN

*CRC Press is an imprint of Taylor & Francis Group, LLC*



**Library of Congress Cataloging-in-Publication Data**

Names: Lin, James C., author.
Title: Noninvasive physiological measurement : wireless microwave sensing / James C. Lin.
Description: First edition. | Boca Raton, FL : CRC Press, 2024. | Includes bibliographical references and index.
Identifiers: LCCN 2023037654 (print) | LCCN 2023037655 (ebook) | ISBN 9781032319155 (hardback) | ISBN 9781032324753 (paperback) | ISBN 9781003315223 (ebook)
Subjects: MESH: Monitoring, Physiologic--methods | Microwaves | Wireless Technology
Classification: LCC RA569.3 (print) | LCC RA569.3 (ebook) | NLM WB 117 |
DDC 612/.014481--dc23/eng/20231113
LC record available at https://lccn.loc.gov/2023037654
LC ebook record available at https://lccn.loc.gov/2023037655

ISBN: 978-1-032-31915-5 (hbk)
ISBN: 978-1-032-32475-3 (pbk)
ISBN: 978-1-003-31522-3 (ebk)

DOI: 10.1201/9781003315223

Typeset in Times
by KnowledgeWorks Global Ltd.

*To my grandsons:*

*Jonah Anderson, Lucas Theodore, and Kai Rong-Zhi*

*and*

*to the bright future that awaits each of them.*

To my grandson

[illegible] Zhi [illegible] Kong-Zhi

[illegible] of them.

# Contents

# List of Figures and Tables

# Preface

It has been known since the early 1970s that Doppler microwave radars can be applied to sense vital signs in humans and animals. The exponential growth of research and development in wireless microwave noninvasive sensing of physiological signatures and volume changes during the past two decades has prompted a special interest in this subject. As a result, there has been a massive outpouring of concepts, technology, and information aimed at achieving, quantifying, and applying connected technological advancements. However, in spite of the tremendous advancement in recent years, there are few textbooks that provide a broad, cohesive treatment in moderate depth of the essential elements of the various aspects of microwave radar sensing in physical fitness, sports medicine, and healthcare delivery. One objective of this book on noninvasive physiological measurement through wireless microwave sensing is to fulfill the need by presenting comprehensive and, amply illustrated coverage of the subject. It is intended for use as a textbook at the graduate or advanced undergraduate level, and as a source of general information for electronic engineers, biomedical scientists, and healthcare professionals interested in research and development of microwave noninvasive physiological sensing to help improve public and patient health.

The book begins with an introduction to the subject and sets off with a historical perspective on pioneering investigations in the subject area. To assist understanding of later materials and discussions, the next four chapters are structured to provide fundamental concepts and methods that underpin the specific themes of application that constitute the last five chapters of the book. Thus, Chapter 3 describes the principles and physical laws governing microwave propagation, reflection, and scattering to augment knowledge of microwave sensing. The two Chapters (i.e., Chapters 4 and 5) that follow are devoted to biophysical topics of the microwave property of biological materials and interactions with biological bodies, with an aim to facilitate an understanding of microwave physiological sensing. Chapter 6 discusses the principles of linear system analysis and signal processing alongside a brief overview of relevant software algorithms to augment detection and extraction of microwave physiological signals. Descriptions of specific algorithms involved in many of the investigations are included with the specific topics discussed in later chapters.

The plans for the rest of the book (i.e., Chapters 7–11) are to describe the leading applications alongside technical advantages and operating principles in each area. These chapters present in-depth discussions of vital-sign detection, monitoring of tissue-volume change and fluid redistribution, arterial pulse wave and pressure determination, wearable sensors, and contemporary applications and advanced topics in noninvasive microwave sensing and measurement. The guiding principles throughout are to start with brief introductions to the specific topics, relevant anatomical structure and physiology, supporting methodologies, and discussions on current state of knowledge, and then progress to incorporation of recent advances within the scope of each topical area. To facilitate an understanding of the measurements and differences in the various organ and tissue systems, essential anatomic and physiological background information is included, where appropriate. It is hoped that this approach will make it unnecessary to refer extensively to the basic textbooks. Nevertheless, specific and general references are given at the end of each chapter. These are provided for the convenience of the readers, who may wish to gain a more detailed knowledge of the subject under discussion, to put the materials in proper perspective, and to overcome potential misunderstanding. Furthermore, to help enhance the pedagogical significance and benefit, the basic and advanced topics described are accompanied by 354 figures and illustrations. I take this opportunity to acknowledge and express my thanks to the many authors for the privilege of reusing published figures, diagrams, or photos in whole or in part, as cited, for illustration in this book.

The many colleagues and students whose contributions to various aspects of the subjects covered in this book are recognized with appreciation. I would like to direct readers to the reference citations for their names that appear in our joint publications. I also wish to express my thanks to the many scientists and researchers for their invaluable suggestions and encouragements in composing the book. Indeed, their scientific works and technical innovations have been an inspiration in the preparation of this book. And importantly, it is with gratitude and love that the author thanks his family for their faith, support, and patience throughout the entire duration in writing this book.

**James Chih-I Lin**
*University of Illinois Chicago*

# Acknowledgments

I would like to express my sincere thanks to those colleagues and fellow scientists and researchers for their magnanimous help in producing and providing various figures for illustration in the book. I am especially obliged to Huei-Ru Chuang, T. S. Jason Horng, Tzuen-Hsi Huang, Jessi Johnson, Asimina Kiourti, Changzhe Li, Lianming Li, Jenshan Lin, Mehrdad Nosrati, Eric Stewart, Toan Khanh Vo Dai, Chao-Hsiung Tseng, Fu-Kang Wang, and Chung-Tse Michael Wu in this regard.

# About the Author

**James C. Lin** is Professor Emeritus at the University of Illinois, Chicago, where he has served as Head of the Bioengineering Department, Director of the Robotics and Automation Laboratory, and Director of Special Projects in Engineering. He held professorships in electrical and computer engineering, bioengineering, physiology and biophysics, and physical and rehabilitation medicine. He received BS, MS and PhD degrees in electrical engineering from the University of Washington, Seattle.

Dr. Lin is a Fellow of American Association for the Advancement of Science (AAAS), American Institute for Medical and Biological Engineering (AIMBE) and the International Scientific Radio Union (URSI), and a Life Fellow of the Institute of Electrical and Electronics Engineers (IEEE). He was recognized in Elsevier's top worldwide scientists in their fields for Career Impact and for Single-Year Impact in 2020. He held a National Science Council Research Chair from 1993 to 1997 and served for many years as an IEEE-Engineering in Medicine and Biology Society distinguished lecturer. He is a recipient of the d'Arsonval Medal from the Bioelectromagnetics Society, IEEE Electromagnetic Compatibility Transactions Prize Paper Award, IEEE COMAR Recognition Award, and CAPAMA Outstanding Leadership and Service Awards. He served as a member of U.S. President's Committee for National Medal of Science (1992 and 1993) and as Chairman of Chinese American Academic & Professional Convention (1993).

Professor Lin has served in leadership positions of several scientific and professional organizations including President of the Bioelectromagnetics Society, Chairman of URSI Commission on Electromagnetics in Biology and Medicine, Co-Chair of URSI Inter-Commission Working Group on Solar Power Satellite, Chairman of the IEEE Committee on Man and Radiation, Vice President US National Council on Radiation Protection and Measurements (NCRP), and member of International Commission on Nonionizing Radiation Protection (ICNIRP). He also served on numerous advisory committees and panels for the U.S. Congress, Office of the U.S. President, National Academy of Sciences, Engineering, and Medicine, National Research Council, National Science Foundation, National Institutes of Health, Marconi Foundation, and the World Health Organization.

He has authored or edited 15 books including the recent book on *Auditory Effects of Microwave Radiation* (Springer, 2021), authored 450 book chapters and journal and magazine articles, and made 300+ conference presentations. He has made many fundamental scientific contributions to electromagnetics in biology and medicine, including microwave auditory effects and microwave thermoacoustic tomography. He has pioneered several medical applications of radio frequency and microwave energies including invention of a minimally invasive microwave ablation treatment for cardiac arrhythmia, and the contact, contactless, and noninvasive microwave sensing of physiological signatures and vital signs. He has chaired several international conferences including IEEE, BEMS and ICST (founding chairman of Wireless Mobile Communication and Healthcare – MobiHealth Conference). He was Editor-in-Chief of the journal *Bioelectromagnetics* from 2006 to 2022, served as a magazine columnist, book series editor, guest editor, and member of the editorial boards of several journals. A member of Sigma Xi, Phi Tau Phi, Tau Beta Pi, and Golden Key honorary societies, and listed in *American Men and Women of Science*, *Who's Who in America*, *Who's Who in Engineering*, *Who's Who in the World*, and *Men of Achievement,* among others.

# 1 Introduction

Monitoring vital signs is an important clinical tool for healthcare practitioners since it can provide a wide range of diagnostic information about the patient with a relatively modest hardware setup. The standard clinical protocol for acquiring vital signs is to apply electrodes and sensors on the patient and wire them to a data acquisition unit, which is typically secured to the patient's body by a strap for continuous ambulatory recordings. For hospitalized patients, the bulky data acquisition unit is placed bedside with cables extending from the body, significantly compromising patient mobility, comfort, and tolerance. While these problems can be considered as inconveniences for adult patients that can be justified by the merits of continuous monitoring, the same experiences can pose as serious challenges for the pediatric population – not only is their physiology significantly different from that of adults, but the physical fragility of neonates and children demands that the vital-sign monitoring technologies intended for children should function as noninvasively as possible and be contactless and unobtrusive, where applicable.

Such technologies would have equally profound applications in monitoring patients with critical burns or victims of hazardous chemical or nuclear contamination. Furthermore, compared to adults, the bundle of cables connecting the electrodes, sensors, and acquisition units can exert excessive force on children's skin and body, restricting the natural movements in both inpatient and outpatient settings. Therefore, there is a great need for vital-sign monitors that are noninvasive, unobtrusive, and noncontact for direct coupling with a patient's body to enable continuous wireless recording and transmission of cardiopulmonary activities. It is desirable that the devices do not require the use of adhesives, gels, and abrasives for minimized impact on the skin, in general, and especially for neonate and children's skin [Ness et al., 2013]. Also, in the context of veterinary healthcare, animals present distinctive vital signs and have radically different skin coverings [Zhou et al., 2020]. Therefore, noninvasive, contactless, and unobtrusive vital-sign sensing would be advantageous. Furthermore, it could bring about a potential microwave radar-based application to differentiate human subjects from animal targets.

In recent years, there has been a dramatic increase in research on the use of microwave and radio frequency (RF) radars for noninvasive physiological measurements. In addition to vital signs, the investigations have involved contact, near-field, contactless, short-range, and remote detection and monitoring of physiological signals and signatures. The signals of interest are associated with physical and physiological movements as well as surface and volume changes in healthy organs and diseased tissues. This interest has been sparked, in part, by pioneering research showing electromagnetic energy, especially in the RF and microwave frequency range, that possesses reasonable dispersion and propagation loss with reliably accurate measurement from outside the body without puncturing or penetrating the skin. The rapid growth in semiconductor electronic fabrication, incredible development of the

DOI: 10.1201/9781003315223-1

cellular mobile communication technology, and the fast-expanding list of miniature chip components, device capabilities, robust engineering designs, and application scenarios have also contributed to the escalation. For example, knowledge of the physiological or pathophysiological status of the heart as a pump for blood and the lungs as a site of gas exchanges is a factor that can greatly assist medical practitioners in the management of patients' cardiovascular and pulmonary conditions and diseases. Indeed, microwave radar technology for sensing vital signs and physiological motions has expanded to sports medicine, fitness sensing, and healthcare monitoring, and, in some cases, it has reached the commercial stage.

Generally, the applicable domains and scenarios include those in which there is an interaction of RF and microwaves with biological matter in gas, fluid, or solid form, both from the inside and outside the human or animal body. They may take the form of wearable, ingestible, or embedded devices, or remote noncontact sensors for physiological signals and signature, vital signs, and motion and location sensing. Moreover, the miniaturization and widespread use of microwave technology and digital processors in Internet of Things (IoT) and common household communication devices makes it feasible to develop low-power, low-cost, and practical radar-type monitors and sensors to help improve the public and personal health status.

These low-power and, in many cases, lightweight RF and microwave sensors function in such a way that they are noninvasive, noncontact, and unobtrusive. They offer convenient real-time measurement without the subject being aware of the presence of the sensor or sensing procedures (i.e., nonintrusive). Microwave and RF technology can transmit through clothing, walls, or other physical barriers and can acquire vital signs from animals with superficial fur or coverings. These unique advantages, capabilities, and features allow the RF and microwave sensors to be used for continuous long-term monitoring, which also makes them amenable to health and safety assessments as well as accessible for covert and security surveillance. They also may be used for vital life-sign detection in support of search-and-rescue missions during emergency and disaster relief. Thus, wireless microwave sensing of physiological signatures and bodily changes could be broadly deployed to encompass wide ranges of human activities and functions encountered in everyday events.

In short, the ability to noninvasively detect and monitor the movement of tissues and organs from outside the body provides many efficient and valuable areas of potential biomedical application. Several noninvasive microwave techniques for contact, contactless, and remote sensing of circulatory and respiratory movements and volume changes have been developed. In general, these systems consist of a microwave generator, a sampling component, a pair of transmitting–receiving antennas, a set of signal conditioning and processing devices, and a display unit. They operate, in general, at continuous wave (CW) frequencies from 1 to 100 GHz and make use of amplitude and/or phase information derived from the received signal. The low average-power density of energy radiated by present systems ranges from approximately 0.01–10 W/m$^2$. These systems can register instantaneous changes in fluid volume, pulse pressure, heartbeat, and respiration rate when in contact with the body surface, at distances from a few millimeters (mm) to greater than 30 m, or behind thick layers of nonconductive structures and walls. In fact, they may be deployed unobtrusively or covertly without knowledge of the participant or targeted individual.

## 1.1 MICROWAVE AND RF RADIATION

The spectra of electromagnetic radiation or waves from low to high frequency begin with electric and magnetic fields to gamma ($\gamma$) rays. Between them are RF, microwave, infrared, and visible light, followed by ultraviolet and X-ray (see Figure 1.1). Electromagnetic waves may be specified in terms of their wavelength or frequency. The speed ($v$) of propagation of electromagnetic waves in a material medium depends on the permittivity ($\varepsilon$) and permeability ($\mu$) properties of the medium. It is given by the product of frequency ($f$) and wavelength ($\lambda$), such that

$$v = f \times \lambda = \frac{1}{\sqrt{\mu\varepsilon}} \tag{1.1}$$

The highest speed at which an electromagnetic wave can travel is $2.998 \times 10^8$ m/s, which is the speed of light traveling in vacuum or free space. In this case, the free space or vacuum permittivity is given by

$$\varepsilon = \varepsilon_0 = 8.854 \times 10^{-12}\, farad/m \tag{1.2}$$

and permeability is given by

$$\mu = \mu_0 = 4\pi \times 10^{-7}\, henry/m \tag{1.3}$$

Wavelength measures the closeness between any two successive peaks or valleys of sinusoidal wave variations or any two successive equivalent points of repetition in a periodic signal, such as zero crossings, as shown in Figure 1.2. Wavelength uses meters (m) as the standard unit of measure. Frequency is defined as any cycle with $2\pi$ variations for the sine wave and is measured in cycles per second (s) or hertz (Hz). It

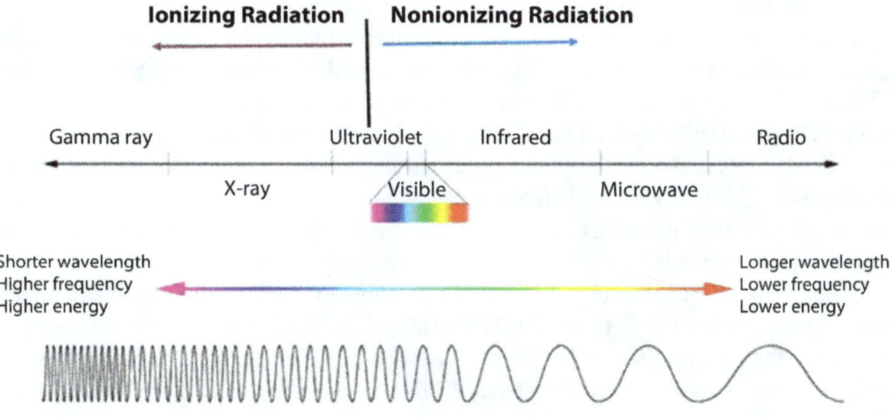


**FIGURE 1.1** A part of the electromagnetic spectrum including microwave and radio frequency radiation.

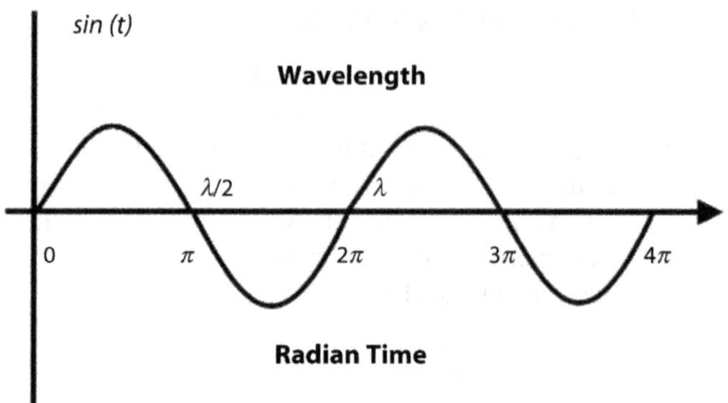


**FIGURE 1.2** The sine wave, sin ($t$), and definition of a wavelength, $\lambda$.

refers to the number of waves that pass a fixed point in unit time. Wavelength and frequency are inversely related, so the higher the frequency, the shorter the wavelength.

### 1.1.1 Frequency Bands and Designations

A list of the wavelengths and frequencies of electromagnetic waves along with some of the common uses and medical applications is provided in Table 1.1. Microwave and RF technology is involved in a wide array of practical, essential, and valuable uses in nearly every aspect of our daily lives. The major areas of application include safety and security, remote monitoring of the Earth's surface, weather surveillance, traffic assistance and control, space exploration, therapeutic intervention, medical and radiological diagnosis, food processing, and others. Simply put, microwave and RF technology enables our connection with others, improves our health and safety, helps us prepare food for our nourishment, and provides for our well-being.

In many of the domestic, industrial, communication, medical, and security applications, common names such as RF, microwave, millimeter wave (mmW), terahertz (THz), or T-wave are used to describe specific regions of the electromagnetic spectrum between 30 kHz and 3 THz (Table 1.2). Also, for the RF region, internationally, the LF, MF, HF, and VHF band designations are often employed to denote the low-, medium-, high-, and very high-frequency bands, respectively. Likewise, microwave radiation may be further divided into UHF (ultrahigh frequency) and SHF (super high frequency) bands.

Another practice is the use of letter designations for various regions of the microwave spectrum from 1 GHz to 110 GHz (Table 1.3). The letter designations starting with L at the low-frequency end run through S, C, X, etc. [IEEE, 2020]. The various letter bands have official frequency limits but are not in any alphabetical order. The K-band has two official subdesignations, the Ku and Ka bands. The lower Ku band describes the frequency range from 12 to 18 GHz, and likewise, the Ka band normally defines frequencies above 27 GHz. However, despite the precise designations, in common usage, the K band is used to represent frequencies above 22 GHz normally designated as the Ka band.

**TABLE 1.1**
**Approximate Wavelength, Frequency, Common Uses, and Some Medical Applications of the Various Regions of the Electromagnetic Spectrum**

| | Wavelength (m) | Frequency (Hz) | Common Uses | Medical Applications |
|---|---|---|---|---|
| **Radio Frequency (RF)** | >1.0 | $<3 \times 10^8$ | Broadcast radio and television; aircraft and ship navigation | MR imaging; cancer treatment; cardiac ablation |
| **Microwave** | $1 \times 10^{-3} - 1 \times 10^{-0}$ | $3 \times 10^8 - 3 \times 10^{11}$ | Telecommunication; microwave oven; radar; Earth sensing | Cardiac ablation; cancer treatment, diathermy |
| **Infrared** | $7 \times 10^{-7} - 1 \times 10^{-3}$ | $3 \times 10^{11} - 4 \times 10^{14}$ | Night vision camera; flame detection | Temperature sensor; infrared sauna |
| **Optical** | $4 \times 10^{-7} - 7 \times 10^{-7}$ | $4 \times 10^{14} - 7.5 \times 10^{14}$ | Optic fiber; lidar; solar cell | Pulse oximeter; laser surgery |
| **Ultraviolet (UV)** | $1 \times 10^{-8} - 4 \times 10^{-7}$ | $7.5 \times 10^{14} - 3 \times 10^{16}$ | Sanitation; disinfection; air purification | Sterilizing bacteria; vitamin B production |
| **X-ray** | $1 \times 10^{-11} - 1 \times 10^{-8}$ | $3 \times 10^{16} - 3 \times 10^{19}$ | X-ray imaging; material inspection; fault detection | Mammography; X-ray tomography |
| **Gamma ray** | $<1 \times 10^{-11}$ | $>3 \times 10^{19}$ | Non-destructive testing; crack detection; astrophysics | Nuclear medicine; cancer radiotherapy |

**TABLE 1.2**
**Internationally Designated Frequency Band of the RF and Microwave Regions of the Electromagnetic Spectrum**

| Common Name | Band Designation | Frequency Range |
|---|---|---|
| **RF** | Low frequency (LF) | 30–300 kHz |
| | Medium frequency (MF) | 300 kHz–3 MHz |
| | High frequency (HF) | 3–30 MHz |
| | Very high frequency (VHF) | 30–300 MHz |
| **Microwave** | Ultrahigh frequency (UHF) | 300 MHz–3 GHz |
| | Super high frequency (SHF) | 3–30 GHz |
| **Millimeter wave (mmW)** | Extremely high frequency (EHF) | 30–300 GHz |
| **Terahertz wave (T-wave)** | Tremendously high frequency (THF) or Terahertz (THz) | 300 GHz–3 THz |

**TABLE 1.3**
**Commonly Used Letter Band Designations of the Microwave Region of the Electromagnetic Spectrum**

| Common Letter Band Designation | Frequency Range |
|---|---|
| L | 1–2 GHz |
| S | 2–4 GHz |
| C | 4–8 GHz |
| X | 8–12 GHz |
| K | 18–27 GHz |
| Ku | 12–18 GHz |
| Ka | 22–36 GHz |
| Q | 36–46 GHz |
| V | 40–75 GHz |
| W | 75–110 GHz |

In addition, there is an industrial, scientific, and medical (ISM) band that is traditionally set aside for unlicensed operations of the named services. They are centered around 6.78, 13.56, 27.12, 40.68, 433.92, and 915 MHz and 2.45, 5.8, and 24.125 GHz. These are exclusively applied to the named bands for their name's sake. However, currently, these frequencies are also being used for cellular and terrestrial communication applications such as Wi-Fi, Bluetooth, and radiolocation services. However, fixed, cellular and mobile communication services operating within these bands must accept any technologically damaging interference that may be caused by other ISM applications.

Microwaves are generated as CW sinusoids or pulses of various forms and are transmitted in CW, baseband, amplitude- or frequency-modulated carrier waves, or pulse-amplitude modulated waves. In some high-power microwave applications, magnetron tubes are the generator of choice, although in some cases, the multiple-beam klystron are favored. For example, an airborne radar based on the magnetron may be used for detecting aircraft or ships at sea, while the klystron is used as a low-power local oscillator for the receiver. However, in many current wireless communication and data transmission systems, solid-state semiconductor devices have replaced both the magnetron and klystron tubes.

Scenarios where sources generate high levels of microwave and RF energy are typically found in food processing plants and medical facilities, such as magnetic resonance imaging (MRI) scanners, or specialized establishments with high-power radars. Some medical diagnostic imaging procedures may involve high levels of microwave and RF radiation at the patient's location or even inside a patient's body. Situations associated with personal use by the public, such as cellular mobile phone, wireless communication, data transmission, or security operations, produce comparably much lower exposures at the position of the user.

## 1.2 MICROWAVE RADAR TECHNOLOGY

The word "radar" was coined in the 1930s as a shortened version of "radio detection and ranging." Initially, the primary purpose of radar was to detect the presence and range of aircraft and ships at sea. Modern radars are used to detect the presence, direction, distance, and speed of objects by sending out RF and microwaves that are reflected off the object back to the source. Doppler radars are typically used to detect moving objects and ascertain their velocity. Current uses of microwave radar have extended to numerous civilian applications where information on relative location and speed of objects of interest is crucial. Common examples include air traffic control, weather monitoring, marine navigation, and autonomous vehicles (self-driving cars) for collision avoidance as well as for proximity of humans, animals, and birds.

The pioneering experiment of radar as a tool for detecting ships and aircraft was conducted with a CW system in 1922 [Skolnik, 1980]. The first pulse radar was designed specifically to detect the conducting layer of the ionosphere [Breit and Tuve, 1926]. The development of pulse radar for detecting objects on Earth began in the 1930s [Taylor et al., 1934]. The first pulse radars operated at a frequency of 60 MHz in the RF range. Radars may be designed to operate in CW, pulse, or Doppler mode, or any combination based on their operational objective, scheme, and configuration.

Today, typical radar operations involve high-power microwave and RF radiation extending from a few kilowatts (kW) to several megawatts (MW). Some military radar installations may have operating power at gigawatt (GW) levels. Most of these operations involve the use of pulse or other modulation techniques to acquire both location and velocity information. Also, many modern radar applications are based on solid-state systems for high- and low-power applications. Furthermore, many small, lightweight, and low-profile modern radar applications use powers that are at or below the milliwatt (mW) level [Balanis, 2008; Michler et al., 2021].

The first steps in realizing the dream of a truly wireless mobility scenario with a completely tether-free electric power supply have been reported [Talla et al., 2017]. A prototype battery-free mobile phone harvesting 3.5 $\mu$W of power was demonstrated by using a combination of analog and digital circuit architectures and a high-efficiency rectenna. The prototype cellular mobile phone was able to place voice calls by harvesting RF power from the laboratory base station. It is significant to note that, at present, the maximum allowable power consumption is 125–250 mW for cellular mobile phones, which are about five orders of magnitude higher than the battery-free prototype's power consumption. Furthermore, the minuscule 3.5 $\mu$W of power consumption suggests that the high levels of currently allowable 125–250 mW RF powers for mobile phones may become unnecessary in the future. Low-power wireless devices may be able to transmit or receive data and voice calls over long distances via energy harvesting without batteries [Lin, 2021b]. It is conceivable that future developments would not only enable mobile phone operations with data transmission via energy harvesting, but also for ultralow power microwave sensing of physiological signals for biomedical applications.

## 1.3 PHYSIOLOGICAL SENSING AND RADIOLOGICAL IMAGING

The sensing and imaging of physiological variables and pathophysiological modifications may be classified into active and passive modes. Of interest in both situations is the energy transfer between a source and a receiver. The fundamental principle of sensing and imaging is to provide necessary and sufficient energy into the propagation channel of interest to enable relevant observations on the human or animal body. To accomplish the objective involves the analysis of energy or waves that propagate from a transmitter to the receiver.

There are several current and potential methods for active microwave sensing and imaging (Figure 1.3). Spatially resolved images may be formed through either projection or tomographic reconstruction processes to display tissue composition differences and depict dielectric permittivity changes associated with tissue structural discontinuities. They include the well-known, clinically efficacious MRI [Bushong and Clarke, 2015] and other modalities under current investigation, such as microwave imaging and microwave thermoacoustic tomography [Lin, 2021a]. Alternatively, time-varying signatures can be detected to permit active interrogation of cutaneous and subcutaneous tissue movements and changes, even though the spatial resolution that can be attained may be restricted.

In the case of reflection measurement, the microwave energy transmitted from the source antenna is backscattered by the biological target and received by the detection system. The backscattered wave provides information on the biological target and on channel factors that govern the propagation to and from the biological target. In contrast, passive measurement involves observation of microwave emissions from subcutaneous tissues, and conversion of those thermally generated microwave emissions to tissue temperatures. This radiometric technique can noninvasively measure

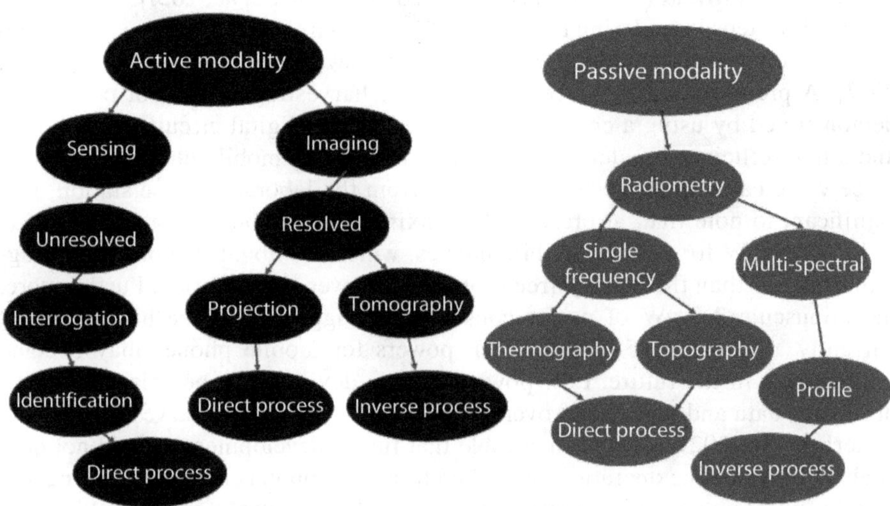


**FIGURE 1.3** Active and passive modalities for noninvasive microwave sensing of physiological changes and conditions.

subcutaneous tissue temperatures to a depth of several centimeters. Furthermore, when medical radiometric measurements are made at several different frequencies or positions, it is possible to retrieve the temperature profiles as a function of depth in tissue. However, a stable and unique mathematical solution to this inverse problem is not guaranteed. Nevertheless, some promising approaches have emerged in recent years.

## 1.4 MICROWAVE SENSING OF PHYSIOLOGICAL SIGNATURES AND MOVEMENTS

Research interests in the use of low-power microwave and RF radar technology for contact and remote detection and monitoring of physiological signals, signatures, movements, and volume changes under physiological and pathophysiological conditions have been growing steadily since the early 1970s. The same principle of detecting the frequency or phase shift in a reflected radar signal can be used to detect small physiological movements and changes using a system such as that shown in Figure 1.4. The ability of Doppler microwave and RF radars to provide location and velocity information of both stationary and moving biological objects without disturbing the subject has attracted considerable attention from researchers, especially in the past decade. Most of the groundbreaking efforts in this area in the 1970s and 1980s have been toward proof-of-concept and prototype development as well as testing through human and animal experimentation. Many of the pioneering contributions to physiological microwave sensing, such as cardiovascular detection, pulmonary–respiratory monitoring, and vital-sign sensing, occurred in this period. Previous summaries and accounts of the investigations that took place in the 1970s and 1980s in developing applications of Doppler microwaves for noninvasive contact, contactless, and remote detection and monitoring of physiological signatures, movements, and volume changes are available in published works [Lin, 1986, 1989, 1992, 1993, 1999; Rozzell and Lin, 1987]. Current interest, progress, and technological innovations demonstrate the tremendous resilience of and enthusiasm for noninvasive microwave physiological sensing technology and application [Li et al., 2013, 2021].

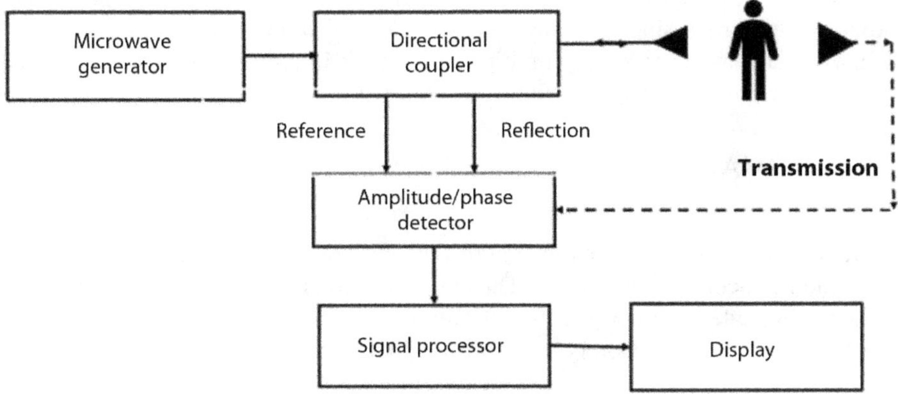


**FIGURE 1.4** Basic functional diagram of a Doppler microwave physiological sensor.

What follows in Chapter 2 is a description in historical context of the remote, noncontact, and noninvasive contact sensing of physiological movements associated with the expansion and contraction of the circulatory and respiratory systems. The noninvasive, contact, noncontact, remotely measured physiological signatures and vital signs are made possible by using the Doppler microwave radar principle and technology. These investigations, first begun in the 1970s and progressed into the 1980s, helped set the stage for much of the research that followed. Around the year 2000, most of the progress in this area was concentrated on improving components, devices, and systems supplemented with signal-processing algorithms to enhance sensor performance. These technology developments pushed toward smaller form factor, better accuracy, lower power, lighter weight, longer detection range, and more robust operation for portable and handheld scenarios [Li et al., 2013]. However, it should be noted that the fundamental approach to and principle of sensing remained steadfast, which is to provide necessary and sufficient source energy into the channel of interest to enable relevant sensing observations on the body channel. Fortuitously, for probing human and animal bodies, RF and microwaves possess frequency ranges with acceptable dispersion and propagation loss for accurate and reliably sensitive measurements. Indeed, the microwave-sensed physiological signals contain significant information about a subject's range, motion, material composition, and surface boundary features that are distinguishable in a heterogeneously complex biological background, which will form the bulk of the discussion in later chapters of this book.

Aside from furthering improvement in components and systems such as the sensing front end and radio frequency identification (RFID) tags, current research efforts have been devoted to more sophisticated signal-processing schemes, including machine learning and artificial intelligence, leveraging other wireless infrastructure, such as Wi-Fi and IoT, and integrated adoptive systems extending to emerging applications to continuous authentication, behavior recognition, occupancy sensing, and search-and-rescue operations [Islam et al., 2022; Li et al., 2021; Thi Phuoc Van et al., 2019]. Thus, a robust research trend is likely to continue going forward. The research and development opportunities associated with accurate, precise, and more sophisticated applications would come with challenges in sensor design, range sensitivity, signal processing, vibration and motion artifact and clutter anomaly reduction, especially when involving multiple subjects or in crowded environments, and complex emergency and search-and-rescue operations, among others.

## 1.5 OPTIMAL MICROWAVE FREQUENCY FOR PHYSIOLOGICAL SENSING

There are two main strategies for microwave physiological sensing: direct-contact and remote noncontact approaches. The remote noncontact strategy is to make observations using reflected microwaves in the air, which permits sensing without disturbing the subject. It may also be accomplished by transmission of microwave signals through physical barriers or obstacles without compromising the integrity of the physiological or anatomical structures [Lin, 1986, 1989]. It includes the contactless near-field scheme, a strategy utilized by many reported studies. The direct-contact strategy is to place the microwave sensor's front end against the skin over the biological target organ or tissue of interest. Thus, the subject is aware of the sensor and measurement process, yet the procedure remains noninvasive. It may not be practical for premature neonates or patients with critical burns or injury to the skin. However, it offers the diagnostic potential of penetrating microwave radiation.

### 1.5.1 Remote, Near-Field, and Noncontact Strategy

The propagation of microwaves in a material medium depend on the permittivity ($\varepsilon$) and permeability ($\mu$) properties of the medium. The wavelength is inversely related to frequency through the equation for speed of propagation, which is constant for a given material (see Eq. 1.1); thus, the higher the frequency, the shorter the wavelength and vice versa (Table 1.4). Furthermore, in general, for sensing applications, a higher frequency and shorter wavelength will provide more accuracy and better spatial resolution in support of more reliable differential sensing.

It should be noted that there is wavelength contraction when going from air to tissue materials with a relative dielectric constant of $\varepsilon_t$, as shown in Eq. (1.4), where $\lambda_0$ and $\lambda_t$ are the wavelengths in a vacuum and tissue, respectively.

$$\lambda_t = \frac{\lambda_0}{\sqrt{\varepsilon_t}} \tag{1.4}$$

The optimal or most viable frequencies for each strategy may vary depending on the microwave propagation differences of in-air and through-tissue operations. They may fundamentally influence the effectiveness, sensitivity, or quality of microwave-detected physiological signals. To date, the frequencies in the 433 MHz to 60 GHz range have been used the most for physiological sensing. However, the question of an optimal frequency for physiological sensing microwaves has been explored only to a limited extent [Lin, 1985].

**TABLE 1.4**
**Frequency and Wavelength in Air, Lungs, and Skin (Muscle) in the RF and Microwave Region of the Electromagnetic Spectrum**

| | Wavelength (mm) | | |
|---|---|---|---|
| Frequency (GHz) | $\lambda_0$ in Air | $\lambda_t$ in Skin and Muscle | $\lambda_t$ in Lungs |
| 0.433 | 693 | 85 | 108 |
| 0.915 | 328 | 44 | 54 |
| 2.450 | 123 | 18 | 22 |
| 5.800 | 52 | 8 | 10 |
| 10.00 | 30 | 5 | 6 |
| 25 | 12 | 2.83 | — |
| 40 | 7.5 | 2.17 | — |
| 60 | 5 | 1.75 | — |

Table 1.4 presents frequency and wavelength in air, lungs, and skin (muscle) in the microwave region of the electromagnetic spectrum from 433 MHz to 60 GHz. For remote noncontact sensing in regions filled with air, the wavelengths vary from a long 123 mm down to 5 mm between 2.45 and 60 GHz, a reduction factor of nearly 25. This fact could potentially help to improve the spatial resolving power down to 0.5 mm using 60 GHz for sensing movements and vibrations at the skin surface. Thus, 60 GHz would be a good choice for using radar reflection measurements in air. For near-zone noncontact sensing with sophisticated signal processing algorithms, the spatial resolution could be reduced by another factor of 2 to 10 to potentially reach 50 microns ($\mu$m). The propagation distance of mmWs is limited at 60 GHz compared to 2.45 GHz. Furthermore, even at 2.45 GHz, the attainable spatial resolution could reach 10% of a wavelength, i.e., 1.2 mm, which is of sufficiently high sensitivity and broad bandwidth to enable noninvasive microwave remote sensing of physiological signals and changes. These observations indicate that there may not be an optimal frequency for remote noncontact sensing. Instead, the efficiency may be dependent on the specific application in target space and frequency.

For near-field noncontact scenarios, antennas are normally spaced at distances of 1.0–5.0 cm from the subject and make use of the scattered field for detection. Depending on the size and wavelength ratio, microwaves reaching a receiving antenna under these circumstances may follow multitudinous pathways in and around the body. The multipath propagation may impose severe limitations, especially on experiments involving transmission measurement [Yamaura, 1977]. Also note that due to the wavelength contraction phenomenon of Eq. (1.2), the wavelength in muscle tissue is nearly 10 times shorter than that in air at 2.45 GHz, while those at 5.8 and 10 GHz are reduced by roughly a factor of six.

However, for contactless Doppler radar vital sign detection, there is another consideration for the optimum microwave frequency. As mentioned, a common understanding of microwave Doppler radar is that the higher the microwave frequency, the shorter the wavelength and, thus, the higher the detection sensitivity. Typical values of human chest-wall movement range from 0.8 to 1.8 mm; the amplitude of heartbeat-induced movement is about 0.08 mm. By modeling the harmonics and the intermodulation interference, simulations have shown that there is an optimum upper carrier frequency for microwave contact vital-sign detection [Li and Lin, 2007]. It was observed that the problem of harmonics is more severe than that of intermodulation. Optimization may be achieved by minimizing the effect of harmonics interference and intermodulation interference on detection accuracy. For typical values of human chest-wall movement, the simulation showed that the upper bound of the microwave frequency as the lower region of the Ka band for improved detection accuracy.

### 1.5.2 Direct-Contact Strategy

There are situations where direct-contact methods that minimize scattered radiation may be preferable over noncontact schemes. In this case, backscattered radiation can be efficiently employed in diagnostic applications using reflection measurement, since multipath propagation contributes less significantly to backscattered or reflected radiation. A vexing design conflict under the direct-contact sensing strategy is the choice of frequency or wavelength of operation because of the diagnostic potential of penetrating microwaves and their propagation characteristics in a tissue medium. This is important from two perspectives, spatial resolution and depth of penetration. The advantage for penetration with deep-lying organs argues for a lower frequency of operation. In contrast, diffraction-limited sensing systems prefer higher operating frequencies for enhanced resolution. These requirements conspire to dictate the decision concerning the optimal frequency of operation.

For simplicity, we assume plane-wave propagation in homogeneous media, which may be characterized in terms of the constants of the medium: wavelength in tissue $\lambda_t$ and the attenuation coefficient $\alpha$ (See Chapter 3). In general, attenuation increases while wavelength decreases with increasing frequency. In the frequency range investigated (up to 10 GHz), especially the range of interest of 915 MHz or higher, the dielectric constants have values of 5–50 for soft tissues (skin, fat, lungs, muscle, etc.) and conductivities have values of 1–500 S/m (See Chapter 4). This wide range of values could provide extremely high reflectivity for microwave radar sensing of biological tissues. The calculated attenuation coefficient and wavelength in tissue for low- (fat) and high-water-content tissues (muscle/skin) are given in Figure 1.5.

While the attenuation coefficient for low-water-content tissue remains relatively constant around 0.5 per cm, it rapidly increases from 0.5 to 3 per centimeter for muscle tissue. Nonetheless, there is significant microwave penetration into the tissue medium. The wavelength in tissue decreases nearly exponentially for both fat and muscle. Note that the wavelength in fat and muscle experiences a contraction from that in air. In fact, it may reduce the effective wavelength by factors of 7.5-to-1 and 7.5-to-3, respectively, for muscle and fat at 4 GHz. This wavelength contraction permits spatial resolutions as small as 0.5 mm (tenth wavelength) for diffraction-limited sensing systems. It can be seen in Figure 1.4 that the shaded region bound by 2–8 GHz represents a frequency span most suited for direct-contact microwave sensing of biological tissue. In this region, the attenuation through tissue is sufficiently

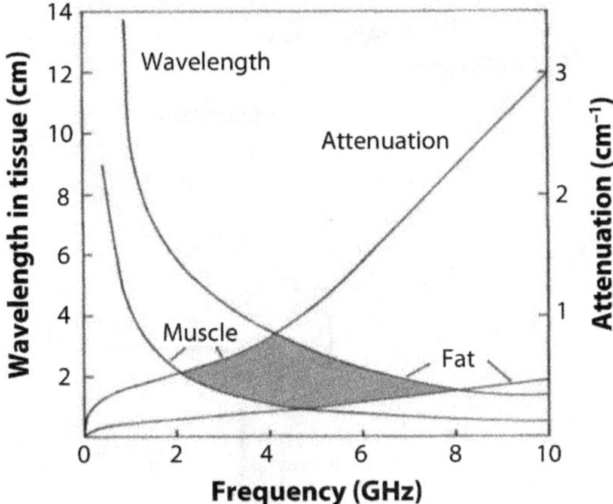


**FIGURE 1.5** Frequencies for minimal attenuation of microwave signals and maximal spatial resolution in skin (muscle) and fat tissues.

low to allow a detectable signal at the front end of a radar receiver, and the spatial resolution is sufficiently short to yield diagnostically useful information. Therefore, 2–8 GHz appears to be optimal for the direct-contact microwave sensing of biological structures in the abdomen, head, and thorax. In fact, in this frequency span, microwaves have acceptable dispersion and propagation loss for accurate contact measurements and are amenable for probing inside human body noninvasively.

It should be noted that for noncontact and remote sensing of physiological parameters, especially through intervening low-loss materials, a lower frequency of operation could become advantageous for a lengthier propagation range and deeper penetration depth through low-loss physical materials.

## 1.6 BENCH-TOP SYSTEMS FOR MICROWAVE PHYSIOLOGICAL SENSING

Most of the efforts in sensing physiological signatures and movements described previously that use microwave Doppler radar date back to the early 1970s. The required architecture for the radar instrumentation was based on general-purpose microwave communication laboratory instruments supplemented with a few custom-designed and built components (see Figure 1.3). This approach is efficient in facilitating exploration and detailed investigations in some cases. The growing research interest in microwave detection of vital signs and physiological events has prompted the development of many experimental systems for dedicated application scenarios [Chan and Lin, 1987; Chen et al. 1986, 2000; Droitcour et al. 2004; Kuo et al., 2016; Lee and Lin, 1985]. The microwave radar systems using fixed RF circuitry can be complicated, limiting, and inefficient for exploratory research. For research that focuses on physiological event detection employing advanced signal analysis, processing algorithms, and pattern-recognition techniques rather than the detection system itself, the hardware instrumentation often can become a formidable challenge.

An experimental setup was proposed that updates the bench-top systems in the block diagram of a microwave physiological sensor given in Figure 1.4. The updated system shown in Figure 1.6 uses more recent general-purpose microwave

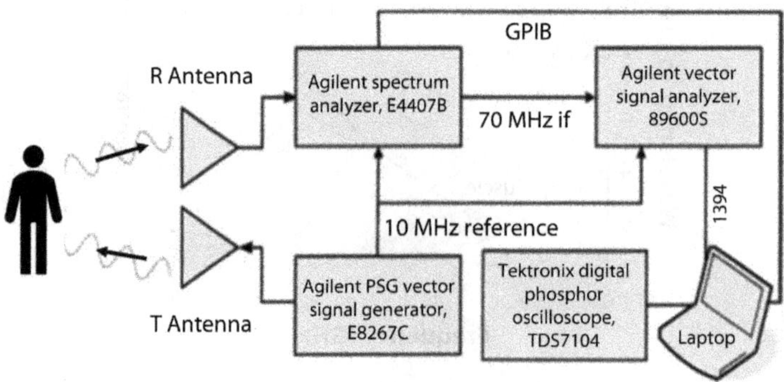


**FIGURE 1.6** System setup of a Doppler microwave radar system for vital-sign measurement.

communication test equipment and instruments [Gu et al., 2010]. It consists of the following laboratory test instruments and components: a signal generator (Agilent E8267C), spectrum analyzer (Agilent E4407B), and vector signal analyzer (Agilent 89600S). The flexible and dependable test setup can be quickly assembled in the laboratory and is easily reconfigurable. It is a flexible approach for prototyping and for conducting investigations in supporting exploratory research to acquire experimental or preliminary data. It can also be used as a foundational instrumentation setup for advanced signal analysis and processing research. It is interesting to note that the bench-top, instrument-based system incorporates a heterodyne digital quadrature demodulation design that helps to mitigate I/Q mismatch occurring in the analog quadrature down converter, which eliminates a potentially performance-limiting imbalance issue. Furthermore, it is a tunable broadband system in which the microwave carrier frequency could be tuned from 1 to 18 GHz. Its performance on detection of vital signs from human subjects has been tested in the laboratory environment with a 2.4 GHz patch antenna array and a broadband antenna. The bench-top instrumentation system offers a quick solution for a prototype to conduct noninvasive microwave measurements of vital signs and signal processing algorithm developments.

## 1.7 TELEMEDICINE AND THE COVID-19 PANDEMIC

The concept of telemedicine was introduced more than 50 years ago. It represents the utilization of telecommunication technology for medical diagnosis, treatment, and patient care. Since then, the enabling technology has grown considerably and is now supported by interactive video, high-resolution monitors, computer networks, smart cellular phones, and a high-speed information infrastructure that includes fiber optics and satellites [Ekeland et al., 2010; Lin, 1999; Su et al., 2016]. Telemedicine enables a physician or specialist at one site to deliver healthcare, patient diagnoses, medical assistance, therapy, or consult with another physician or paramedical personnel at a remote site [Baer et al., 1997; Lin, 1999]. Thus, the aim of telemedicine is to provide expert-based healthcare to distant sites and to provide advanced care through modern telecommunication and information technologies. Note that the definition of telemedicine is different from telehealth [HRSA, 2022]. While telemedicine refers specifically to delivery of remote clinical services, telehealth can refer to remote nonclinical services, such as provider training, administrative conferences, and continuing medical education, in addition to clinical services.

Telemedicine practice has increased dramatically, especially over the past few years. The use of telemedicine is likely continue to increase even after the return of face-to-face patient interactions following the coronavirus disease 2019 (COVID-19) pandemic, as healthcare providers are frequently be tasked with managing telemedicine and remote patient monitoring. Microwave radar-based contactless sensing techniques can facilitate the remote automatic transfer of heartbeat and breathing rate information to provide quick diagnoses and to assist healthcare professionals to make clearer judgments on patient management and appropriate treatment. The advent of the once-in-a-century COVID-19 pandemic has caused the routine practice of taking a patient's vital signs to become an arduous assignment. Interestingly, microwave radar-based noninvasive contactless vital-sign sensing for COVID-19 is being explored for potential applications in detecting COVID-19 cases and assisting healthcare workers to care for COVID-19 patients [Islam et al., 2021; Taylor et al., 2020]. Specifically, the detection of irregular breathing patterns, which is a major manifestation of COVID-19, and the sensing of heartbeats can provide a monitoring system for the patient's cardiovascular system functions. Furthermore, it is conceivable that microwave sensors could be incorporated into a handheld device (such as a smartphone) for wireless healthcare applications and remote physiological monitoring.

More and more, telemedicine is considered a service to provide increased access to high-quality healthcare that is efficient and cost effective. There is solid evidence supporting the use of telemedicine for management, counseling, and interventions including remote monitoring of chronic conditions such as cardiovascular and respiratory diseases. For clinical applications, virtual care has been shown to be equivalent to in-person care in some cases. The recent reviews conducted to examine the current state of the application of telemedicine amid the COVID-19 pandemic have been encouraging. The benefits of continuing telemedicine usage in the future speak to the advantages of telemedicine going forward, which include the ability to extend access to specialty services and the potential to help mitigate the looming physician and healthcare personnel shortages [Hincapié (Chincapin) et al., 2020; Kichloo et al., 2020]. The COVID-19 pandemic has accelerated the use of telemedicine. As a tool, it has transformed the provision of medical services and overcome difficulties for patient care during the pandemic. Its benefits are specific to different fields of medical practice. For example, compared to conventional care, telemedicine is more effective in improving treatment outcomes for diabetes patients, especially for those with type 2 diabetes [Su et al., 2016]. However, comprehensive and effective implementation of telemedicine may vary according to specialties. It is important to engage telemedicine services into the healthcare landscape, to reap the benefits of this service in the future, and, perhaps, to be prepared for future pandemics.

## 1.8 PROTECTION LIMITS FOR HUMAN EXPOSURE TO MICROWAVES

There are two U.S. government agencies that have issued exposure rules and regulations concerning the health and safety of RF and microwave radiation: the Federal Communications Commission (FCC) and Occupational Safety and Health Administration (OSHA). The FCC evaluates the effect of emissions from FCC-regulated RF and microwave transmitters on the quality of the human environment. It recently reaffirmed the exposure limits that it had first adopted in 1996 [FCC, 2019; Lin, 2020]. The RF and microwave exposure rules established by the FCC are based on specific absorption rate (SAR) and maximum permissible exposure (MPE) limits [FCC, 2022]. SAR is the accepted metric or quantity that corresponds to the relative amount of RF and microwave power deposition (energy absorption) in a portion of the body (i.e., any part of a user of a wireless device), or the entire body in the radiation domain of a Wi-Fi antenna or base station. The basic restrictions for human exposure are defined by SAR limits. MPE limits are derived from the SAR limits in terms of free-space field strength and power density. Specifically, it established a quantity of local tissue SAR of 1.6 W/kg, as determined in any 1 g of body tissue. Also, an average value of 0.08 W/kg in any 1 g of body tissue was set for whole-body exposures for the general population. A whole-body average SAR of 0.4 W/kg was chosen as the restriction to provide protection for occupational exposure.

The MPE applicable to both the general population and to occupational exposures in terms of power density are 10 and 50 W/m$^2$ for 1.5–100 GHz, respectively. These limits are for whole-body continuous exposure for indefinite time periods. Exposure levels higher than these limits are permitted by the FCC for shorter exposure times, as long as the average exposure is over a period not more than (or equal to) the specified averaging time of 30 minutes and 6 minutes, respectively, for the general population and occupational exposure.

OSHA, by statute, sets standards and regulations for RF and microwave radiation as a part of a larger nonionizing radiation safety program. Currently, there are no specific OSHA standards for RF and microwave radiation. Its voluntary exposure limit of 100 W/m$^2$ is a guideline but not a requirement for application to various occupational exposure situations [OSHA, 2022]. It does not create additional employer obligations and it is unenforceable as a government law. However, although the limit is not within OSHA regulations, it does provide guidance related to worker protection. Furthermore, from time to time, OSHA can update its guidance in response to new scientific information. Note that vital-sign radar sensors have power density ranging from 0.01–1.10 W/m$^2$ [see Sections 2.2 and 8.2; Johnson et al., 2019; Kagawa et al., 2016]. Clearly, these radar sensors can function at levels well below those permitted by the FCC microwave safety rules and OSHA guidelines. Further discussions on standards and guidelines for safety levels with respect to human exposure to electric, magnetic, and electromagnetic fields including microwave and RF radiation are given in the references [Lin, 2022; 2023a,b].

## 1.9 ORGANIZING PRINCIPLES OF THE BOOK

The motivation for writing this book is to present coherently, in a single volume, many of the multidisciplinary research studies of the wireless microwave noninvasive sensing of physiological signatures that have undergone exponential growth in recent years. The research and development approaches range from putative applications to prototype realizations. The objective is to provide a clearer understanding and better appreciation of pioneering investigations, recent accomplishments, and future advances in microwave noninvasive physiological sensing. It will begin with a historical perspective on pioneering investigations in the subject area. From that point, the book is substantively divided into two parts. The four chapters that immediately follow are structured to provide fundamental concepts and methodologies that underpin the specific application topics that constitute the last five chapters of the book. Thus, Chapter 3 discusses the physical laws governing RF and microwave propagation, reflection, and scattering to enrich the knowledge of wireless microwave sensing. Chapters 4 and 5 are devoted to the biophysical topics of the microwave properties of biological materials and microwave interaction with biological bodies for better understanding of the sensing phenomena. They are followed by

Chapter 6, which discusses the principles of linear system analysis and signal processing alongside a brief overview of relevant software algorithms to augment signal detection and extraction. It is noted that brief descriptions of specific algorithms involved in many of the investigations are included with the specific topics to be discussed in subsequent chapters.

Chapters 7 through 11 will describe the leading applications alongside technical advantages and operating principles under various situations. These chapters present in-depth discussions of vital-sign detection, monitoring of tissue-volume change and redistribution, arterial pulse wave and pressure determination, wearable sensors and sensing, and contemporary applications and advanced topics in noninvasive microwave sensing and measurement. The guiding principles throughout are to start with brief introductions to the specific topics at hand, their supporting methods, and a discussion of the current state of knowledge, and then progress to incorporate recent advances within the scope of each topical area. To facilitate understanding and appreciation of the measurements and differences of the various organ and tissue systems, relevant information on anatomy and physiology is included, where appropriate. It is hoped that this approach will make it unnecessary to refer extensively to basic textbooks. Nevertheless, specific and general references are given at the end of each chapter. These are intended for the convenience of the reader who wishes to obtain a more detailed knowledge of the subject areas.

## REFERENCES

Baer, L., Elford, D. R., Cukor, P., 1997. Telepsychiatry at forty: What have we learned? Harv. Rev. Psychiatry, 5(1):7–17

Balanis, C., Ed. 2008. Modern Antenna Handbook. Hoboken: Wiley

Breit, G., Tuve, M., 1926. A test of the existence of the conducting layer. Phys. Rev., 28:554

Bushong, S. C., Clarke, G., 2015. Magnetic Resonance Imaging, 4th ed, St Louis: Mosby

Chan, K. H., Lin, J. C., 1987. Microprocessor based cardiopulmonary rate monitor. Med. Biol. Eng. Comput., 25:41–44

Chen, K. M., Huang, Y., Zhang, J., Norman, A., 2000. Microwave life detection systems for searching human subjects under earthquake rubble and behind barrier. IEEE Trans. Biomed. Eng., 47(1):105–114

Chen, K. M., Misra, D., Chuang, H. R., Postow, E., 1986. An X-band microwave life-detection system. IEEE Trans. Biomed. Eng., 33(7):697–701

Droitcour, A. D., Boric-Lubecke, O., Lubecke, V. M., Lin, J., Kovac, G. T. A., 2004. Range correlation and I/Q performance benefits in single-chip silicon Doppler radars for noncontact cardiopulmonary monitoring. IEEE Trans. Microw. Theory Tech., 52(3):838–848

Ekeland, A. G., Bowes, A., Flottorp, S., 2010. Effectiveness of telemedicine: A systematic review of reviews. Int. J. Med. Inform, 79(11):736–771

FCC, 2019. Resolution of notice of inquiry, second report and order, notice of proposed rulemaking, and memorandum opinion and order, U.S. Federal Communications Commission (FCC), Washington, D.C., FCC 19-126. Adopted: Nov. 27, 2019; Released: Dec. 4, 2019. [Online]. https://docs.fcc.gov/public/attachments/FCC-19-126A1.pdf

FCC, 2022. Radiofrequency radiation exposure limits. Displaying title 47, up to date as of 10/20/2022. U.S. Federal Communications Commission (FCC), Washington, D.C. https://www.ecfr.gov/current/title-47/chapter-I/subchapter-A/part-1/subpart-I/section-1.1310. (Displaying title 47, up to date as of 10/20/2022)

Gu, C., Li, C., Lin, J., Long, J., Huangfu, J., Ran, L., 2010. Instrument-based noncontact Doppler radar vital sign detection system using heterodyne digital quadrature demodulation architecture. IEEE Trans. Instrum. Meas., 59(6):1580–1588

Hincapié (Chincapin), M. A., Gallego, J. C., Gempeler, A., Piñeros, J. A., Nasner, D., Escobar, M. F., 2020. Implementation and usefulness of telemedicine during the COVID-19 pandemic: A scoping review. J. Prim. Care Community Health. doi: 10.1177/2150132720980612

HRSA, 2022. The Health Resources Services Administration, https://www.healthit.gov/faq/what-telehealth-how-telehealth-different-telemedicine# Last accessed July 2022

IEEE, 2020. Standard Letter Designations for Radar-Frequency Bands, IEEE Std 521-2019, 1–15. doi: 10.1109/IEEESTD.2020.8999849

Islam, S. M. M., Boric-Lubecke, O., Lubecke, V. M., Moadi, A. K., Fathy, A. E., 2022. Contactless radar-based sensors: Recent advances in vital-signs monitoring of multiple subjects. IEEE Microw. Mag., 23(7):47–60. doi: 10.1109/MMM.2022.3140849

Islam, S. M. M., Fioranelli, F., Lubecke, V. M., 2021. Can radar remote life sensing technology help combat COVID-19? Front. Comms. Net., 2:648181. doi: 10.3389/frcmn.2021.648181

Johnson, J. E., Shay, O., Kim, C., Liao, C., 2019. Wearable millimeter-wave device for contactless measurement of arterial pulses. IEEE Trans. Biomed. Circuits Syst., 13(6):1525–1534

Kagawa, M., Tojima, H., Matsui, T., 2016. Non-contact diagnostic system for sleep apnea-hypopnea syndrome based on amplitude and phase analysis of thoracic and abdominal Doppler radars. Med. Biol. Eng. Comput., 54(5):789–798

Kichloo, A., Albosta, M., Dettloff, K., Wani, F., El-Amir, Z., Singh, J., Aljadah, M., Chakinala, R. C., Kanugula, A. K., Solanki, S., Chugh, S., 2020. Telemedicine, the current COVID-19 pandemic and the future: A narrative review and perspectives moving forward in the USA. Fam. Med. Community Health, 8(3):e000530

Kuo, H. C., Lin, C. C., Yu, C. H., Lo, P. H., et al., 2016. A fully integrated 60-GHz CMOS direct-conversion Doppler radar RF sensor with clutter canceller for single-antenna noncontact human vital-signs detection. IEEE Trans. Microw. Theory Tech., 64(4):1018–1028

Lee, J. Y., Lin, J. C., 1985. Microprocessor based non-invasive pulse wave analyzer. IEEE Trans. Biomed. Eng., 32:451–455

Li, C., Lin, J., 2007. Optimal carrier frequency of non-contact vital sign detectors. Proceedings of the IEEE Radio and Wireless Symposium, Long Beach, CA, 281–284. doi: 10.1109/RWS.2007.351823

Li, C., Lubecke, V. M., Boric-Lubecke, O., Lin, J., 2013. A review on recent advances in doppler radar sensors for noncontact healthcare monitoring. IEEE Trans. Microw. Theory Tech., 61(5):2046–2060

Li, C., Lubecke, V. M., Boric-Lubecke, O., Lin, J., 2021. Sensing of life activities at the human-microwave frontier. IEEE J. Microw., 1 (1): 66–78. doi: 10.1109/JMW.2020.3030722

Lin, J. C., 1985. Frequency optimization for microwave imaging of biological tissues. Proc. IEEE, 72:374–375

Lin, J. C., 1986. Microwave propagation in biological dielectrics with application to cardiopulmonary interrogation. In: Larsen, L. E., Jacobi, J. H., Eds., Medical Applications of Microwave Imaging (pp. 47–58), New York: IEEE Press

Lin, J. C., 1992. Microwave sensing of physiological movement and volume change: A review. Bioelectromagnetics, 13:557–565

Lin, J. C., 1993. Diagnostic applications of electromagnetic fields. In: Stone, R., Ed., Review of Radio Science 1992 (pp. 771–778), Oxford University Press

Lin, J. C., 1999. Application of telecommunication technology to health-care delivery. IEEE Eng. Med. Biol., 18:28–31

Lin, J. C., 2020. FCC announces its existing RF exposure limits apply to 5G. IEEE Microw. Mag., 21(4):15–17

Lin, J. C., 2021a. Microwave thermoacoustic tomographic (MTT) imaging. Physics in Medicine and Biology, 66(10):10–30

Lin, J. C., 2021b. Safety of wireless power transfer. IEEE ACCESS, 9:125342–125347

Lin, J. C., 2022. Health Safety Guidelines and 5G Wireless Radiation, IEEE Microwave Magazine, v23/1, 10–13

Lin, J. C., 2023a. Incongruities in recently revised radiofrequency exposure guidelines and standards. Environmental Research, 222, April 2023. https://doi.org/10.1016/j.envres.2023.115369

Lin, J. C., 2023b. RF health safety limit recommendations. IEEE Microwave Magazine, 24(6): 18–22

Michler, F., Scheiner, R., Reissland, T., Weigel, R., Koelpin, A., 2021. Micrometer sensing with microwaves: Precise radar systems for innovative measurement applications. IEEE Journal of Microwaves, 1(1):202–217

Ness, M. J., Davis, M. R., Carey, W. A., 2013. Neonatal skin care: A concise review. Int. J. Dermatol, 52(1):14–22

OSHA, 2022. Safety and Health Topics: Radiofrequency and Microwave Radiation. https://www.osha.gov/radiofrequency-and-microwave-radiation/standards

Rozzell, T., Lin, J. C., 1987. Biomedical applications of electromagnetic energy. IEEE Eng. Med. Biol. Mag., 6:52–56

Skolnik, M. I., 1980. Introduction to Radar Systems, 2nd ed, McGraw-Hill

Su, D., Zhou, J., Kelley, M. S., Michaud, T. L., Siahpush, M., Kim, J., Wilson, F., Stimpson, J. P., Pagán, J. A., 2016. Does telemedicine improve treatment outcomes for diabetes? A meta-analysis of results from 55 randomized controlled trials. Diabetes Res. Clin. Pract., 116:136–148

Talla, V., Kellogg, B., Gollakota, S., Smith, J. R., 2017. Battery-free cell phone, Proc. ACM Interact. Mobile, Wearable Ubiquitous Technol. 1(2):1–20. doi: 10.1145/3090090

Taylor, A. H. L., Young, L. C., Hyland, I. A., 1934. System Detecting Objects by Radio, U.S. Patent 1,981,884

Taylor, W., Abbasi, Q. H., Dashtipour, K., Ansari, S., et al., 2020. A review of the state of the art in non-contact sensing for COVID-19. Sensors, 20 (19), 5665. doi:10.3390/s20195665

Thi Phuoc Van, N., Tang, L., Demir, V., Hasan, S. F., Duc Minh, N., Mukhopadhyay, S., 2019. Review-microwave radar sensing systems for search and rescue purposes. Sensors, 19(13), 2879. doi: 10.3390/s19132879

Yamaura, I., 1977. Measurement of 1.8-2.7-GHz microwave attenuation in the human torso. IEEE Trans. Microw. Theory Tech., 25:707–710

Zhou, J., Sharma, P., Hui, X., Kan, E. C., 2020. A wireless wearable RF sensor for brumation study of chelonians. IEEE J. Electromagn. RF Microw. Med. Biol., 5(1):17–24

# 2 Pioneering Investigations

The backscattering of Doppler-shifted microwaves from humans and animals has been effectively employed in sensing, monitoring, and diagnostic applications since the early 1970s. This chapter begins with a brief narrative account of a scientific journey that guided me to the subject of research discussed in this book—microwave noninvasive physiological measurement and sensing. An expanded but succinct technical description of the early research and development efforts during the first two decades of their advancement follows in Sections 2.2 and 2.3 from a historical perspective. The purpose is to bring pioneering research on the subject to the attention of interested readers who may have joined the effort at different junctures in this exciting endeavor.

## 2.1 A SCIENTIFIC RESEARCH JOURNEY

In 1968, the U.S. Congress enacted the Radiation Control for Health and Safety Act [U.S. Senate, 1968]. The deliberations that preceded it had highlighted a general lack of current scientific knowledge on the biological effects and health implications of exposure to both ionizing radiation, such as X-rays, and nonionizing radiation, such as microwaves. The deliberations revealed the considerable amount of unnecessary radiation people were exposed to each year. The U.S. Congress declared that the public's health and safety must be protected against the dangers of radiation from electronic products, including microwaves. The act authorized the federal government to set radiation standards, monitor compliance, and undertake research. It directed the U.S. Department of Health, Education, and Welfare (HEW) to establish and carry out an electronic product radiation control program designed to protect the public from radiation emitted by electronic products. HEW was renamed the Department of Health and Human Services (HHS) in 1979 to reflect its new mandates, without the education portfolio.

It was the first time the health and safety issues of microwave radiation struck my consciousness. This chapter begins with a brief personal journal of the historical events that steered me to the theme of scientific research on microwave noninvasive physiological sensing. The possibility that, aside from intended telecommunication uses, microwaves could exert influence on biology and may evoke physiological responses became a subject of personal interest and an intriguing matter for research. Nevertheless, telecommunications application of electromagnetic radiation remained the focus of research for my dissertation, which was on microwave and millimeter wave propagation in discrete random media. The advisor of my doctoral dissertation, Professor Akira Ishimaru at the University of Washington in Seattle, is one of those professors who is genuinely appreciated by his students. His example of blending rigorous analysis with imaginative research and his willingness to pay close attention to the works of his students have been a tremendous influence on my academic career. He not only launched me into university teaching and research, but

DOI: 10.1201/9781003315223-2

he also started a tradition that set the tone for my intellectual pursuit and service to my chosen profession.

The nascent interest in the health and safety of microwave radiation culminated in an appointment as a junior bioengineering faculty member in the Department of Rehabilitation Medicine at the University of Washington School of Medicine upon completion of my graduate school education in the summer of 1971. The topics of my research were the health and safety of microwaves and therapeutic microwave diathermy treatments as part of the physical medicine protocol. It was a privilege to work with the group leader, Dr. Arthur W. Guy, as a junior faculty member in the rehabilitation medicine department. It was an exciting time. We worked hard and accomplished a lot in the process. Several topics of research conducted during that period were covered in the d'Arsonval Medal Award Lecture given in Maui, Hawaii [Lin, 2004].

### 2.1.1 Respiratory Measurement and Microwave Cardiography

During a scientific conference in the early 1970s, a conversation with Professor Charles Susskind, Department of Electrical Engineering and Computer Science (EECS), University of California, Berkeley, made me aware of his interest in bioengineering research. Later, I learned he was a cofounder of Berkeley's bioengineering program. The discussions centered on the application of microwaves to record volume changes in biological subjects and, specifically, the use of changes of microwave reflectance and transmittance as a measure of circulatory and respiratory volume changes. Indeed, a brief theoretical discussion of the possibilities for applying microwaves in detection and mapping of lung diseases characterized by the presence of excess water was published later [Susskind, 1973]. The discussions caused me to realize the potential application of microwaves for measuring physiological signals associated with cardiopulmonary movements in humans and animals.

An invitation from Wayne State University (WSU) in 1974 allowed me to become a professor in the departments of electrical and computer engineering and physical medicine and rehabilitation. The appointment at WSU prompted the launch of several research projects, among them, contactless microwave sensing and monitoring of physiological signatures. The investigations began with noninvasive measurement and remote monitoring of the respiratory movement of humans and animals. The technique involved the use of continuous wave (CW) Doppler microwave radar for measuring the respiratory movements of human and animals including cats, rabbits, and rats [Lin, 1975; Lin and Salinger, 1975]. It provided a novel approach to detecting respiratory movements without compromising the integrity of the underlying physiological phenomena. It is noted in the short paper reporting the use of a microwave Doppler radar setup for novel respiratory monitoring in humans and animals, that the results from a rabbit were presented because data from rabbits as a laboratory animal were less common, but the cat drawing was kept in the illustration [Lin, 1975]. Furthermore, a contactless microwave apnea monitor based on CW microwave radar was designed and tested [Lin et al., 1977]. The Doppler microwave apnea monitor was able to detect instantaneous changes in respiration, including artificially induced apnea and hyperventilation in an anesthetized cat (3 kg) positioned in recumbency in an incubator. It is noteworthy that continuous monitoring of respiratory activities during the first days of life, especially of low-birth weight infants, is especially beneficial. Stimuli, such as a timely touch, that are sufficient to wake the infant are usually strong enough to re-establish breathing to avert infant death due to sudden infant death syndrome (SIDS) in many cases.

Shortly thereafter, a contactless noninvasive Doppler microwave cardiography technique was developed to detect changes in the backscattered microwaves caused by precordial displacements of the chest wall and the vibrations in response to ventricular contraction [Lin et al., 1979]. The noncontact sensing approach eliminated any change in sensitivity and discomfort caused by attaching sensors to the chest. The microwave technique was given the name of microwave apexcardiography (MACG), in recognition of MACG detecting variations in the backscattered microwave signal using an antenna positioned over the apex of the heart. Microwave apexcardiograms reflect the hemodynamic events within the left ventricle. It is comparable to the conventional seismocardiography (SCG) signal typically recorded by attaching an accelerometer to the skin over the apex, near the sternum. Also, the salient features of MACG measurements echo the familiar electrocardiogram (ECG). However, in contrast both to ECG and SCG sensors, MACG measurements do not involve any radar sensor attached to the chest. As mentioned later in the chapter, noninvasive Doppler microwave sensors can successfully and reproducibly measure cardiovascular signal waveforms of diagnostic quality [Papp et al., 1987].

When microwaves impinge on a biological target, a strong scattering phenomenon takes place such that roughly one-half of the incident microwave is reflected by the biological target. Moreover, the reflected microwaves experience a Doppler effect, which shifts their frequency either up or down from the frequency of the impinging microwave, depending on the direction of the movement with respect to the microwave source [Lin, 1986, 1989, 1992]. Because the chest, heart, and lungs are in constant motion, microwaves bounced back from these organs provide a method to sense vital signs, such as heartbeat and respiration, remotely and noninvasively without the need for cooperation by the subject or when conventional detection or monitoring is not possible. The advantage afforded by remote sensing suggests the potential use of this technology for monitoring frail and elderly patients or patients with premature development or the detection of unauthorized personnel or intruders. It also has the potential to monitor persons who fall prey to hazardous scenarios such as explosion, fire, chemical or nuclear contamination, or natural and other human-made disasters. Furthermore, the approach can be used to monitor unrestrained animals in cages, holding areas, or in their natural habitats, in addition to veterinary clinics.

### 2.1.2 Vital-Sign Sensing

The conversations that began some years ago with Susskind led to an invitation to spend a year in the Autumn of 1980 at Berkeley's EECS department and to conduct research with scientists at the Lawrence Berkely National Laboratory, with the support of a grant award from the National Institutes of Health (NIH). However, other events intervened. When informed about my new appointment at the University of Illinois Chicago (UIC) as professor and chair of the bioengineering department, Susskind graciously remarked, "you got your professorship at Illinois, and I am happy about it." A gentleman and scholar, indeed! Fortunately, the research on microwave interaction with biological systems that was to be initiated at Berkeley continued at UIC.

Theoretical research at UIC showed that for remote sensing of vital signs, microwave frequencies between 2 and 10 GHz are preferable [Lin, 1985]. Indeed, heart and respiratory rates have been detected and monitored at distances of a few to tens of meters in human subjects, with or without intervening physical (nonmetallic) barriers [Chan and Lin, 1987]. Microwaves at these frequencies can penetrate layers of clothing and do not require direct sensor contact with the subject. Problems such as skin irritation, restriction of breathing, and electrode connections are eliminated. For longer distances, a higher sensitivity with low levels of radiated power can be achieved by using a directive and higher gain antenna and by minimizing various noise sources.

A portable microprocessor-based remote noninvasive Doppler microwave heartbeat and respiration sensor was developed for use without physical contact with the subject when direct contact is either impossible or undesirable [Chan and Lin, 1985, 1987; Lin et al., 1984; Popovic et al., 1984]. The front end consisted of a low-power (10.5 GHz, 5–10 mW) microwave transceiver connected to a horn antenna. The output from the transceiver is proportional to the displacement of the chest-wall movement associated with expansion and contraction of the heart and lungs. The signal was processed using analog circuits for amplification and filtration. A software algorithm was designed to successfully extract both the heart and respiration signals and to separate the higher-frequency heart signal from the lower-frequency breathing signal.

### 2.1.3 Arterial Pressure Pulse Wave and Cerebral Edema

For centuries, physicians have used palpation of the arterial pulse as a diagnostic tool. In modern times, noninvasive recording of the arterial pulse has been used to evaluate cardiovascular function and monitor arterial pressure. A Doppler microwave technique was implemented to measure arterial pulse waves and the characteristics of arterial-wall movements. The Doppler microwave pulse wave sensor consisted of a low-power, solid-state source, a signal-processing module, and a sensing head (probe) operating at 25 GHz that can be used to perform measurement with either no contact or in direct contact with the skin. Experimental validations of the noninvasive Doppler microwave pulse measurement were conducted at a variety of arterial sites, including the carotid, brachial, and radial arteries in human participants [Lee et al., 1983; Lee and Lin, 1985; Lin, 1989, 1992]. The waveforms obtained by the microwave sensor in direct contact with skin over the arteries compared favorably with invasively obtained arterial blood pressure waveforms. For example, the clinical efficacy of the noninvasive Doppler microwave arterial pulse wave sensor was assessed with human participants [Papp et al., 1987]. Specifically, the ability to detect pathological conditions in patients with known diseases was evaluated by obtaining microwave-sensed carotid pulse waveforms using contact application of the noninvasive sensor along with simultaneously recorded intra-aortic pressure waves. There was remarkable resemblance of the microwave-sensed arterial pulse wave and the invasively recorded pressure wave ("the gold standard" for arterial pressure measurement). The recordings were used to calculate, for example, left ventricular ejection time (LVET) and the time required for the aortic pressure to reach one half of its maximum amplitude (T1/2). The results confirmed that the noninvasive Doppler microwave sensor can successfully and reproducibly detect pressure pulse waveforms of diagnostic quality [Papp et al., 1987].

In an alternative approach, a noninvasive microwave transmission system applied at close range to a human-head model demonstrated the capability for continuous monitoring and quantifying time-dependent changes in intracranial fluid volume, such as cerebral edema, with minimal interference to the integrity of the pathophysiological events from the measurement instrumentation [Clarke and Lin, 1983; Lin and Clarke, 1982]. Note that the increase or decrease in cerebral fluid volume is correlated with intracranial pressure (ICP). By recording the phase of a transmitted microwave signal, increases in intracranial fluids of about 1% are detectable *in vivo.* These findings indicate that the noninvasive microwave technique may be a potentially viable approach in assessing the progression of cerebral edema on a long-term basis.

Thus, the investigations that first began in the 1970s and grew in the 1980s helped to set the stage for the microwave noninvasive physiological sensing research and development that followed. A summary and a review of the advancements in the microwave monitoring of physiological movement and volume change were published [Lin, 1989, 1992], and an updated account on the history of wireless microwave sensing was also presented [Lin, 2011]. Sections 2.2 and 2.3 provide succinct descriptions of scientific advancements made during those periods. Additional discussions will appear alongside appropriate topics in subsequent chapters.

### 2.1.4 Translational Research

There are three salient instances where laboratory investigations developed into translational research through differing degrees of collaboration with the industrial sector—the thread traces back to the 1980s. The transcatheter minimally invasive surgical procedure was recognized increasingly as a treatment of choice for chronic cardiac and vascular diseases. Therapeutic options for managing a variety of cardiovascular diseases were concentrated on pharmacologic agents and surgical interventions. Beginning in the 1980s, there was growing interest in nonpharmacological therapy and minimally invasive procedures.

In a modest but significant fraction of patients with ventricular tachycardias—unusually high heart rhythms — available drug therapy was found unsatisfactory because of a lack of meaningful response or due to unacceptable side effects [Aliot and Lazzara, 1987; Breithardt et al., 1988; Scheinman and Davis, 1986]. Transvenous catheter electrical ablation of the atrioventricular (AV) junction to effect complete AV block became an increasingly accepted technique for treating patients with drug-resistant supraventricular arrhythmias [Breithardt et al., 1988; Fontaine et al., 1987; Gallagher et al., 1982; Josephson, 1984; Nathan et al., 1984; Scheinman and Davis, 1986]. During that same period, percutaneous transluminal balloon angioplasty became a viable method in treating arteriosclerotic diseases [Chokshi et al., 1987; Kent et al., 1984]. Unlike ablation, angioplasty is a palliative treatment procedure. Its primary goal lies in the dilatation and recanalization of obstructions in arteries to achieve maximum function for a prolonged period of time. Percutaneous transluminal coronary angioplasty developed into a frontline treatment of symptomatic patients with silent ischemia and abnormal exercise stress-test results. However, problems of abrupt closure and late restenosis of the dilated segment prompted the investigation of thermal techniques to prevent occlusion and restenosis. The advantages of microwave heating technology for transluminal catheter treatment of tachyarrhythmias and arteriosclerotic diseases were proposed and investigated in dogs [Beckman et al., 1987; Lin, 1989, 1990, 1993b; Lin et al., 1988, 1989]. Note that, aside from microwaves, other energy sources such as lasers, electrical, and radio frequency currents have been used both for angioplasty and cardiac ablation [Huang and Wilber, 2000; Lin, 2000]. The major limitations of those techniques include perforation of heart and vessel walls as well as unfocused damage to cardiovascular tissues [Anand et al., 1988; Isner and Clarke, 1989; Prince et al., 1987; Spears, 1987, 1989].

Novel catheter antennas were developed for percutaneous cardiovascular applications using flexible micro- or miniature coaxial cables (2 mm diameter) beginning in the 1980s [Lin, 1990, 1993b; Lin et al., 1996; Lin and Wang, 1987a,b, 1995, 1996]. These novel catheter antennas represented state-of-art breakthroughs. The design advantages of these catheter antennas compared to conventional monopole or helical antennas are that they produce higher and broader energy depositions in the tip (or distal) region of the antenna, low-power absorptions along the transmission cable, and minimal reflected power or unwanted tissue heating. In the late 1980s, at the invitation of Arye Rosen and Fred Sterzer, I presented a seminar to members of the RCA Sarnoff Laboratories in Princeton, New Jersey. The design, performance, and applications of these novel catheter antennas were discussed at length. Rosen and Sterzer's ensuing work on the microwave angioplasty technique, which combined transluminal microwave antenna heating to soften the blood-vessel occlusions induced by plaque, followed by customary balloon angioplasty for vascular expansion, is noteworthy [Rosen et al., 1990; Rosen and Rosen, 1995].

Minimally invasive cardiac ablation became a widely used procedure for the treatment of cardiac arrhythmias—irregular heart rhythms [Huang and Wilber, 2000]. In the case of atrial fibrillation, minimally invasive microwave ablation is a safe and effective procedure that may be applied to a wide variety of patients [Saltman et al., 2003; Williams et al., 2002]. Minimally invasive intervention offers several benefits: long incisions are replaced with a puncture wound, major cardiac and pulmonary complications are sidestepped, and the need for postoperative intensive care is significantly reduced. In the case of cardiac ablation, minimally invasive intervention offers a "cure" without major surgery. In addition, it replaces chronic drug therapy and reduces its accompanying side effects and inconvenience. My team first proposed and used microwave energy as an ablative energy source for the experimental treatment of cardiac arrhythmias in a canine model in 1987 [Beckman et al., 1987; Lin, 1999a,b, 2000; Lin, 2003; Lin et al., 1988, 1989, 1995, 1996].

An important aspect of these developments was the production of adequate temperature rise and distribution in the target tissue, superficial or deep-seated. Moreover, successful ablative therapies require not only a suitable radiation energy source for heat production, but an understanding of the underlying pathological condition being treated to define the critical target tissue temperature and the ability of the therapeutic microwave energy to reach the target organ or tissue. Thus, in addition to innovative engineering design, the characterization of the proper performance of antennas for ablation therapy entails analytic and numerical solutions of electromagnetic and thermal problems [Cavarnaro and Lin, 2019; Lin, 2018a]. The process involves solving both Maxwell's equations and the bioheat equation to analyze and simulate microwave radiation patterns and temperature distributions inside target biological tissues. Computational algorithms, such as the finite-difference time-domain (FDTD) formulation, have been applied to simulate the effectiveness and performance of transcatheter intraluminal antennas [Bernardi et al., 2004; Lin et al., 2008; Pisa et al., 2001]. In this regard, several innovative catheter antennas were developed, analyzed, and tested both in phantom models and in experimental animals including cap-choke antennas, dipole antennas with coaxial choke, and sleeved-slot antennas [Lin, 1999a; Lin and Wang, 1987a,b, 1995, 1996; Lin et al., 1995, 1996, 2008].

The pioneering demonstration and studies of catheter microwave ablation therapy for treating cardiac arrhythmias caught the interest of a startup company in the late 1990s. Fred Seddiqui, CEO/President of AFx and its predecessor Fidus of Fremont, California, was engaged in an extensive series of exchanges concerning our novel microwave systems and technologies. Our ground-breaking research was successfully translated, and the startups turned out to be lucrative. In 2004, Guidant Cardiac Surgery acquired AFx for $45 million plus predetermined milestone payments. It was satisfying to receive an unsolicited email from Rick O'Connor (Director, Product Development, Guidant Cardiac Surgery, Santa Clara, California), dated Aug 23, 2004, which stated, "Your widely published research in the field of medical microwave therapy has been a resource to us."

During the 1990s, engaging meetings were convened in San Francisco for a startup to develop a product based on microwave noncontact vital-sign sensing technologies for driver drowsiness detection. The successful product would have the potential to render timely driver assistance by alerting the driver for accident prevention. However, while the in-depth discussion recognized the demand and identified the impact of this technology and service, the startup did not get off the ground.

Also, a proposal to Microsoft Research on using cellphones as a platform for healthcare did not gain their support [Lin et al., 2007]. In this case, the microwaves transmitted by a phone's antenna bounced back from the chest of the user would be picked up by the antenna and processed to yield the Doppler frequency shift in the reflected signal to extract the user's heartbeat and respiration. The project was deemed extremely competitive and that there were clear indications of expanding worldwide interest in the proposed research.

Just prior to the turn of the century in 1999, by arrangement of Olga Boric-Lubecke and Jenshan Lin, I gave a seminar to members of the technical staff at Bell Laboratories in Murray Hill, New Jersey, on the topic of the remote sensing of vital signs with microwave signals. The group of scientists who were conducting research on radio frequency (RF) integrated circuit (RFIC) technology for telecommunications became interested in research on the biomedical applications of wireless systems. An informal collaboration was initiated to integrate the remote vital-sign monitoring function with existing telecommunications infrastructures, and to make the remote vital-sign monitoring technology applicable to a broad portion of the population in an efficient manner. The objective was to be realized using personal wireless devices, cellular mobile handsets, or other wearable RF devices. The vital-sign data would be channeled to a remote location through a mobile telephone or wireless connection [Boric-Lubecke et al., 1999; Lubecke et al., 2000].

Further experimentations at Bell Laboratories using a radio system with frequencies and powers typical in mobile phones and silicon BiCMOS RFICs developed for DCS 1800/PCS1900 mobile phone base station applications showed that signals from such consumer electronics could provide readily extractable data on heart and respiration activity [Droitcour et al., 2001, 2002]. In the case of cellular mobile telephones, the microwaves transmitted by a phone's antenna bounce back to the phone from the chest, heart, and lungs of the user. The handset can then send this signal, picked up by its antenna, to the base station, where further signal processing would detect the Doppler frequency shift in the reflected signal and extract the user's heartbeat and respiration rate. On a different approach alongside the route of CW microwave Doppler radar, advancements in wireless technologies have made it feasible to integrate such microwave radar on a single chip. Accordingly, a microwave Doppler radar transceiver was fully integrated in 0.25 $\mu$m silicon CMOS and BiCMOS technologies for the first time by the Boric-Lubecke-Lin team [Droitcour et al., 2003, 2004]. The single-chip radar sensor was compact, lightweight, and, significantly, the miniaturized circuitry consumed less power. The development took the lead in low-cost, compact, modern radar systems capable of being integrated in sensor networks and of delivering highly accurate measurements of vital signs.

In the 2000s, an interdisciplinary research team was recruited from UIC's departments of emergency medicine, computer science, and electrical and computer engineering to explore the use of wireless vital-sign sensing and mobile communication technology with an aim to enhance healthcare delivery through health promoters in rural regions and underserved communities [Lin, 2004, Lin et al., 2010]. The objectives of the project included: (1) to develop and test biosensors to be attached to cellphones and develop protocols to facilitate the transfer and use of objective patient data between health promoters and physicians for decision support; (2) to demonstrate the ability to train health promoters on the use of the enhanced cellphones and transmission of data; (3) to ensure the quality of the data transmission; and (4) to show an ability to make clinical decisions remotely based on information transmitted through established wireless mobile communication networks. The project would demonstrate its vision via a prototype test-bed application, where the telemedicine solution would be test deployed and evaluated in a rural region within a recognized health-promoter program. It was anticipated that the objectives and quantitative measures of patient data and experiences would facilitate the continued development and implementation of greater technological sophistication in concordance with the philosophy of "start small, think big," as advocated in a review article on telemedicine implementation [Broens et al., 2007].

Most efforts were aimed at the research and development of sophisticated technologies to better enable telemedicine to serve the needs of highly developed healthcare systems [Lin, 1999]. However, this research additionally focused on wireless noncontact sensing and monitoring of vital signs [Lin, 1992, 1993a; Lin and Lin, 2009]. Currently, health monitors with a variety of sensing features are commonly installed in the latest model of smartphones. Many advances have permitted critical-access hospitals in developed countries to gain access to knowledge and consultative services with clinical specialties that are not immediately or locally available. While the advanced technology is not available universally, cellphone technology is changing rapidly in the global communication environment. In developing countries and regions where healthcare is unreliable, extremely limited, or unavailable, telemedicine solutions remain an option to provide access to a service that would otherwise be impossible.

Furthermore, telemedicine and telehealth practices have increased dramatically over the past few years [Hincapié (Chincapin) et al., 2020; Koonin et al., 2020; Nitiema, 2022; Shave, 2022]. As their use increased even after the return of face-to-face patient interactions during the coronavirus (COVID-19) pandemic, healthcare and medical technology innovations would likely be concerned, encouraged, and tasked with more efficacious management of telemedicine and telehealth including remote patient monitoring. The opportunity also invites a vast spectrum of medical and healthcare technology challenges. Wireless microwave sensing and monitoring of physiological and pathophysiological signatures alongside the mobile wireless transfer of healthcare data could play a crucial role in a successful telehealth program.

In summary, research in microwave noninvasive physiological sensing has undergone seemingly exponential growth since 2000. The calendar year 2000 did not merely mark the start of a new century, as significant as it may be—it was a watershed year. What set out as an informal collaboration led to the blossoming of one of the most exciting research areas for microwaves in biology and medicine. The pioneering investigations provided inspiration to the Boric-Lubecke-Lin team at Bell Laboratories for their studies and investigations. It is fair to say that their innovative research inspired others to explore and advance applications of the remote contactless microwave sensing of physiological signatures and vital signs, worldwide. Metaphorically, it is hoped that the humble specks planted would succeed in producing gems and jade to be unearthed in the years to come.

### 2.1.5 DARPA Workshop on Noninvasive Blood Pressure Monitoring

A U.S. Defense Advanced Research Project Agency (DARPA) workshop on the continuous, noninvasive monitoring of blood pressure in Coronado, California, in June 2009 provided the opportunity to demonstrate and discuss our research on the noninvasive microwave technique for continuously monitoring and quantifying time-dependent changes along the cardiovascular tree, including arterial blood pressure [Lin and Lin, 2009]. The discussion showed that microwaves can provide a viable approach to noninvasively detect and continuously monitor physiological signatures, movements, and volume changes without compromising the integrity of the underlying physiological events. It involved several application scenarios in which noninvasive microwave-contact approaches held promise, including the sensing of heartbeat, pressure pulse waves in central and peripheral circulations, and ventricular movements related to the cardiovascular system that replicate the hemodynamic events within the tissues and organs [Chan and Lin, 1987; Lee and Lin, 1985; Lin et al., 1979; Papp et al., 1987]. Examples consist of the Doppler microwave interrogation of arterial-wall properties and pressure-pulse characteristics at a variety of arterial sites, such as the carotid, brachial, radial, and femoral arteries, specifically microwave-sensed continuous carotid pulse waveforms obtained in patients using contact application 24 GHz microwave energy along with simultaneously recorded intra-aortic pressure waves. The resemblance of the microwave-sensed arterial pulse and the invasively recorded pressure wave was remarkable. These results confirm that a noninvasive Doppler microwave sensor can successfully and reproducibly detect pressure pulse waveforms of diagnostic quality.

The need for noninvasive and continuous monitoring of both systolic and diastolic blood pressure is pervasive across all medical environments, but most especially on the military battlefield where rapid triage, stabilization, and evacuation are critical to the survival of the wounded. The objective of this DARPA program was to develop capabilities to perform continuous, noninvasive monitoring of blood pressure for battlefield triage and casualty transport. In general, there is a critical medical need for the continuous monitoring of blood pressure that is noninvasive and flexible enough to be implemented, regardless of the injury, and that interferes minimally with other essential medical procedures.

### 2.1.6 DARPA RadioBio—A Sensing Challenge

An interesting but different electromagnetic sensing challenge was announced in 2017 through a new DARPA research initiative: "RadioBio: What Role Does Electromagnetic Signaling Have in Biological Systems?" [DARPA, 2017]. The goal of this project is to "determine if purposeful signaling via electromagnetic waves between biological systems exists, and, if it does, determine what information is being transferred." The request for proposal called for clearly identified hypotheses for communication channel(s) with specific predictions and experimental tests that could definitively prove each hypothesis. The goal of RadioBio is innovative and intriguing, especially given DARPA's well-earned reputation for creating breakthrough technologies for national security and beyond. The far-reaching Internet project is an obvious case in point. The task of discovering, studying, and comprehending how electromagnetic fields and waves affect the intricate biology of living cellular organisms is not only of fundamental scientific importance, but also has practical and technological value. Once electromagnetic signaling and communication in living organisms have been harnessed, the possibilities and potential applications in data transfer, information delivery, and communication for command and control are enormous.

The challenge of RadioBio is simple and complex at the same time. The challenge is simple because living biological cells and organisms have long been known to emit electromagnetic fields and waves. As mentioned, suitable sensors and instrumentation may be applied to detect these signals noninvasively, near the organism or at a close distance. Macroscopically, organized cells can generate and emit detectable electromagnetic signals in the noisy, cluttered environment of living bodies. These signals have been successfully applied to create tools for the medical diagnosis modern medical practice relies on. Aside from the title of this book, abundant examples include electrocardiography and magnetocardiography for the heart, electroencephalography and magnetoencephalography for the brain, electromyography for neuromuscular tissues, and electroretinography for the eye, to name a few. Those signals are supported by the electromagnetic fields and the waves emitted by living cells, tissues, or organs, which are detectable from the human-body surface with specific sensors and electronic instrumentations.

In cardiology, minimally invasive endocardioelectrophysiology of the myocardium is often performed to help assess sources of cardiac arrhythmias inside the heart. Moreover, many biomedical research laboratories regularly use miniature penetrating and patch-clamp microelectrodes to record currents from the efflux and influx of biochemical ions, both intracellularly and extracellularly [Arber and Lin, 1985a,b; Smith et al., 2013]. However, the spectra of the recordings mentioned are typically low—well below 1 kHz—and definitely not in the RF region above 3 kHz, the band commonly used for noninvasive microwave physiological sensing. These types of low-frequency signals can support only limited informational content for wireless communication purposes. This is not to imply that they are incapable of transmitting meaningful or purposeful messages. Even a low-frequency signal with only 1 bit of information can convey a meaningful message in a purposefully designed wireless communication system under specialized circumstances and for special purposes or operational requirements.

The challenge is also complex, and not merely because researchers have yet to report direct measurements of electromagnetic radiation involving kilohertz to terahertz signals from a single cell or cluster of living cells close in or far away. There is a total lack of knowledge about any communication-relevant electromagnetic channel between biological cells or systems or any understanding of what biologically significant information may be transferred intracellularly or extracellularly. The properties and behaviors of ion channels located at cell membranes are subjects presented in basic textbooks on physiology. Ion channels are critical to regulating the life processes of biological cells and, by extension, in the functioning of higher organs and structures. Some explicit examples include voltage-gated ion channels with their exquisite sensitivity to transmembrane potential difference [Purves et al., 2001] and mechanically gated ion channels with their unique sensitivity to mechanical cells' deformations, stretches, and movements [Ranade and Syeda, 2015].

Thus, the phenomena of biochemical ionic exchanges through channels at cell membranes, ligands, or neurotransmitters through synaptic junctions in neural cells are well established. These exchanges represent movements of electronic charge-carrying ions (or charge flow). The flow of electrons forms electric currents, which generate electromagnetic radiation by Ampere's law (an integral part of Maxwell's classic theory of electromagnetism, see Chapter 3). The emitted and received electromagnetic waves may embed or encode information or signaling for cell-to-cell communication; in addition, they may be involved in intracellular and/or extracellular communication under normal or physiologically stressed conditions. These electromagnetic fields and waves should be amenable to noninvasive detection. Thus, the detected electromagnetic fields and waves would be clearly purposeful; they might also play some essential roles in signaling and communication alongside biochemical ions.

One project proposed was to design and execute controlled laboratory-cell biology experiments using isolated cells and cell clusters in culture, e.g., isolated, identifiable, and viable snail esophageal neurons and neuron pairs [Lin, 2018b, 2019]. The snail neuronal cell preparations were selected for the enhanced repeatability of results and the ability to maintain cell viability over an extended period of time at room temperature [Arber and Lin, 1985a,b]. These experiments may be followed up with other single cells and cell clusters in culture, which potentially may transmit and receive signals via electromagnetic fields and waves. Of course, it would be important to conduct computational modeling to assess the electronic signaling behaviors of as many intracellular and extracellular components as practicable, with the aim of specifying unique features, signal levels, and bandwidths from ionic current flow and concomitant electromagnetic radiation.

The goal would be to define electromagnetic effects that are purposeful and not just side effects of ionic exchanges. The working hypothesis was the characterization of a kHz-to-MHz communication channel derived from acquired data and known facts, such as time constants from microelectrode-recorded electrophysiological signals and their fading behavior. A related goal would be to develop sensitivity-enhanced passive microsensors, nanoscale biosensors, graphene antennas, and instrumentations exhibiting the proper bandwidth and sensitivity to detect anticipated weak fields in extracellular space noninvasively.

### 2.1.7 A Side Bar—Microwave and Blood–Brain Barrier (BBB) Interactions: A Different Kind of Sensing

The blood–brain barrier (BBB) is an anatomic and physiologic complex associated with the cerebral vascular system [Banks, 2016; Begley, 2004; Neuwelt et al., 2008; Sweeney et al., 2019]. It is composed of a network of astrocytic pseudopodia, which envelope the tight junctions of the vascular endothelium. The cell layers constituting the barrier form a regulatory system that maintains the physiochemical environment of the brain within certain narrow limits that are essential for life. It functions as a differential filter that permits the selective passage of biological substances from blood to the brain. For instance, amino acids, anesthetics, and glucose may gain access to brain cells, while carbohydrates, proteins, and most microorganisms and antibiotics are excluded from brain tissues by the BBB. Even so, it is interesting to note that while the hydrophobic barrier is readily crossed by small lipid-soluble molecules, certain other lipid-insoluble molecules, such as glucose, can also cross the barrier. The intact BBB protects the brain from damage, whereas a disrupted BBB may subject the central nervous system (CNS) to assault from extraneous microorganisms and allow an influx of normally excluded hydrophilic molecules into the brain tissue.

Many investigators have reported the detection of microwave interactions on the BBB of experimental animals with varying results since 1980. Studies showing or not showing a microwave-induced increase in rat BBB permeability have used both high and low levels of microwave exposure. A preponderance of the studies did not report local specific absorption rates (SARs) inside the head. The relationship between incident power density and the specific rate of microwave energy absorption was not defined in many cases. It was difficult to draw a definitive conclusion based on these studies. In addition, nearly all the investigations used protocols that involved whole-body exposure of the experimental animal. Nevertheless, the reported microwave-induced disruption of the BBB at lower levels of microwave exposure has attracted considerable attention.

To quantify the relationship between incident power density and SAR, and to assess any correlation between BBB permeation and the distribution of SAR inside the rat brain, we implemented an experimental approach that employed partial exposure of one side of the rat brain using a small antenna applied directly to the scalp of an anesthetized rat (see Figure 3.19). The head of the rat was held in a stereotaxic head frame, which was constructed using a nonperturbing dielectric material (Delrin). A series of studies was performed in the laboratory using visual dye markers such as Evans blue and sodium fluorescein. It was observed that a 20-minute exposure to 2450 MHz microwaves of average incident power densities that ranged between 5 W/m$^2$ and 26 kW/m$^2$ and SARs between 0.04 and 200 W/kg did not produce staining in the brain, except in regions that normally are highly permeable. The highest temperature measured in the brain was less than 42°C in this case [Lin and Lin, 1980, 1981]. But the results indicated that when the applied microwave power was high enough to elevate the temperature of the brain to 43°C or higher, BBB permeability increased for normally excluded Evans blue dye [Lin and Lin, 1982] and $^{86}$Rb [Goldman et al., 1984]. Moreover, microwave hyperthermia-induced BBB disruption was shown to be reversible within 30–45 minutes following microwave treatment.

To further delineate the mechanism for BBB–microwave interaction, we studied the combined effects of ethanol and microwaves on the permeation of Evans blue through the BBB in rats. It was found that intravenous infusion of ethanol prior to microwave irradiation resulted in the cooling of the brain, thereby mitigating against an excessive increase in brain temperature, and it could attenuate the observed changes in BBB permeation [Neilly and Lin, 1986]. In particular, this result showed that as the quantity of alcohol was increased, the degree of staining was decreased or eliminated. The steady-state temperature of the irradiated area of the brain was highest in animals receiving saline or the smallest dose of alcohol. As the quantity of alcohol was increased, the brain temperature was reduced below 42°C. These results indicate that ethanol inhibits microwave-induced permeation of the BBB through reduced heating of the brain. These studies have helped to reach a general consensus that reliably demonstrable increases of BBB permeability are associated with microwave-induced hyperthermia and that the observed changes are not due to microwave-specific interaction.

The reliability and reversibility of the microwave hyperthermia-induced increases of BBB permeability encouraged us to initiate an investigation to explore its potential as a modality using microwave selective hyperthermia to facilitate the chemotherapeutic treatment of brain tumors. For example, methotrexate (MTX) is a widely prescribed antifolate used in chemotherapy for a variety of neoplasms. It is the drug often used for high-dose chemotherapy. However, the BBB permeability of MTX is among the lowest among the agents that are currently in clinical use. In this study of the effect of selective microwave hyperthermia on the transport of MTX across the BBB, standard high-pressure liquid chromatography (HPLC) analysis was applied to determine the drug concentration in rat brain tissue [Lin et al., 1998]. The MTX concentration in brain tissue was assayed for conditions with or without microwave hyperthermia. Also, we correlated the amount of MTX uptake by the brain after microwave hyperthermia treatment as a function of time. The results indicated that MTX uptake was substantially increased (roughly 20-fold) in rat brains subjected to a noninvasive microwave hyperthermia treatment. Furthermore, the increase was reversible within 45 minutes, post-microwave treatment.

Hyperthermia cancer therapy is a treatment procedure in which the tumor temperature is elevated to the range of 43–45°C. The technique is mostly used in conjunction with radiotherapy and chemotherapy to which it works as a sensitizer. The ability of ionizing radiation to kill tumor cells and the anticancer action of drugs are enhanced by hyperthermia[Datta et al., 2015; Lin, 1999c; Mei et al., 2020; Oei et al., 2020; Watmough and Ross, 1986]. Furthermore, as noted previously, microwave hyperthermia can increase BBB permeability to certain anticancer drugs. However, its efficacy depends on the production of temperatures in excess of 42°C throughout the tumor volume without overheating the adjacent normal tissue, i.e., maintaining the surrounding area's temperature at or below 42°C to avoid collateral thermal damage of normal cells and tissues.

## 2.2 MICROWAVE SENSING OF PHYSIOLOGICAL SIGNATURES AND VOLUME CHANGES IN THE 1970s

The two fundamental schemes for coupling microwave energy into biological bodies and tissues include noncontact and direct-contact methods. The viability of both noncontact and direct-contact schemes was demonstrated, however, there have been fewer investigations exploring the direct-contact method compared to the contactless, noncontact, or remote approach. Noncontact sensing may take place either in near-field or under far-field conditions at distances of meters or more between the microwave source and target. What follows in this section are succinct descriptions, in historical context, of the noninvasive contactless and contact sensing of physiological signatures and movements associated with the expansion and contraction of the cardiovascular and pulmonary systems. Specific and more detailed discussions of these subjects are presented in later chapters alongside the topic under discussion. The noninvasively measured physiological signatures and vital signs are first enabled by using the Doppler microwave radar principle and technology. These investigations that first began in the 1970s and continued in the 1980s helped to launch a tremendous amount of related research at the start of the 21$^{st}$ century.

As mentioned previously, research interests in the use of low-power microwave and RF radar technology for noninvasive detection and monitoring of physiological signals, signatures, movements, and volume changes have been growing since the early 1970s. The same principle of detecting the frequency or phase shift in a reflected radar signal can be used to detect small physiological movements and changes using a system such as that shown in Figure 2.1. The ability of Doppler microwave and RF radars to provide location and velocity information of stationary and moving biological objects unobtrusively has attracted considerable attention, especially in the past decade. Most of the earlier groundbreaking efforts in this area have been toward proof-of-concept and prototype development alongside human and animal testing. Many of the pioneering contributions to microwave physiological sensing, such as cardiovascular detection, pulmonary–respiratory

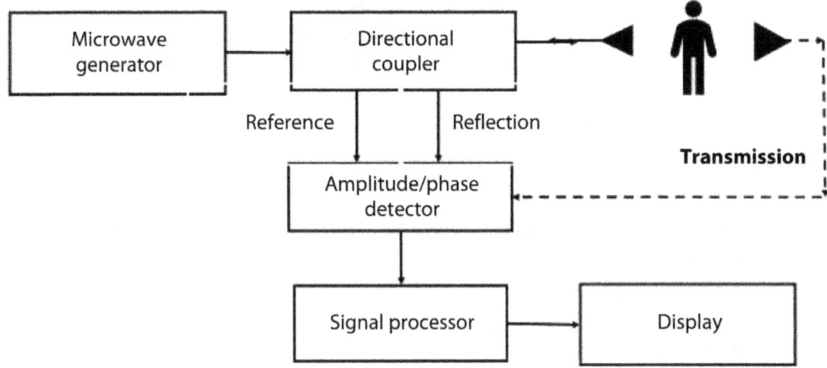


**FIGURE 2.1** A basic functional diagram of a Doppler microwave physiological sensor.

monitoring, and vital-sign sensing, occurred within this period. Summaries and accounts of the investigations that took place in the 1970s and 1980s in developing applications of Doppler microwaves for noninvasive contact, contactless, and remote sensing and monitoring of physiological signatures and volume changes are available [Lin, 1986, 1989, 1992, 1999; Boric-Lubecke et al., 1999]. Current interest, growth in development, and technological innovations demonstrate the tremendous resilience of and enthusiasm for noninvasive microwave physiological sensing technology and application.

The year 2000 was an important year. For the decade that followed, much of the progress in this area concentrated on improving components, devices, and systems supplemented with signal processing algorithms to enhance sensor performance. These technology developments pushed toward smaller form factor, better accuracy, lower power, lighter weight, longer detection range, and more robust operation for portable and handheld scenarios [Li et al., 2013]. However, it should be noted that the fundamental approach and principle of sensing remained steadfast, which are to provide necessary and sufficient sources energy into the domain of interest to enable relevant sensing observations on the body-centered channel. Fortuitously, for probing the human and animal bodies, RF and microwaves possess the frequency ranges with acceptable dispersion and propagation loss for accurate and reliably sensitive measurements. Indeed, the microwave sensed physiological signals contain significant information about a subject's range, motion, material composition, and surface boundary features that are distinguishable in a heterogeneously complex biological background, which will inform the discussion in later chapters of this book.

### 2.2.1 Respiratory Activity Measurement

As mentioned previously, the investigation of microwave Doppler radar techniques to measure and remotely monitor respiratory activity began in the 1970s [Lin, 1975; Lin and Salinger, 1975]. The technique involved the use of CW microwave radar for measuring the respiratory movements of humans and animals (for example, cats, rabbits, and rats). The noncontact or remote sensing technique is based on the backscattering of microwave radiation. A beam of microwave radiation is directed toward the upper torso of the subject, the reflection from the chest is compared to the transmitted energy, and the resultant signal is measured to provide respiratory information. The method is direct, noninvasive, and does not require any direct skin contact or electrode attachment to the subject.

A basic functional diagram of a Doppler microwave radar sensor is shown in Figure 2.1. The system consists of a source of microwave radiation, a signal sampling device (directional coupler), a pair of transmitting and receiving antennas, an amplitude or phase detector, a set of appropriate low-pass and high-pass frequency filters as the signal processor, and a visual display unit.

#### 2.2.1.1 Respiration in Rabbits

In one series of experiments, an albino rabbit was confined to a cardboard box. The distance between the 10 GHz horn antenna and the rabbit in the box was 30 cm [Lin, 1975]. The receiving horn was located either right next to the transmitting horn, or at an angle, but was aimed at the upper torso of the rabbit. The received signal was fed to a ratio meter for signal detection, where the amplitude was compared with a portion of the forward microwave signal. The ratio meter provided the instantaneous ratio between the scattered and the reference signals, and the output is a voltage whose fundamental frequency corresponds to the rate of respiration. A strip chart recording is shown in Figure 2.2. In addition to respiration rate, the resultant signal can be analyzed to give additional respiratory and body movement information. The method is simple, noninvasive, and does not require any skin contact through the rabbit's fur.

#### 2.2.1.2 Breathing of a Seated Human Subject

An example of the experimental results obtained using the same setup as in Figure 2.1 for a seated human subject breathing purposefully at 47 times a minute is given in Figure 2.3. The subject was fully clothed. The distance between the subject and the X-band horn antenna was 30 cm and the incident power density was about 1 microwatt per square centimeter (or 10 mW/m$^2$) [Lin, 1975]. It is seen that the respiratory waveform resembles that of a sinusoid without clutter noise. The noninvasive measurement suggests that the technique can be used for reliably sensing and monitoring human respiration.

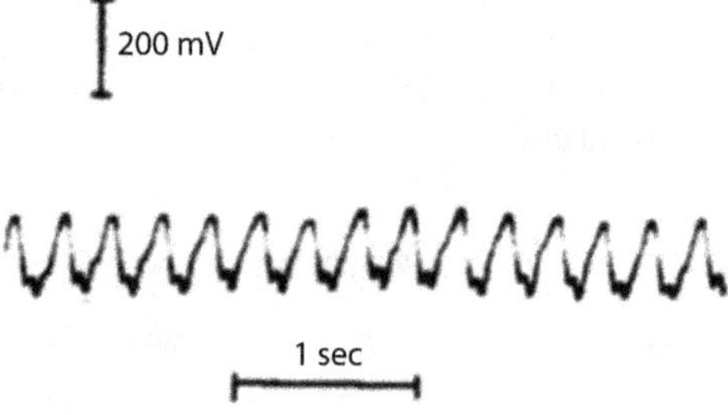


**FIGURE 2.2** Microwave measurement of respiration of an unanesthetized but calm rabbit inside of a cardboard box.

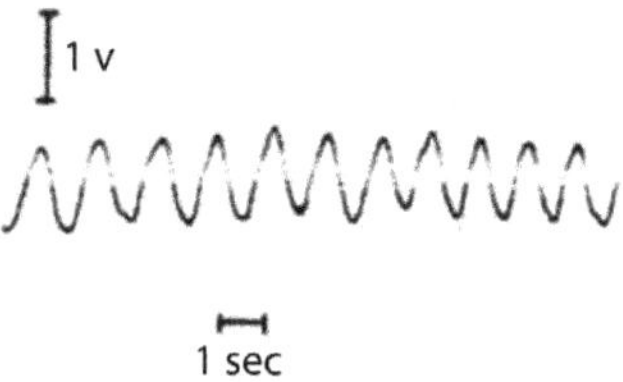


**FIGURE 2.3** Microwave respiratory measurement for a seated human subject breathing at 47 times per minute.

#### 2.2.1.3 Microwave Apnea Detection

Continuous monitoring of respiratory activities during the first days of life of low-birth-weight infants is especially helpful because stimuli sufficient to waken the infant are usually strong enough to re-establish breathing. A contactless microwave apnea monitor based on microwave CW Doppler radar was designed, fabricated, and evaluated in cats [Lin et al., 1977]. In this case, a transceiver horn antenna directed microwaves at 10 GHz toward the upper torso of the cat (Figure 2.4). As Figure 2.5 shows, the Doppler microwave apnea monitor can detect instantaneous changes in respiration including artificially induced hyperventilation and apnea in an anesthetized cat (3 kg) positioned in recumbency in an incubator, and the return of the cat's respiration to normal, in real time. The remote microwave-sensing approach is advantageous over more conventional techniques because it does not require any physical contact with the subject. Furthermore, the results are especially supportive of current interest in the use of noninvasive and contactless microwave Doppler monitoring for sleep research.

#### 2.2.1.4 Respiratory Record of Cats Under Stress

A continuous record of the Doppler radar-sensed respiratory record of an anesthetized cat under heat stress by subjecting it to differential heating of the head is shown in Figure 2.6. A 10 GHz standard gain horn antenna is aimed toward the

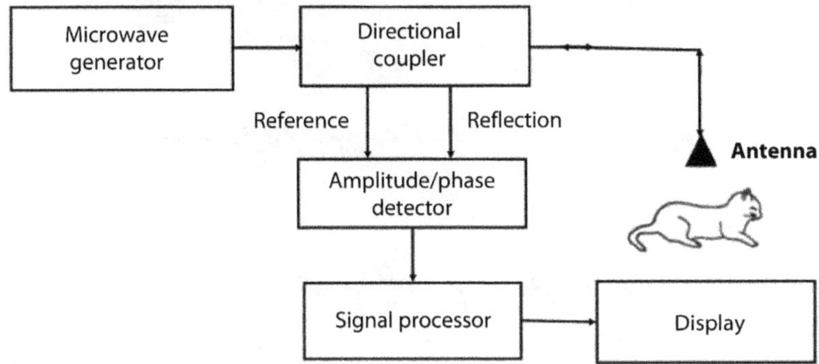


**FIGURE 2.4** A transceiver horn antenna directed microwaves at 10 GHz toward the upper torso of the cat.

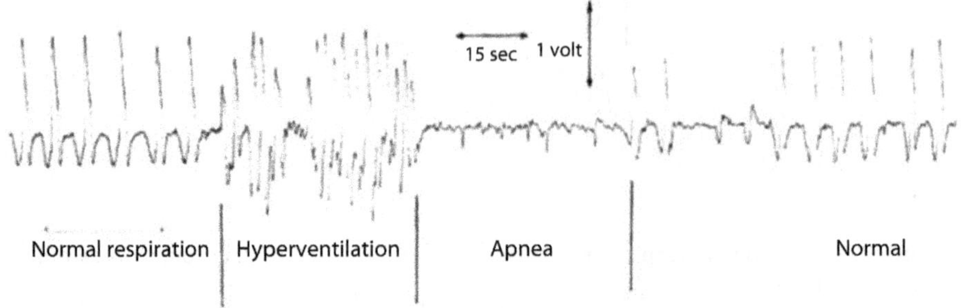


**FIGURE 2.5** A microwave apnea detector recorded respiratory activity of an anesthetized cat showing apneic episode and recovery.

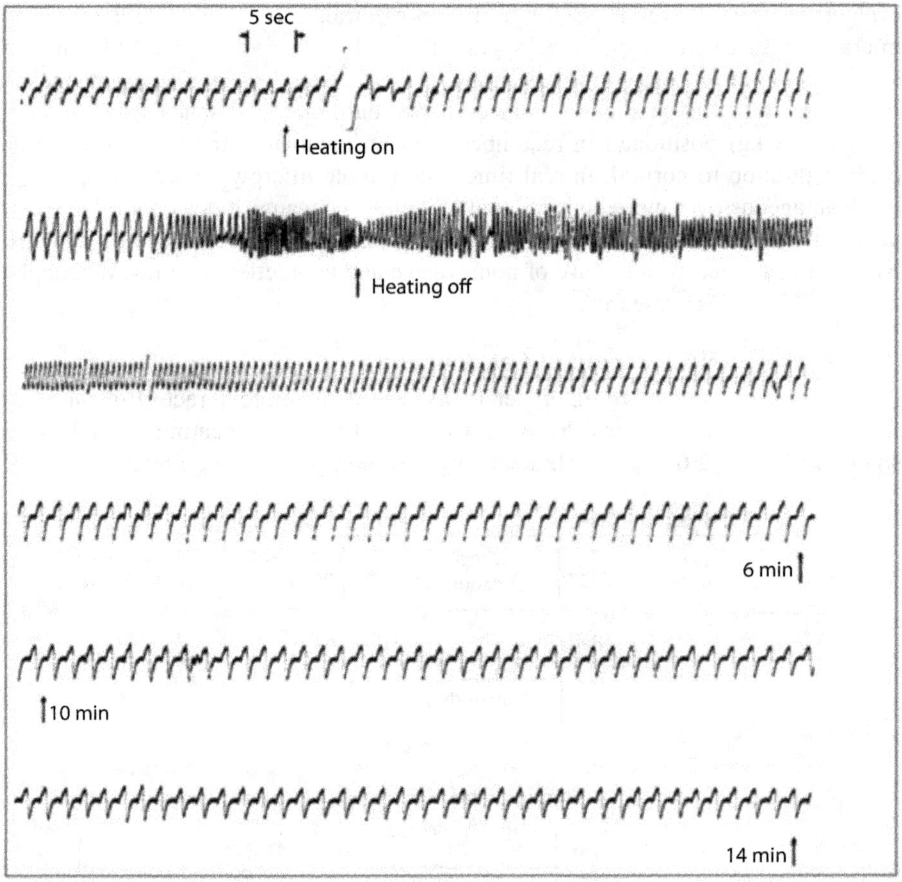

5 sec
Heating on
Heating off
6 min
10 min
14 min

**FIGURE 2.6** Continuous tracing of microwave sensor-monitored respiratory record of a cat subjected to a brief period (heating on and off) of selective heating of the head and brain.

thorax of the animal at 2 meters. The figure shows that the Doppler microwave sensor can register sudden and rapid changes in respiratory activity. The respiration rate increases simultaneously with brain heating. A period of hyperventilation is followed by an intense tachypnea or panting respiration. The rapid panting gradually ended about 14 minutes after cession of brain heating to return to normal. In this case, the 10 GHz X-band source had a maximum output of 10 mW. The incident power density is 10 mW/m$^2$.

### 2.2.2 Measurement of Heart Rate and Sensing of Cardiac Events

Movements and vibrations on the chest wall can manifest events generated by the beating heart inside the chest. These physiological mechanical events are measurable using Doppler microwaves and, as mentioned previously, are referred to as microwave apexcardiography. MACG can be recorded as in ECG to provide an index for assessment of cardiac performance. The principle of operation is based on detection of the changes in the reflected microwaves caused by displacements and vibrations of the chest wall in response to ventricular contraction [Lin et al., 1979]. The functional schematic for the low-power noncontact microwave technique (Figure 2.7) is comparable to the microwave system shown in Figure 2.1. Microwave energy is derived from a signal generator operating at 2450 MHz. The incident power is fed through a 20 dB directional coupler and emitted through a coaxial antenna. The reflected microwave signal is modulated both in amplitude and phase by the moving chest wall. Using the forward signal as a reference, both the amplitude and phase of the reflected signal can be measured as a function of small chest-wall displacement over the heart with a vector voltmeter (instead of a ratio meter mentioned, which works on the signal amplitude). Since the linear phase

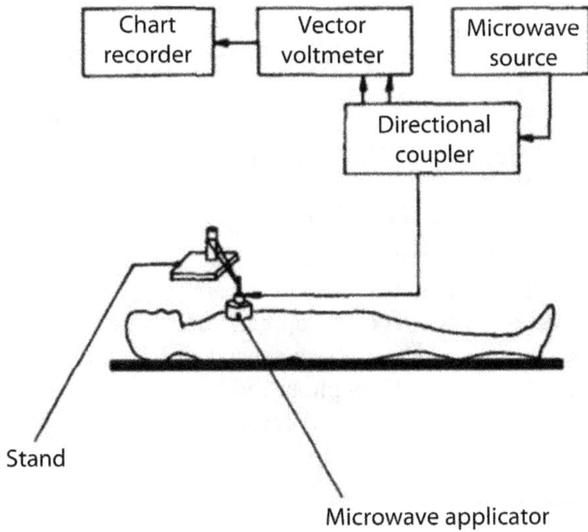


**FIGURE 2.7** A human participant lying on a table in the supine position.

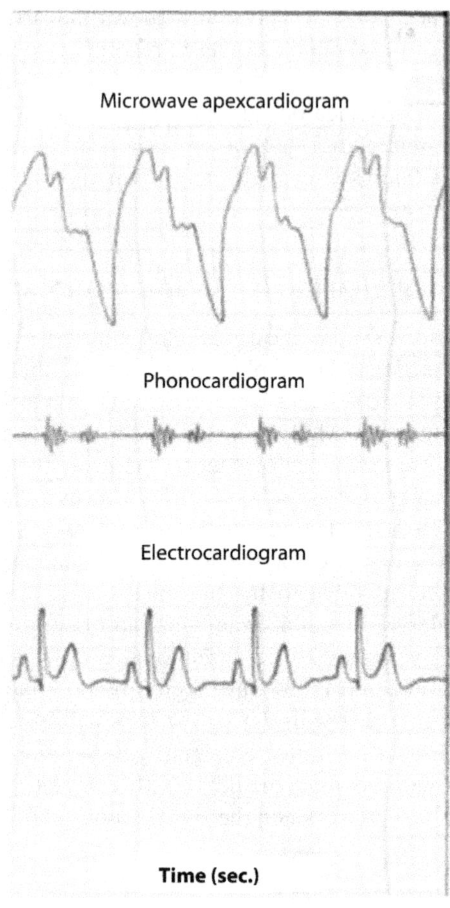


**FIGURE 2.8** Microwave apexcardiography or Doppler radar sensing of a healthy young male participant's cardiac events.

variation yields a stronger signal, the output voltage corresponding to phase variation is chosen for detection.

For the experimental results shown in Figure 2.8, the human subject lies on a table in the supine position. The coaxial circular antenna applicator (see Lin et al., 1982) is located over the left side of heart (i.e., over the apex of the heart, near the sternum) with a separation of 3 cm between the applicator's front end and the chest wall. Figure 2.7 presents the microwave phase-sensed pulsatile response for a healthy young male who held his breath throughout the measurement. The ECG and heart-sound tracings for the same subject are recorded simultaneously. It is seen that the same heart rate is provided by the ECG, heart sound, and pulsatile microwave tracings. As the description in Chapter 7 shows, noninvasive Doppler microwave sensing can replicate the hemodynamic events within the heart during each cardiac cycle [Lin et al., 1979] and successfully and reproducibly measure cardiovascular signal waveforms and timing characteristics in the cardiac cycle of sufficient diagnostic quality to assist contactless noninvasive assessment of cardiovascular performance [Papp et al., 1987].

The Doppler microwave images of the hemodynamic events within the left ventricle give distinctly different characteristics from a conventional chest-attached, microphone-sensed phonocardiogram (PCG), which records the mechanical vibrations associated with the opening and closing of the heart valves. Furthermore, MACG resembles the conventional SCG signal, since both are related to the precordial displacements or vibrations. However, SCG is typically recorded by attaching an accelerometer to the skin, near the sternum. This difference represents a unique feature offered by the noncontact microwave technique. Doppler microwave radar has the advantage of not requiring any mechanical contact with the subject. It also has a very wide frequency response, limited only by the bandwidth (1 kHz) of the vector voltmeter. It can reproduce the heart signal such as the precordial movement of the chest wall caused by left ventricular contraction more faithfully than other competing techniques. The technique is simple, uses low power, and is noninvasive and noncontact.

Heart rate and respiratory rate along with temperature and blood pressure are the four most important clinical vital-sign measurements that indicate the general state of physical health of a person. The results shown in Figures 2.3 and 2.6 for a Doppler microwave-measured respiratory pattern and in Figure 2.8 for a heart rate signal demonstrate separately and collectively the ability of the Doppler microwave technique for noninvasive and contactless sensing of these important vital signs. Their usefulness in assessing the status of the body's vital functions was furthered through the development of systems for extracting heart and respiration rates simultaneously using a single sensor in the decade to follow (see Section 2.3.1).

### 2.2.3 Noninvasive Monitoring Fluid Buildup in the Lungs

The application of microwaves to record volume changes in biological subjects was first suggested a few decades ago [Moskalenko, 1960]. In particular, the paper mentioned the use of changes of microwave reflectance and transmittance as a measure of circulatory and respiratory volume changes. A dozen years later, a theoretical discussion of the possibilities for applying microwaves in detection and mapping of lung diseases characterized by the presence of excess water was presented [Susskind, 1973]. Subsequently, microwave technology was explored to assess pulmonary edema using radar reflection and microwave transmission approaches some years later [Durney et al., 1978; Iskander and Durney, 1980; Pedersen et al., 1978].

When fluid builds up in and around the lungs, it makes it difficult to breathe. This may happen with pulmonary edema or pleural effusion. Pulmonary edema is caused by excessive fluid collection in the air sacs (the tiny alveoli) in the lungs. Pleural effusion occurs when fluid builds up in the layers of tissue that cover or line the outside of the lungs. The pleura are thin membranes that line the lungs. The accumulated fluid has a considerably higher dielectric constant or permittivity compared to lung tissue and, thus, can be detected using microwave techniques.

The experimental setup for the measurement is essentially the same as what is shown in Figure 2.1, except for the use of a network analyzer and a two-channel

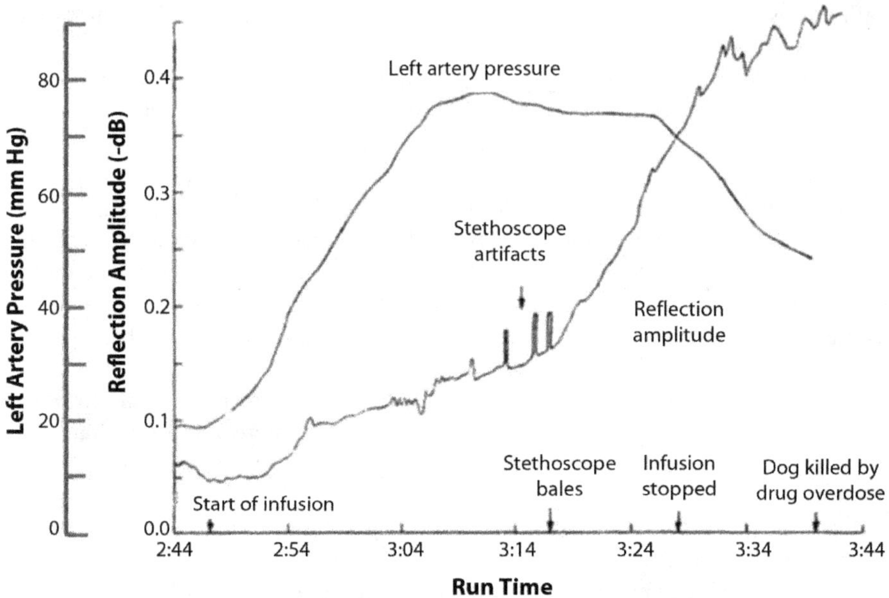


**FIGURE 2.9** Changes in the baseline of the amplitude of the microwave reflection coefficient and in left atrial pressure during development of pulmonary edema in an anesthetized 25 kg dog on a respirator.

strip chart recorder. The 13 cm × 13 cm square direct-contact microwave applicator was strapped to the right side of the chest just below the right forelimb. The frequency used was 915 MHz and the power density from the applicator was limited to less than 0.1 W/m$^2$. Figure 2.9 shows the change in the baseline of the amplitude of microwave reflection coefficient and left atrial pressure during development of pulmonary edema in a 25 kg dog that was anesthetized and placed on a respirator.

Pulmonary edema was induced by inserting a balloon catheter into the left atrium of the anesthetized dog. Fluids (2000 mL of isotonic saline solution) were infused over a 22-minute period with no significant changes in either left atrial pressure or microwave reflection. At 2:47 pm (see Figure 2.9), an infusion of Dextran 40 was initiated, which immediately produced a steadily increasing left atrial pressure and, 5 minutes later, a steadily changing baseline of the amplitude of reflection coefficient. At 3:17 pm, crackles were heard with a stethoscope and, subsequently, the amplitude of reflected microwave was rapidly increasing. At 3:28 pm, the infusion of Dextran 40 was stopped, at which time a total of 2600 mL had been administered. The experiment was terminated at 3:40 pm. Autopsy revealed a grossly enlarged heart and severe edema of the lower lobes of the lungs. The amplitude change accompanying the progression of edema is clear and gives supportive evidence to the monitoring potential of the microwave reflection technique. Thus, the experimental results demonstrated the feasibility for real-time microwave measurement of fluid buildup in and around the lungs inside the chest.

## 2.3 MICROWAVE SENSING OF VITAL SIGNS AND ARTERIAL PULSES IN THE 1980s

Research on the noninvasive microwave approach for measuring cardiopulmonary parameters continued and expanded to pulse pressure waves, arterial-wall or blood-vessel motion, as well as for cerebral edemas and cerebral vascular extravasations in the 1980s. The investigations and proposals have also included vital-sign monitoring of patients with critical burns and premature developments, and heartbeat and respiration-rate detection in victims of environmental contamination or disasters such as earthquakes or building collapses [Chan and Lin, 1985, 1987; Chen et al., 1986; Lin, 1986, 1989].

### 2.3.1 Remote Contactless Sensing of Vital Signs

The ability to detect remotely such vital signs as heartbeat and respiration rate is particularly useful when direct contact with the subject is either impossible or undesirable. Also, this approach can overcome artifacts and variabilities in sensitivity that result when electrodes are attached to or strapped on the subject. In some situations, remote contactless measurements can be more advantageous. Indeed, microwave detection was obtained at distances of a few to tens of meters, with or without intervening nonconducting physical barriers.

The most often used frequencies are 2 and 10 GHz microwaves. The potential applications are wide, including patient health assessment, health fitness sensing, neonatal monitoring, burn management, rescue operations necessitated by fire, chemical, or nuclear accidents, and natural disasters such as an earthquake [Chan and Lin, 1985, 1987; Chen et al., 1986; Popovic et al., 1984, Sharpe et al., 1986]. Both heartbeat and respiration rate have been detected from chest movements by 10 GHz microwaves at a distance of a few centimeters from subjects [Byrne et al., 1986; Chan and Lin, 1985; 1987; Popovic et al., 1984]. Furthermore, remote contactless sensing was reported at distances as far as 30 meters with millimeter-wavelength microwaves [Sharpe et al., 1986].

#### 2.3.1.1 Microprocessor-Based Remote Contactless Vital-Sign Sensing

By the early 1980s, contactless microwave sensing of the frequency and regularity of heart and respiration rates was increasingly recognized as a promising technique for assessing the functional status of cardiopulmonary organs. Computers (known then as minicomputers) were used for processing and enhancing the measurements through off-line signal analysis and cardiopulmonary rate extraction. The approaches involved considerable manual data handling in addition to the processing done by computers. Later, the process of analyzing and extracting cardiopulmonary signals from chest movements became more automated through the development of microprocessor-enabled pattern recognition algorithms.

A portable microprocessor-based noninvasive contactless Doppler microwave heart rate and respiration monitor was developed for use in short-range situations where direct contact with the subject is either impossible or undesirable [Chan and Lin, 1985; 1987; Popovic et al., 1984]. The front end consisted of a low-power (10.5 GHz, 5–10 mW)

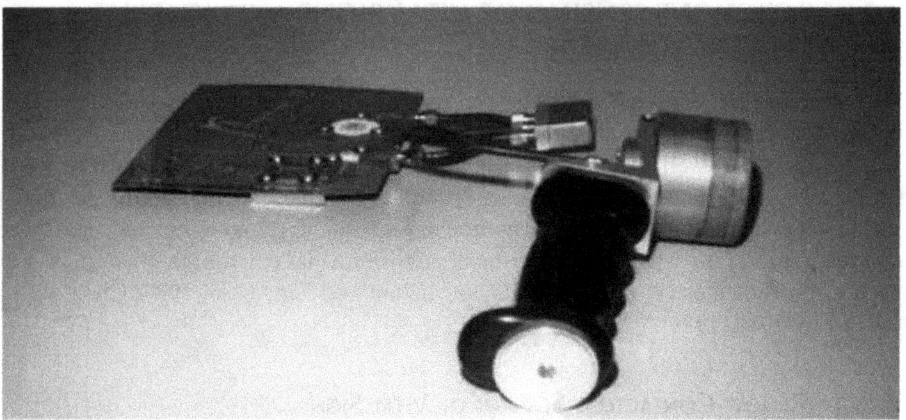

**FIGURE 2.10** A microprocessor-based contactless 10.5 GHz microwave vital sign monitor showing a circuit board and handheld circularly polarized antenna.

microwave transceiver and a circularly polarized X-band antenna (Figure 2.10). The output from the transceiver, which is proportional to the displacement of the chest-wall movement associated with expansion and contraction of the heart and lungs, fed into an analog signal processing circuit for amplification and filtration.

A software algorithm was designed to assist detect both heartbeat and respiration signals and to separate the higher-frequency heartbeat signal from the lower-frequency breathing signal. Figure 2.11 displays typical heartbeat- and breathing-signal waveforms recorded from a healthy young adult male. As expected, the two signals have clearly distinguishable characteristics. The typical breathing signal resembles a sinusoid-like respiration signal, while the heartbeat signal displays the recurrent and usual complex characteristics. The performance of the vital heartbeat rate and respiration monitor was evaluated on human subjects. A comparison of monitor-detected and visually determined heartbeat and respiration rates gave maximum errors between the sensor and visual determinations of 7% and 9%, respectively, with 0.98

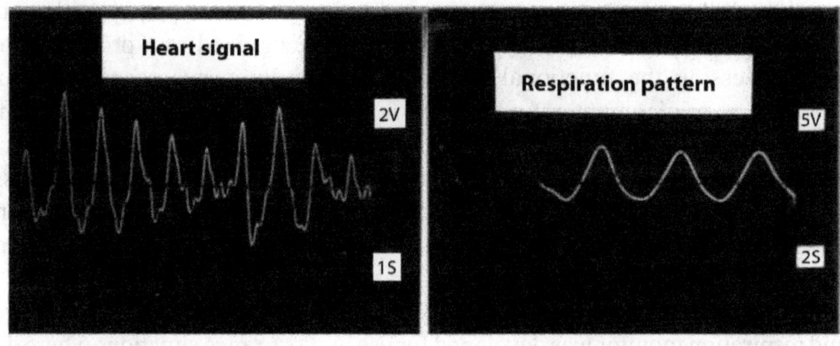


**FIGURE 2.11** Heart and respiration channel records of a healthy human subject from a microprocessor-based contactless 10.5 GHz microwave vital sign monitor.

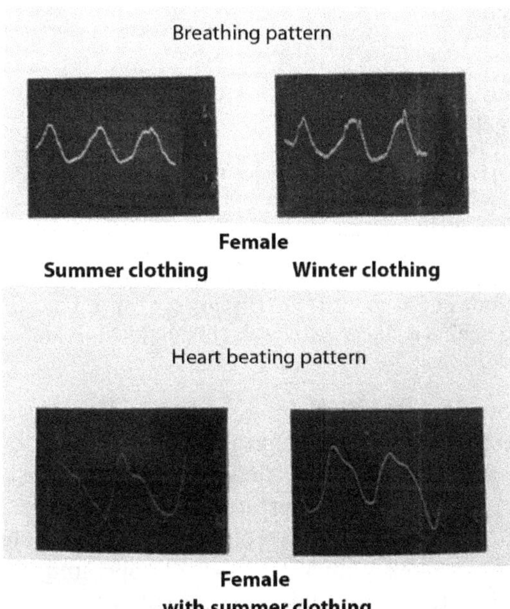


**FIGURE 2.12** Contactless remote microwave sensing of vital signs of a human subject wearing summer or winter clothing.

and 0.99 calculated correlation coefficients. Note that remote noncontact Doppler microwave radar sensors can penetrate layers of clothing to detect the vital signs of human subjects. Figure 2.12 shows the contactless sensed vital signs (respiration and heartbeat) of human subjects wearing summer or winter clothing.

#### 2.3.1.2 Through-Wall Detection and Remote Sensing of Vital Signs

In remote sensing of vital signs, the returned microwave signal received by the antenna consists of a large clutter and a weak Doppler signal scattered from the body. Aside from more directive and higher-gain antennas, system designs that minimized various noise sources to achieve high sensitivity with low levels of radiated microwave power were some of the important considerations in further efforts during this period. A manual clutter-cancellation subsystem, in which the clutter signal was cancelled by a reference signal whose amplitude and phase are adjusted by a variable attenuator and a phase shifter in a 10 dB directional coupler, successfully demonstrated capabilities to detect the heartbeat and respiration rate of human subjects lying on the ground at 30 meters and through nonconducting physical fences [Chen et al., 1986; Sharpe et al., 1986]. Figure 2.13 shows that a 10 GHz microwave system with manual clutter cancellation was able to detect the heartbeat and respiration rate of subjects hidden behind a 15 cm thick cinder block wall [Chen et al., 1986]. It is noteworthy that a microprocessor-controlled automatic clutter-cancellation subsystem consisting of a programmable microwave attenuator and a programmable microwave phase-shifter was developed subsequently for microwave

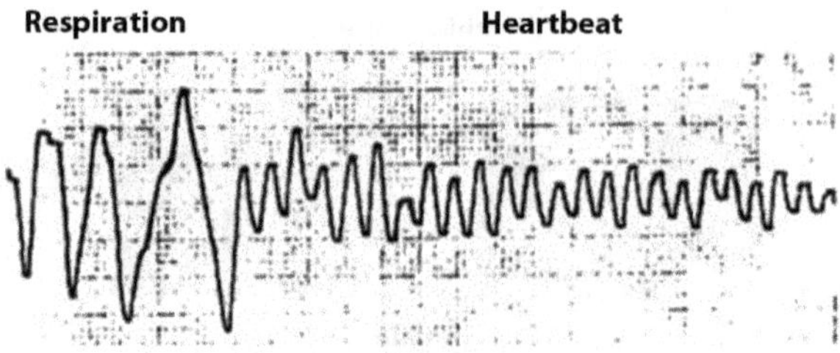


**FIGURE 2.13** Microwave (20 mW, 10 GHz) sensing of heartbeat and respiration from a human subject sitting behind a cinder block wall (15 cm thick) at 3 m.

life-detection systems (L-band 2 GHz or X-band 10 GHz). A series of experiments demonstrated the applicability of the improved microwave life-detection system for rescue purposes with the automated clutter-cancellation subsystem [Chuang et al., 1991]. Furthermore, a 2 GHz system performed well for remotely detecting human breathing and heartbeat signals through a pile of 1 m thick rubble.

Moreover, a lower-frequency microwave system operating at 450 or 1150 MHz was evaluated for detection of breathing and heartbeat signals of human subjects through obstacles as thick as 3 meters of earthquake rubble or collapsed building materials. As shown in Figure 2.14, the breathing and heartbeat signals can be extracted from a human subject buried in a field test environment of simulated earthquake rubble [Chen et al. 2000]. The utility of similar systems was demonstrated for use in a variety of rescue-related operations where direct physical contact with the subject is impractical or not possible.

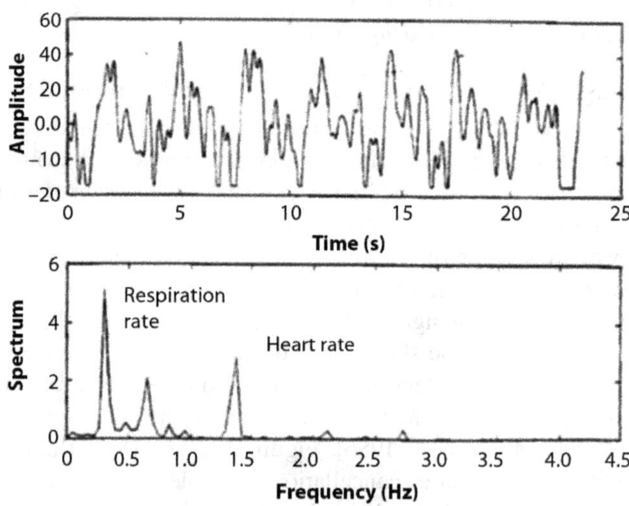


**FIGURE 2.14** Heartbeat and respiration signals of a female human subject recorded from the top of simulated rubble with a 450 MHz reflector antenna. The subject is lying within a cavity among the rubble. The peak at 0.6 Hz is the second harmonic of the respiration signal.

### 2.3.2 Arterial Pulse Wave and Pressure Sensing

Doppler microwaves were applied to investigate the wall properties and pressure-pulse characteristics at a variety of arterial sites such as the carotid, brachial, radial, and femoral arteries [Lee and Lin, 1985; Papp et al., 1987; Stuchly et al., 1980; Thansandote et al., 1983]. Typically, microwave reflection measurements were performed using a waveguide antenna (probe) placed in direct contact with the skin over the artery of interest (Figure 2.15). An oscilloscope record of brachial artery motion measured using a 25 GHz Doppler microwave sensor in contact with the skin over the artery is shown in Figure 2.16. Likewise, a set of experimental tracings obtained from 10 GHz waveguide antennas is given in Figure 2.17 for arteries in the upper and lower extremities [Stuchly et al., 1980]. The Doppler microwave tracings are proportional to the arterial-wall movements and closely resemble the well-known arterial waveform for these arteries. They can provide information about the regularity and frequency characteristics of arterial-wall movement, as well as the physiological condition and patency of the artery. Evaluation with human participants conducted with 3 and 10 GHz systems found that the 3 GHz Doppler radar is significantly less sensitive to changes of arterial-wall movement than the 10 GHz system [Thansandote et al., 1983].

An example of a microwave-sensed carotid-pulse waveform in a patient measured by the contact application of 25 GHz microwaves is shown in Figure 2.18, where the simultaneously recorded intra-aortic pressure waves are also displayed for comparison. Note the resemblance of the Doppler microwave-sensed arterial pulse and the invasively recorded pressure waves. The similarity between the two sets of waveforms clearly shows a large segment of the two waveforms has the same

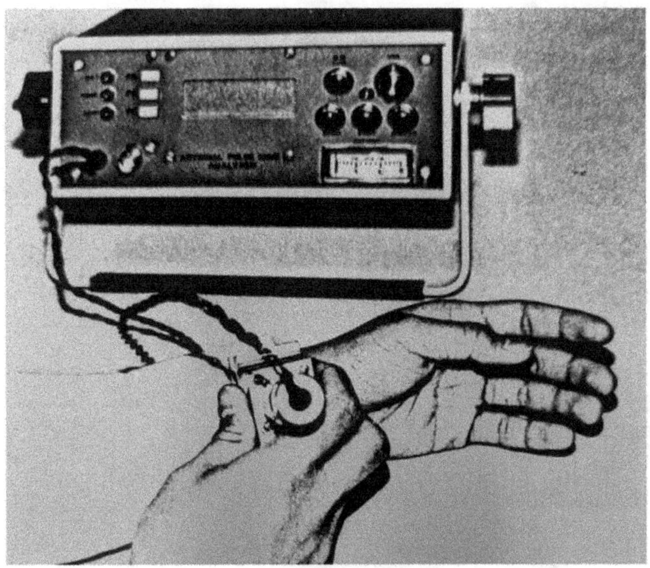

**FIGURE 2.15** A direct contact Doppler microwave arterial pulse wave sensor.

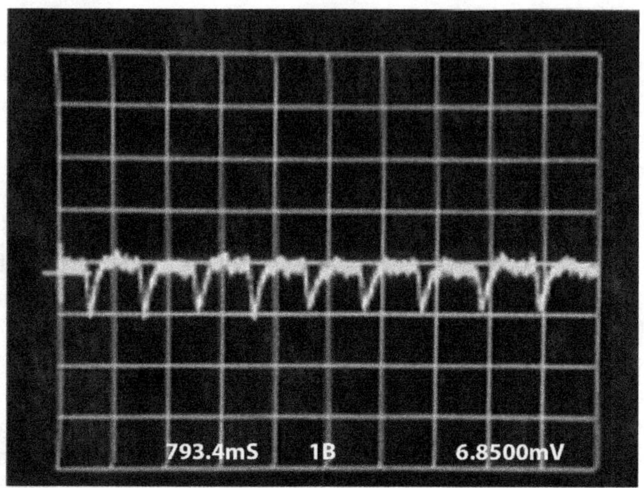


**FIGURE 2.16** Oscilloscope tracings of brachial artery motion measured using a 25 GHz Doppler microwave sensor in contact with the skin on the arm over the artery.

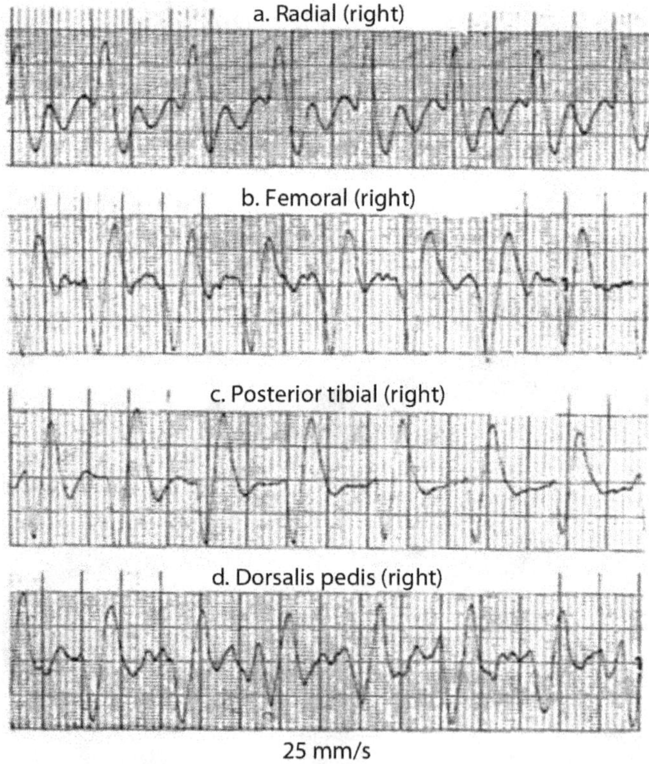


**FIGURE 2.17** Tracings of arterial-wall motion measured using 10 GHz Doppler microwaves: (a) radial artery in the arm; (b) femoral; (c) posterior tibial; and (d) dorsalis pedis arteries in the leg of a human subject.

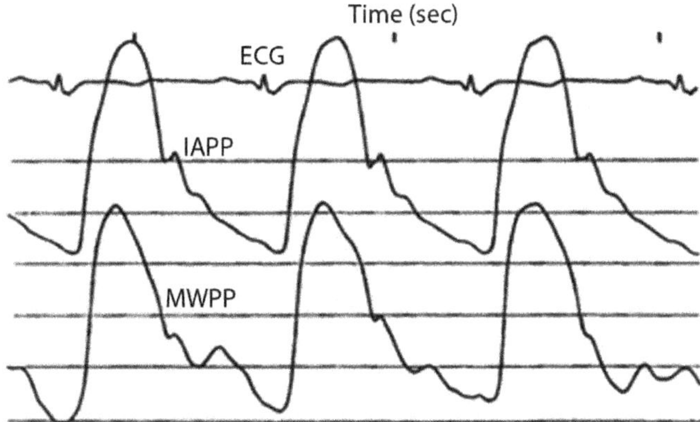


**FIGURE 2.18** Microwave sensing of the carotid pressure pulse wave (MWPP) and invasively recorded intra-aortic pressure pulse wave (IAPP) from a human subject.

characteristics. However, because of its mode of motion detection, the Doppler microwave sensor will detect other motions within its space. For example, the microwave tracings in Figure 2.18 have a distinctive positive wave before each carotid upstroke, which results from jugular venous expansion, which is not present in the corresponding intra-aortic pressure pulse waves.

The consistency of the Doppler microwave pulse waves with respect to the intra-aortic pressure measurements was evaluated by sequential pulse waves from five patients. The results confirm that a noninvasive Doppler microwave sensor can successfully and reproducibly detect pressure-pulse waveforms of diagnostic quality [Papp et al., 1987]. However, the pulse waves obtained by the microwave sensor are relative and cannot be interpreted on an absolute scale since they are derived from the relative expansion of the target artery. Therefore, if used alone, microwave Doppler cannot provide numeric values for systolic and diastolic blood pressure. However, the microwave sensor can be used in conjunction with a calibrated blood pressure measuring device such as an automatic blood pressure cuff, which would provide the necessary calibration for the Doppler microwave measure pressure waves [Lin and Lin, 2009].

### 2.3.3 Cerebral Edemas and Extravasations

A microwave-sensing technique to monitor brain edema investigated the use of transmitted microwave energy to detect the increased content of intracranial water [Clarke and Lin, 1983; Lin and Clarke, 1982]. By recording the phase of a transmitted microwave signal (see Figure 2.19), increases in intracranial saline of about 1% are detectable in rats. Figure 2.20 shows the recordings of relative phase change and ICP for an injection of an aliquot of saline (0.07 mL), followed by another injection (0.05 mL). A sharp increase in ICP is paralleled by a negative increase in phase. These findings indicate that the progression of brain edema on a long-term basis may be assessed using the microwave technique. Furthermore, phase changes that are related to small intracranial variations of pressure are observed, indicating that detection of

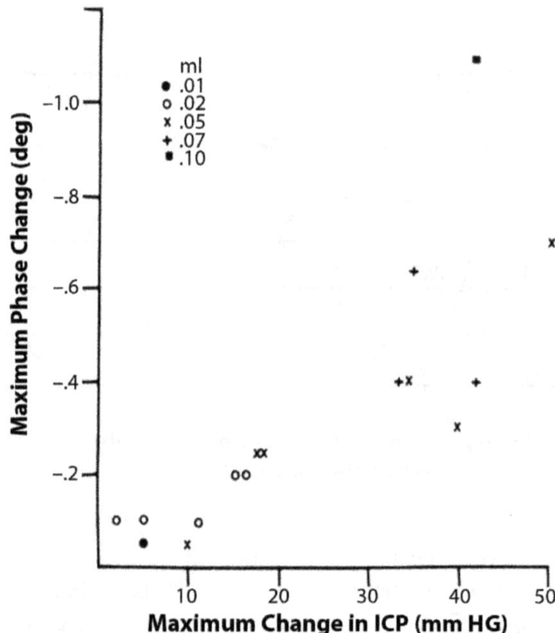


**FIGURE 2.19** Microwave sensing of intracranial pressure (ICP) in rats. Maximum phase change versus ICP change for injections of aliquots (symbols represent volume of aliquots).

pathologic pressure variations such as Traube-Hering-Mayer waves and plateau waves [Bumstead et al., 2017; Cerutti et al., 1994; Julien, 2006; Nelson et al., 2001; Rieger et al., 2018] is possible by the noninvasive microwave technique. Indeed, reports have shown typical increased water content of white brain matter of 9% [Penn, 1980]. This level of increased water content is well within the range of detectability by microwave sensing. The water content of white and gray matter in a normal human brain are 0.71 and 0.01 and 0.83 and 0.03 g/mL, respectively [Whittall et al., 1997].

## 2.4 A SUMMARY

In summary, Sections 2.2 and 2.3 presented brief historical accounts of the pioneering investigations that took place in the 1970s and 1980s in developing applications of Doppler microwaves for noninvasive contact, contactless, and remote detection and monitoring of physiological signatures, movements, and volume changes. The growing current interest and expanding applications in noninvasive microwave-sensing present the scientific community with unprecedented research and development opportunities. It is also clear that each of the application scenarios is accompanied by its own technology challenges and unique sets of potential and critical limitations that would preclude an overall solution for all the scenarios. Much work remains to be done in enhancing and extending the capabilities of these Doppler microwave-sensing modalities. Note that the average power levels of microwave energy emitted by these sensors are 3 or 20 mW, which are one to two orders of magnitude lower

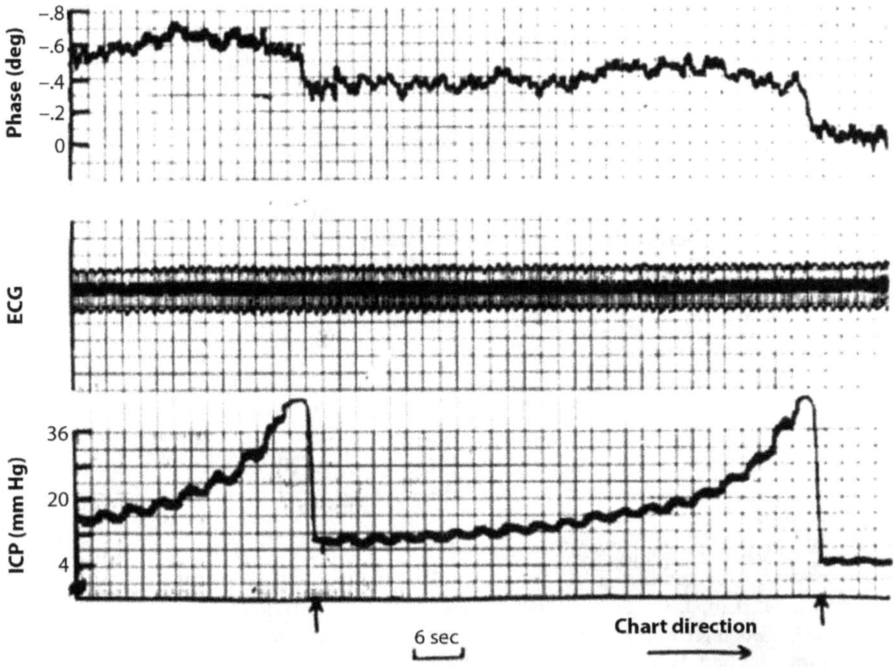


**FIGURE 2.20** Intracranial pressure (ICP) in rats (bottom), electrocardiogram (ECG) (middle), and microwave phase change (top) following aliquot injection of 0.07 and 0.05 mL aliquots of saline (arrows).

than the power consumption levels of the 125–250 mW currently permitted for cellular mobile telephone operations. Thus, noninvasive microwave Doppler physiological sensing systems, as low-power devices, would conveniently sidestep any wireless radiation safety regulations or simply render it a moot issue.

## REFERENCES

Aliot, E., Lazzara, R., Eds., 1987. Ventricular Tachycardias from Mechanism to Therapy. Dordrecht: Martinus Nijhoff

Anand, R. K., Sinclair, I. N., Jenkins, R. D., Hiechle, J. F. Jr, James, L., Spears, J. R., 1988. Laser balloon angioplasty: Effect of constant temperature versus constant power on tissue weld strength. Laser Surg. Med., 8:40–44

Arber, S., Lin, J. C., 1985a. Microwave-induced changes in nerve cells: Effects of modulation and temperature. Bioelectromagnetics, 6:257–270

Arber, S., Lin, J. C., 1985b. Extracellular calcium and microwave enhancement of conductance in snail neurons. Radiat. Environ. Biophys, 24:149–156

Banks, W. A., 2016. From blood-brain barrier to blood-brain interface: New opportunities for CNS drug delivery. Nat. Rev. Drug Dis., 15:275–292

Beckman, K. J., Lin, J. C., Wang, Y., Illes, R. W., Papp, M. A., Hariman, R. J., 1987. Production of reversible and irreversible atrioventricular block by microwave energy. 60th Scientific Sessions, Anaheim, CA: American Heart Association; also in Circulation 1987. Abstract. 16:1612

Begley, D. J., 2004. Delivery of therapeutic agents to the central nervous system: The problems and the possibilities. Pharmacol. Therap., 104:29–45

Beckman, K.J.K. J., Lin, J.C.J. C., Wang, Y., Illes, R.W.R. W., Papp, M.A.M. A., Hariman, R.JR. J., 1987. Production of reversible and irreversible atrioventricular block by microwave energy. 60th Scientific Sessions, American Heart Association, Anaheim, CA; also in Circulation 1987. Abstract. 16:1612

Bernardi, P., Cavagnaro, M., Lin, J. C., Pisa, S., Piuzzi, E., 2004. Distribution of SAR and temperature elevation induced in a phantom by a microwave cardiac ablation catheter. IEEE Trans. Microwave Theory and Techniques, 52:1978–1986

Boric-Lubecke, O., Nikawa, Y., Snyder, W., Lin, J., Mizuno, K., 1999. Novel microwave and millimeter-wave biomedical applications. Electronics, 3:46–53

Breithardt, G., Borggrefe, M., Zipes, D. P., 1988. Nonpharmacological Therapy of Tachyarrhythmias. Mount Kisco, NY: Futura Publishing

Broens, T. H., Veld, R. M., Vollenbroek-Hutten, M. M., Hermens, H. J., van Halteren, A. T., Nieuwenhuis, L. J., 2007. Determinants of successful telemedicine implementations: A literature study. J. Telemed. Telecare, 13(6):303–309

Bumstead, J. R., Bauer, A. Q., Wright, P. W., Culver, J. P., 2017. Cerebral functional connectivity and Mayer waves in mice: Phenomena and separability. J. Cereb. Blood Flow Metab., 37:471–484

Byrne, W., Flynn, R., Zapp, R., Siegel, M., 1986. Adaptive filter processing in microwave remote heart monitors. IEEE Trans. Biomed. Eng., 33:717–722

Cavarnaro, M., Lin, J. C., 2019. Importance of exposure duration and metrics on correlation between RF energy absorption and temperature increase in a human model. IEEE Trans. Biomed. Eng., 66(8):2253–2258

Cerutti, C., Barres, C., Paultre, C. Z., 1994. Baroreflex modulation of blood pressure and heart rate variabilities in rats: Assessment by spectral analysis. Am. J. Physiol., 266:H1993–H2000

Chan, K. H., Lin, J. C., 1985. An algorithm for extracting cardiopulmonary rates from chest movement. Proc. IEEE Eng. Med. Biol. Conf., IEEE, 466–469

Chan, K. H., Lin, J. C., 1987. Microprocessor based cardiopulmonary rate monitor. Med. Biol. Eng. Comput., 25:41–44

Chen, K. M., Huang, Y., Zhang, J., Norman, A., 2000. Microwave life detection systems for searching human subjects under earthquake rubble and behind barrier. IEEE Trans. Biomed. Eng., 47(1):105–114

Chen, K. M., Misra, D., Chuang, H. R., Postow, E., 1986. An X-band microwave life-detection system. IEEE Trans. Biomed. Eng., BME-33(7):697–701

Chokshi, S. K., Meyers, S., Abi-Mansour, P., 1987. Percutaneous transluminal coronary angioplasty: Ten years' experience. Prog. Cardiovas. Dis., 3:147–210

Chuang, H. R., Chen, Y. F., Chen, K. M., 1991. Automatic clutter canceller for microwave life-detection system. IEEE Trans. Instrum. Meas., 40:747–750

Clarke, M. J., Lin, J. C., 1983. Microwave sensing of increased intracranial water content. Invest. Radiol., 18:245–248

DARPA (Defense Advanced Research Projects Agency), 2017. RadioBio: What role does electromagnetic signaling have in biological systems? [Online]. Available: www.darpa.mil/news-events/2017-02-07

Datta, N. R., Ordonez, S. G., Gaipl, U. S., Paulides, M. M., Crezee, H., Gellermann, J., Marder, D., Puric, E., Bodis, S., 2015. Local hyperthermia combined with radiotherapy and-/or chemotherapy: Recent advances and promises for the future. Cancer Treat. Rev., 41:742–753

Droitcour, A. D., Boric-Lubecke, O., Lubecke, V., Lin, J., Kovacs, G. T. A., 2002. 0.25 m CMOS and BiCMOS single-chip direct-conversion Doppler radars for remote sensing of vital signs. in Int. Solid-State Circuits Conf. Dig., vol. 1, San Francisco, CA, 348

Droitcour, A. D., Boric-Lubecke, O., Lubecke, V., Lin, J., Kovacs, G. T. A., 2003. Range correlation effect on ISM band I/Q CMOS radar for noncontact sensing of vital signs. in IEEE MTT-S Int. Microwave Symp. Dig., vol. 3, Philadelphia, PA, 1945–1948

Droitcour, A. D., Boric-Lubecke, O., Lubecke, V. M., Lin, J., Kovac, G. T. A., 2004. Range correlation and I/Q performance benefits in single-chip silicon Doppler radars for noncontact cardiopulmonary monitoring. IEEE Trans. Microw. Theory Tech., 52(3):838–848

Droitcour, A., Lubecke, V., Lin, J., Boric-Lubecke, O., 2001. A microwave radio for Doppler radar sensing of vital signs. IEEE IMS Digest, 175–178

Durney, C. H., Iskander, M. F., Bragg, D. G., 1978. Noninvasive microwave methods for measuring changes in lung water content. Proc. IEEE Electro/78 30/6, Boston, 1–7

Fontaine, G., Lechat, P. H., Cansell, A., Guiraudon Cruz-Linares, E., Koulibali, M., Chomette, G., Auriol, M., Grosgogeat, Y., 1987. Advances in the treatment of cardiac arrhythmias in the last decade: Definition and role of ablative techniques. In: Fontaine, G., Scheinman, M. M., Eds., Ablation in Cardiac Arrythmias, Mount Kisco, New York: Futura Publishing Company, Inc, 5–19

Gallagher, J. J., Svenson, R. H., Kasell, J. H., German, L. D., Bardy, G. H., Broughton, A., Critelli, G., 1982. Catheter technique for closed-chest ablation of the atrioventricular conduction system. N. Engl. J. Med., 306(4):194–200

Goldman, H., Lin, J. C., Murphy, S., Lin, M. F., 1984. Cerebrovascular Permeability to 86Rb in the rat after exposure to pulsed microwaves. Bioelectromagnetics, 5: 323–330

Hincapié (Chincapin), M. A., Gallego, J. C., Gempeler, A., Piñeros, J. A., Nasner, D., Escobar, M. F., 2020. Implementation and usefulness of telemedicine during the COVID-19 pandemic: A scoping review. J Prim Care Community Health. doi: 10.1177/2150132720980612

Huang, S. K. S., Wilber, D. J., Eds., 2000. Radiofrequency Catheter Ablation of Cardiac Arrhythmias: Basic Concepts and Clinical Applications, 2nd ed, Armonk, New York: Futura

Iskander, M. F., Durney, C. H., 1980. Electromagnetic techniques for medical diagnosis: A review. Proc. IEEE, 68:126–132

Isner, J. M., Clarke, R. H., Eds., 1989. Lasers in Cardiacvascular Disease. Boston: Martinus Nijhoff

Josephson, M. E., 1984. Catheter ablation of arrythmias. Ann. Int. Med., 101:234

Julien, C., 2006. The enigma of Mayer waves: Facts and models. Cardiovasc. Res., 70:12–21

Kent, K. M., Butiroglia, L. G., Black, P. C., Bourassa, M. G., Cowley, M. J., Dorros, G., Detre, K. M., Gossalin, A. J., Gruentzig, A. R., Kelsey, S. F., Mock, M. D., Mullin, S. M., Passamani, E. R., Myler, R. K., Simpson, J., Stertzer, S. M., van Raden, M. J., Williams, D. O., 1984. Long term efficacy of percutaneous transluminal coronary angioplasty (PTCA): Report from the National Heart, Lung and Blood Institute PTCA registry. Amer. J. Cardiol., 53:27c

Koonin, L. M., Hoots, B., Tsang, C. A., et al., 2020. Trends in the use of telehealth during the emergence of the COVID-19 pandemic—United States, January–March 2020. MMWR Morb. Mortal. Wkly. Rep. 69:1595–1599

Lee, J. Y., Lin, J. C., 1985. Microprocessor based non-invasive pulse wave analyzer. IEEE Trans. Biomed. Eng., 32:451–455

Lee, J. Y., Lin, J. C., Popovic, M. A., 1983. Microprocessor-Based Arterial Pulse Wave Analyzer. Conference of IEEE Eng. Columbus, OH: Medicine and Biology Society

Li, C., Lubecke, V. M., Boric-Lubecke, O., Lin, J., 2013. A review on recent advances in Doppler radar sensors for noncontact healthcare monitoring. IEEE Trans. Microw. Theory Tech., 61(5):2046–2060

Lin, J. C., 1975. Noninvasive microwave measurement of respiration. Proc. IEEE, 63:1530

Lin, J. C., 1985. Frequency optimization for microwave imaging of biological tissues. Proc. IEEE, 72:374–375

Lin, J. C., 1986. Microwave propagation in biological dielectrics with application to cardiopulmonary interrogation. In: Larsen, L. E., Jacobi, J. H., Eds., Medical Applications of Microwave Imaging (pp. 47–58), New York: IEEE Press

Lin, J. C., 1989. Microwave noninvasive sensing of physiological signatures. In: Lin, J. C., Ed., Electromagnetic Interaction with Biological Systems (pp. 3–25), Plenum

Lin, J. C., 1990. Transcatheter microwave technology for treatment of cardiovascular diseases. In: O'Connor, M. E., Bentall, R. H. C., Monahan, J. C., Eds., Emerging Electromagnetic Medicine (pp. 125–134), New York: Springer-Verlag

Lin, J. C., 1992. Microwave sensing of physiological movement and volume change: A review. Bioelectromagnetics, 13:557–565

Lin, J. C., 1993a. Diagnostic applications of electromagnetic fields. In: Stone, R., Ed., Review of Radio Science 1992 (pp. 771–778), Oxford University Press

Lin, J. C., 1993b. Microwave technology for minimally invasive interventional procedures. Chinese J. Med, Biol. Eng., 13:293–304

Lin, J. C., 1999a. Catheter microwave ablation therapy for cardiac arrhythmias. Bioelectromagnetics, 20(Suppl):120–132

Lin, J. C., 1999b. Biomedical applications of electromagnetic fields and waves: Radio frequencies and microwaves. In: Stone, R., Ed., Review of Radio Science 1996–1999 (pp. 959–970), Oxford, UK: Oxford University Press

Lin, J. C., 1999c. Hyperthermia therapy. In: Webster, J. G., Ed., Encyclopedia of Electrical and Electronics Engineering (vol. 9, pp. 450–460), New York: Wiley

Lin, J. C., 2000. Biophysics of radiofrequency ablation. In: Huang, S. K. S., Wilber, D. J., Eds., Radiofrequency Catheter Ablation of Cardiac Arrhythmias: Basic Concepts and Clinical Applications (pp. 13–24), 2nd ed, Armonk, New York: Futura

Lin, J. C., 2003. Minimally invasive medical microwave ablation technology. In: Hwang, N. H. C., Woo, S. L. Y., Eds., New Frontiers in Biomedical Engineering (pp. 545–562), New York: Kluwer/Plenum

Lin, J. C., 2004. Studies on microwaves in medicine and biology: From snails to humans. Bioelectromagnetics, 25:146–159

Lin, J. C., 2011. History of Wireless microwave sensing. IEEE Radio and Wirel. Symp., Pahoenix, AZ

Lin, J. C., 2018a. Computational methods for predicting electromagnetic fields and temperature increase in biological bodies, chapt 9. Bioengineering and Biophysical Aspects of Electromagnetic Fields (pp. 299–397), 4th ed

Lin, J. C., 2018b. DARPA's RadioBio and recent US bioelectromagn. Etic research programs. URSI Radio Sci. Bull., 365:49–51

Lin, J. C., 2019. RadioBio and other recent U.S. Bioelectromagnetics research programs. IEEE Microw. Mag., 20(1):14–16

Lin, J. C., 2021. Microwave thermoacoustic tomographic (MTT) imaging. Phys. Med. Biol., 66(10):10–30

Lin, J. C., Beckman, K. J., Hariman, R. J., 1989. Microwave ablation for tachycardia. Proc. IEEE Eng. Med. Biol. Soc., Seattle, WA

Lin, J. C., Beckman, K. J., Hariman, R. J., Bharati, S., Lev, M., Wang, Y. J., 1995. Microwave ablation of the atrioventricular junction in open heart dogs. Bioelectromagnetics, 16:97–105

Lin, J. C., Bernardi, P., Pisa, S., Cavagnaro, M., Piuzzi, E., 2008. Antennas for medical therapy and diagnostics. In: Balanis, C., Ed., Modern Antenna Handbook (pp. 1377–1428), Wiley

Lin, J. C., Chan, K. H., Popovic, M. A., 1984. Dual Frequency Cardiorespiratory Rate Monitor. Ann. Meeting of Bioelectromagnetics Society, Atlanta, GA

Lin, J. C., Clarke, M. J., 1982. Microwave Imaging of Cerebral Edema, Proc. IEEE, 70:523–524

Lin, J. C., Dawe, E., Majcherek, J., 1977. A Noninvasive Microwave Apnea Detector. Proc. 1977 San Diego Biomed. Symp., Academic Press, 441–443

Lin, J. C., Hariman, R. J., Beckman, K. J., 1988. Transcatheter cardiac ablation using microwave energy, Bioelectromagnetics Soc. Anual Meeting, Stamford, CT

Lin, J. C., Hariman, R. J., Wang, Y. G., Wang, Y. J., 1996. Microwave catheter ablation of the atrioventricular junction in closed-chest dogs. Med. Biol. Eng. Comput., 34:295–298

Lin, J. C., Kiernicki, J., Kiernicki, M., Wollschlaeger, P. B., 1979. Microwave apexcardiography. IEEE Trans. Microw. Theory Tech., 27:618–620

Lin, J. C., Lin, M. F., 1980. Studies on microwave and blood-brain barrier interaction. Bioelectromagnetics, 1:313–323

Lin, J. C., Lin, M. F., 1981. Temperature-time profile in rats subjected to selective microwave irradiation of the brian. IEEE Trans. Biomed. Engg., 28:29–31

Lin, J. C., Lin, M. F., 1982. Microwave hyperthermia-induced blood-brain barrier alterations. Radiat. Res., 89:77–87

Lin, J. Y., Lin, J. C., 2009. Contact microwave noninvasive continuous monitoring of blood pressure, DARPA Workshop on Continuous, Non-Invasive Monitoring of Blood Pressure, Coronado, California

Lin, J. C., Salinger, J., 1975. Microwave Measurement of Respiration, IEEE S-MTT Int. Microw. Symp., Palo Alto, CA

Lin, J. C., Wang, Y. J., 1987a. Interstitial microwave antennas for thermal therapy. Int. J. Hyperthermia, 3:37–47

Lin, J. C., Wang, Y. J., 1987b. An implantable microwave antenna for interstitial hyperthermia. Proc. IEEE, 75(8):1132–1133

Lin, J. C., Wang, Y. J., 1995. Catheter antenna for percutaneous microwave therapy. Microw. Opt. Tech. Lett., 8:70–72

Lin, J. C., Wang, Y. J., 1996. The cap-slot catheter antenna for microwave ablation therapy. IEEE Trans. Biomed. Eng., 43:657–660

Lin, J. C., Lin, J. C., Wolfson, O., 2007. Microsoft research on cell phone as a platform forhealthcare. MS submission code 2182. University of Illinois, Chicago

Lin, J. C., Yuan, P. M. K., Jung, D. T., 1998. Enhancement of anticancer drug delivery to the brain by microwave induced hyperthermia. Bioelectrochem. Bioenerg., 47:259–264

Lin, J. Y., Chamberlin, S., Lin, J. C., Wolfson, O., Schonfeld, D., 2010. Smartphone assisted healthcare delivery in rural, resource-poor regions. NIH proposal 1 RC4 LM010970-01. University of Illinois, Chicago

Lubecke, V. M., Boric-Lubecke, O., Gammel, P. L., Yan, R. H., Lin, J. C., 2000. Remote sensing of vital signs with telecommunications signals. World Congress on Medical Physics and Biomedical Engineering, Chicago

Mei, X., Ten Cate, R., Van Leeuwen, C. M., Rodermond, H. M., De Leeuw, L., Dimitrakopoulou, D., Stalpers, L. J. A., Crezee, J., Kok, H. P., Franken, N. A. P., et al., 2020. Radiosensitization by hyperthermia: The effects of temperature, sequence, and time interval in cervical cell lines. Cancers, 12:582

Nathan, A. W., Ward, D. E., Bennett, D. H., Bexton, R. S., 1984. Catheter ablation of atrioventricular conduction. Lancet, 1:1280

Neilly, J. P., Lin, J. C., 1986. Interaction of ethanol and microwaves on the blood-brain barrier of rats. Bioelectromagnetics, 7:405–414

Nelson, K. E., Sergueef, N., Lipinski, A. R., Chapman, A. R., Glonek, T., 2001. Cranial rhythmic impulse related to the traube-hering-mayer oscillation: Comparing laser-Doppler flowmetry and palpation. JAOA, 101(3):163–173

Neuwelt, E., Abbott, N. J., Abrey, L., Banks, W. A., Blakley, B., Davis, T., et al., 2008. Strategies to advance translational research into brain barriers. Lancet. Neurol., 7:84–96

Nitiema, P., 2022. Telehealth Before and during the COVID-19 pandemic: Analysis of health care Workers' opinions. J. Med. Internet Res., 24(2):e29519

Oei, A. L., Kok, H. P., Oei, S. B., Horsman, M. R., Stalpers, L. J. A., Franken, N. A. P., Crezee, J., 2020. Molecular and biological rationale of hyperthermia as radio- and chemosensitizer. Adv. Drug Deliv. Rev., 163–164:84–97

Papp, M. A., Hughes, C., Lin, J. C., Pouget, J. M., 1987. Doppler microwave: A clinical assessment of its efficacy as an arterial pulse sensing technique. Invest. Radiol., 22:569–573

Pedersen, P. C., Johnson, C. C., Durney, C. H., Bragg, D. G., 1978. Microwave reflection and transmission measurements for pulmonary diagnosis and monitoring. IEEE Trans. Biomed. Eng., BME-25:40–48

Penn, R. D., 1980. Cerebral edema and neurological function: CT, evoked responses, and clinical examination. In Cervos-Navarro, J., Ferszt, R., Eds., Advances in Neurology (Vol. 29), New York: Raven

Popovic, M. A., Chan, K. H., Lin, J. C., 1984. Microprocessor-based noncontact heart rate/respiration monitor, IEEE Eng. Med. Biol. Conf., Los Angeles, 754–757

Pisa, S., Cavagnaro, M., Bernardi, P., Lin, J. C., 2001. A 915-MHz antenna for microwave thermal ablation treatment: Physical design, computer modeling and experimental measurement. IEEE Trans. Biomed. Eng., 48:599–601

Prince, M. R., La Muraglia, G. M., Teng, P., Deutsch, T. F., Anderson, R. R., 1987. Preferential ablation of calcified plaque with laser induced lasmas. IEEE J. Quantum Electron., QE-23:1783–1786

Purves, D., Augustine, G. J., Fitzpatrick, D., Katz, C., Samuel, A., LaMantia, J. O., McNamara, M. A., Williams, S. M., Eds., 2001. Neuroscience, 2nd ed, Sunderland, MA: Sinauer Associates

Ranade, S. S., Syeda, R., 2015. Mechanically activated ion channels. Neuron, 87:1162–1119. doi: 10.1016/j.neuron.2015.08.032

Rieger, S., Klee, S., Baumgarten, D., 2018. Experimental characterization and correlation of Mayer waves in retinal vessel diameter and arterial blood pressure. Front. Physiol., 9:892. doi: 10.3389/fphys.2018.00892

Rosen, R., et al., 1990. Percutaneous transluminal microwave balloon angioplasty," IEEE Trans. Microw. Theory Tech., 38(1):90–93

Rosen, A., Rosen, H., 1995. New Frontiers in Medical Device Technology. New York, NY, USA: Wiley

Saltman, A. E., Rosenthal, L. S., Francalancia, N. A., Lahey, S. J., 2003. A completely endoscopic approach to microwave ablation for atrial fibrillation. Heart Surg. Forum., 6(3):E38–E41

Scheinman, M. M., Davis, J. C., 1986. Catheter ablation for treatment of tachyarrhythmias: Present role and potential promise. Circulation, 73:10

Sharpe, S. M., MacDonald, A., Seals, J., Crowgey, S. R., 1986. An electromagnetic-based non-contact vital signs monitor, Georgia Tech. Res. Inst., Biomed. Div., Atlanta

Shave, J., 2022. The state of telehealth before and after the COVID-19 pandemic. Prim Care, 49:517–530. doi: 10.1016/j.pop.2022.04.002

Smith, T. G., Lecar, H., Redman, S. J., Eds., 2013. Voltage and Patch Clamping With Microelectrodes. New York: Springer

Spears, J. R., 1987. PTCA restenosis: Potential prevention with laser balloon angioplasty. Amer. J. Cardiol., 60:61B–64B

Spears, J. R., 1989. Thermal remodelling of the arterial wall and lumen with laser balloon angioplasty. In: Isner, J. M., Clarke, R. H., Eds., Lasers in Cardiacvascular Disease, Boston: Martinus Nijhoff

Stuchly, S. S., Goldberg, M., Thansandote, A., Carraro, B., 1979. Monitoring of arterial wall movement by microwave Doppler radar. Proc. 1978 Symp. Electromagn. Fields Biol. Syst., Ottawa, Canada, pp. 229–242, IMPI, Edmonton

Stuchly, S. S., Smith, A., Goldberg, M., Thansandote, A., Menard, A., 1980. A microwave device for arterial wall motion analysis. Proc. 33rd Annual Cpnf. Eng. Med. Biol., 22:47

Susskind, C., 1973. Possible use of microwaves in the management of lung disease, Proc. IEEE, 61: 673
Sweeney, M. D., Zhao, Z., Montagne, A., Nelson, A. R., Zlokovic, B. V., 2019. Blood-Brain barrier: From physiology to disease and back. Physiol. Rev., 99:21–78
Thansandote, A., Stuchly, S. S., Smith, A. M., 1983. Monitoring variations of biological impedances using microwave Doppler radar. Phys. Med. Biol., 28(8):983
U.S. Senate, 1968. 90th Congress, H.R. 10790, (1968, Oct. 18). Public Law 90602, An Act to Amend the Public Health Service Act to Provide for the Protection of the Public Health from Radiation Emissions from Electronic Products. https://www.gpo.gov/fdsys/granule/STATUTE82/STATUTE82Pg1173/contentdetail.htm
Watmough, D. J., Ross, W. M., Eds., 1986. Hyperthermia. Glasgow: Blackie
Whittall, K. P., MacKay, A. L., Graeb, D. A., Nugent, R. A., Li, D. K., Paty, D. W., 1997. In vivo measurement of T2 distributions and water contents in normal human brain. Magn. Reson. Med., 37(1):34–43
Williams, M. R., Argenziano, M., Oz, M. C., 2002. Microwave ablation for surgical treatment of atrial fibrillation. Semin. Thorac. Cardiovasc. Surg., 14(3):232–237

# 3 Microwave Propagation, Reflection, and Scattering

The objective and principle of sensing with radiative energy is to couple sufficient power to the target of interest and make an observation via the channel or communication medium. The specific aim of this book is to noninvasively probe the human or animal body using microwave radiation. As mentioned in Chapter 1, the radio frequency (RF) and microwave frequency ranges offer acceptable dispersion and propagation loss, but sufficient spatial resolution, for reliably accurate measurement from outside the body.

The physical fundamentals of microwave and RF radiation are presented in this chapter for an understanding of the essential elements of microwave propagation in a material medium. The propagation, reflection, and transmission are functions of the source configuration and its frequency, composition, shape, and size of the targeted object, as well as orientation and position of the object with respect to the source. The approach of this chapter is to develop yet confine the coverage to the most relevant topics, rather than provide a comprehensive discussion of the interactions and phenomena describable by physical laws of electromagnetic theory.

An understanding of the interaction of microwave and RF radiation with biological systems is facilitated through knowledge of the physical laws describing the behavior and characteristics of microwave and RF radiation in space and time. The physical principles of microwave and RF radiation are prescribed by a set of physical laws called Maxwell's equations of electromagnetic theory. The equations represent mathematical expressions of experimentally validated observations. They are applicable for linear or nonlinear, isotropic or anisotropic, homogeneous or heterogeneous media. Maxwell's equations are macroscopic laws that define the relationship between space- and time-averaged electric and magnetic fields. They apply to regions or volumes whose dimensions are larger than atomic dimensions. Time intervals of observation are assumed to be long enough to allow for an averaging of atomic fluctuations.

From the four laws of electromagnetics, one may deduce all macroscopic electromagnetic characteristics and behavior, including microwave and RF propagation from source to target or object, exposure of biological subjects, reflection, refraction, and transmission at tissue interfaces, and dosimetry, which is the quantification of microwave and RF radiation's distribution and dispersion and attenuation in biological bodies and materials. This knowledge is important for the comprehension and interpretation of experimental results using microwave and RF radiation, as well as to applying them to health and safety assessments and biomedical applications.

Microwave and RF radiation consist of oscillating electric and magnetic fields propagating through free space at the speed of light, $2.998 \times 10^8$ m/s. This speed varies depending on the material medium through which the wave travels. It is a


DOI: 10.1201/9781003315223-3

function of the permittivity and permeability of the material media. In addition to being radiated through a transmitting antenna, microwave and RF radiation may be transported from the source by coaxial transmission lines or waveguides. Microwave and RF radiation may be detected and measured by diodes, bolometers, or similar devices, and their associated instruments and systems.

## 3.1 THE MAXWELL EQUATIONS

Maxwell's four mathematical equations may be stated in either integral or differential equation form. Each formulation provides a distinct description of electromagnetic radiation in space. In integral forms, they specify the electric and magnetic fields along lines, through surfaces and over volumes, and lend the equations to easy physical interpretation. In contrast, the differential equations depict the radiation's behavior at points in space. These formulations are mathematically equivalent since they may be derived from each other using Stokes' and divergence theorems from vector analysis.

The integral forms of Maxwell's equations are given by

$$\oint \boldsymbol{E} \cdot \boldsymbol{dl} = -\int_{s} \frac{\partial \boldsymbol{B}}{\partial t} \cdot \boldsymbol{ds} \qquad \text{(Faraday's law)} \tag{3.1}$$

$$\oint \boldsymbol{H} \cdot \boldsymbol{dl} = \int_{s} \left( \boldsymbol{J} + \frac{\partial \boldsymbol{D}}{\partial t} \right) \cdot \boldsymbol{ds} \qquad \text{(Ampere – Maxwell's law)} \tag{3.2}$$

$$\oint \boldsymbol{D} \cdot \boldsymbol{ds} = \int_{v} \rho \, dv \qquad \text{(Gauss electric law)} \tag{3.3}$$

$$\oint \boldsymbol{B} \cdot \boldsymbol{ds} = 0 \qquad \text{(Gauss magnetic law)} \tag{3.4}$$

where

**E** = electric field strength in volt/meter (V/m)
**H** = magnetic field strength in ampere/meter (A/m)
**D** = electric flux density in coulomb/square meter ($C/m^2$)
**B** = magnetic flux density in weber/square meter ($Wb/m^2$)
**J** = conduction current density in ampere/square meter ($A/m^2$)
$\rho$ = charge density in coulomb/cubic meter ($C/m^3$)

According to Faraday's law (Eq. 3.1), the total voltage induced in an arbitrary closed path in space is equal to the total time rate of decrease of magnetic flux through the area bounded by the closed path. Therefore, a time-varying magnetic field generates an electric field. There is no restriction on the nature of the medium.

Ampere's law (Eq. 3.2) asserts that the line integral or sum of the magnetic field strength around a closed path is equal to the total current enclosed by the path. The total current may consist of two parts: a conduction current with density **J** and a displacement or dielectric current with density $\partial \boldsymbol{D}/\partial t$. Thus, Ampere's or Ampere-Maxwell's law implies that a magnetic field can only be produced by currents or movement of charges. The displacement current was first introduced by Maxwell and allowed him to unify the separate laws governing electricity and magnetism into a unified electromagnetic theory. It also led to the postulate of electromagnetic waves that can transport energy, and the concept that light is an electromagnetic wave.

Eq. (3.3) is Gauss's electric law, which declares that the net outward flow of electric flux through a closed surface is equal to the charge contained in the volume enclosed by the surface. Gauss's law for the magnetic field (Eq. 3.4) states that the net outward flow of magnetic flux through a closed surface is zero. Therefore, magnetic flux lines are always continuous and form closed loops.

Although Eqs (3.1) through (3.4) lend to ready physical interpretation of electromagnetic phenomena associated with macroscopic surface and volumes, they are not in forms most suitable for the mathematical analysis of physical events taking effect at or surrounding a point in space. It is often expedient to solve differential equations to obtain the field quantities. The desired differential equations may be derived by using Stokes's and divergence theorems from vector analysis. As a result, Maxwell's equations in differential form are given by,

$$\nabla \times \boldsymbol{E} = -\frac{\partial \boldsymbol{B}}{\partial t} \quad \text{(Faraday's law)} \tag{3.5}$$

$$\nabla \times \boldsymbol{H} = \boldsymbol{J} + \frac{\partial \boldsymbol{D}}{\partial t} \quad \text{(Ampere} - \text{Maxwell's law)} \tag{3.6}$$

$$\nabla \cdot \boldsymbol{D} = \rho \quad \text{(Gauss electric law)} \tag{3.7}$$

$$\nabla \cdot \boldsymbol{B} = 0 \quad \text{(Gauss magnetic law)} \tag{3.8}$$

Eq. (3.5) says that the curl or circulation of an electric field around a point in space equals the time rate of decrease of magnetic flux density at that point. Conversely, a time-varying magnetic field generates an electric field around it.

Eq. (3.6) states that a curl or circulation of a magnetic field around a point in space equals the total current passing through that point. The total current may consist of two parts: a conduction current with density **J** and a displacement current with density $\partial \boldsymbol{D}/\partial t$. Again, Ampere's law holds, and a magnetic field is produced by currents or movement of charges.

The Gauss electric law of Eq. (3.7) says that the divergence or outward flow of electric flux from a point in space is equal to the charges located at that point, thus indicating that electric fields are associated with electric charges.

The companion Gauss law for the magnetic field (Eq. 3.8) states that the net outward flow of magnetic flux at any point is zero. Therefore, magnetic flux lines converging at a point are always equal to the number of fluxes leading away from the same point in space. This is consistent with the statement of Eq. (3.4) that magnetic flux lines are always continuous and form closed loops. It suggests that there is no net accumulation of magnetic charges at any point in space and allows the well-known conclusion that, unlike electric charges, magnetic charges do not exist.

It is seen from the right-hand side of Eqs (3.6) and (3.7) that the sources of electromagnetic fields and waves are electrical charges and current flow. In fact, the conservation of charge principle gives rise to an equation of continuity for current flow in differential form,

$$\nabla \cdot \boldsymbol{J} = -\frac{\partial \rho}{\partial t} \tag{3.9}$$

which indicates that the outward flow of electric current is equal to the time rate of decrease of electric charge density at that point.

When the electromagnetic fields are harmonically oscillating functions with a single frequency $f$, all field quantities may be assumed to have a time variation represented by $e^{j\omega t}$, where $\omega = 2\pi f$ in radians is the angular frequency. Under this assumption, the $j\omega t$ derivatives in Maxwell's equations may be replaced by a multiplier $j\omega$, and the common factor $e^{j\omega t}$ may be omitted from these equations. Maxwell's equations can be reduced to the time harmonic form and written as,

$$\nabla \times \boldsymbol{E} = -j\omega \boldsymbol{B} \tag{3.10}$$

$$\nabla \times \boldsymbol{H} = \boldsymbol{J} + j\omega \boldsymbol{D} \tag{3.11}$$

$$\nabla \cdot \boldsymbol{D} = \rho \tag{3.12}$$

$$\nabla \cdot \boldsymbol{B} = 0 \tag{3.13}$$

Note the use of boldface letters for the vectors that are complex functions of spatial coordinates.

A set of auxiliary equations relating the fields and flux densities is required to determine the electric and magnetic fields produced by a given current or charge distribution. For a linear, isotropic, and homogeneous medium, the field quantities are related as follows:

$$\boldsymbol{D} = \varepsilon \boldsymbol{E} \tag{3.14}$$

$$\boldsymbol{B} = \mu \boldsymbol{H} \tag{3.15}$$

$$\boldsymbol{J} = \sigma \boldsymbol{E} \tag{3.16}$$

Eqs (3.14) through (3.16) are commonly referred to as the constitutive relations. The free space or vacuum is a medium in which the permittivity is given by

$$\varepsilon = \varepsilon_0 = 8.854 \times 10^{-12}\, \mathit{farad/m}\ (\mathrm{F/m}) \tag{3.17}$$

permeability is given by

$$\mu = \mu_0 = 4\pi \times 10^{-7}\, \mathit{henry/m}\ (\mathrm{H/m}) \tag{3.18}$$

and conductivity, $\sigma = 0$. For other media, it is conventional to introduce the dimensionless ratios,

$$\varepsilon_r = \frac{\varepsilon}{\varepsilon_0} \tag{3.19}$$

$$\mu_r = \frac{\mu}{\mu_0} \tag{3.20}$$

which are usually labeled as relative dielectric constant and relative permeability, respectively. Biological materials generally have relative permeabilities close to that of free space and relative dielectric constants that show characteristic dependence on material and frequency.

## 3.2 THE WAVE EQUATION

Eqs (3.10) and (3.11) are a set of coupled equations both containing electric and magnetic field quantities. If we assume that the conduction current density is zero in the region of interest, these two equations may be combined to give two second-order differential equations, one containing the electric field strength and the other containing the magnetic field strength:

$$\nabla^2 \boldsymbol{E} + \omega^2 \mu\varepsilon \boldsymbol{E} = 0 \tag{3.21}$$

$$\nabla^2 \boldsymbol{H} + \omega^2 \mu\varepsilon \boldsymbol{H} = 0 \tag{3.22}$$

where we also have taken the charge density as zero for a source-free region. It is customary to let $k^2 = \omega^2\mu\varepsilon$, where $k$ is the wave number and has the following relationships:

$$k = \omega\sqrt{\mu\varepsilon} = \frac{\omega}{v} = \frac{2\pi}{\lambda} \tag{3.23}$$

Eqs (3.21) and (3.22) are wave equations in harmonic form. Their solutions represent electromagnetic waves propagating with velocity $v$ equal to $(\mu\varepsilon)^{-1/2}$. The wavelength $\lambda$ is equal to $\frac{v}{f}$, where $f$ is the frequency. In free space, $v$ is equal to the speed of light, $c = 2.998 \times 10^8$ m/s, as mentioned previously.

In a medium with finite electrical conductivity $\sigma$, a conduction current density $\boldsymbol{J} = \sigma\boldsymbol{E}$ will exist and this will give rise to energy loss, such as Joule heating. The wave equations in media of this type have a loss term given by $j\omega\mu\sigma$, such that

$$\left(\nabla^2 + \omega^2\mu\varepsilon - j\omega\mu\sigma\right)\boldsymbol{E} = 0 \tag{3.24}$$

$$\left(\nabla^2 + \omega^2\mu\varepsilon - j\omega\mu\sigma\right)\boldsymbol{H} = 0 \tag{3.25}$$

It should be mentioned that a finite conductivity is equivalent to an imaginary component in the permittivity $\varepsilon$. Comparing Eqs (3.21) and (3.22) with (3.24) and (3.25), it is seen that the equivalent permittivity is given by $(\varepsilon - \frac{j\sigma}{\omega})$.

## 3.3 BOUNDARY CONDITIONS AT MATERIAL INTERFACES

The behavior of electric and magnetic fields in situations where the physical or biological properties of the medium change abruptly across one or several interfaces is governed by certain boundary conditions to be satisfied at the interfaces. These conditions must be satisfied by any solution to the electric and magnetic fields and the wave equation. They may be derived by applying Maxwell's Eqs (3.1) through (3.4) to infinitesimal regions containing these interfaces (Figure 3.1). If medium 1 and medium 2 are separated by a common boundary, the boundary conditions at the interface may be summarized as follows for tangential and normal components with respect to the boundary:

1. The tangential components of the electric field strengths are continuous across the boundary, such that

$$E_{t1} = E_{t2} \tag{3.26}$$

2. The normal components of the electric flux densities differ by an amount equal to the surface charge density $\rho_s$, such that

$$D_{n1} - D_{n2} = \rho_s \tag{3.27}$$

   If there is no surface charge on the boundary, $\rho_s = 0$, which is the usual case of dielectric materials, then

$$D_{n1} = D_{n2} \tag{3.28}$$

3. The tangential components of magnetic field strength differ by an amount equal to the surface current density $J_s$, such that

$$H_{t1} - H_{t2} = J_s \tag{3.29}$$

   In all cases except that of a perfect conductor, the surface current density is vanishingly small, then

$$H_{t1} = H_{t2} \tag{3.30}$$

4. The normal components of magnetic flux density are continuous across a boundary, such that

$$B_{n1} = B_{n2} \tag{3.31}$$

When considering fields in an infinite region of space, the radiation condition — a boundary condition equivalent — requires that the field at infinity must be an outward-propagating wave with a finite amount of energy. Alternatively, electric and magnetic fields must vanish rapidly so that the energy stored in the fields and the energy flow at infinity are zero.

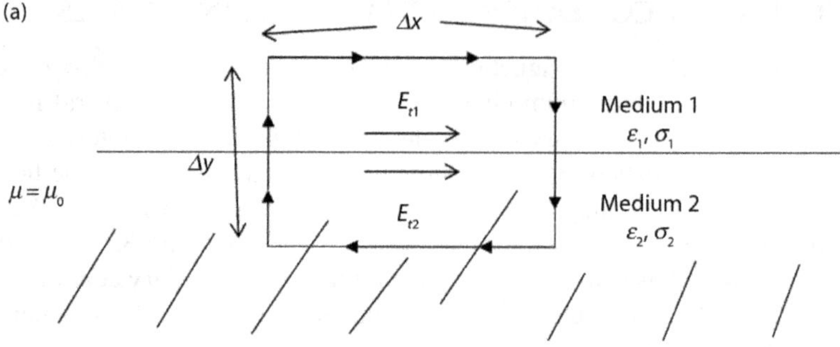


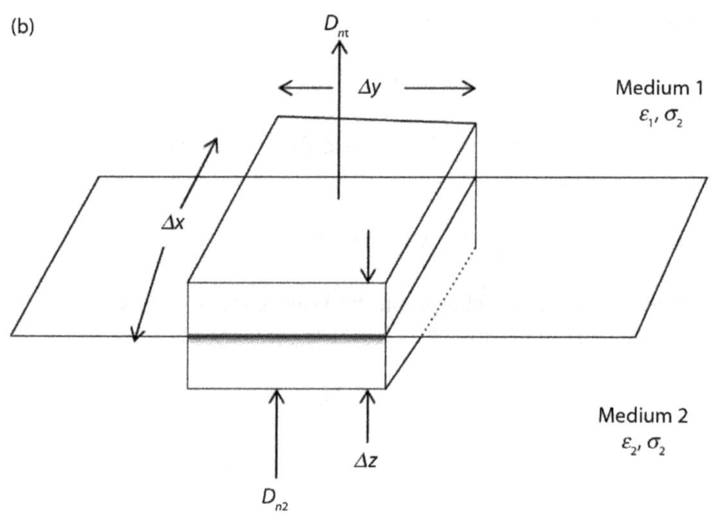


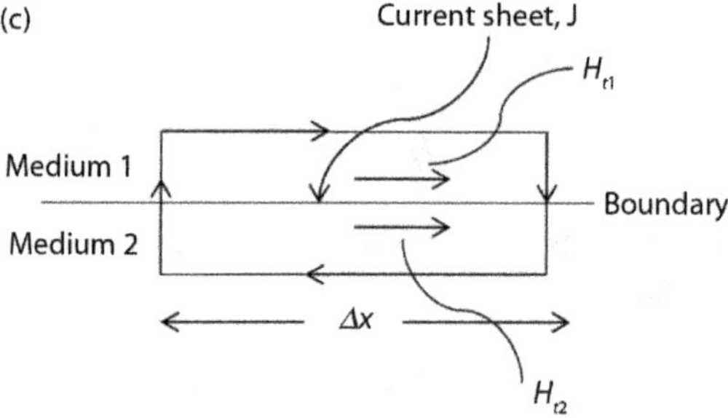


**FIGURE 3.1** Boundary conditions and schematics for evaluating tangential and normal electric and magnetic field components at interface between two different material media. (a) tangential components of the electric field strength; (b) Normal components of the electric flux density; (c) Tangential components of magnetic field strength; (d) Normal components of magnetic flux density. *(Continued)*

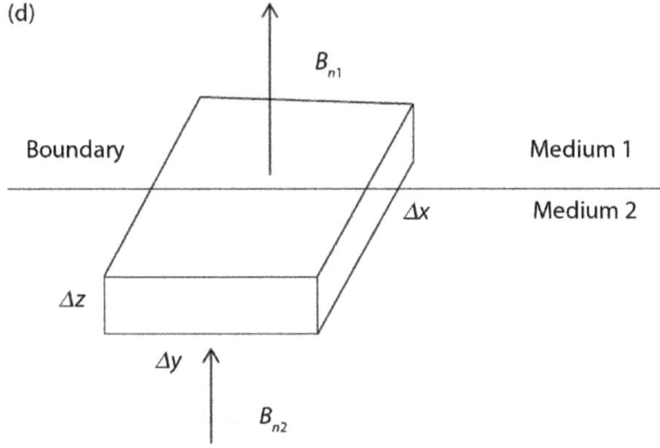


**FIGURE 3.1** *(Continued)*

## 3.4 ENERGY STORAGE AND POWER FLOW

Electromagnetic energy is either stored in the electric and magnetic fields or radiated away in the form of electromagnetic waves. For a region in which permittivity and permeability are functions of position but not time, the energy density at a point is given by

$$W = \left(\frac{1}{2}\right)\left(\varepsilon E^2 + \mu H^2\right) \tag{3.32}$$

where $(1/2)\varepsilon E^2$ is the energy stored per unit volume in the electric field and $(1/2)\mu H^2$ is the energy stored per unit volume in the magnetic field. The stored energy is partitioned between electric and magnetic fields and is transferred from electric to magnetic fields and back again as a function of time.

In regions with finite conductivity, part of the electromagnetic energy may be extracted by (lost to) the conducting medium or dissipated as Joule heat as a function of time. The equation

$$P_a = \left(\frac{1}{2}\right)\sigma E^2 \tag{3.33}$$

represents the absorbed power density, power loss, or dissipated power; the absorbed power may be converted to heat energy over time. The absorbed power density also equals the specific rate of energy absorption or specific absorption rate (SAR), which is generally accepted as the metric for quantifying microwave and RF energy deposition in biological systems. In this case, $SAR = P_a$, in units of watts per kilogram (W/kg). Note that SAR is independent of time. The determination of SAR and its distribution in biological tissues is commonly referred to as dosimetry.

The instantaneous density of power that flows across a surface bounding a region in space is given by the Poynting vector **P**,

$$\boldsymbol{P} = \boldsymbol{E} \times \boldsymbol{H} \tag{3.34}$$

Thus, the direction of power flow is perpendicular to **E** and **H**, and is in the direction of Poynting vector **P**. It can be shown by an application of the Poynting theorem that the total power flowing into a region is equal to the total power loss or power dissipated within the region plus the time rate of increase of energy stored within the region. The power density that impinges on a surface area normal to the direction of propagation is proportional to the square of the electric or magnetic field and is expressed in watts per square meter ($W/m^2$) or milliwatt per square centimeter ($mW/cm^2$). Note that 1 $mW/cm^2$ = 10 $W/m^2$. For sensing applications, typically very low powers are involved; thus, the unit of microwatt per square meter ($\mu W/m^2$) may also be used.

For electric and magnetic fields that vary sinusoidally with time, the time-averaged power flow or rate of energy flow per unit area is

$$P_d = \left(\frac{1}{2}\right) Re\left(\boldsymbol{E} \times \boldsymbol{H}^*\right) \tag{3.35}$$

where $\boldsymbol{H}^*$ is the complex conjugate of **H** and $P_d$ is given by the real (Re) part of the product of two sinusoidal quantities.

## 3.5 PLANE WAVES AND FAR-ZONE FIELD

The radiated energy of a small antenna (a point source or dipole) in free space takes the form of a spherical wave in which the wave fronts are concentric spherical shells. The spherical wave fronts expand as the wave propagates outward from the source. At points far from the source, the wave front would essentially appear as a plane. This is analogous to the situation of an observer on earth who sees the Earth's surface as a plane (flat), since the person can view only a small portion of the global surface. Both the electric and magnetic fields of the wave lie in the plane of the wave front. They vary only in the direction of propagation. Such a wave is called a plane wave. It is a very important practical case since fields radiated by any transmitting antenna appear as plane waves at distances far from the source. Moreover, through Fourier analysis, a suitable combination of plane waves may be made to represent a wave of any desired form in space and time.

At distances far from the source or transmitting antenna (the far zone), typically 10 wavelengths or more, RF and microwaves may be considered as plane waves whose electric and magnetic fields are perpendicular from each other and both are perpendicular to the direction of wave propagation. Moreover, the electric and magnetic field maximum occur at the same location in space at any given moment in time, as depicted in Figure 3.2. In this case, the electric field strength in volts per meter (V/m) is related to the magnetic field strength in amperes per meter (A/m) through a constant known as intrinsic impedance, which is medium dependent and is approximately 376.7 ohms for air or free space. In all other dielectric media including biological materials, the intrinsic impedance is always smaller than that of free space.

For distances less than 10 wavelengths from the transmitting antenna (the near zone), the maxima and minima of electric and magnetic fields do not occur at the

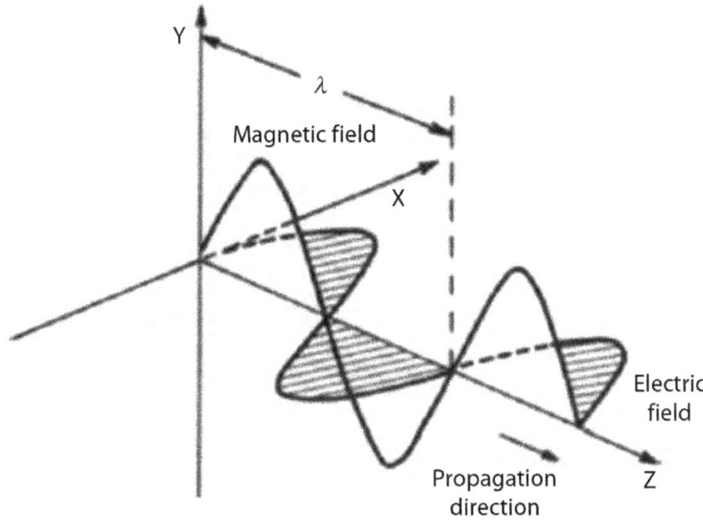


**FIGURE 3.2** The direction of plane-wave propagation, electric field, and magnetic field orientation in space at a given moment in time.

same location along the direction of propagation. That is, the electric and magnetic fields are out of time phase. The ratio of electric and magnetic field strengths is no longer constant; it varies from point to point. The direction of propagation is also not uniquely defined as in the far zone case, making the situation complicated (more details are given later in the chapter). It should be noted that various field regions generally do not affect the basic mechanisms by which RF and microwaves act on a biological system, although the quantitative aspects of the interaction may differ due to changes in energy coupling. In general, when plane-wave microwave and RF radiation impinge from the air on a planar biological structure, a large fraction of the incident energy may be reflected. Furthermore, the transmitted fraction is attenuated exponentially as it propagates in the tissue. Thus, there will be energy loss associated with the channel (fading channel).

## 3.6 POLARIZATION AND PROPAGATION OF PLANE WAVES

The polarization of a plane wave refers to the time-varying characters of the electric field at a given location in space. To specify the orientation of microwaves and RF radiation in space, it is necessary to specify the orientation of one of the field vectors. Since the magnetic field vector is always perpendicular to the electric field vector, knowledge of the orientation of the latter is sufficient to describe the orientation of the wave. If the electric field of the waves always lies in a specific location, the wave is said to be linearly polarized. An example would be a linearly polarized plane wave in the $x$ direction of a rectangular coordinate system. If both $E_x$ and $E_y$ are present and in time phase, the resultant electric field has a direction dependence on the relative magnitude of $E_x$ and $E_y$. The angle that this direction makes with the

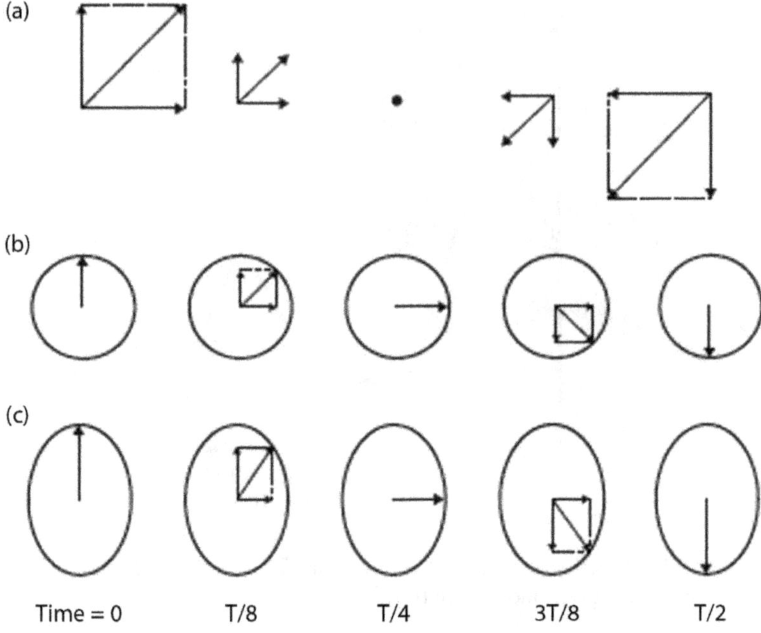


**FIGURE 3.3** Polarization of electromagnetic plane waves: (a) linear polarization; (b) circular polarization; (c) elliptical polarization. Arrows indicate directions of electric field and its coordinate components.

$x$ axis, however, is constant with time. The wave is, therefore, also linearly polarized (Figure 3.3).

If $E_x$ and $E_y$ are equal in magnitude and $E_y$ leads $E_x$,

$$\boldsymbol{E} = E_x\mathbf{x} + jE_y\mathbf{y} \tag{3.36}$$

$E_x$ and $E_y$ reach their maximum values at different instants of time, the direction of the resultant electric field will vary with time. It can be shown that the locus of the endpoint of the resultant electric field will be a circle. The wave is said to be circularly polarized. Moreover, it may be seen that looking in the direction of propagation, the rotation of the electric field vector is that of a left-handed screw advancing in the direction of propagation. The wave is, therefore, also said to be left circularly polarized (Figure 3.3). If the $x$ component of the electric field leads the $y$ component instead, a reversal of the direction of rotation is obtained.

The most general form of polarization is elliptical polarization. This happens when $E_x$ and $E_y$ differ in magnitude as well as time phase. Assuming again $E_y$ leads $E_x$ by 90°, since $E_x$ and $E_y$ are not equal in magnitude, the endpoint of the resultant field traces out an ellipse in the plane normal to the direction of propagation (see Figure 3.3). The circular polarization is in fact a special case of elliptical polarization.

A wave propagating in any direction has no field variations in planes normal to the direction of propagation in a linearly polarized plane wave. In this section, we shall describe the properties of plane-wave propagation in free space, lossy (biological) media, and media involving plane boundaries.

### 3.6.1 Plane Waves in Free Space

Assume that the electric field is polarized in the $x$ direction and the wave is propagating in the $z$ direction, the wave equation, Eq. (3.24) reduces to

$$\frac{d^2E_x}{dz^2}+k_0^2E_x=0 \tag{3.37}$$

where $k_0=\omega(\mu_0\varepsilon_0)^{1/2}$ is the free space wave number or propagation constant. The solution to this equation is

$$E_x=E_0e^{-jk_0z} \tag{3.38}$$

The associated magnetic field is related to the electric field through Maxwell's equation (Eq. 3.10), thus

$$H_y=\sqrt{\frac{\varepsilon_0}{\mu_0}}E_x \tag{3.39}$$

The ratio of $E_x$ to $H_y$ has the dimension of impedance and is called the intrinsic impedance. The intrinsic impedance of free space is

$$\eta_0=\sqrt{\frac{\mu_0}{\varepsilon_0}}=120\pi\simeq 377\text{ ohms} \tag{3.40}$$

Figure 3.2 shows the electric and magnetic fields as a function of distance at some instant of time. The wavelength $\lambda$, in general, or $\lambda_0$ in free space is defined as the distance over which the sinusoidal waveform passes through a full cycle of $2\pi$ radians. Note that the electric and magnetic fields are in time phase but in space quadrature.

The time-averaged power flow or average power density associated with this wave is

$$P_d=\left(\frac{1}{2}\right)\left(\frac{E_0^2}{\eta_0}\right) \tag{3.41}$$

The direction of power flow is normal to both electric and magnetic field vectors and is in the direction of wave propagation.

### 3.6.2 Plane Waves in Lossy or Biological Media

In the case of a plane wave propagating through a homogeneous isotropic medium with dielectric loss or finite conductivity, such as biological materials, the governing equation (Eq. 3.24) becomes

$$\left(\frac{d^2E_x}{dz^2}\right)-\gamma^2E_x=0 \tag{3.42}$$

where $\gamma$ is the propagation factor given by

$$\gamma = \sqrt{j\omega\mu(\sigma + j\omega\varepsilon)} \tag{3.43}$$

The solution of Eq. (3.42) for a wave propagating along the positive $z$ direction is

$$E_x = Ee^{-\gamma z} \tag{3.44}$$

The corresponding solution for the magnetic field is

$$H_y = \left(\frac{\gamma}{j\omega\mu}\right) Ee^{-\gamma z} \tag{3.45}$$

The intrinsic impedance of a medium was previously defined as the ratio of electric field to magnetic field. Thus,

$$\eta = \frac{E_x}{H_y} = \frac{j\omega\mu}{\gamma} = \sqrt{\frac{j\omega\mu}{\sigma + j\omega\varepsilon}} \tag{3.46}$$

For a lossless dielectric medium $\sigma = 0$, the intrinsic impedance reduces to

$$\eta = \sqrt{\frac{\mu}{\varepsilon}} \tag{3.47}$$

As shown earlier, $\eta$ has a value of about 377 ohms for free space. Since dielectric media have approximately the same permeability of free space and have permittivity greater than free space, it follows that the intrinsic impedance of free space is the upper limit of the attainable value for dielectric materials.

The real and imaginary parts of complex propagation factor $\gamma$ may be represented by $\alpha$ and $\beta$ such that

$$\gamma = \alpha + j\beta \tag{3.48}$$

and

$$\alpha = \omega\sqrt{\frac{\mu\varepsilon}{2}\left(\sqrt{1 + \frac{\sigma^2}{\omega^2\varepsilon^2}} - 1\right)} \tag{3.49}$$

$$\beta = \omega\sqrt{\frac{\mu\varepsilon}{2}\left(\sqrt{1 + \frac{\sigma^2}{\omega^2\varepsilon^2}} + 1\right)} \tag{3.50}$$

where $\alpha$ and $\beta$ are referred to as the attenuation coefficient and propagation coefficient, respectively. It is clear from Eqs (3.44), (3.45), and (3.48) that the amplitude of the wave decreases as it advances in the lossy medium and the reduction is exponential in nature. Furthermore, since $\alpha$ is related to $\omega$ and $\sigma$, the rate of attenuation is proportional to frequency and conductivity. The factor, $\frac{\sigma}{\omega\varepsilon}$, is known as the loss tangent. It is the ratio of the magnitude of conduction current density to the magnitude of displacement current density in a material medium. It is a useful way to classify the transitional behavior of materials at different frequencies by the loss tangent. The medium acts as a dielectric material for smaller loss tangents (less than unity). Conversely, it behaves more like a conducting material. When $\sigma \gg \omega\varepsilon$, such as for a good conductor, $\alpha$ and $\beta$ may be simplified to yield

$$\alpha = \beta = \sqrt{\frac{\omega\mu\sigma}{2}} \tag{3.51}$$

The time average power density associated with a plane wave propagating through a lossy media is

$$P_d = \left(\frac{1}{2}\right) Re\left[\frac{E^2 e^{-2\alpha z}}{\eta}\right] \tag{3.52}$$

It is easily seen from Eq. (3.52) that the average power density decreases according to $e^{-2\alpha z}$ as the wave propagates in the lossy medium or channel. This is as expected since the field decreases exponentially ($e^{-\alpha z}$) as it travels in the medium. At $z = \delta$, both electric and magnetic field strengths decrease to $1/e$, or 36.8% of their value at the surface—the point of entry into the lossy medium (the term conducting medium is also used to mean lossy medium).

The quantity $\delta$ is known as the depth of penetration or skin depth and is given by

$$\delta = \frac{1}{\alpha} \tag{3.53}$$

Therefore, the depth of penetration is inversely proportional to conductivity and frequency. It should be mentioned that the fields do not fail to penetrate beyond the depth of $\delta$; this is merely the point at which they have decreased to about 37% of their initial value. The power density will decrease to about 14% accordingly.

The concept as presented here applies strictly to planar media or planar-like structures. It may be extended, however, to bodies of other geometry, so long as the depth of penetration is much smaller than the radius of curvature of the body surfaces.

## 3.7 REFLECTION AND TRANSMISSION AT INTERFACES

When microwave and RF radiation propagating in one medium impinges on a second medium with different dielectric properties, partial reflection occurs at the boundary between the two media. A portion of the incident radiation may also be transmitted into the second medium. If the intrinsic impedances of the two media are approximately equal, most of the energy is transmitted into the second medium, and the reflected radiation is relatively small. Conversely, if intrinsic impedances differ greatly, the transmitted radiation is small, and the reflected radiation is relatively large. If the wave impinges normally on the boundary

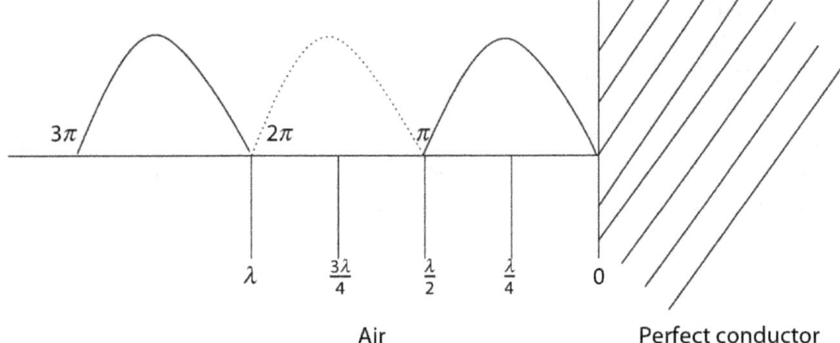


**FIGURE 3.4** A standing wave created when a plane wave impinges normally on a perfect conductor. The fields are shown at time, t = T/8, where T is the period of the wave.

surface, the resulting reflected wave propagating back toward the source combines with the incident wave to form a standing wave in the first medium. An example of the standing wave created by a perfect conductor is shown in Figure 3.4. The term standing wave ratio (SWR) is defined as the ratio of maximum to minimum electric field strength in a standing wave. It is used as a measure of the degree of impedance mismatch or of the differences between the electromagnetic properties of the two media.

The essential features of the behavior of microwave and RF radiation at the surface between two media may be deduced from an analysis of the simple equation of a plane-wave incident perpendicularly upon a plane surface between two media (see Figure 3.5). Both media are assumed to be infinite in extent in all directions except at the boundary ($z = 0$). At any plane $z$, we may define a wave impedance $Z(z)$ as the ratio of total electric to total magnetic fields at that plane:

$$Z(z) = \frac{E_x(z)}{H_y(z)} \tag{3.54}$$

for the wave propagating along the positive $z$ direction in medium 2, such as a tissue layer, $Z = \eta_2$ is the intrinsic impedance. Similarly, for the incident plane wave traveling positively in medium 1, $Z = \eta_1$; however, there is also a negatively traveling wave

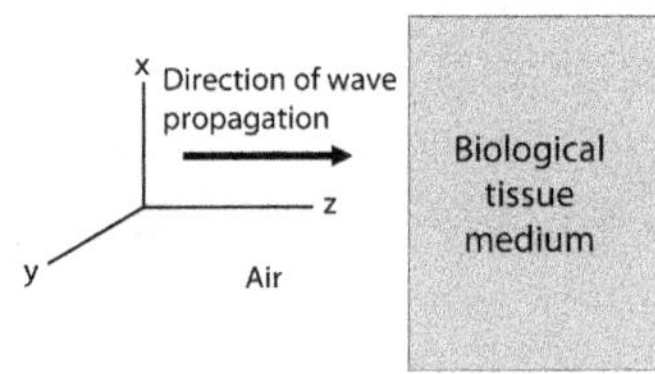


**FIGURE 3.5** Plane wave impinging on two-layered media: medium 1 (air) and medium 2 (a tissue layer).

having a $Z = -\eta_1$. The combination of the incident and reflected components gives rise to a wave impedance that varies with $z$ in medium 1, such that

$$Z(z) = \eta_1 \left( \frac{\eta_2 - \eta_1 tanh\ \gamma_1 z}{\eta_1 - \eta_2 tanh\ \gamma_1 z} \right) \tag{3.55}$$

where $\gamma_1$ is the propagation factor in medium 1, or air, if that is the case.

The reflected radiation is characterized by the reflection coefficient $R$, which is defined as the ratio of the reflected electric field strength to the incident field strength at the boundary and is given by

$$R = \frac{\eta_2 - \eta_1}{\eta_2 + \eta_1} \tag{3.56}$$

In a similar manner, the transmission coefficient $T$ is defined as the ratio of the transmitted electric field strength to that of the incident field at the boundary,

$$T = \frac{2\eta_2}{\eta_2 + \eta_1} \tag{3.57}$$

It is seen from Eqs (3.56) and (3.57) that when $\eta_2 = \eta_1$, i.e., the electrical properties of the media are approximately equal, there is no reflection and transmission is maximal. On the other hand, there is complete reflection when $\eta_2$ is zero. As shall be seen later in the chapter, for biological materials, microwave reflection and transmission behaviors fall between the two extremes. The latter of the two extremes may be encountered when metallic components are involved in research on biomedical aspects of microwave and RF radiation.

The SWR may be expressed in terms of the magnitude of the reflection coefficient as

$$SWR = \frac{1 + |R|}{1 - |R|} \tag{3.58}$$

It can be shown using the results of the previous paragraph that the SWR = 1 when there is matching equality of media. Any mismatch of the two media will result in an SWR greater than unity.

For the situation illustrated in Figure 3.5, the electric and magnetic fields may be expressed as

$$E_{1x} = E_i \left( e^{-\gamma_1 z} + R e^{\gamma_1 z} \right) \tag{3.59}$$

$$H_{1y} = \left( \frac{E_i}{\eta_1} \right) \left( e^{-\gamma_1 z} - R e^{\gamma_1 z} \right) \tag{3.60}$$

$$E_{2x} = E_i T e^{-\gamma_2 z} \tag{3.61}$$

$$H_{2y} = \left( \frac{E_i}{\eta_2} \right) T e^{-\gamma_2 z} \tag{3.62}$$

where the reflection coefficient $R$ and transmission coefficient $T$ are as defined previously. $E_i$ is the incident electric field strength.

The time-averaged density of power transmitted across the interface is

$$P_t = \frac{1}{2}\frac{E_i^2}{\eta_1}\left(1-|R|^2\right) \tag{3.63}$$

The difference between the incident and transmitted power must be that reflected, or

$$P_r = \frac{1}{2}\frac{E_i^2}{\eta_1}\left(|R|^2\right) \tag{3.64}$$

Let us consider, for example, the case of a metal conductor ($\eta_2 = 0$); according to Eq. (3.56), the reflection coefficient $R = -1$. There will not be any transmitted energy. The incident and reflected components of the electric and magnetic fields will combine in medium 1, as indicated in Eqs (3.59) and (3.60), such that

$$E_x = -2jE_i sin\beta z \tag{3.65}$$

$$H_y = \left(\frac{2E_i}{\eta}\right) cos\beta z \tag{3.66}$$

These equations represent a wave that is stationary in space. The values of $E$ and $H$ are sine and cosine functions of $z$, respectively. The maxima and minima do not move in the $z$ direction but remain at a fixed position as time passes (Figure 3.4). Also note that $E_x$ is 90° apart in time phase from $H_y$ and the peak values of $E$ do not occur at the same point in space as $H$ field. In other words, the electric and magnetic energies of a standing wave are in space and time quadrature. The energy is not transferred but oscillates back and forth from the electric field to the magnetic field over a distance of $\lambda/4$.

The situation involving a plane-wave incident upon several parallel layers of dielectric materials is also of practical interest. The problem may be treated by considering quantities in each medium and use of an impedance formulation like Eq. (3.55). Examples of wave propagation in multiple layers of biological material are given in Chapter 5.

## 3.8 REFRACTION OF MICROWAVE AND RF RADIATION

The refraction and transmission of a plane wave at a plane interface depends on the frequency, polarization, and angle of incidence of the wave, and on the dielectric constant and conductivity of the medium. A wave of general polarization usually is decomposed into its orthogonal linearly polarized components, whose electric and magnetic fields are parallel to the interface [Ishimaru, 2017]. These components are called $E$ and $H$ polarizations, respectively, and can be treated separately and combined afterward. The reflection coefficients for $H$ and $E$ polarizations are given by

$$R_h = \frac{-\left(\frac{\varepsilon_2}{\varepsilon_1}\right)cos\theta + \sqrt{\left(\frac{\varepsilon_2}{\varepsilon_1}\right) - \sin^2\theta}}{\left(\frac{\varepsilon_2}{\varepsilon_1}\right)cos\theta + \sqrt{\left(\frac{\varepsilon_2}{\varepsilon_1}\right) - \sin^2\theta}} \quad (3.67)$$

$$R_e = \frac{cos\theta - \sqrt{\left(\frac{\varepsilon_2}{\varepsilon_1}\right) - \sin^2\theta}}{cos\theta + \sqrt{\left(\frac{\varepsilon_2}{\varepsilon_1}\right) - \sin^2\theta}} \quad (3.68)$$

and the corresponding transmission coefficients are given by

$$T_h = (1 + R_h)\frac{cos\theta}{\sqrt{1 - \left(\frac{\varepsilon_1}{\varepsilon_2}\right)\sin^2\theta}} \quad (3.69)$$

$$T_e = 1 + R_e \quad (3.70)$$

where $\theta$ is the angle of incidence (Figure 3.6) and $\varepsilon_1$ *and* $\varepsilon_2$ are the complex permittivity of the medium in front of and behind the interface, respectively. In particular, $\varepsilon = \varepsilon_0[\varepsilon_r - j(\frac{\sigma}{\omega\varepsilon_0})]$ with free-space permittivity $\varepsilon_0$ and radian frequency $\omega = 2\pi f$. It is noted that the angle of reflection is equal to the angle of incidence, while the angle of transmission is given by Snell's law of refraction.

$$sin\theta_t = \sqrt{\frac{\varepsilon_1}{\varepsilon_2}}sin\theta \quad (3.71)$$

An examination of Eq. (3.67) shows that, for $H$ polarization, it is possible to find an angle so that $R_h = 0$ and the wave is totally transmitted. This angle, referred to as

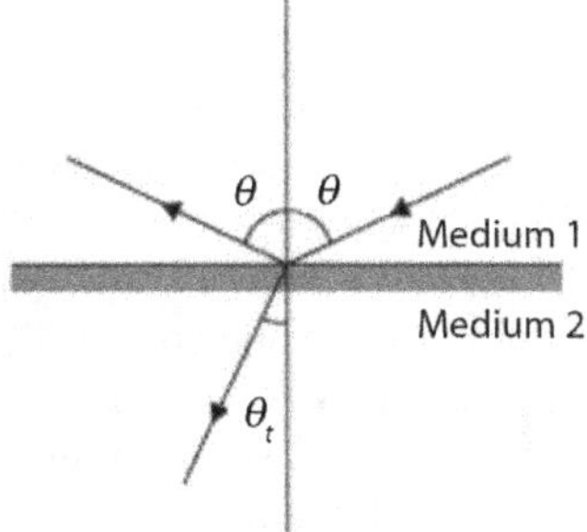


**FIGURE 3.6** Plane wave incident upon a boundary surface at an angle of incidence $\theta$.

the Brewster angle $\theta_B$, can be obtained by setting the numerator of Eq. (3.67) equal to zero such that

$$\theta_B = \tan^{-1}\sqrt{\frac{\varepsilon_2}{\varepsilon_1}} \tag{3.72}$$

Note that a Brewster angle exists for either $\varepsilon_1 > \varepsilon_2$ *or* $\varepsilon_1 < \varepsilon_2$. Thus, a circularly polarized wave incident at $\theta_B$ becomes linearly polarized upon reflection since there will be no reflection for the *H*-polarized component.

There is a second phenomenon that applies to both polarizations. For a wave that is incident from a medium with a higher permittivity onto a medium with a lower permittivity, total reflection can take place at the interface between the two dielectric media. This incident angle is called the critical angle

$$\theta_c = \sin^{-1}\sqrt{\frac{\varepsilon_2}{\varepsilon_1}} \tag{3.73}$$

Under these conditions, the incident wave is totally internally reflected. The wave in the medium with smaller permittivity will decay exponentially away from the interface.

Note that other important topics of propagation and coupling of RF and microwave energy with respect to the human body, such as frequency dependence, orientation and polarization effects on scattering, the Doppler effect from target motion, and range and velocity resolution, are discussed in Chapter 5.

## 3.9 RADIATION OF ELECTROMAGNETIC ENERGY

RF and microwaves are radiated into space or material media through antennas or radiators that serve as transitions between the transmission system and space or material medium. Furthermore, an antenna can also be used as a device to receive microwave and RF radiation. The distribution of radiated energy from an antenna as a function of direction or orientation is given by the antenna radiation pattern. The pattern usually consists of several lobes or sectors. The lobe with the largest maximum is referred to as the main lobe, while the smaller lobes are called minor or side lobes. If the pattern is measured sufficiently far from the antenna so that there is no change in pattern with distance, the pattern is called the far-zone or radiation pattern. Measurement at lesser distances gives near-zone patterns, which are functions of both angle and distance.

In general, antennas involved in biomedical applications are of the order of 1 wavelength in size, and include such diverse types as dipoles, slots, horns, and apertures [Balanis, 2008; Lin et al., 2008]. Most of these are designed for near-zone operations. Therefore, these antennas are referred to as broad-beam antennas. Consequently, their far-zone-radiated energy may be distributed broadly in space, if they reach that far. Another class of antennas, called narrow-beam antennas, focus radiate energy into confined regions and are mostly used in communication and target acquisition situations, such as search radars used for astronomy and military operations.

Another important parameter of an antenna is the power gain, or simply the gain, G, of an antenna; this may be defined as the ratio of the maximum radiation intensity to the radiation intensity from a lossless isotropic antenna radiating the same total power. In this case, the radiation intensity is the average power radiated per unit solid angle. An isotropic antenna is one that radiates uniformly in all directions. It should be noted that the gains of an antenna may also be defined with respect to any reference antenna. Furthermore, the gain of an antenna is applicable to all antennas regardless of its function. Specifically, the gain of an antenna, when it is used for transmitting, is the same as its gain when used for receiving purposes—reciprocity property.

The near- and far-zone characteristics of microwave and RF antennas will be briefly discussed using the example of a short dipole. The short dipole is a simple antenna, but a very important one theoretically. For example, any linear antenna may be regarded as a series of short dipoles, and large antennas of other shapes may be regarded as being composed of many short dipoles. Thus, knowledge of the properties of the short dipole is useful in determining the properties of large antennas of complex shape.

### 3.9.1 The Short Dipole Antenna

For the short dipole illustrated in Figure 3.7, the length $l$ is short compared with a wavelength ($l \ll \lambda$), and the width or diameter is small compared with its length. It is energized by a transmission line that does not radiate. Hence, for purposes of analysis, the short dipole may be considered simply as a thin conductor of length $l$ carrying a uniform current $\boldsymbol{I}$. It can be shown [Jordan and Balmain, 1968] that the electric and magnetic fields from the dipole have only three components $E_\theta, E_r$, and $H_\phi$ in the spherical coordinate system and they are given by

$$E_r = \frac{\eta \boldsymbol{I} l e^{j(\omega t - \beta r)} cos\theta}{2\pi}\left(\frac{1}{r^2} + \frac{1}{j\beta r^3}\right) \tag{3.74}$$

$$E_\theta = \frac{\eta I l e^{j(\omega t - \beta r)} sin\theta}{4\pi}\left(\frac{j\beta}{r} + \frac{1}{r^2} + \frac{1}{j\beta r^3}\right) \tag{3.75}$$

$$H_\phi = \frac{I l e^{j(\omega t - \beta r)} sin\theta}{4\pi}\left(\frac{j\beta}{r} + \frac{1}{r^2}\right) \tag{3.76}$$

Also, the other components $E_\phi, H_r$, *and* $H_\theta$ are zero at all points. At points far from the dipole antenna, $r$ is large; the terms involving $\frac{1}{r^2}$ and $\frac{1}{r^3}$ in Eqs (3.74) through

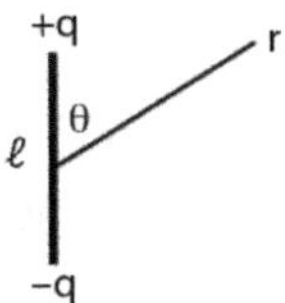


**FIGURE 3.7** An elementary dipole antenna of length $l$ which is short compared with a wavelength, ($\lambda \gg l$), and the width or diameter is small compared with its length.

(3.76) can be neglected in comparison with terms involving $\frac{1}{r}$. Thus, in the far field, there are only two field components given by

$$E_\theta = j\frac{\eta I\beta l}{4\pi r}e^{j(\omega t-\beta r)}sin\theta \tag{3.77}$$

$$H_\phi = j\frac{I\beta l}{4\pi r}e^{j(\omega t-\beta r)}sin\theta \tag{3.78}$$

The wave impedance in the far field, i.e., the ratio of $E_\theta$ to $H_\phi$ as given by Eqs (3.77) and (3.78), is the same as the intrinsic impedance of the medium. Also, $E_\theta$ and $H_\phi$ in the far field are in time phase and at right angles to each other. Thus, the electric and magnetic fields in the far field of a short dipole are related in the same fashion as in a plane wave. Furthermore, the direction and time-averaged flow of energy per unit area are given by Poynting vector (Eqs 3.34 and 3.35),

$$\boldsymbol{P} = \eta\left(\frac{I\beta l}{4\pi r}\right)^2 \sin^2\theta\hat{r} \tag{3.79}$$

Clearly, energy flow in the far field is real, outgoing, and is entirely in the radial direction. The energy is, hence, radiated and the term radiation field is synonymous with far field. In the far field, the intensity of radiated energy decreases as $\frac{1}{r^2}$ with increasing distance.

It is instructive to take apart the far-field expression of Eqs (3.77) and (3.78) into seven basic physical quantities to gain some important physical insights. For example, $E_\theta$ may be written as

$$E_\theta = \left(\frac{1}{2}\right)(\boldsymbol{I})\left(\frac{l}{\lambda}\right)\left(\frac{1}{r}\right)(\eta)\left[je^{j(\omega t-\beta r)}\right]sin\theta \tag{3.80}$$

where $\frac{1}{2}$ is a constant (magnitude) factor, $\boldsymbol{I}$ is the dipole current, $\frac{l}{\lambda}$ is the dipole length expressed in wavelengths, $\frac{1}{r}$ is the distance factor, $\eta$ is the intrinsic impedance of the medium, $je^{j(\omega t-\beta r)}$ is the phase factor, and $sin\theta$ is the pattern factor specifying the field variation with angle. Accordingly, the radiated electric field behavior or performance characteristics of the simple dipole antenna is a function of the seven physical parameters. Indeed, in general, the far-field description of any antenna will involve all seven of these factors, regardless how complex the antenna structure becomes.

### 3.9.2 Near-Zone Radiation

Examination of the expressions for $E_r$, $E_\theta$, and $H_\phi$ shows that, at points close to the short dipole antenna where $r$ is small, the $\frac{1}{r^2}$ and $\frac{1}{r^3}$ terms become predominant and Eqs (3.74) through (3.76) are reduced to

$$E_r = -j\frac{\eta Il}{2\pi\beta r^3}e^{j(\omega t-\beta r)}cos\theta \tag{3.81}$$

$$E_\theta = -j\frac{\eta Il}{4\pi\beta r^3}e^{j(\omega t-\beta r)}sin\theta \tag{3.82}$$

$$H_\phi = \frac{Il}{4\pi r^2}e^{j(\omega t-\beta r)}sin\theta \tag{3.83}$$

Consequently, both components of the electric field are in time quadrature with the magnetic field. Thus, the electric and magnetic fields in the near field are related as in a standing wave. The maxima and minima of electric and magnetic field do not occur at the same point in space. The ratio of electric to magnetic field strength varies from point to point, giving rise to widely divergent field impedance.

Furthermore, the terms that vary as $\frac{1}{r^3}$ in the expression for $E_r$ and $E_\theta$ correspond exactly to the field of an oscillatory electrostatic dipole; these $\frac{1}{r^3}$ terms are referred to as electrostatic fields. The terms that vary inversely as $r^2$ are just the fields that would be obtained by a direct application of Ampere's law. Thus, the field represented by the $\frac{1}{r^2}$ term is called the induction field and becomes predominant at points close to the dipole.

If the Poynting vector is invoked, it will be clear that the electrostatic and induction terms contribute to energy that is stored in the field during one-quarter of a cycle and return to the dipole during the next cycle without any net or average outward energy flow. In the near field, the energy flow is largely reactive; only the $\frac{1}{r}$ terms contribute to an average outward flow of energy. The energy transfer characteristics are illustrated in Figure 3.8, where the arrows represent the direction of energy flow at successive instants of time [Kraus and Carver, 1973].

The criterion of distance most used to demarcate near and far fields is that the phase variation of the field from the antenna does not exceed $\frac{\lambda}{16}$ [Silver, 1949]. This boundary occurs at a conservative distance of

$$R = \frac{2D^2}{\lambda} \tag{3.84}$$

where $D$ represents the largest dimension of the antenna aperture. In the far field, the field strengths decrease as $\frac{1}{r}$ and only transverse field components appear.

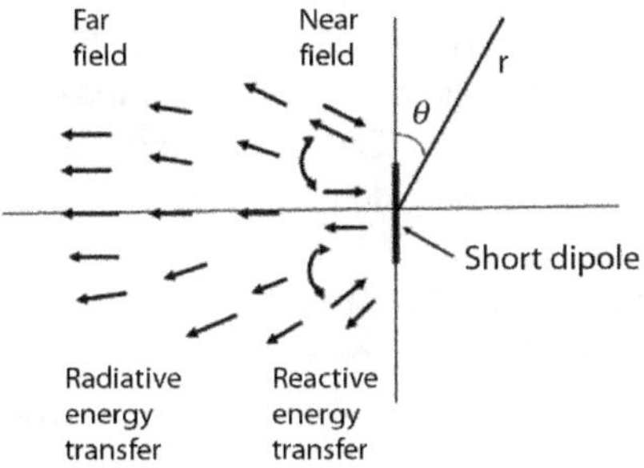


**FIGURE 3.8** Flow of electromagnetic energy from a dipole antenna where the arrows represent the direction of energy flow at successive instants of time. The same flow pattern is on both sides of the dipole antenna.

The near field can be divided into two subregions: the radiative near-field region and the reactive near-field region. In the radiative near-field region, the region closer than $\frac{2D^2}{\lambda}$, the radiation pattern varies with the distance from the antenna. The region of space surrounding the antenna in which the reactive components predominate is known as the reactive near-field region. The extent of this region varies for different antennas. For most antennas, however, the outer limit is a few wavelengths or less. For the special case of the short dipole, the reactive components predominate to approximately $\frac{\lambda}{2\pi}$, where the radiating and reacting components are equal.

For the three field regions illustrated in Figure 3.8, the boundary between the radiative and reactive near-field regions has been conservatively assumed to be $1\lambda$ away from the antenna. It should be noted that at low frequencies, the wavelengths are long and the induction field may extend to very large distances from the source. The corresponding wavelengths at high frequencies are quite short, and the induction field may not exist at all.

In the far-field region, the electric and magnetic fields are outgoing waves with plane-wave fronts, and the power density along the axis of the antenna in free space is given by

$$P_c = \frac{PG}{4\pi r^2} \tag{3.85}$$

where $P$ is the total radiated power, $G$ is the gain of the antenna, and $r$ the distance from the antenna [Balanis, 2008]. Clearly, in the far field, the power density along the beam axis falls off inversely with the square of the distance.

Power density in the near field is not as uniquely defined as in the far field, since the electric and magnetic fields and their ratio vary from point to point. Furthermore, the angular distribution is dependent on the distance from the antenna. Therefore, it is necessary to individually arrive at a quantitative estimate of the power density even along the axis. In general, the near-field power density depends on the antenna shape and aperture field distribution. Analyses have been reported for various types of antennas.

The calculated on-axis power density for a square antenna is shown in Figure 3.9, where the dashed line indicates the envelope of maximum power density obtained [Hansen, 1964]. It is seen that at points close to the antenna ($\frac{2D^2}{\lambda} < 0.1$), the power density oscillates at about a normalized value of 4.5. It reaches a peak normalized value of 13.3 at $\frac{0.18D^2}{\lambda}$ in the radiative near-field region. But the power density falls below the $\frac{1}{R^2}$ value for distances less than $\frac{D^2}{\lambda}$. The on-axis power density for a circular aperture is given in Figure 3.10. The normalized value at a point close to the antenna is about 16. The peak power density occurs at about $\frac{0.2D^2}{\lambda}$ and is nearly 42 times the value of $\frac{2D^2}{\lambda}$.

These results indicate that the transition point between reactive and radiative near-field regions occur from 0.2 to $\frac{0.4D^2}{\lambda}$. Moreover, they give average and maximum near-field power densities as follows:

1. Square aperture antenna with uniform field distribution:

$$P_d = \frac{0.88P}{A}, \text{ average} \tag{3.86}$$

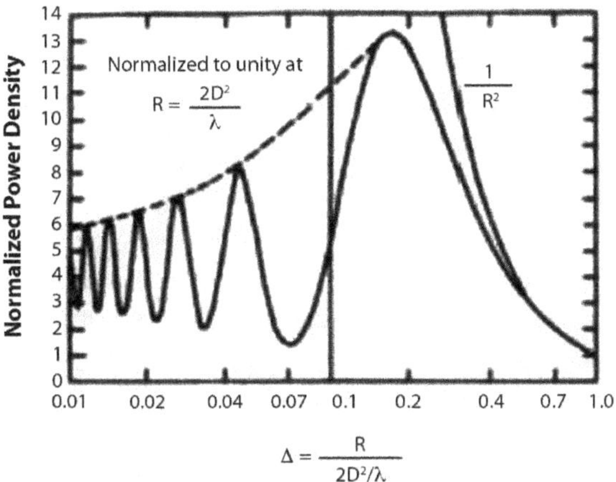


FIGURE 3.9 The on-axis power density of a uniform square antenna.

$$P_d = \frac{3.61P}{A}, \text{ maximum} \tag{3.87}$$

2. Circular aperture antenna with uniform field distribution:

$$P_d = \frac{3.01P}{A}, \text{ average} \tag{3.88}$$

$$P_d = \frac{4.86P}{A}, \text{ maximum} \tag{3.89}$$

where $P$ is the total radiated power and $A$ is the area of the antenna. Thus, the maximum near-field power density that can exist on the axis of a practical aperture

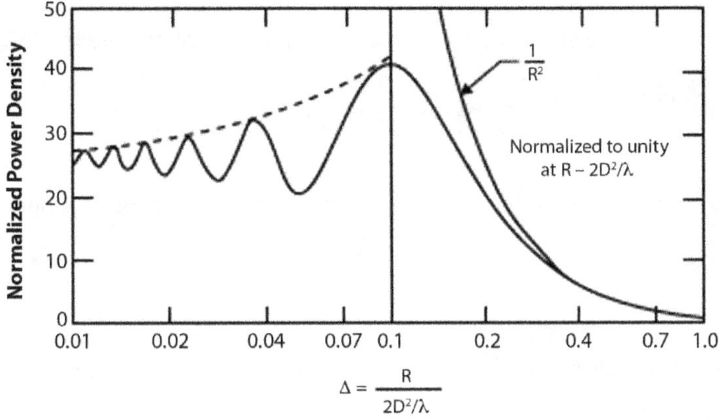


FIGURE 3.10 The on-axis power density of a tapered circular aperture antenna.

antenna is about $\frac{5P}{A}$. It should be noted that these formulas do not include the effect of ground reflections, which could cause a value of power density that is four times the free-space value [Mumford, 1961]. Thus, the electromagnetic radiation in the far field is quite different from that in the near field, although there is a smooth transition from one to the other. It is important to note that radiation is largely confined to within a cylinder whose cross section is the antenna aperture until the distance from the antenna approaches the transition range. This characteristic is also indicated by the on-axis power density, which, at large distances, varies inversely as the square of the distance, but in the near field, oscillates about a constant value.

### 3.9.3 Antenna Receiving Characteristics

Thus far, we have been mainly concerned with transmitting antennas that radiate energy. As mentioned earlier, an antenna can also be used to receive RF and microwave radiation. This is because the performance of an antenna when used for transmitting is the same as its performance when used for receiving, according to the reciprocity theorem [Balanis, 2008; Ishimaru, 2017]. However, a more direct characterization of receiving-antenna performance is effective cross section or effective area. The effective cross section is defined as the area of an ideal antenna that absorbs the same amount of energy from an incident plane wave as the actual antenna. The effective cross section has significance when applied to horns and reflector antennas that have well-defined physical apertures. For these antennas, the ratio of the effective cross section to the actual aperture is a direct measure of the antenna's effectiveness in radiating or receiving the energy to or from the desired direction. Normal values of this ratio for reflector antennas vary from 45% to 75%, depending on antenna type and design, with 65% considered as rather good for the commonly used parabolic reflector antenna [Jordan and Balmain, 1968].

The total power or rate of energy extracted by a receiving antenna with the effective cross section $S$ from an incident plane wave is therefore given by

$$P = P_d S \tag{3.90}$$

Since the effective cross section is related to the gain of an antenna through

$$S = \frac{\lambda^2}{4\pi} G \tag{3.91}$$

the total power received in the field of impinging plane wave for any antenna is

$$P = \frac{\lambda^2}{4\pi} P_d G \tag{3.92}$$

The rate of energy extraction for the short dipole antenna illustrated in Figure 3.7 is

$$P = 1.5 \frac{\lambda^2}{4\pi} P_d \tag{3.93}$$

For this special case of a thin dipole antenna of finite length $l$, the maximum gain is [Harrington, 1961]

$$G = \frac{\eta}{\pi R_r}\left(1 - cos\frac{\beta l}{2}\right)^2 \tag{3.94}$$

where $\eta$ is the intrinsic impedance of the medium and $R_r$ is the radiation resistance of an antenna defined by analogy to Ohm's law as

$$R_r = \frac{P}{|I|^2} \tag{3.95}$$

where $I$ is the antenna current. The total received power is found using Eq. (3.92) as

$$P = \frac{\eta\lambda^2 P_d}{4\pi^2 R_r}\left(1 - cos\frac{\beta l}{2}\right)^2 \tag{3.96}$$

Because of the cosine term and the $R_r$ term in the denominator of Eq. (3.96), the total power received, or rate of energy extracted by a thin dipole antenna, reaches a peak as a function of the antenna length expressed in terms of wavelength. That is, the antenna exhibits resonant receiving characteristics. The total energy extracted from an impinging plane wave peaks for selected antenna lengths. The first of the resonant lengths occurs at a length $l$ equals $0.9\lambda$.

### 3.9.4 Radar Cross Section

In radar operations, the parameter radar cross section (RCS) is commonly used to characterize the scattering property of a radar target. It is the effective size of the target in reflection. It is the functional equivalent to the projected area of a sphere that intercepts an amount of the incident power and then reflects to the transmitter (receiver) [Skolnik, 2008]. It is conceptually related to the scattered and incident electric fields and can be expressed as

$$RCS = (\lim R \to \infty)\ 4\pi R^2 \left(\left|\frac{E_s^2}{E_i^2}\right|\right) \tag{3.97}$$

where $R$ is the range of the target to the receiver, $E_s$ is the scattered or reflected electric field by the target in the direction of the receiver, and $E_i$ is the electric field incident on the target.

In general, the RCS of a target is a function of the frequency and polarization of the incident wave, the angles of incidence and observation, and the geometrical shape and material composition of the object. However, the resolution of targets and specificity in target property pose challenges. Large signal-to-noise ratios are necessary for good resolution. RCS values of common objects are listed in Table 3.1 for X-band radar under monostatic or reflection mode operation when the transmitter

**TABLE 3.1**
**Typical Radar Cross Section of Common Objects**

| Object | Radar Cross Section ($m^2$) |
|---|---|
| Jumbo jet airliner | 100 |
| Passenger automobile | 100 |
| Commercial jet | 40 |
| Cabin cruiser boat | 10 |
| Small four-passenger jet or fighter aircraft | 2 |
| Adult human male | 1 |
| Large bird | 0.5 |
| Insects | 0.00001 |

and receiver are the same or at the same location [Balanis, 2008]. Larger and metallic targets with higher reflected fields tend to yield higher RCS values. As seen in Table 3.1, objects in different scenarios may have comparable RCS depending on the radar's range, beam width, and frequency of operation.

### 3.9.5 Conventional Antenna Configurations and Radiation Patterns

A large variety of antenna designs is available for various applications. In addition to the dipole and aperture antennas mentioned previously, antennas commonly applied for physiological sensing, especially in prototyping investigation, are briefly discussed in this section. Each antenna's performance characteristics are distinguished by its radiation pattern — two- (2-D) or three-dimensional (3-D) spatial distribution of radiated energy as a function of position and orientation. These properties include the on-axis power density, distribution of radiated power density, and radiation pattern, which, in most cases, are determined in the far-field region. The design and performance characteristics of these antennas can be specific to the applications, and their use under various physiological sensing scenarios is discussed in later chapters along with their application.

Dipole antennas (see Figure 3.7) are simple in construction, consisting of two straight metal wires or rods with a feed point at the center. It is a fundamental antenna element and the most used because of the radiation pattern's symmetry over the transverse plane of the dipole, and independence of the angles surrounding the dipole, as shown in Figure 3.11. It has low directivity because the ratio of radiated power in each direction from the antenna to the radiated power averaged over all directions is low. Thus, the dipole antenna is known to offer an omnidirectional (i.e., donut or toroidal-shaped) radiation pattern.

Aperture antennas may have circular and rectangular configurations; their variations include open-ended waveguides and horns (Figure 3.12), circular dish and parabolic reflectors (Figure 3.13), and slot antennas [Lin, 1974; Lin et al., 1979] (Figure 3.14). In general, aperture antennas are used in applications to directly point the source at a target of interest. Also, the circular parabolic reflector antenna is

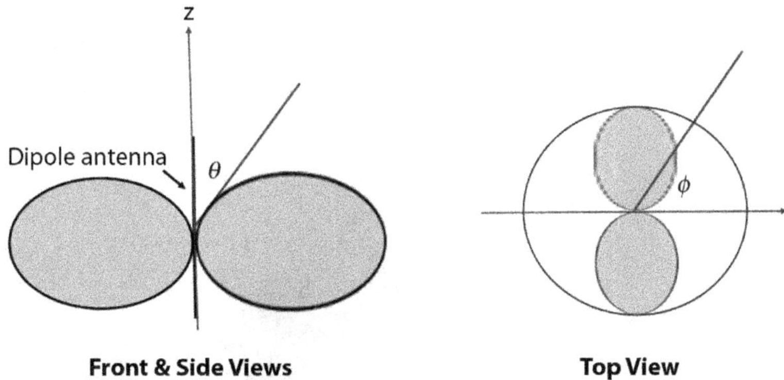


**FIGURE 3.11** An 3-D sketch of a donut shaped or toroidal radiation pattern for a typical linear dipole antenna with its length along the z-axis.

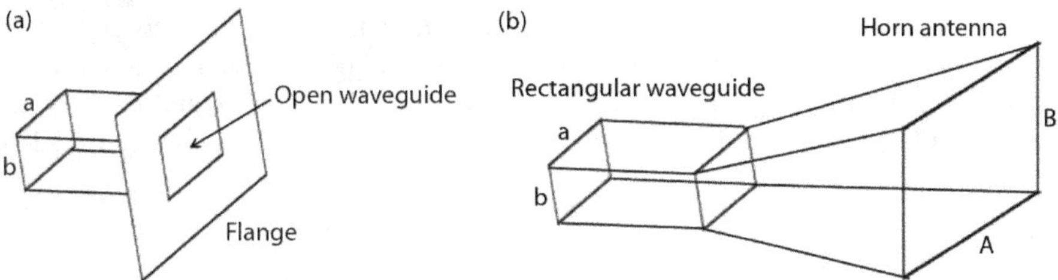


**FIGURE 3.12** Configuration for open-ended waveguide (a) and rectangular horn (b) antenna: (A and a) and (B and b) indicating width and height of horn and waveguide sections, respectively.

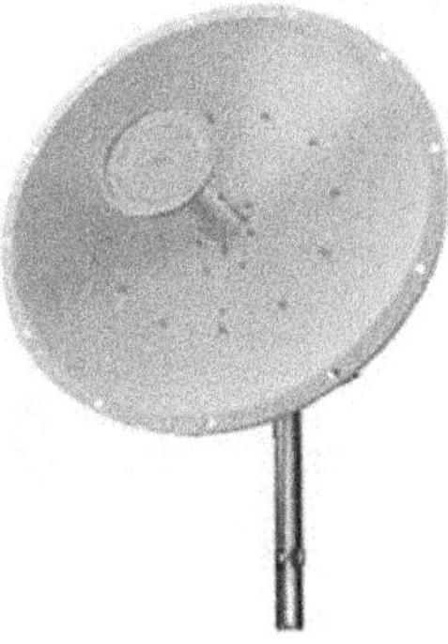

**FIGURE 3.13** Shape of circular dish and parabolic reflector antennas.

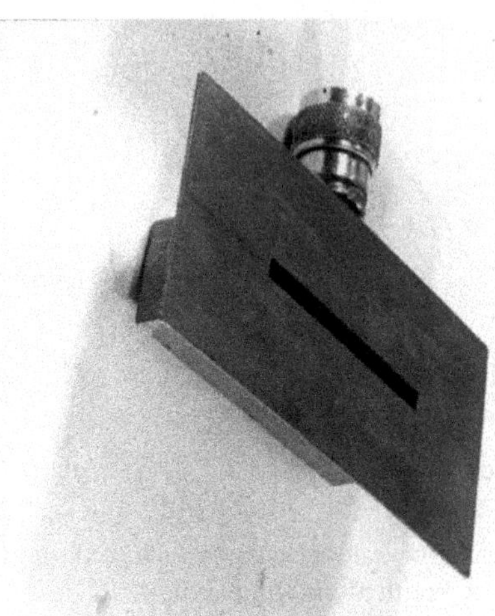

**FIGURE 3.14** Photograph of a cavity-backed microwave slot antenna.

a common antenna found in direct television, and it is the antenna configuration used for many microwave communication systems. Its performance characteristics are typically defined by its focal length $f$, the aperture diameter $D$, and its $f/D$ ratio [Balanis, 2008]. For a circular parabolic antenna with a given $f/D$ ratio (Figure 3.15), the subtended angle ($\theta$) at the feed point is given by

$$\theta = \arctan\left[\frac{8\left(\dfrac{f}{D}\right)}{16\left(\dfrac{f}{D}\right)^2 - 1}\right] \tag{3.98}$$

Most circular reflector antenna designs feature values of $f/D$ between 0.35 and 0.65 with $42° < \theta < 71°$. A representative 2-D radiation pattern is shown in Figure 3.16. It can be seen that the pattern is highly directional. The maximum antenna gain may be greater than 29 dB, ~850 in some cases.

The directivity of a standard gain horn antenna is typically above 12 dB. A diagram of the radiation pattern for a waveguide-fed rectangular horn antenna showing

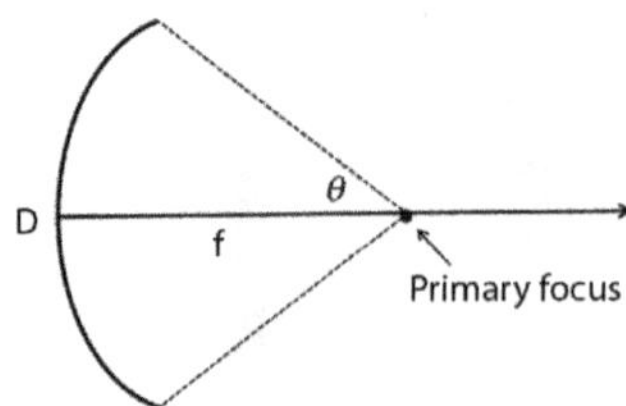


**FIGURE 3.15** Schematic diagram of a circular or parabolic reflector antenna.

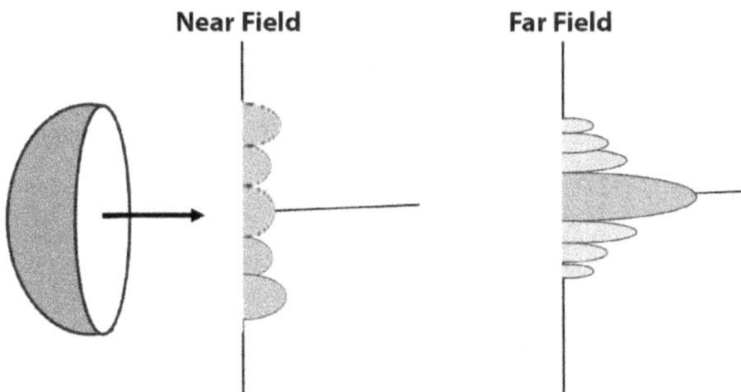


**FIGURE 3.16** Radiation pattern for a circular dish antenna with a main and multiple minor or side lobes.

main and side lobes is given in Figure 3.17. The gain of this horn antenna is 18 dB. Note that the rectangular horn antenna is essentially a flared open waveguide. The waveguide feed acts as a high-pass filter; it blocks microwave propagation below the waveguide's cutoff frequency and passes frequencies above this level. Since horn antennas generally operate over a wide frequency band, they are often designed to have optimal aperture field at the lowest (cutoff) frequency in the band. However, the horn's physical aperture becomes electrically larger at higher frequencies. Consequently, the antenna gain actually increases as the frequency increases.

An associated aperture type antenna is the coaxial circular waveguide applicator [Lin et al., 1982] which was used for microwave apexcardiography (Figure 3.18). Furthermore, conical horns as conceptual extensions from the rectangular to circular waveguide configuration can provide a better directivity — about 15 dB for standard gain — compared to rectangular horns. Aside from open-ended waveguide antenna applicators, a related aperture antenna with a circular matching dielectric plate for direct-body-contact applications is shown in Figure 3.19. The small (15 mm

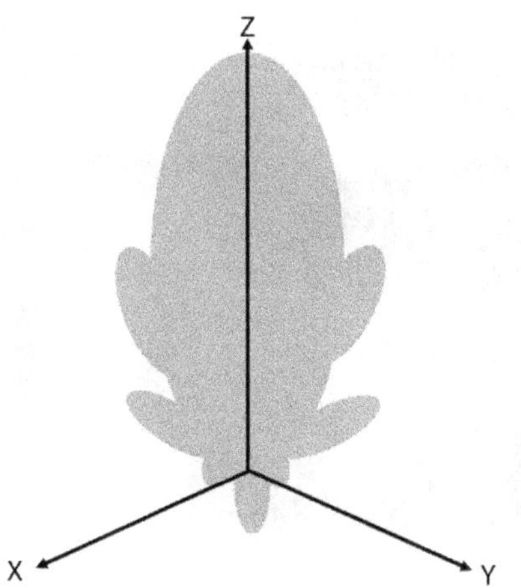


**FIGURE 3.17** Radiation pattern for a horn antenna with main and side lobes.

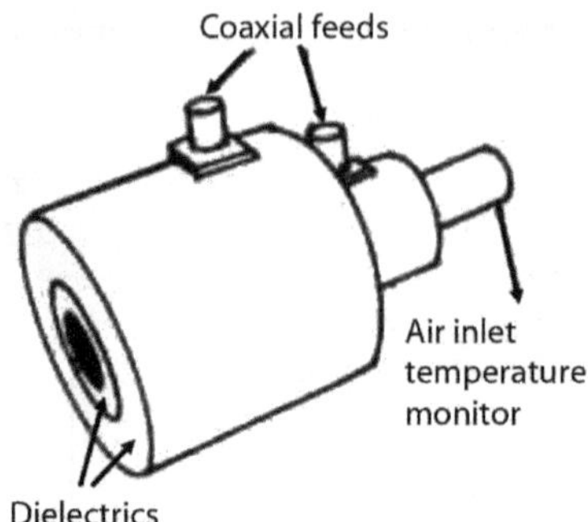


**FIGURE 3.18** A coaxial circular waveguide aperture antenna.

diameter) antenna can provide a convenient narrow beam microwave antenna for noninvasive contact applications.

### 3.9.6 Microstrip Patch and Array Antennas

A class of antennas of special importance to recent developments in microwave physiological sensing is the microstrip patch antenna. Microstrip antennas are made of thin patches of metal on a grounded dielectric substrate and are often designed for use in array form (Figure 3.20). Different types of microstrip patch antennas and arrays of multiple antenna elements have been designed for operation at different frequencies and for use with various noninvasive physiological sensing and monitoring applications. Figures 3.21 and 3.22 present three microstrip patch antenna arrays designed with improved gain and radiation characteristics for noncontact sensing at the 60 GHz frequency band.

Since the patch antenna synthesizes its radiation pattern in the far-field region, its radiation efficiency is degraded when the patch antenna is operated in a near-field zone close to the body. Therefore, patch antennas or arrays may not be efficient for sensing tiny physiological movements such as arterial pulse waves. Nonetheless,

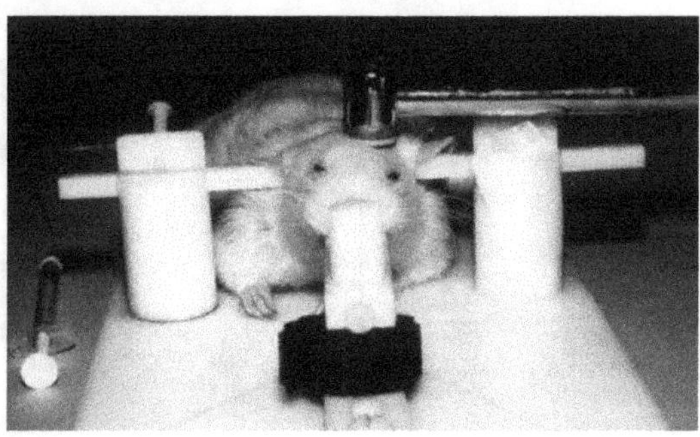

**FIGURE 3.19** A 2450 MHz aperture antenna with circular matching dielectric plate for direct-contact applications.

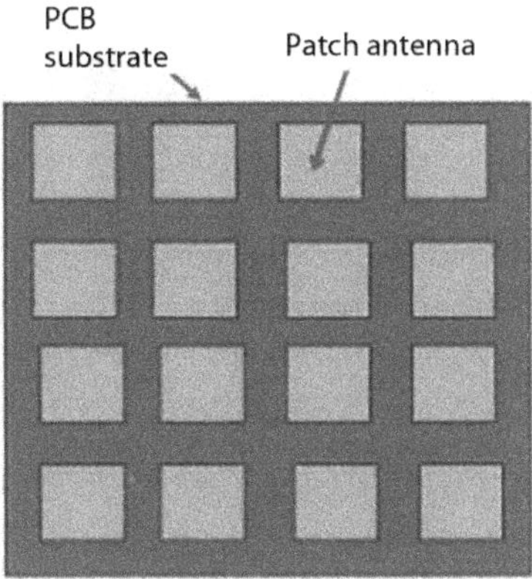


**FIGURE 3.20** The design of a 4 × 4 element patch antenna array.

they can be small and flexible with a low profile and light weight, and can serve as patch antennas and arrays to be wearable on the body. However, the design and characteristics of wearable antennas are specific to the application domain. The performance requirements may include suitability for body-worn applications at various locations on the body with nonplanar surfaces. Also, some wearable antenna designs are integrated into fabric and clothing to be fashionable and inconspicuous. Some of the textile antennas use conductive threads to stitch the antenna design onto the textile substrate to maintain flexibility and conformity [Alharbi et al., 2018] or use metallized fabrics or conductive inks for textile antennas [Hubalek et al., 2016]. Furthermore, patch antennas have been designed that would support either on- or off-body operation with a unique omnidirectional radiation pattern for on-body information transfer and a unidirectional radiation pattern for off-body communication [Hu et al., 2017; Tong et al., 2018].

The design of a four-element 24 GHz antenna array for contactless vital-sign monitoring was reported [Kathuria and Seet, 2020, 2021]. The light-weight, compact

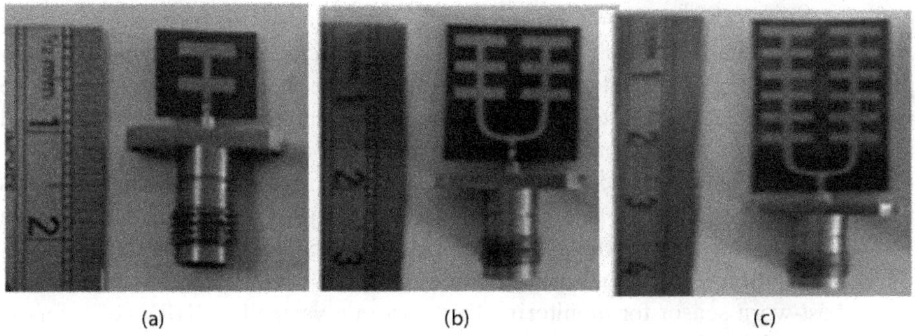


**FIGURE 3.21** Patch antenna arrays with 2×1 elements (a), 3×2 elements (b); and 6×2 elements (c). Dimensions in millimeters.

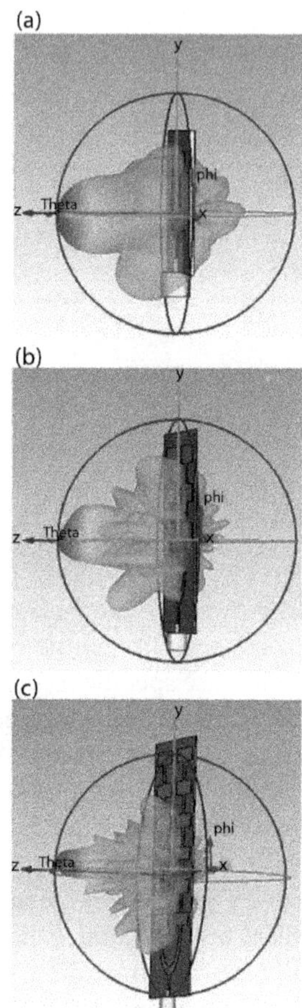


**FIGURE 3.22** Simulated 3-D far-field patterns (FFP) of patch antenna arrays shown in Figure 3.21(a), (b), and (c). (From Rabbani and Ghafouri-Shiraz, 2017.)

27 × 53 mm antenna array was fabricated on a flexible 100 $\mu$m thick liquid crystal polymer (LCP) substrate ($\varepsilon_r = 3.35$) and demonstrated a relatively high gain of 6.2 dB. A wideband antenna in the shape of a button with a circular patch antenna and complementary split-ring resonator radiating element on the short edge of a ground plane was shown to be optimal because the electric field is maximized. Clothing material is placed between the button and ground plane [Yan and Vayesndenbosch, 2018]. Furthermore, a button-shaped dual-mode wearable antenna showed characteristics that may make the antenna a sensor suitable for on-body information transmission and off-body energy harvesting [Zhang et al., 2021]. Figure 3.23 illustrates a prototype of the button-shaped dual-use wearable antenna.

A chest-worn sensor for monitoring the heart rate variability (HRV) of a person in motion without direct contact with the skin was developed to operate at 5.8 GHz with circular polarization to reduce motion-related clutter noise. It involves a self-injection-locked oscillator (SILO) and a microstrip patch tag antenna [Arif et al.,

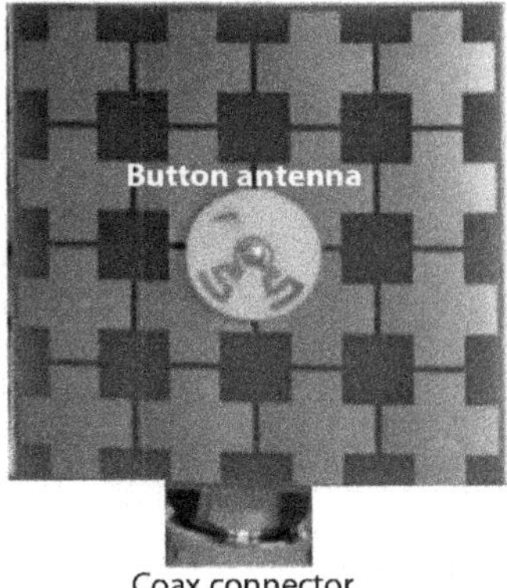


**FIGURE 3.23** A prototype dual-band wearable button antenna sensor.

2022]. The 45 × 34 × 0.8 mm tag antenna consists of a ring slot antenna and a split-ring resonator array in a stack to enhance sensor directivity while reducing the motion clutter for combined sensing and data communication functions (see Figure 3.24). The performance of the microstrip tag antenna was computer simulated and experimentally validated by monitoring the HRV of a wearer engaged in various walking and running activities. Note that the results presented in Figure 3.25 show that the use of the outer ring slot improves the fractional bandwidth (FBW) of the antenna from 2.1% to 9.6% and axial ratio FBW toward the receiver (in the +z direction) from 1.7% to 3.3%. For this design, the E- and H-plane radiation patterns are increased by 7.5 and 8.6 dB, respectively, toward the body (in the −z direction) through the addition of the outer ring slot, which lessens the blocking of the radiated field by the gourd-shaped patch.

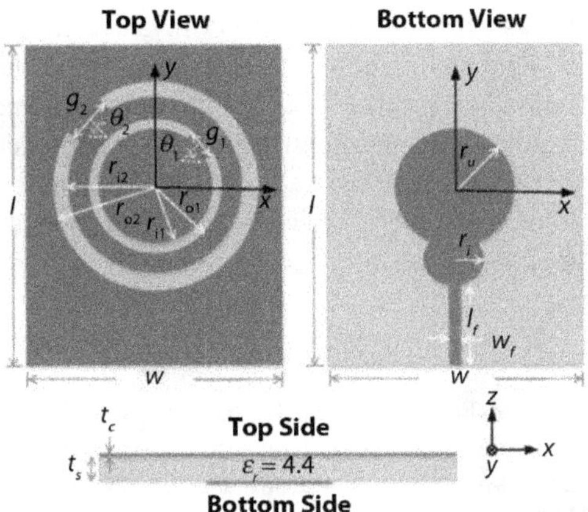


**FIGURE 3.24** Design configuration of circularly polarized patch antenna: $r_{i1}$ = 6 mm, $r_{o1}$ = 7.5 mm, $r_{i2}$ = 10.5 mm, $r_{o2}$ = 13 mm, $g_1$ = 1 mm, $g_2$ = 8 mm, $\theta_1$ = 45°, $\theta_2$ = 157.5°, $r_u$ = 10 mm, $r_l$ = 4 mm, $l_f$ = 10 mm, $w_f$ = 1.5 mm, 1 = 45 mm, $w$ = 34 mm, $t_s$ = 0.8 mm, and $t_c$ = 27 μm.

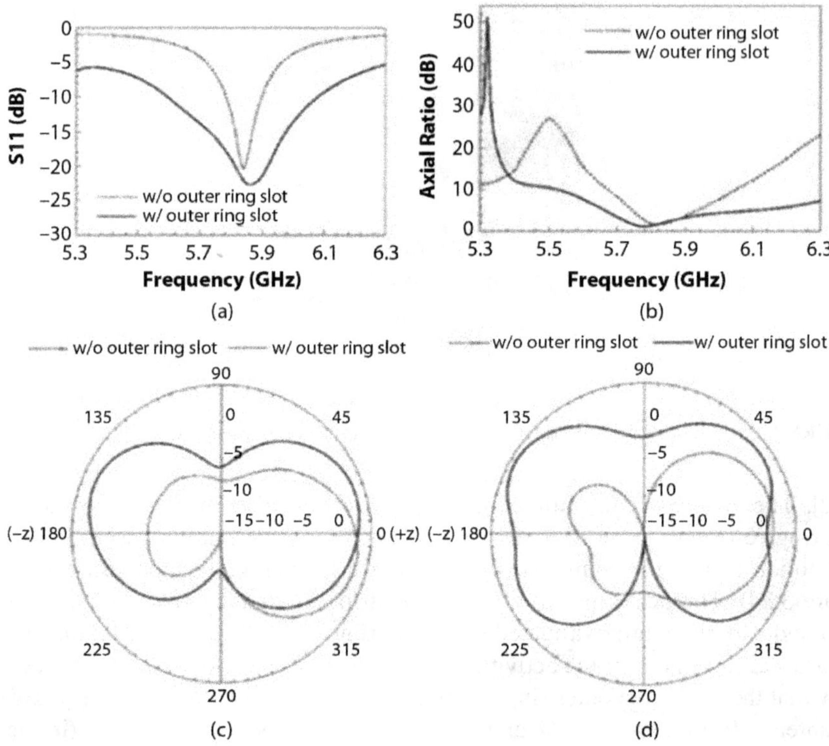


**FIGURE 3.25** Simulated performance of circular polarized patch antenna with and without the outer ring slot shown in Figure 3.22: (a) S11 transmission parameter, (b) axial ratio parameter, (c) E-plane radiation pattern, and (d) H-plane radiation pattern.

In summary, antennas are important for noninvasive microwave physiological sensing. Whether as a single element or an array of multiple elements, their performance in the transmission and reception of signals with minimum losses is essential for success. Aside from the examples mentioned in this chapter, a variety of antennas of different designs for operation at different frequencies that meet the requirements of noninvasive physiological sensing will be described alongside various applications and scenarios in later chapters.

## REFERENCES

Alharbi, S., Chaudhari, S., Inshaar, A., Shah, H., Zou, C., Harne, R. L., Kiourti, A., 2018. E-textile origami dipole antennas with graded embroidery for adaptive RF performance. IEEE Antennas Wirel. Propag. Lett., 17:2218–2222

Arif, R. E., Su, W. C., Horng, T. S., 2022. Chest-worn heart rate variability monitor with a self-injection-locked oscillator tag. IEEE Trans. Microw. Theory Tech., 70(5):2851–2860. doi: 10.1109/TMTT.2022.3155185

Balanis, C., Ed., 2008. Modern Antenna Handbook. Wiley

Hansen, R. C., Ed., 1964. Microwave Scanning Antennas (Vol. I). Academic Press

Harrington, R. F., 1961. Time Harmonic Electromagnetic Fields. McGraw-Hill

Hu, X., Yan, S., Vandenbosch, G. A. E., 2017. Wearable button antenna for dual-band WLAN applications with combined on and off-body radiation patterns. IEEE Trans. Antennas Propag., 65:1384–1387

Hubalek, J., Lacik, J., Puskely, J., Prasek, J., Raida, Z., Vasina, P., 2016. Wearable antennas: Comparison of different concepts. In: 10th Eur. Conf. Antennas Propag., IEEE. 1–4

Ishimaru, A., 2017. Electromagnetic Wave Propagation, Radiation, and Scattering: From Fundamentals to Applications. Wiley

Jordan, E. C., Balmain, K. G., 1968. Electromagnetic Waves and Radiating Systems. Prentice-Hall

Kathuria, N., Seet, B. C., 2020. 24 GHz Flexible LCP Antenna Array for Radar-based Noncontact Vital Sign Monitoring. Asia-Pacific Signal and Information Processing Association Annual Summit and Conference (APSIPA ASC), 1472–1476

Kathuria, N., Seet, B. C., 2021. 24 GHz flexible antenna for Doppler radar-based human vital signs monitoring. Sensors, 21:3737

Kraus, J. F., Carver, K. R., 1973. Electromagnetics. McGraw-Hill

Lin, J. C., 1974. A cavity-backed slot radiator for microwave biological effect research. J. Microw. Power 9: 63–67

Lin, J. C., Bernardi, P., Pisa, S., Cavagnaro, M., Piuzzi, E., 2008. Antennas for medical therapy and diagnostics. In: Balanis, C., Ed., Modern Antenna Handbook (pp. 1377–1428), Hoboken, NJ: Wiley

Lin, J. C., Kantor, G., Ghods, A., 1982. A class of new microwave therapeutic applicators. Radio Sci., 17:119S–123S

Lin, J. C., Kiernicki, J., Kiernicki, M., Wollschlaeger, P. B., 1979. Microwave apexcardiography. IEEE Trans. Microw. Theory Tech., 27:618–620

Mumford, W. W., 1961. Some technical aspects of microwave radiation hazards. Proc. IRE, 49:427

Rabbani, M. S., Ghafouri-Shiraz, H., 2017. Ultra-wide patch antenna array design at 60 GHz band for remote vital sign monitoring with Doppler radar principle. J. Infrared Milli. Terahz. Waves, 38:548–566

Silver, S., Ed., 1949. Microwave Antenna Theory and Design. McGraw-Hill

Skolnik, M. I., 2008. Radar Handbook, 3rd ed, McGraw-Hill

Tong, X., Liu, C., Liu, X., Guo, H., Yang, X., 2018. Switchable on-/off-body antenna for 2.45 GHz WBAN applications. IEEE Trans. Antennas Propag., 66:967–971

Yan, S., Vandenbosch, G. A. E., 2018. Design of wideband button antenna based on characteristic mode theory. IEEE Trans. Biomed. Circuits Syst., 12:1383–1391

Zhang, J., Meng, J., Li, W., Yan, S., Vandenbosch, G. A. E., 2021. A wearable button antenna sensor for dual-mode wireless information and power transfer. Sensors, 21(17):5678. doi: 10.3390/s21175678. PMID: 34502570; PMCID: PMC8433973

# 4 Microwave Property of Living Matter

Biological materials are heterogeneous and consist of molecules, organelles, cells, organs, tissues, and water. There are also various ions, polar molecules, membranes, and membrane-bound components. These are the components that form the structure of the biological body, including humans. These substances are often called dielectric materials, owing to the similarity of the electric, magnetic, chemical, and physical nature of such materials.

Water forms a major portion of the substance of living bodies. Thus, biological materials may be classified into three major groups according to their water content. The first group is of high water content (90% or more), consisting of fluids containing electrolytes, macromolecules, and other cellular materials, and includes blood, vitreous humor, and cerebrospinal fluid (CSF). The second group is of moderate water content (80% or less) and consists of skin, muscle, brain, and internal organs. The last group is made up of tissues with low water content (less than 40%) such as fat, bone, and tendons.

The frequency-dependent property characteristics of biological dielectric materials may be described by the relaxation processes associated with many dielectric materials that display a time-dependent response to sudden excitations. This chapter presents a succinct description of the dielectric relaxation processes and gives a brief summary of the measured tissue dielectric permittivity data known also as dielectric constant and electrical conductivity for different frequencies and temperatures.

## 4.1 FREQUENCY DEPENDENCE OF DIELECTRIC PERMITTIVITY

The electromagnetic properties of biological materials have been extensively studied [Gabriel et al., 1996a,b; Schwan, 1957, 1963; Schwan et al., 1976; Schwan and Foster, 1980]. A basic understanding has been achieved of the structures and mechanisms that determine the radio frequency (RF) and microwave properties of biological materials [Lin, 2021; Michaelson and Lin, 1987].

Biological materials have magnetic permeability values close to that of free space or vacuum and are independent of frequency. It is noted, however, that biological tissues are not free of ferromagnetic particles. They exhibit very high dielectric constants compared with many other types of homogeneous solids and liquids. This is because biological tissues are heterogeneous and consist of ions, macromolecules, cells, and other membrane-bound substances. An example of the frequency-dependent character of biological tissue material is given in Figure 4.1 for muscle. There are three principal regions of dispersions, described as $\alpha, \beta$, and $\gamma$ dispersions, respectively. Each dispersion is defined either by a single relaxation frequency or a small group of relaxation frequencies.


DOI: 10.1201/9781003315223-4

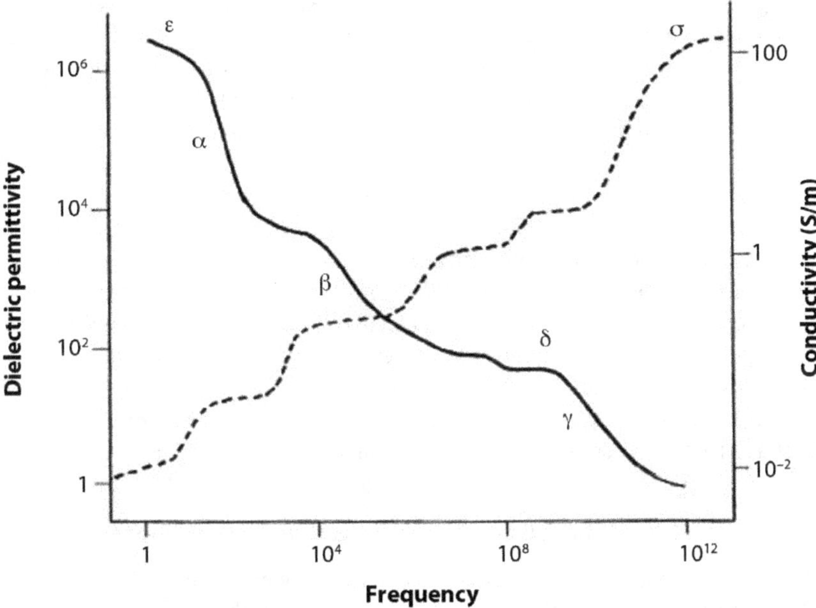


**FIGURE 4.1** Dielectric permittivity and electrical conductivity of muscle-like biological materials as a function of frequency from 1 Hz to 1 THz.

The $\alpha$ dispersion at an extremely low frequency (<10 kHz) is the result of cell membrane capacitance variations with frequency. The membrane capacitance undergoes a pronounced decrease from 10 $\mu f/cm^2$ to 1 $\mu f/cm^2$ as the frequency increases. The $\beta$ dispersion originates from the heterogeneous nature of biological tissues (proteins and macromolecules). At frequencies between 1 kHz and 10 MHz, the applied electric field causes electric charges to accumulate at boundaries separating tissue regions of different dielectric property, for example, membranes separating intra- and extracellular fluids. Finite durations of time are required before the boundaries can reach charge neutrality, giving rise to the relaxation phenomenon.

As the frequency increases, insufficient time is available during each cycle to allow complete charging of the cell membranes. The total charges per cycle must decrease, along with the membrane capacitance, as the frequency is increased. This is manifested as a decrease in the dielectric constant.

For still higher frequencies, the membrane capacitance change stabilizes until the rotational and vibrational properties of polar molecules of water become significant. This dispersion is characterized by a single relaxation frequency slightly lower than that of pure water.

There is a minor relaxation termed the $\delta$ dispersion, occurring between the $\beta$ and $\gamma$ dispersions (Figure 4.1). This is caused by the relaxation of water molecules bound to the surface of macromolecules, and the rotation of amino acids as well as charged side groups of proteins [Grant et al., 1978; Schwan, 1977].

The conductivities of biological materials change in a similar manner. Cell membranes have a relatively high capacitance (about 1 $\mu f/cm^2$) at frequencies near the $\beta$ dispersion. They become progressively short-circuited for frequencies above the $\beta$ dispersion, permitting the intracellular fluid to participate in current conduction. This causes the conductivity to increase as the frequency increases. In the $\gamma$ dispersion region, the rotation of water molecules is accompanied by viscous loss, which accounts for the principal mechanism for increased conductivity.

It can be seen from the dispersion behavior of muscle tissue summarized earlier that the dielectric and conductivity properties of biological materials in the RF and microwave frequency range are largely determined by the relaxation properties of the biological membrane, protein macromolecule, and tissue water. More detailed descriptions may be found in other studies [Daniel, 1967; Debye, 1929; von Hipp, 1954].

For additional information about dielectric permittivity properties of biological materials, the reader is referred to other works [Cole, 1968; Gabriel et al., 1996a,b; Grant et al., 1978; Hill et al., 1969; Michaelson and Lin, 1987; Schwan, 1957].

## 4.2 DIELECTRIC RELAXATION PROCESSES

The frequency-dependent nature of the electrical properties of biological materials may be described by relaxation processes associated with many dielectric materials displaying a time-dependent response to sudden excitation. Polar molecules and cellular components rotate in response to an applied electric field. This rotation is impeded by inertia and viscous forces. Therefore, the reorientation of polar molecules does not occur instantaneously, giving rise to the time-dependent behavior (relaxation). Moreover, cells and tissues composed of structural components of different properties, when subjected to a step-function electrical stimulation, require a finite duration of time for charges to accumulate at the interfaces. The accumulation of charges at interfaces continues until a condition of charge equilibrium is re-established; thus, the relaxation. Many types of relaxation processes can occur in tissue material (see Figure 4.1), owing to dipoles and charges existing in the material.

For isotropic media, the permittivity $\varepsilon$ is represented by

$$\varepsilon = \varepsilon_0 \left( 1 + \frac{\omega_p^2}{\omega_s^2 - \omega^2 + j\omega v} \right) \tag{4.1}$$

where

$$\omega_p^2 = \frac{\rho q^2}{m\varepsilon_0} \tag{4.2}$$

and $\varepsilon_0$ is the free-space permittivity, $q$ and $m$ are the particle charge and mass, respectively, $\omega_s$ is the characteristic frequency of the elastic spring-mass system, and $v$ is the particle collision frequency [Lin, 2021; Michaelson and Lin, 1987]. Clearly, $\varepsilon$ is a complex quantity and can be denoted as

$$\varepsilon = \varepsilon' - j\varepsilon'' \tag{4.3}$$

where $\varepsilon'$ *and* $\varepsilon''$ are the real and imaginary parts of the permittivity. It can be obtained by equating the real and imaginary parts of Eqs (4.1) and (4.3), respectively.

As mentioned, the relaxation phenomenon is exhibited by all biological tissues and many dielectric materials. In general, there are two types of dielectric materials of interest to the biophysical aspects of electromagnetic interactions with biological systems.

### 4.2.1 Low-Loss Dielectric Materials

For low-loss dielectric materials characterized by low collision frequency, $v$, $\varepsilon'$, *and* $\varepsilon''$ can be derived from Eq. (4.1) for $\omega \neq \omega_s$

$$\frac{\varepsilon'}{\varepsilon_0} = 1 + \left[\frac{\omega_p^2}{\omega_s^2 - \omega^2}\right] \tag{4.4}$$

$$\frac{\varepsilon''}{\varepsilon_0} = \frac{\omega v \omega_p^2}{\left(\omega_s^2 - \omega^2\right)^2} \tag{4.5}$$

A graphical representation of this result is shown in Figure 4.2. The real part of permittivity is usually high at low frequencies, increasing to extremely high values at the characteristic frequency $\omega_s$ and returning to $\varepsilon_0$ at higher frequencies. The imaginary part of permittivity is small at all frequencies, except near $\omega_s$. Permittivity is high because of the large particle displacement at the characteristic frequency, giving rise to large collisional and, thus, absorption effects. For most solid dielectric materials of practical interest to microwave biophysics (e.g., Plexiglas), the frequency $\omega_s$ is in the optical spectrum or above. Thus, they are characterized by low loss and a slowly increasing dielectric constant with frequency. Values of $\frac{\varepsilon'}{\varepsilon_0}$ and $\frac{\varepsilon''}{\varepsilon'}$ for some low-loss materials are given in Table 4.1, as a function of frequency.

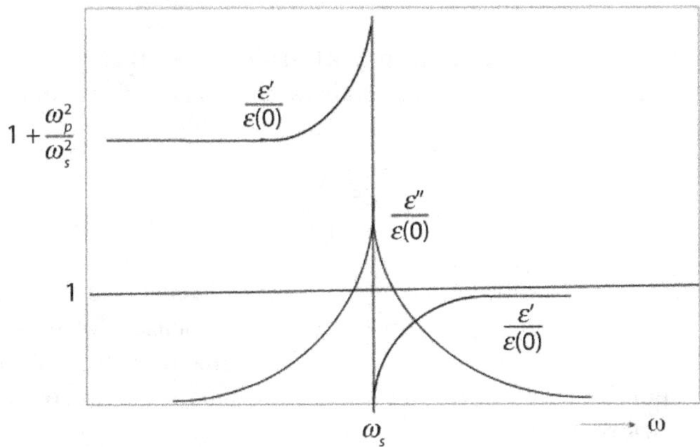


**FIGURE 4.2** Frequency dependence of permittivity of typical or common low-loss dielectric materials.

**TABLE 4.1**
**Permittivity of Common Low-Loss Dielectric Materials at 25°C**

| | $\frac{\varepsilon'}{\varepsilon_0}$ | | | | $\frac{\varepsilon''}{\varepsilon'}$ | | | |
|---|---|---|---|---|---|---|---|---|
| | **Frequency (Hz)** | | | | | | | |
| | **$10^6$** | **$10^8$** | **$3\times10^9$** | **$2.5\times10^{10}$** | **$10^6$** | **$10^8$** | **$3\times10^9$** | **$2.5\times10^{10}$** |
| Beeswax | 2.53 | 2.45 | 2.39 | | $9.2\times10^{-3}$ | $9\times10^{-3}$ | $7.5\times10^{-3}$ | |
| Fused quartz | 3.78 | 3.78 | 3.78 | 3.78 | $1\times10^{-4}$ | $2\times10^{-4}$ | $6\times10^{-5}$ | $2.5\times10^{-4}$ |
| Glass – soda borosilicate | 4.84 | 4.84 | 4.82 | 4.63 | $3.6\times10^{-3}$ | $3\times10^{-3}$ | $5.4\times10^{-3}$ | $9\times10^{-3}$ |
| Foamed polystyrene | 1.03 | 1.03 | 1.03 | 1.03 | $2\times10^{-4}$ | $2\times10^{-4}$ | $1\times10^{-4}$ | $1\times10^{-4}$ |
| Polystyrene | 2.26 | 2.26 | 2.26 | 2.26 | $2\times10^{-4}$ | $2\times10^{-4}$ | $3.1\times10^{-4}$ | $6\times10^{-4}$ |
| Teflon (polytetrafluoroethylene) | 2.21 | 2.21 | 2.21 | 2.08 | $2\times10^{-4}$ | $2\times10^{-4}$ | $1.5\times10^{-4}$ | $6\times10^{-4}$ |

### 4.2.2 Lossy Dielectrics at Low Frequencies

At frequencies considered low compared to the characteristic frequency ($\omega \ll \omega_s$), Eq. (4.1) reduces to

$$\frac{\varepsilon}{\varepsilon_0} = 1 + \frac{\dfrac{\omega_p^2}{\omega_s^2}}{1 + \dfrac{j\omega v}{\omega_s^2}} \tag{4.6}$$

This equation may be expressed in terms of the permittivity at zero frequency,

$$\varepsilon(0) = \varepsilon_0\left(1 + \frac{\omega_p^2}{\omega_s^2}\right) \tag{4.7}$$

and the permittivity at infinite frequency $\varepsilon(\infty) = \varepsilon_0$. Note that both these limiting values of complex permittivity are real numbers. Thus, Eq. (4.6) written in the Debye form becomes

$$\varepsilon = \varepsilon(\infty) + \frac{\varepsilon(0) - \varepsilon(\infty)}{1 + j\omega\tau} \tag{4.8}$$

where $\tau = v/\omega_s^2$ is the relaxation time and is inversely related to the relaxation frequency $\omega_r$. Relaxation time $\tau$, proportional to $v$, is a measure of how fast charges move in response to an applied electric field. A low value of $v$ means fewer collisions and a faster response, giving rise to a shorter relaxation time $\tau$. From Eq. (4.8), the real and imaginary parts of $\varepsilon$ may be written as

$$\varepsilon' = \varepsilon(\infty) + \frac{\varepsilon(0) - \varepsilon(\infty)}{1 + (\omega\tau)^2} \tag{4.9}$$

$$\varepsilon'' = \frac{\omega\tau\left[\varepsilon(0)-\varepsilon(\infty)\right]}{1+(\omega\tau)^2} \tag{4.10}$$

The loss mechanism described earlier applies to a model in which there are only bound charges. In biological materials and many other liquids and solids, there exist an appreciable number of free charges. The loss mechanisms in these materials are described by the conductivity relating the current density to the applied field (see Chapter 3, Eqs 3.9 and 3.16). This may be visualized as free charges moving randomly because of their thermal velocities and frequently colliding with other particles making up the material. The applied electric field produces a general drift in the direction of the applied field with a nonzero average velocity. This component of velocity and the resulting current are in phase with the applied field at low frequencies, compared with the collision frequency, and represent an ohmic or Joule loss. At any frequency, this loss and that of the bound charge add directly. If one is interested only in the macroscopic behavior, it is customary to include the conduction loss in the imaginary part of the permittivity or vice versa. If one is to be concerned with microscopic properties, it would then be necessary to keep the two mechanisms separate.

Furthermore, in biological materials, it is impossible to separate the two contributions from measurements made at a given frequency. Therefore, the presence of a finite $\varepsilon''$ has the effect of producing a total electrical conductivity $\sigma$, and a finite conductivity is equivalent to a total imaginary part of the permittivity as $\varepsilon''$. The relationship between $\sigma$ *and* $\varepsilon''$ may be derived from two of Maxwell's equations, (3.10) and (3.11) (see Chapter 3), or

$$\sigma = \omega\varepsilon'' \tag{4.11}$$

where $\sigma$, an equivalent conductivity representing all losses, is given by

$$\sigma = \frac{\omega^2\tau\left[\varepsilon(0)-\varepsilon(\infty)\right]}{1+(\omega\tau)^2} \tag{4.12}$$

This equation for conductivity can be expressed in an alternate fashion such as

$$\sigma = \sigma(0)+\left[\sigma(\infty)-\sigma(0)\right]\frac{(\omega\tau)^2}{1+(\omega\tau)^2} \tag{4.13}$$

where $\sigma(0)$ and $\sigma(\infty)$ are conductivity values far below and above the relaxation frequency $\omega_s$. The conductivity term $\sigma(0)$ has been added to account for the ionic and frequency-independent contribution to Eqs (4.8) and (4.13), which are special cases of the Kramers-Kronig relationship [Böttcher, 1952]. They show that the frequency response of the permittivity determines that of the conductivity and vice versa.

It is also convenient to define a relative dielectric constant through dividing $\varepsilon'$ by the free-space permittivity $\varepsilon_0$:

$$\varepsilon_r = \frac{\varepsilon'}{\varepsilon_0} \tag{4.14}$$

This notation will be used often in this book, as this notation is simple and facilitates mathematical manipulations. It should be mentioned that $\varepsilon_r$ is usually referred to simply as the dielectric constant and it is dimensionless (see also Chapter 3, Eq. 3.19). For example, the dielectric constants for common building materials vary between 2 and 5 for fiber, glass, wood, and dry bricks.

The ratio $\varepsilon''/\varepsilon'$ is also a commonly used parameter for dielectric materials and is called the loss tangent. For low-loss materials such as those given in Table 4.1, the loss tangent is much less than unity. On the other hand, biological materials are characterized by the considerable number of losses and, therefore, have loss tangents close to or greater than 1.

The variation with frequency of the real and imaginary parts of permittivity and electrical conductivity is illustrated in Figure 4.3. It is seen that the dielectric constant $\varepsilon'$ falls from a higher value of $\varepsilon(0)$ to $\varepsilon(\infty)$ as the frequency increases through the dispersion region, while the conductivity rises from a small value of $\sigma(0)$ *to* $\sigma(\infty)$. The imaginary part of the permittivity $\varepsilon''$ peaks at $\omega\tau = 1$ and falls off for both higher and lower frequencies.

### 4.2.3 Biological Materials

The results summarized in Eqs (4.9), (4.10), and (4.12) depict the dielectric properties of biological tissues in most RF and microwave frequency regions. For a particular range of frequencies, the value of $\varepsilon(\infty)$ *and* $\varepsilon(0)$ may be considered the permittivity at frequencies far above and below the relaxation frequency $\omega_s$.

Since the dielectric properties of biological materials are complex, they require a distribution of relaxation processes for representation throughout the RF and microwave frequencies [Cole and Cole, 1941]. In this case, the dielectric behavior may be modeled as the sum of relaxation processes, with each process being a noninstantaneous exponential relaxation from one state to another, as depicted in Eqs (4.9),

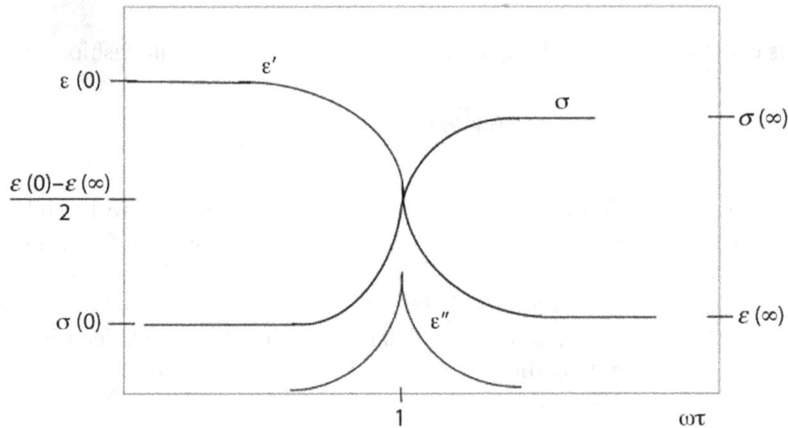


**FIGURE 4.3** Frequency-dependent characteristics of permittivity and conductivity of lossy dielectric materials.

(4.10), and (4.12). The corresponding responses in the frequency domain are of the form often called the Debye equation:

$$\varepsilon = \varepsilon_0 + \sum_{n=1}^{N} \frac{\Delta\varepsilon_n}{1 + j\omega\tau_n} \tag{4.15}$$

where $\Delta\varepsilon_n$ is the difference between the permittivity far below and far above the relaxation frequency, and $\tau_n$ is the relaxation time associated with each relaxation process.

As presented earlier, the dielectric properties of biological materials can often be characterized by using three distinct relaxation processes. The relaxation times are well separated such that $\tau_1 \gg \tau_2 \gg \tau_3$. The corresponding relaxation frequencies for each region are about 100 Hz, 50 kHz, and 25 GHz at body temperature (37°C) for most biological materials.

## 4.3 TEMPERATURE DEPENDENCE OF DIELECTRIC PROPERTIES

It was indicated previously that the electrical properties of biological tissues throughout the RF and microwave frequency ranges are governed by structural and rotational relaxation phenomena. There are abundant layers of tissues and membranes with different dielectric constants and conductivities in biological materials. When an electric field is applied, surface charges build up at the interface between two adjacent layers, thus generating varying permittivity values. Furthermore, molecular dipoles tend to orient in an applied electric field. Since the reorientation of polar molecules does not occur instantaneously, it gives rise to a rotational relaxation effect.

The movement of charges, whether to accumulate at tissue interface or to realign through rotation, is hindered by collisions with particles in the surrounding medium. The speed of movement depends, therefore, on temperature, among other factors. Thus, both dielectric constants and conductivities are temperature-sensitive [Lin, 1988].

A mathematical treatment of the temperature dependence of the dielectric constant and conductivity, however, is not straightforward. The few studies concerned with the temperature dependence of dielectric constants and conductivities have shown that the temperature dependence of conductivity is much more pronounced than that of the dielectric constant. Near a relaxation frequency, the relationship

$$\frac{d\varepsilon}{\varepsilon} = \frac{d\sigma}{\sigma} \frac{\varepsilon(0) - \varepsilon(\infty)}{\varepsilon(0) + \varepsilon(\infty)} \tag{4.16}$$

may be derived for the relative change in dielectric constant to relative change in conductivity [Schwan and Foster, 1980]. Since $\varepsilon(0)$ and $\varepsilon(\infty)$ are fairly independent of temperature, and $\varepsilon(0)$ is much larger than $\varepsilon(\infty)$, the change of the dielectric constant with temperature must be smaller than that of the conductivity.

In general, the dielectric properties of biological materials are characterized by three distinct dispersion regions. For each dispersion, the temperature coefficient reflects those of $\varepsilon(0), \varepsilon(\infty),$ *and* $\omega_s$. The dispersion may be due to frequency-dependent membrane capacitance arising from ionic gating currents through or counter ions surrounding membranes. These ionic activities have temperature coefficients similar to that of the conductivity of electrolytes; i.e., about 2% per °C. The dispersion is caused by polarization effects in which the cellular membranes are charged through electrolytes. Hence, the temperature coefficient is equal to that of the conductivity of electrolytes. The dispersion originates from the rotational relaxation of water molecules. Hence, its temperature dependence is equal to that of water, which again is close to 2% per °C. Thus, the temperature coefficient of the conductivity for biological materials has a maximum value of about 2% per °C for tissues with higher water content, such as blood, CSF, and most organs.

### 4.3.1 Temperature Dependence of Measured Tissue Dielectric Permittivity

The temperature dependence of the dielectric properties of biological tissues in the microwave frequency range has only been studied more vigorously since about 2000, although there were some discussions on the topic, especially regarding water and electrolytes, around 1980. It is interesting to observe this in the context of scientific investigations of therapeutic heating of deep-seated tissues like muscle by microwave radiation that began in mid-1940s. Further clinical studies of microwave diathermy led to its acceptance as a therapeutic instrument by the American Medical Association in 1947. Microwave diathermy's therapeutic effectiveness in traumatic conditions such as sprains and stresses, especially when combined with massage, is clearly indicated and remains an integral part of the treatment modalities in physical and sports medicine.

Microwave hyperthermia as a clinical treatment for localized malignant disease began in the late 1970s. The objective of this controlled temperature elevation is the treatment of tumors directly, by microwave-induced irreversible biological damage, or indirectly, by enhancing the therapeutic effectiveness of other treatment regimens such as ionizing radiation or chemotherapy [Lin, 1999; Watmough and Ross, 1986]. There has been a steady stream of publications over the past 40 years on all aspects of hyperthermia therapy, showing hyperthermia is gaining wider use in clinical practice in treating a variety of malignant tumors.

Microwave and RF catheter ablation for cardiac arrhythmias was first announced in 1987 for tachyarrhythmia [Huang and Wilber, 2000; Lin, 2003]. Shortly thereafter, this minimally invasive microwave technique was adopted to help ablate malignant liver nodules. Microwave catheter ablation, along with the use of RF energy, has become an important therapy in the management of related diseases.

As mentioned, scientific attention has mostly been directed toward the frequency-dependence of dielectric permittivity properties. Since about 2000, perhaps given the momentum of the successful applications of minimally invasive ablation techniques in the RF and microwave frequency range, there has been much to stimulate interest in the temperature dependence of dielectric permittivity of biological tissues. However, only limited data on temperature-dependent dielectric permittivity are available.

Table 4.2 summarizes published papers on measured temperature-dependent microwave dielectric permittivity, relative dielectric constant and conductivity of freshly excised animal tissues ranging in temperatures from 5 to 90°C, and their

**TABLE 4.2**
**Measured Temperature-Dependent Dielectric Permittivity of Animal Tissues at Microwave Frequencies**

| Frequency (MHz) | Tissue Type | Temp Range (°C) | $\varepsilon$ | $\varepsilon$ Coeff. (%/°C) | $\sigma$ (S/m) | $\sigma$ Coeff. (%/°C) | Reference |
|---|---|---|---|---|---|---|---|
| 400 | Human blood | 25–45 | — | –0.10 | 0.7 | 1.13 | Jaspard and Nadi, 2002 |
| 468 | Porcine muscle | 36–60 | 65.03 | –0.30 | 1.11 | 0.92 | Fu, 2014 |
| 468 | Porcine kidney | 36–60 | 58.36 | –0.42 | 1.04 | 1.30 | Fu, 2014 |
| 468 | Porcine liver | 36–60 | 51.43 | –0.35 | 0.80 | 1.03 | Fu, 2014 |
| 915 | Bovine liver | 50–80 | 48.10 | –0.13 | 1.03 | 1.82 | Chin and Sherar, 2001 |
| 915 | Bovine liver | 10–90 | 52.56 | –0.04 | 0.88 | 1.14 | Stauffer et al., 2003 |
| 915 | Bovine/Porcine liver | 37–60 | 49.50 | –0.20 | 0.99 | 1.33 | Lazebnik et al., 2006 |
| 915 | Animal liver | 5–50 | 48.0 | –0.22 | 0.94 | 1.29 | Brace, 2008 |
| 1000 | Human blood | 25–45 | — | –0.11 | 0.70 | 0.98 | Jaspard and Nadi, 2002 |
| 2450 | Bovine/Porcine liver | 37–60 | 47.60 | –0.17 | 1.77 | 0.20 | Lazebnik et al., 2006 |
| 2450 | Animal liver | 5–50 | 45.50 | –0.18 | 1.62 | –0.20 | Brace, 2008 |
| 2450 | Bovine liver | 15–80 | 43.52 | –0.15 | 1.74 | –0.13 | Lopresto et al., 2012 |

coefficients of temperature dependence. The tissue types tested include blood, kidney, liver, and muscle from several different species. These data corroborate the decrease of dielectric constants and increase of conductivity as a function of frequency in the microwave spectrum region. Most of the data were obtained for liver in the 25 to 80°C temperature range, clearly displaying the contemporary interest in liver ablation. While the permittivity values are derived from tissues of many different species, there is little variation among the measured values for a given tissue type, except for the well-known frequency-dependent drop in dielectric constant and rise in conductivity.

The data in Table 4.2 shows a slight average decrease (–0.20% per °C) of dielectric constant with increasing temperature for frequencies from 400 to 2450 MHz. In contrast, the conductivity increases by 1.01% per °C on average. These results are consistent with the general notion that dielectric constants are independent of temperature, and the change of the dielectric constant with temperature is smaller than that of the conductivity. Unexpectedly, two reports indicated slight decreases of 0.13% to 0.20% per °C in conductivity at 2450 MHz.

It is interesting to note the temperature coefficients of the dielectric constant and conductivity (–0.10 and 1.13%/°C) at 400 MHz and (–0.11 and 0.98%/°C) at 1000 MHz, respectively, for blood. As anticipated, the dielectric constants show very minor changes, but conductivity showed an increase about 1% per °C. The $\delta$ and $\gamma$ dispersions, over which 400 and 1000 MHz reside, are prone to membrane capacitance,

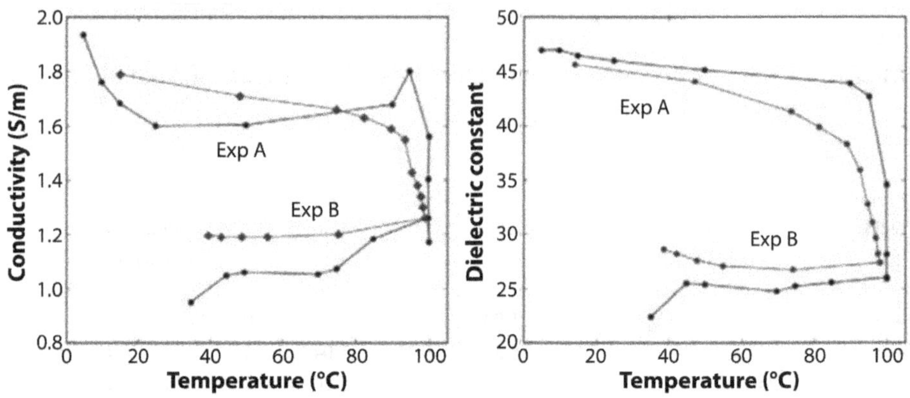


**FIGURE 4.4** Temperature dependence of relative permittivity and conductivity of animal liver tissue at 2450 MHz.

arising from ionic gating currents through or counterions surrounding membranes (Figure 4.1). These ionic activities have temperature coefficients that are expected to be like that of the conductivity of electrolytes, i.e., about 2% per °C. The dispersions are also caused by polarization effects and the rotational relaxation of water molecules in which cellular membranes are charged through the electrolytes. Hence, the temperature coefficient should be equal or close to that of the conductivity of electrolytes and its temperature dependence is equal to that of water, which again is close to 2% per °C. Thus, the temperature coefficient of conductivity for blood materials would have a maximum value of about 2% per °C, as for most tissues with higher water content.

A graph of the temperature dependence of relative permittivity and conductivity of animal liver tissue at 2450 MHz [Rossmanna and Haemmerich, 2014] is presented in Figure 4.4. While the basic data derived from Brace [2008] and Lopresto et al. [2012] were limited, they demonstrate modest changes with temperatures from below 25°C to near 100°C. The severe irreversible decrease of dielectric permittivity and electrical conductivity at 2450 MHz is expected as the temperatures approached a high of 100°C. Protein denaturation and other cellular and molecular damage obviously have already taken effect at 65°C or below, well ahead of the boiling point of water at 100°C. So, what happens to tissue damage at 100°C is a non sequitur. Note that aside from temperature, the extent of tissue change depends also on exposure duration.

Further discussions on the temperature dependence of dielectric constant and conductivity for water are given in Section 4.4.1.

## 4.4 MEASURED AND MODELED TISSUE PERMITTIVITY DATA

This section presents some of the measured tissue permittivity data or dielectric constants and conductivities of biological materials most relevant to the aims and objectives of this book. It will be seen that the dielectric properties of biological materials are indeed described by the relaxation processes detailed previously. It is emphasized that although the permittivity values are derived from tissues of many different species, there is little variation among the measured values for a given tissue type. An exception is fatty tissue, which is characterized by low dielectric constant and conductivity and by low electrolyte content. The water content in fatty tissue ranges from a few percent to more than 40%, depending on the animal species [Schwan, 1957]. Since the dielectric constant and conductivity of water are high, the permittivity of fatty materials may differ significantly with variations in water content.

### 4.4.1 Permittivity of Water

Water, by far, is the most abundant component of animals and constitutes approximately 60% of the total body mass in humans. For example, water makes up 93% of blood, about 80% of skeletal muscle, and approximately 70% of brain matter. The fluid nature of water allows both the dissolved electrolytes and the suspended substances to diffuse to different parts of the cell or tissue. When the cell or tissue loses its water, life is endangered or extinguished.

Of the total body water, about 62% is in the intracellular space and 38% in the extracellular space. Thus, water content exerts major influence on the permittivity properties (dielectric constant and conductivity) of biological materials. Next is a brief discussion of the permittivity properties of water as a function of frequency and temperature.

It is well known that dielectric constant and conductivity display characteristic dispersions at microwave frequencies. A graph showing the frequency dependence of the dielectric constant and conductivity of water at 37°C is given in Figure 4.5. A relaxation frequency is seen at 32 GHz. Both the dielectric constant and conductivity are constant and invariant from DC to 1 GHz. At frequencies above 3–5 GHz, water starts to disperse. The dielectric constant falls from a value of 74 at 10 MHz to about 28 at 35 GHz before reaching a lower limit near 4.5. Conversely, conductivity increases

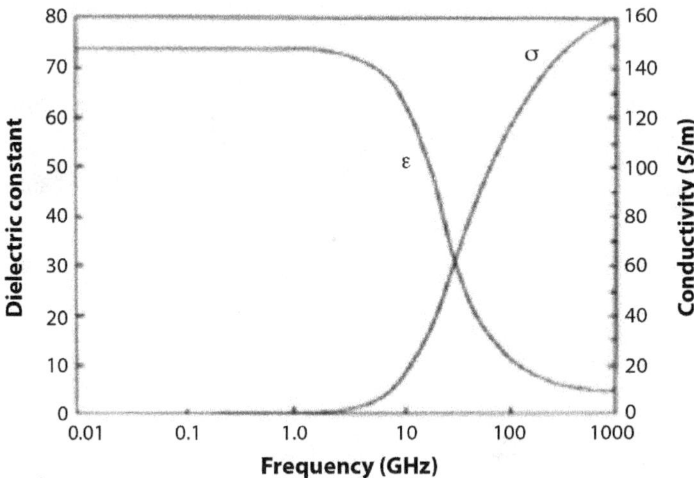


**FIGURE 4.5** Permittivity (dielectric constant and conductivity) of free water at 37 °C from 0.01 to 1000 GHz (10 MHz to 1 THz).

monotonically for frequencies beyond the microwave range. Clearly, the dielectric behavior of water is characterized by a single relaxation process between DC and microwave frequencies, which is governed by the induced rotations of individual water molecules as polar dipoles in a viscous fluid. Furthermore, the variations of water permittivity are represented by the simple Debye equations of (4.9 and 4.12), where $\tau$ is the relaxation time constant and $\sigma(0)$ is the DC conductivity, essentially zero for water.

The temperature dependence of the dielectric permittivity of water for six frequencies [Grant et al., 1978] is given in Figure 4.6 These graphs indicate that the

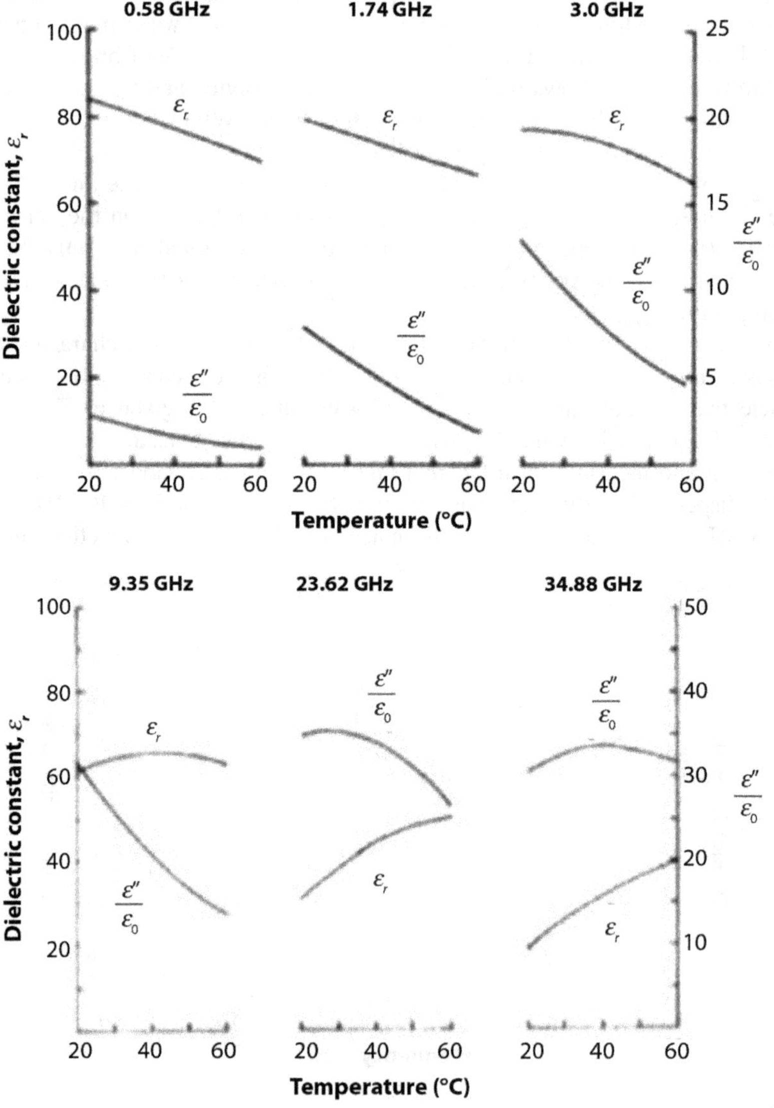


**FIGURE 4.6** Temperature dependence of dielectric permittivity (dielectric constant and conductivity) at six microwave frequencies.

dielectric constants and conductivity ($\sigma = \omega\varepsilon''$) of water at 0.58, 1.74, and 3.00 GHz decrease with increasing temperature, while those at 9.4, 23.7, and 34.9 GHz may increase, peak, and decrease with increasing temperature. These subtleties in the response to temperature change at higher frequencies probably stem from the fact that water starts to disperse above 5 GHz.

Note that the relaxation frequency of water increases with temperature in an exponential fashion. In particular, the relaxation frequency at 0°C is 8.84 GHz and becomes 39.8 GHz at 60°C. Furthermore, in the presence of polar solute molecules, the relaxation frequency shifts to lower frequencies because the dispersion of the solute molecules takes place at frequencies far below that for water. This will give rise to second or third regions of dispersion, which are usually well separated from that of water.

### 4.4.2 Measured Tissue Permittivity

The availability of accurate information about the permittivity properties of biological tissues is important for the study of both macroscopic and microscopic interactions of RF and microwave radiation with biological systems. On a macroscopic level, these properties govern the coupling and power deposition in tissue upon exposure to RF and microwave radiation. On a microscopic level, they suggest mechanisms that may underlie the absorption of RF and microwave energy by mammalian tissues. This quantitative information is also essential for analyzing the relationships among various responses from RF and microwave interactions and to help assess potential applications such as diagnostic usefulness of RF and microwave radiation, as well as for applications in safety and security situations.

Over the years, a large body of experimental data about dielectric permittivity of mammalian tissues has been accumulated through *in situ*, *ex vivo*, and *in vivo* laboratory studies by many researchers. A rigorous effort has been devoted to consolidating the data by using modern measurement techniques to provide new data to fill gaps in knowledge with respect to tissue types and frequency ranges [Gabriel et al., 1996a,b; Gabriel and Gabriel, 1996].

The following sections discuss representative data of measured tissue dielectric permittivity. They also include results for modeled data on dielectric constants and conductivities, principally from studies performed by the Gabriel group.

#### 4.4.2.1 Permittivity Data of Tissues in the Human Head

The relative permittivity and conductivity values for the 25 tissue types represented in the human head are listed in Table 4.3. They include skin, bone, CSF, fat, gray matter, white matter, muscle, teeth, etc. A Cole and Cole [1941] extrapolation technique was used to determine dielectric permittivity values for the tissues at the RF and microwave frequencies of 64, 300, and 400 MHz [Gabriel et al., 1996a]. Note that, in general, the relative permittivity and conductivity of blood, brain, eyes, CSF, muscle, and other tissues with higher water content are an order of magnitude higher than the corresponding parameters for bone, fat, tooth, and others tissue with low water content. The values of dielectric constant and conductivity for tissues with intermediate water content such as cartilage,

**TABLE 4.3**
**Relative Permittivity (Dielectric Constant) and Conductivity of Tissues in the Human Head at 37°C**

| | 64 MHz | | 300 MHz | | 400 MHz | | Density |
|---|---|---|---|---|---|---|---|
| **Tissue Type** | $\sigma$ (S/m) | $\varepsilon_r$ | $\sigma$ (S/m) | $\varepsilon_r$ | $\sigma$ (S/m) | $\varepsilon_r$ | $\rho$ (kg/m$^3$) |
| Blood | 1.206 | 86.51 | 1.316 | 65.69 | 1.350 | 64.18 | 1058 |
| Blood vessel | 0.429 | 68.69 | 0.537 | 48.36 | 0.562 | 47.00 | 1040 |
| Body fluid | 1.503 | 69.13 | 1.517 | 69.02 | 1.529 | 69 | 1010 |
| Bone (cancellous) | 0.161 | 30.89 | 0.215 | 23.18 | 0.235 | 22.44 | 1920 |
| Bone (cortical) | 0.059 | 16.69 | 0.083 | 13.45 | 0.091 | 13.15 | 1990 |
| Bone marrow | 0.021 | 7.215 | 0.027 | 5.76 | 0.029 | 5.67 | 1040 |
| Cartilage | 0.452 | 62.96 | 0.552 | 46.81 | 0.587 | 45.47 | 1097 |
| Cerebellum | 0.718 | 116.5 | 0.972 | 59.82 | 1.030 | 55.99 | 1038 |
| CSF | 2.065 | 97.35 | 2.224 | 72.79 | 2.251 | 70.99 | 1007 |
| Eye (aqueous humor) | 1.503 | 69.13 | 1.517 | 69.02 | 1.529 | 69 | 1009 |
| Eye (cornea) | 1.000 | 87.45 | 1.150 | 61.43 | 1.193 | 59.28 | 1076 |
| Eye (lens) | 0.586 | 60.57 | 0.647 | 48.97 | 0.669 | 48.15 | 1053 |
| Eye (retina) | 0.883 | 75.35 | 0.975 | 58.93 | 1.004 | 57.67 | 1026 |
| Eye (sclera/wall) | 0.883 | 75.35 | 0.975 | 58.93 | 1.004 | 57.67 | 1026 |
| Fat | 0.035 | 6.511 | 0.039 | 5.635 | 0.041 | 5.579 | 916 |
| Glands | 0.778 | 73.98 | 0.851 | 62.47 | 0.877 | 61.55 | 1050 |
| Gray matter | 0.511 | 97.54 | 0.691 | 60.09 | 0.738 | 57.43 | 1038 |
| Ligaments | 0.474 | 59.52 | 0.537 | 48.00 | 0.560 | 47.29 | 1220 |
| Lymph | 0.778 | 73.98 | 0.851 | 62.47 | 0.877 | 61.55 | 1040 |
| Mucous membrane | 0.488 | 76.80 | 0.630 | 51.96 | 0.669 | 49.89 | 1040 |
| Muscle | 0.688 | 72.27 | 0.770 | 58.23 | 0.796 | 57.13 | 1047 |
| Nerve (spine) | 0.312 | 55.11 | 0.418 | 36.95 | 0.447 | 35.41 | 1038 |
| Skin/dermis | 0.435 | 92.29 | 0.640 | 49.90 | 0.688 | 46.78 | 1125 |
| Tooth | 0.059 | 16.69 | 0.083 | 13.45 | 0.091 | 13.15 | 2160 |
| White matter | 0.291 | 67.91 | 0.413 | 43.82 | 0.445 | 42.07 | 1038 |

lens, ligaments, and nerves are lower by 30–40% from the respective values for high-water-content tissues.

#### 4.4.2.2 Brain Tissue Permittivity Data

Dielectric permittivity and conductivity of gray and white matter in the brain from reported studies at 37°C are presented in Figures 4.7 and 4.8 for frequencies from 100 Hz to 100 GHz. The dispersion behaviors are obvious and rather broad, suggesting an overlap of individual relaxation processes in brain materials. Some measurements have shown slight variations in permittivity between *in vivo* and *in vitro* tissue preparations [Burdette et al., 1980]. Changes in dielectric permittivity and conductivity are quite large and are in opposite directions. For example, the dielectric permittivity for brain tissue (average of gray and white

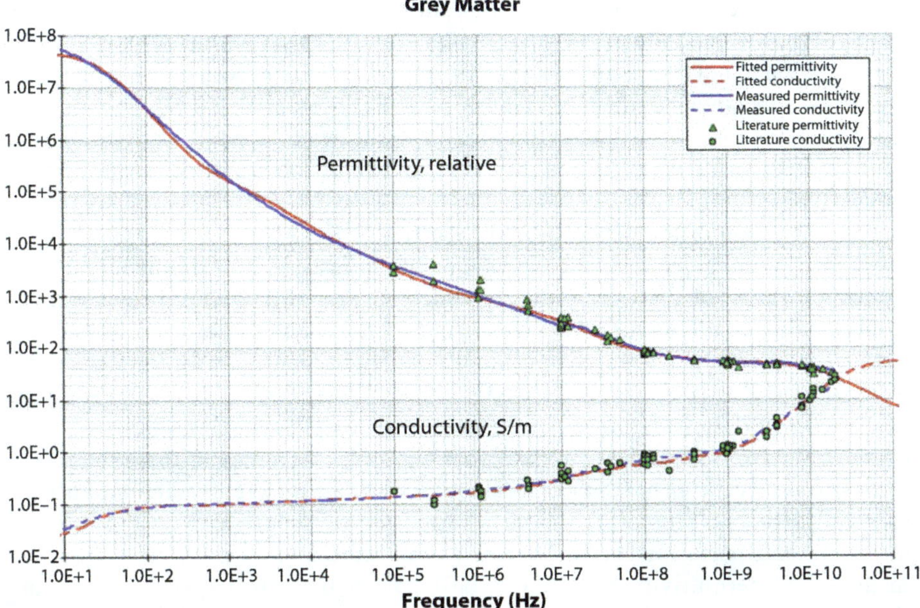


**FIGURE 4.7** Dielectric permittivity and conductivity of gray matter in the brain at 37°C. (From Gabriel and Gabriel, 1996.)

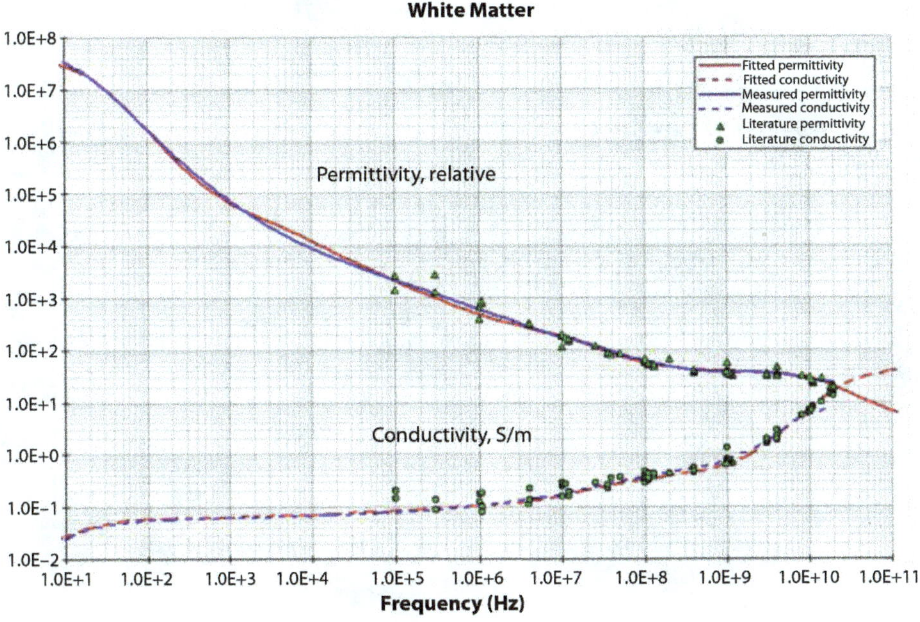


**FIGURE 4.8** Dielectric permittivity and conductivity of white matter in brain at 37°C. (From Gabriel and Gabriel, 1996.)

matter) $\varepsilon_r$ decreases from 110 to 30 as the frequency increases from 10 MHz to 10 GHz, while conductivity $\sigma$ increases from 0.3 to 6.0 S/m. As depicted in Figures 4.7 and 4.8, there are differences in permittivity between gray and white matter — a fact measurement has clearly shown [Foster et al., 1979]. The disparities mostly resulted from the difference in tissue water content as the apparent volume fraction of water is roughly 0.70 and 0.55 for gray and white matter, respectively.

A comparison of the permittivity properties of fresh human brain tissue with those for canine, ovine, primate, and swine brain tissue at 37°C in the microwave frequency range of 2 to 4 GHz is provided in Figure 4.9. The dielectric constant remains unaltered for all species listed within the test microwave frequency range [Lin, 1975]. However, in addition to the slight increase with frequency, the measured conductivity values showed a greater variability in the composite representation of data from brains of different species. Nevertheless, the similarity between the two sets of data suggests that within the accuracy of these measured data, the dielectric properties of brain tissues from different mammalian species are identical. This observation is supported by mouse and rat brain-tissue measurements performed at 37°C, which again showed no significant differences in dielectric permittivity of brain tissue between these two species of rodents [Steel and Sheppard, 1985]. Indeed, the validity of this conclusion prevails to date. Although the available permittivity values are derived from tissues of different mammalian species, there is little variation among the measured values for a given tissue type.

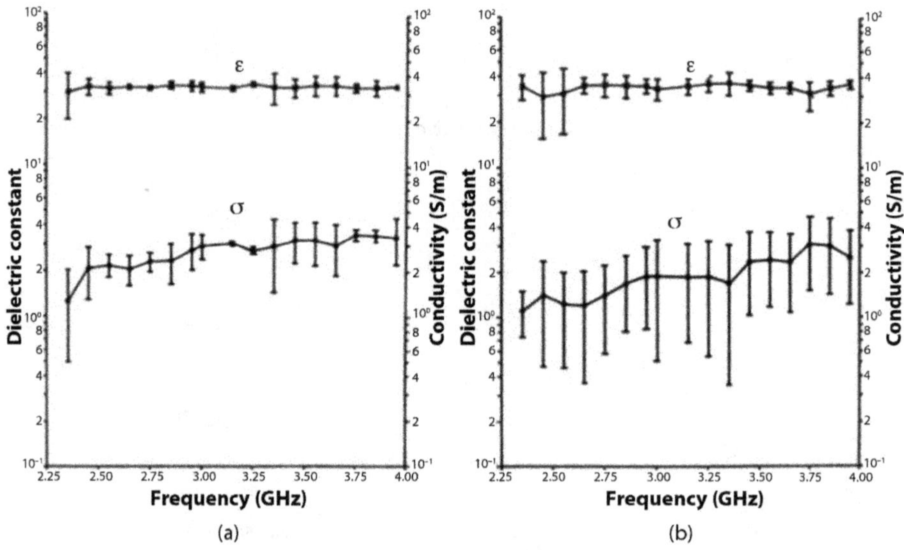


**FIGURE 4.9** Permittivity properties of homogenized fresh brain tissues at 37°C in the microwave frequency range 2–4 GHz. Fresh human data (a) and combined fresh canine, ovine, primate, swine, and human (b).

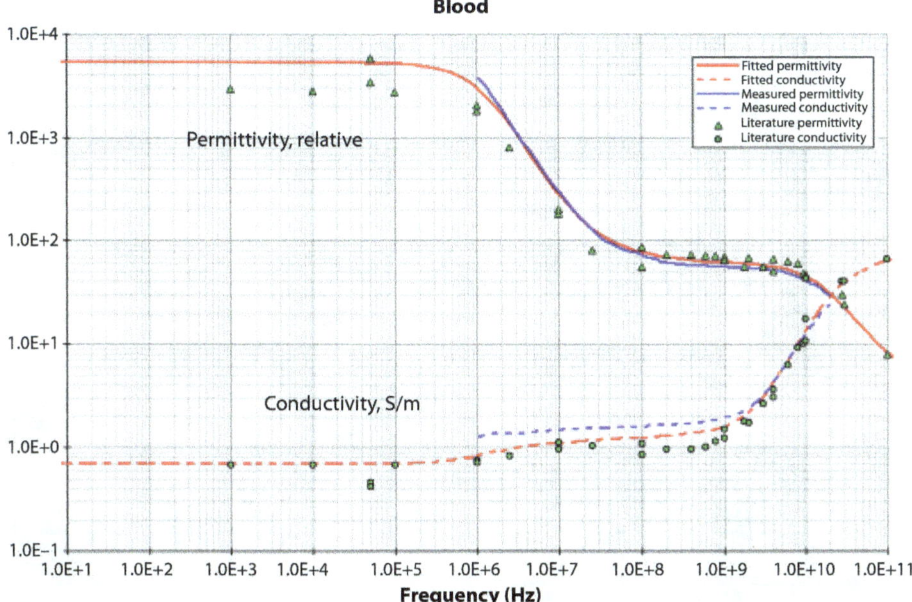


**FIGURE 4.10** Dielectric constant $\varepsilon_r$ and conductivity $\sigma$ for blood at 37°C as a function of frequency. (From Gabriel and Gabriel, 1996.)

#### 4.4.2.3 Blood, Heart, Aorta, Lung, CSF, and Fat Tissue Permittivity Data

The dielectric constant $\varepsilon_r$ and conductivity $\sigma$ for blood at 37°C as a function of frequency are given in Figure 4.10. The values and changes of dielectric constant and conductivity are quite large, principally due to the presence of cell membrane-associated substances. It is interesting to note the close agreement between measured *in vivo* and *in vitro* data and between measured and modeled data on dielectric permittivity and conductivity. Blood displays two distinctive relaxation zones. In the major dispersion, as the frequency increases from 1 MHz to 10 GHz, $\varepsilon_r$ decreases from greater than 3000 to less than 40, while $\sigma$ increases from 0.7 to 20 S/m.

The frequency dependence of relative permittivity and conductivity for heart, aorta, and CSF tissues in the frequency range of 10 Hz to 100 GHz are presented in Figures 4.11–4.13, respectively. It is seen in Figure 4.11 that the permittivity for heart muscle slowly decreases from 2000 to less than 15 as the frequency rises from 1 MHz to 10 GHz, while conductivity $\sigma$ increases from 0.5 to 2.0 S/m. The dielectric constants and conductivities for skin and muscle are known to be nearly identical [Cook, 1951] and have $\varepsilon_r$ and $\sigma$ values between those for blood and brain tissue. They are comparable to that of heart tissue, thus revealing the intermediate water content in their composition. The dielectric constant declines and conductivity rises with increasing frequency. The dielectric properties of the aorta have not been extensively investigated. Hence, measured data for the aorta is limited. The available information shown in Figure 4.12 suggests a single relaxation dispersion in the frequency region between 1 MHz and 10 GHz, where $\varepsilon_r$ decreases from

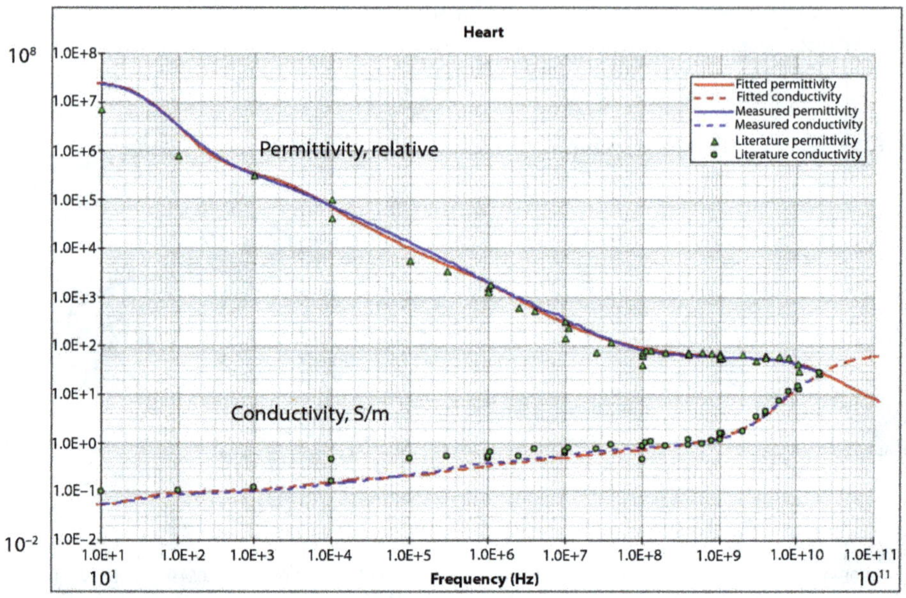


**FIGURE 4.11** Relative permittivity and conductivity for the heart muscle in the frequency range of 10 Hz to 100 GHz. (From Gabriel and Gabriel, 1996.)

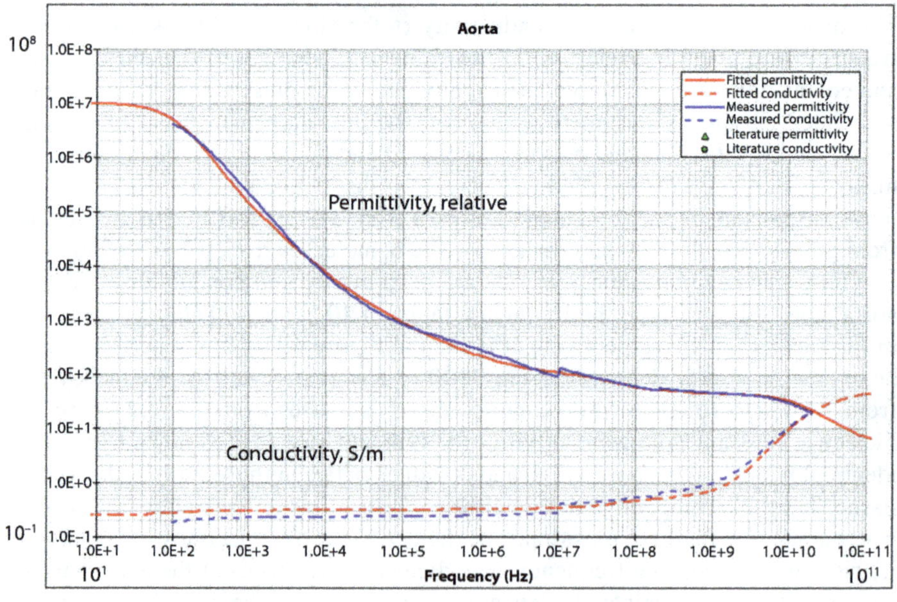


**FIGURE 4.12** Relative permittivity and conductivity for the aorta in the frequency range of 10 Hz to 100 GHz. (From Gabriel and Gabriel, 1996.)

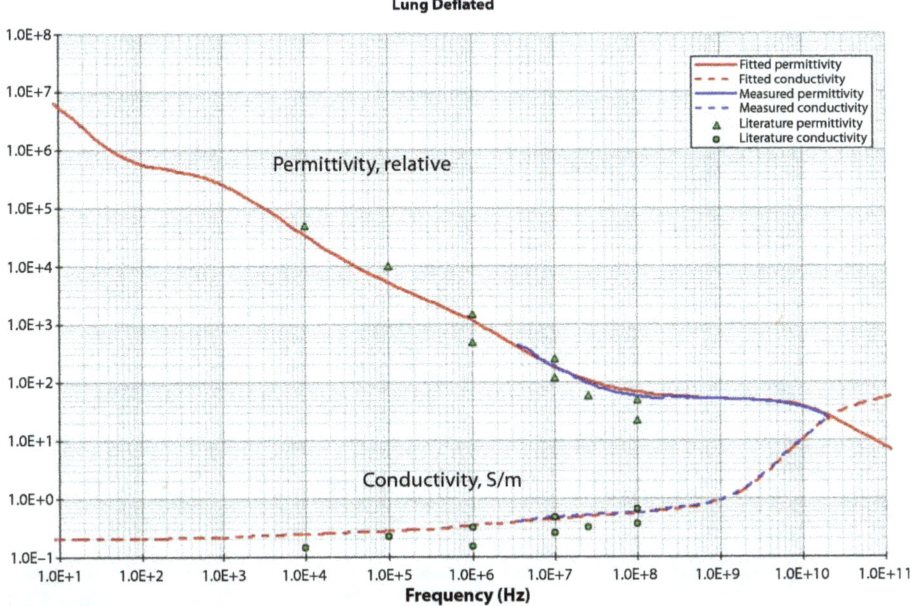


**FIGURE 4.13** Frequency dependence of the dielectric constant and conductivity for deflated lungs. (From Gabriel and Gabriel, 1996.)

250 to 2.0, while $\sigma$ increases from 0.3 to 10 S/m as the frequency increases from 1 MHz to 10 GHz. It is noteworthy that the dielectric constant and conductivity are independent of frequencies between 100 and 1000 MHz for many tissues with intermediate water content. They are reduced by roughly 30–40% from the respective values for high-water-content tissues; for example, a value of 50 for $\varepsilon_r$ and a value of 1.0 S/m for $\sigma$ at 1000 MHz. Specifically, the lungs, as an intermediate-water-content tissue of interest, have average values of about 50 and 0.5 S/m for $\varepsilon_r$ and $\sigma$, respectively, between 100 and 1000 MHz (see Figures 4.13 and 4.14 for frequency dependence of dielectric constant and conductivity for inflated and deflated lungs).

The behavior of relative permittivity and conductivity for CSF, shown in Figure 4.15, as a function of frequency is consistent with its material constituents. CSF is a clear, colorless, watery fluid that fills the ventricles of the brain and the subarachnoid space around the brain and spinal cord. CSF is mainly derived from blood (80%), while the remainder consists of brain-derived and intrathecally produced molecules (20%). The molecular constituents of CSF include an abundance of water alongside a limited quantity of hormones, metabolites, and other substances [Sakka et al., 2011; Tumani et al., 2017]. Accordingly, the values of dielectric constant and conductivity tend to be flanked by blood and pure water. Thus, $\varepsilon_r$ and $\sigma$ of CSF, necessarily of high water content, decreases from 100 to 50 and increases from 0.4 to 35 S/m, respectively, in the frequency range of 1.0 MHz to 10 GHz.

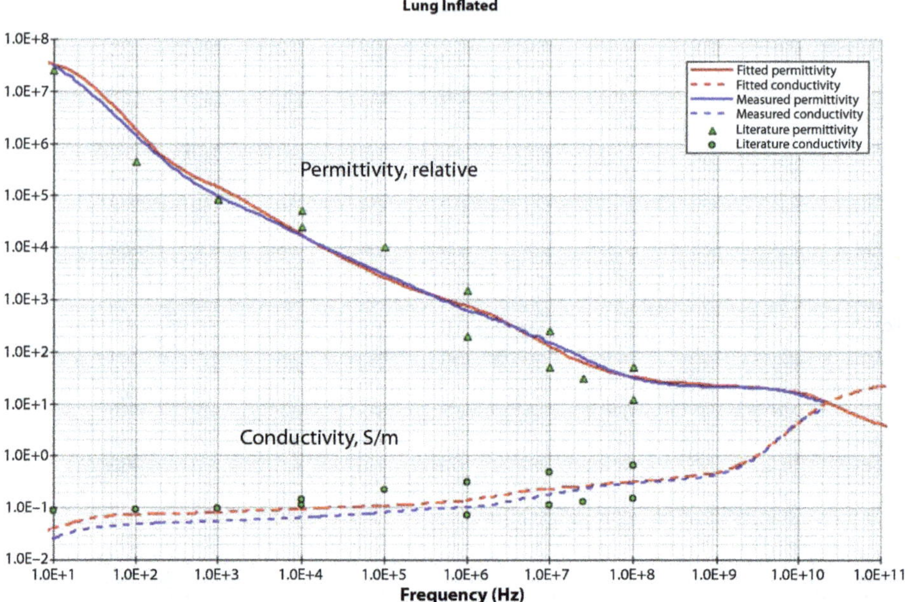


**FIGURE 4.14** Frequency dependence of the dielectric constant and conductivity for inflated lungs. (From Gabriel and Gabriel, 1996.)

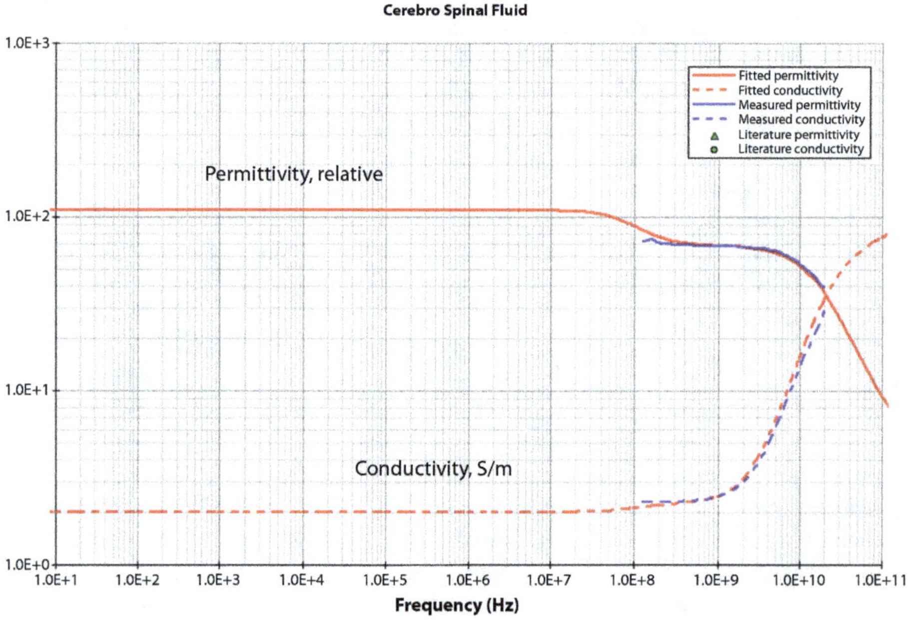


**FIGURE 4.15** Relative permittivity and conductivity for cerebrospinal fluid tissues in the frequency range of 10 Hz to 100 GHz. (From Gabriel and Gabriel, 1996.)

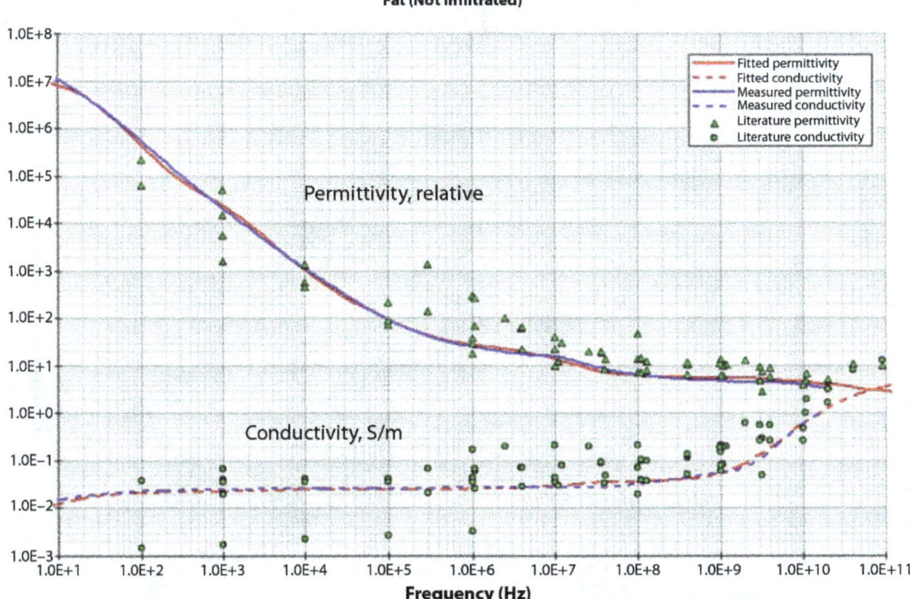


**FIGURE 4.16** Dielectric permittivity and conductivity for fat tissues in the frequency range of 10 Hz to 100 GHz. (From Gabriel and Gabriel, 1996.)

The permittivity properties of low-water-content tissues, especially for fatty tissues, tend to exhibit large variations in the measured dielectric constant and conductivity (see Figure 4.16). This is partially caused by the difficulty in handling fatty tissue *in vitro* without changing the fat and water content, but it is also due to variations in fatty-tissue composition among different mammalian species, including humans [Schwan and Li, 1953, 1956]. Indeed, the water content of fatty tissues can vary from a few percent to roughly 40%. Furthermore, as an exception, fatty tissues are characterized by low electrolyte content. In general, the $\varepsilon_r$ and $\sigma$ of tissues of low water content are an order of magnitude lower than the corresponding values for tissues of higher water content. Specifically, the relative permittivity $\varepsilon_r$ for not infiltrated fat tissue decreases from 15 to 0.4 and conductivity $\sigma$ increases from 0.02 to 0.15 S/m in the frequency range of 1.0 MHz to 10 GHz.

### 4.4.3 Debye Modeling of Biological Tissue Permittivity Data

As an example of modeling the frequency-dependent permittivity properties of various tissues using measured permittivity values by the Debye equation (Eq. 4.15), permittivity for frequencies between 10 and 3000 MHz may be modeled as the sum of two relaxation processes with two constants such that Eq. (4.15) becomes

$$\varepsilon^*(\omega) = \varepsilon_0\left[\varepsilon_\infty + \frac{\varepsilon_{s1} - \varepsilon_\infty}{1 + j\omega\tau_1} + \frac{\varepsilon_{s2} - \varepsilon_\infty}{1 + j\omega\tau_2}\right] \tag{4.17}$$

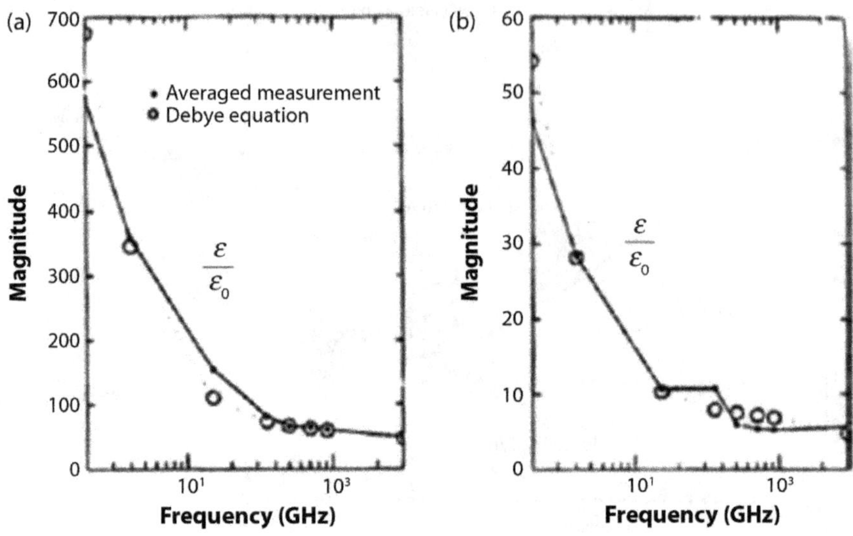


**FIGURE 4.17** Measured and modeled tissue properties using two Debye relaxation constants for (a) muscle and (b) fat.

where $\varepsilon_\infty$ is the high frequency permittivity and the static (or low frequency) permittivity is given by

$$\varepsilon_s = \varepsilon_{s1} + \varepsilon_{s2} - \varepsilon_\infty \tag{4.18}$$

For the results shown in Figure 4.17, the measured properties of biological tissues (muscle and fat) were obtained from the literature. Optimized values for $\varepsilon s_1$, $\varepsilon s_2$, $\varepsilon(\infty)$, $\tau_1$, and $\tau_2$ in Eq. (4.17) were obtained by nonlinear least squares fitting to the measured data for fat and muscle (Table 4.3), with $\tau_1$ and $\tau_2$ being the average of the optimized values for fat and muscle, respectively [Lin and Gandhi, 1996]. Many other tissues have properties between these two types of tissues.

## REFERENCES

Böttcher, C. J. F., 1952. Theory of Electric Polarization. Amsterdam: Elsevier

Brace, C. L., 2008. Temperature-dependent dielectric properties of liver tissue measured during thermal ablation: Toward an improved numerical model. Conf. Proc. IEEE Eng. Med. Biol. Soc. 230–233

Burdette, E. C., Cain, F. L., Seals, J., 1980. In vivo probe measurement technique for determining dielectric properties at VHF through microwave frequencies. IEEE Trans. Microw. Theory Tech., 28(4):414–427

Chin, L., Sherar, M., 2001. Changes in dielectric properties of ex vivo bovine liver at 915 MHz during heating. Phys. Med. Biol., 46(1):197–211

Cole, K. S., 1968. Membranes, Ions, and Impulses. University of California Press

Cole, K. S., Cole, R. H., 1941. Dispersion and absorption in dielectrics: Alternating current characteristics. J. Phys., 9:341–351

Cook, H. F., 1951. Dielectric behaviors of some types of human tissues at microwave frequencies. Br. J. Appl. Phys., 2:295

Daniel, V. V., 1967. Dielectric Relaxation. New York: Academic Press
Debye, P., 1929. Polar Molecules. New York: Reinhold
Foster, K. R., Schepps, J. L., Stoy, R. D., Schwan, H. P., 1979. Dielectric properties of brain tissue between 0.01 and 10 GHz. Phys. Med. Biol., 24(6):1177–1187
Fu, F., Xin, S. X., Chen, W., 2014. Temperature- and frequency-dependent dielectric properties of biological tissues within the temperature and frequency ranges typically used for magnetic resonance imaging-guided focused ultrasound surgery. Int. J. Hyperthermia, 30(1):56–65
Gabriel, C., Gabriel, S., 1996. Compilation of the dielectric properties of body tissues at RF and microwave frequencies. AFOSR/NL Bolling AFB, DC
Gabriel, S., Lau, R. W., Gabriel, C., 1996a. The dielectric properties of biological tissues: II. Measurements in the frequency range 10 Hz to 20 GHz. Phys. Med. Biol., 41:2251–2269
Gabriel, S., Lau, R. W., Gabriel, C., 1996b. The dielectric properties of biological tissues: III. Parametric models for the dielectric spectrum of tissues. Phys. Med. Biol., 41:2271–2293
Grant, E. H., Sheppard, R. J., South, G. P., 1978. Dielectric Behavior of Biological Molecules in Solution. Oxford, UK: Clarendon
Hill, N. E., Vaughan, W. E., Price, A. H., Davies, M., 1969. Dielectric Properties and Molecular Behavior D. Princeton, NJ: Van Nostrand
Huang, S. K. S., Wilber, D. J., Eds., 2000. Radiofrequency Catheter Ablation of Cardiac Arrhythmias: Basic Concepts and Clinical Applications, 2nd ed, Armonk, New York: Futura
Jaspard, F., Nadi, M., 2002. Dielectric properties of blood: An investigation of temperature dependence. Physiol. Meas., 23(3):547–554
Lazebnik, M., Converse, M. C., Booske, J. H., Hagness, S. C., 2006. Ultrawideband temperature-dependent dielectric properties of animal liver tissue in the microwave frequency range. Phys. Med. Biol., 51(7):1941–1955
Lin, J. C., 1975. Microwave properties of fresh mammalian brain tissues at body temperature. IEEE Trans. Biomed. Eng., 22:74–76
Lin, J. C., 1988. Electromagnetic Heating Techniques for Organ Rewarming, Biophysics of Organ Cryopreservation, Eds. Pegg, D., Karow, A. (pp. 315–335), Plenum Press
Lin, J. C., 2021. Auditory Effects of Microwave Radiation. Springer
Lin, J. C., 1988. Electromagnetic Heating Techniques for Organ Rewarming, Biophysics of Organ Cryopreservation, Eds. David Pegg and Armand Karow (pp. 315–335), Plenum Press
Lin, J. C., 1999. Hyperthermia therapy. In: Webster, J. G., Ed., Encyclopedia of Electrical and Electronics Engineering (Vol. 9, pp. 450–460), New York: Wiley
Lin, J. C., 2003. Minimally invasive medical microwave ablation technology. In: Hwang, N. H. C., Woo, S. L. Y., Eds., New Frontiers in Biomedical Engineering (pp. 545–562, Chapter 36). New York: Kluwer/Plenum
Lin, J. C., Gandhi, O. P., 1996. Handbook of biological effects of electromagnetic fields. In: Polk, C., Postow, E., Eds., Handbook of Biological Effects of Electromagnetic Fields (pp. 337–402), CRC Press
Lopresto, V., Pinto, R., Lovisolo, G. A., Cavagnaro, M., 2012. Changes in the dielectric properties of ex vivo bovine liver during microwave thermal ablation at 2.45 GHz. Phys. Med. Biol., 57(8):2309–2327
Michaelson, S. M., Lin, J. C., 1987. Biological Effects and Health Implications of Radiofrequency Radiation. New York: Plenum Press
Rossmanna, C., Haemmerich, D., 2014. Review of temperature dependence of thermal properties, dielectric properties, and perfusion of biological tissues at hyperthermic and ablation temperatures. Crit. Rev. Biomed. Eng., 42(6):467–492
Sakka, L., Coll, G., Chazal, J., 2011. Anatomy and physiology of cerebrospinal fluid. Eur. Ann. Otorhinolaryngol. Head Neck Dis., 128(6):309–316

Schwan, H. P., 1957. Electrical properties of tissues and cell suspensions. Advances in Biological and Medical Physics (pp. 147–209). New York: Academy Press
Schwan, H. P., 1963. Electric characteristics of tissues. Biophysik J., 1:198–208
Schwan, H. P., 1977. Field interaction with biological matter. Ann. NY Acad. Sci., 303:198–213
Schwan, H. P., Foster, K. R., 1980. RF-field interactions with biological systems: Electrical properties and biophysical mechanisms. Proc. IEEE, 68(1):104–113
Schwan, H. P., Li, K., 1953. Capacity and conductivity of body tissues at ultrahigh frequencies. Proc. IRE, 41:1735–1740
Schwan, H. P., Li, K., 1956. Hazards due to total body irradiation by radar. Proc. IRE, 44:572–1584
Schwan, H. P., Sheppard, R. J., Grant, E. H., 1976. Complex permittivity of water. J. Chem. Phys., 64:2257–2258
Stauffer, P. R., Rossetto, F., Prakash, M., Neuman, D. G., Lee, T., 2003. Phantom and animal tissues for modelling the electrical properties of human liver. Int. J. Hypertherm., 19(1):89–101
Steel, M. C., Sheppard, R. J., 1985. Dielectric properties of mammalian brain tissue between 1 and 18 GHz. Phys. Med. Biol., 30:621–630
Tumani, H., Huss, A., Bachhuber, F., 2017. The cerebrospinal fluid and barriers - anatomic and physiologic considerations. Handb. Clin. Neurol., 146:21–32
von Hipp, A. R., 1954. Dielectric Materials and Applications. MA: MIT Cambridge
Watmough, D. J., Ross, W. M., Eds., 1986. Hyperthermia. Blackie, Glasgow

# 5 Microwaves in Biological Systems

Regardless of the mode of interaction, the communication channel created for signal and information transfer by the incident radio frequencies (RF) and microwaves must be linked to the biological system. Microwave energy must be coupled to the biological body for the system to respond in some manner. Wireless sensing requires the transmission and reception of RF and microwave radiation near and through the body. Therefore, it is important to consider and evaluate the power and field strength associated with the energy transfer between sensors and exposed subjects or target tissues for healthcare applications and efficacy considerations. While sufficient energy is required for effectiveness, excessive levels of exposure may lead to unintended consequences on target organs or surrounding tissues. Thus, knowledge of biological responses to the RF and microwave radiation used in physiological sensing and monitoring must be quantified and correlated with the observed changes and responses.

This chapter discusses the coupling, reflection, transmission, distribution, and dosimetry of RF and microwaves in biological bodies, especially in humans. It describes plane-wave propagation in biological media and the reflection and refraction by layered tissues. It considers the reflection and transmission of plane waves at tissue boundaries. It gives specific examples of the microwave and RF radiation fields propagating in biological systems and their distributions based on the fundamental principles of electromagnetic theory. This chapter also discusses the influence of the microwave properties of tissue media, namely, dielectric permittivity, on the interaction of microwave radiation with biological media.

These topics are complex functions of not only microwave sources and application scenarios, but also the shape, size, composition, and structure of the exposed subjects, as well as orientation and position of the subject with respect to the source. Thus, the channel for microwave propagation in and around the body presents unique challenges. There are shadowing effects from variations in location and the motion of tissues and body elements. An especially challenging dynamic aspect to all these problems comes from variations in body posture and movement that may occur. Signal losses are increased for on-body compared with free-space wave propagations. Furthermore, antennas designed to operate in free space may function differently when operating in or placed on the body.

## 5.1 METRICS FOR EXPOSURE AND DOSIMETRY

### 5.1.1 Exposure Quantities and Units

The exposure metrics include incident electric field and magnetic field, induced electric field, and incident power density. As mentioned in Chapter 3, plane-wave

DOI: 10.1201/9781003315223-5

propagation is defined by electric and magnetic fields that are perpendicular to each other and to the direction of wave propagation. Furthermore, the electric and magnetic field maxima occur at the same location in space at any given moment in time. In this case, the electric field strength in volts per meter (V/m) is related to the magnetic field strength in amperes per meter (A/m) through intrinsic impedance, which is medium dependent and is approximately 376.7 ohms for air or free space. In all other dielectric media including biological materials, the intrinsic impedance is smaller than that of free space.

For a plane wave propagating in air with electric field strength $E_o$ and intrinsic impedance $\eta_0$, the average power density $P_d$ in watts per square meter (W/m$^2$) associated with the plane wave is given by Eq. 5.1 (see also Eq. 3.41 and associated discussions in Chapter 3).

$$P_d = \left(\frac{1}{2}\right)\left(\frac{E_0^2}{\eta_0}\right) \tag{5.1}$$

Also, the units for power densities may be expressed in terms of milliwatts per square centimeter (mW/cm$^2$) or microwatt per square meter ($\mu$W/m$^2$) for lower exposure levels; note that 1 mW/cm$^2$ = 10 W/m$^2$. Likewise, the electric field strength may be expressed in mV/m as a unit for lower levels of exposures.

### 5.1.2 Dosimetry Quantities and Units

Dosimetry may be defined as the quantification of RF and microwave radiation distribution and absorption in biological materials or animal bodies under exposure [Cavagnaro and Lin, 2019; Guido and Kiourti, 2020; Lin, 2007]. The commonly employed metrics for dosimetry quantities include transmitted and induced power density, specific absorption rate (SAR), and specific absorption (SA) in biological bodies or tissue materials. The metric SAR (in W/kg) referred to in Chapter 3, Section 3.4 is a derived quantity and is given by the time derivative of the incremental energy absorbed by (or deposited in) an incremental mass contained in a volume of a given density [Chou et al., 1996; Lin, 2007; NCRP, 1981]. This definition allows SAR to be used as a metric for RF and microwaves in both the near and far field. SA (in J/kg or W-s/kg) is the amount of energy deposited or absorbed and is given by the integral of SAR over a finite interval of time. Information on SA and SAR is of interest because it can serve as an index for extrapolation of experimental results from cell-to-cell, cell-to-tissue, tissue-to-animal, animal-to-animal, and animal-to-human exposures. It is also useful in analyzing relationships among various observed biological responses in different experimental models and subjects.

The induced field is of primary interest because it relates the RF and microwave radiation to specific responses of the body, it facilitates understanding of biological phenomena, and is independent of mechanisms of interaction. Once the induced field is known, quantities such as SAR can be derived by a simple conversion formula. For example, from an induced electric field $E$ in V/m

$$SAR = \frac{\sigma E^2}{\rho} \tag{5.2}$$

where $\sigma$ is the bulk electrical conductivity and $\rho$ is the mass density (kg/m$^3$) of tissue. At present, the smallest isotropic implantable electric field probe available with sufficient sensitivity for practical use is about 0.1–1 mm in diameter and quite expensive. Consequently, a common practice in experimental dosimetry relies on the use of temperature rise produced under a short-duration (<30 seconds) high-intensity exposure condition. The duration should be sufficiently short to prevent significant convective or conductive heat contribution to rising tissue temperature and the intensity should be sufficient to produce a measurable temperature elevation. This condition is sometimes referred to as thermal containment. In this case, the time rate of initial rise in temperature (slope) can be related to SAR through an alternative, empirical, or secondary method, so that

$$SAR = c\frac{\Delta T}{\Delta t} \tag{5.3}$$

where $c$ is the specific heat capacity of tissue (J/kg-°C), $\Delta T$ is the temperature increment (°C), and $\Delta t$ is the short-exposure duration(s) over which $\Delta T$ is measured.

It is important to distinguish the use of SAR and its alternative derivation from temperature-based measurements. The quantity of SAR is merely a metric for power deposition or energy absorption, and it should not be construed to imply any mechanism of interaction, thermal, or otherwise. However, it is a quantity that pertains to a macroscopic phenomenon through the use of bulk electrical conductivity and mass density in the derivation of Eq. (5.2) and the use of specific heat capacity of tissue in Eq. (5.3).

It is essential to note the use of bulk electrical conductivity, specific heat capacity, and mass density (kg/m$^3$) of tissue in the derivation of SAR from electric field strength and temperature elevation. Their use in the definition means that the size of the tissue mass must be selected, over which SAR is determined [Lin, 2007]. In common usage, 1 or 10 g of tissue in the form of a cubic volume are specified. Obviously, the numerical value of SAR would be the same regardless of what mass or volume is chosen if the induced field and power deposition are uniform. Variances arise when the absorption is nonuniform or tissues with differing properties are within the same volume of averaging mass. In principle, a 10 g averaging mass could underestimate SARs of nonuniform fields by up to a factor of 10 compared with a 1 g averaging mass. It is emphasized that recent advances suggest that spatial resolutions comparable to 0.01 g or less are routinely obtainable using available computational algorithms and resources to provide higher spatial precision in SAR determination.

An investigation on the influence of absorption metrics and averaging schemes on the correlation between microwave energy and induced temperature elevation for plane-wave exposures using voxel-based anatomic models of the human body suggests that exposure duration also can play a major role [Cavagnaro and Lin, 2019]. Correlation of microwave-induced SAR and temperature increases were evaluated at several frequencies. The results showed that the best correlation with temperature increase occurs for exposure durations between 1 and 2 minutes for SAR at 700–2700 MHz frequencies. In this case, a 1 g mass appears to be optimal. For longer exposures, the maximum correlation coefficient is reduced, and the correlation favors a larger averaging mass. At steady state (about 30 minutes), the correlation of temperature increase with SAR is maximum for a mass of 9 g for the frequencies considered. In general, SAR provides a better correlation with temperature elevation for short exposures. Knowledge of the correlation between microwave exposure and temperature increases has implications and can help guide microwave applications in biomedical applications such as imaging and sensing.

Clearly, a complex biological structure like the human body consists of multiple layers of tissue, curved surfaces with different dielectric properties, and organs of different dimensions, alongside cylindrical limbs and a spheroidal head would all affect the scattered and transmitted microwave distribution. Furthermore, the distribution of scattered and transmitted microwave energy depends on the antenna type and geometry and the tissues surrounding the antenna. Thus, the dosimetry in general becomes even more complex and highly application-specific. This discussion begins with quantification of plane-wave-induced microwave distribution and absorption at planar tissue boundaries and progresses to include anatomical human body models.

## 5.2 REFLECTION AND TRANSMISSION AT PLANAR TISSUE SURFACES

At boundaries separating regions of different biological materials, including air, microwave energy is reflected and transmitted (Figure 5.1). For a plane wave impinging normally from a medium, the reflection coefficient R, and transmission coefficient T, given in Eqs (3.56) and (3.57) (see Chapter 3), provide measures of microwave energy coupling; R and T are related through $R = T - 1$. The fraction of incident power reflected by the discontinuity is $R^2$ and the transmitted fraction is $R^2 = (1 - T^2)$. Table 5.1 gives the calculated reflection coefficient for several air–tissue and tissue–tissue interfaces. Clearly, about one half of the incident power is reflected at these boundaries. Furthermore, the reflection coefficient for tissue–tissue interfaces generally is smaller than air–tissue interfaces. The percent reflected power for tissue–tissue interfaces ranges from a low of 5 for muscle–blood to a high of 50 for bone–biological fluid interfaces. This suggests that the closer the dielectric properties on both sides of the interface, the smaller the power reflection [Lin and Bernardi, 2007].

The data from Table 5.1 suggest the power transmitted, $T^2 = (1 - R^2)$, at air–tissue interfaces is variable, but can be quite substantial at RF and microwave

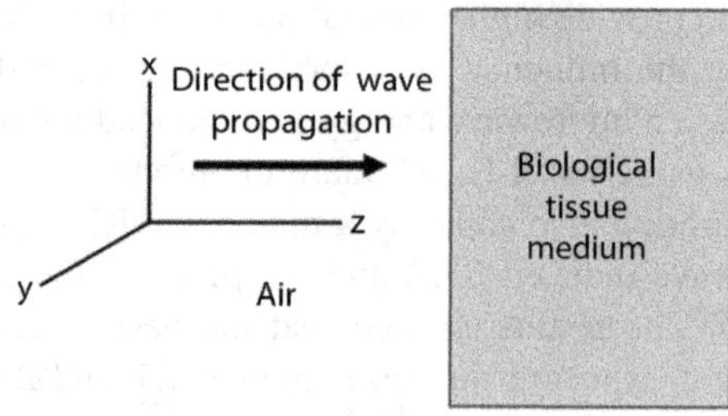


**FIGURE 5.1** A plane wave impinging normally on a planar tissue medium.

**TABLE 5.1**
**Magnitude of Reflection Coefficient (in Percent) between Air and Tissue and between Biological Tissues at 37°C**

| | Frequency (MHz) | Air | Fat B | Lung | Muscle (Skin) | Blood | Saline |
|---|---|---|---|---|---|---|---|
| Air | 433 | 0 | 46 | 76 | 82 | 81 | 83 |
| | 915 | 0 | 43 | 73 | 78 | 79 | 80 |
| | 2450 | 0 | 41 | 71 | 76 | 77 | 79 |
| | 5800 | 0 | 39 | 70 | 75 | 76 | 78 |
| | 10,000 | 0 | 37 | 70 | 74 | 76 | 78 |
| Fat (Bone) | 433 | | 0 | 46 | 56 | 56 | 60 |
| | 915 | | 0 | 43 | 52 | 54 | 57 |
| | 2450 | | 0 | 42 | 50 | 53 | 57 |
| | 5800 | | 0 | 42 | 50 | 53 | 56 |
| | 10,000 | | 0 | 45 | 52 | 54 | 58 |
| Lung | 433 | | | 0 | 14 | 13 | 19 |
| | 915 | | | 0 | 12 | 14 | 18 |
| | 2450 | | | 0 | 10 | 15 | 19 |
| | 5800 | | | 0 | 10 | 14 | 19 |
| | 10,000 | | | 0 | 10 | 13 | 18 |
| Muscle (Skin) | 433 | | | | 0 | 4 | 6 |
| | 915 | | | | 0 | 4 | 7 |
| | 2450 | | | | 0 | 5 | 10 |
| | 5800 | | | | 0 | 4 | 9 |
| | 10,000 | | | | 0 | 3 | 9 |
| Blood | 433 | | | | | 0 | 6 |
| | 915 | | | | | 0 | 4 |
| | 2450 | | | | | 0 | 5 |
| | 5800 | | | | | 0 | 5 |
| | 10,000 | | | | | 0 | 6 |
| Saline | 433 | | | | | | 0 |
| | 915 | | | | | | 0 |
| | 2450 | | | | | | 0 |
| | 5800 | | | | | | 0 |
| | 10,000 | | | | | | 0 |

frequencies. Figure 5.2 shows that the power transmission coefficient is frequency dependent, more so at lower microwave frequencies for air–muscle and fat–muscle interfaces.

As the transmitted microwaves propagate in tissue medium, microwave energy is extracted from the electromagnetic field and absorbed by the medium, resulting in a progressive reduction of microwave power density as it advances in the tissue. This reduction is quantified by the penetration depth (see Chapter 3, Eq. 3.53), which is the distance through which the power density decreases by a factor of $e^{-2}$. Table 5.2

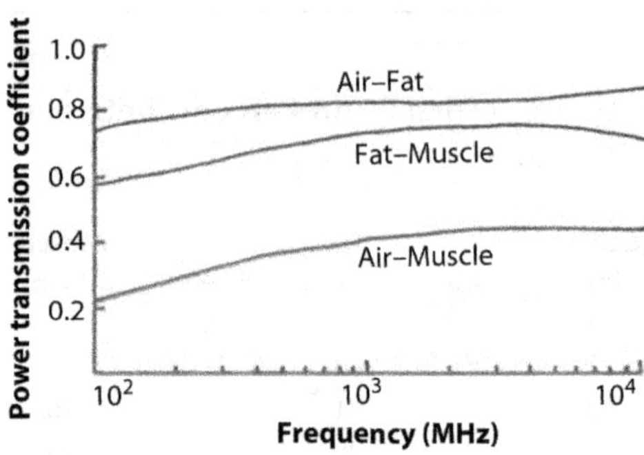


**FIGURE 5.2** Power transmission coefficients at different tissue interfaces as functions of frequency. The power reflection coefficient is equal to 1 – the power transmission coefficient.

presents the calculated depth of penetration in selected tissues. It is seen that the penetration depth depends inversely on frequency, the higher the frequency the lower the penetration depth. The depth takes on different values for different tissues. In particular, the penetration depth for fat and bone is nearly five times greater than for higher-water-content tissues.

Table 5.3 presents the calculated skin depth, reflection coefficient, and transmission coefficient for plane-wave incidents from air using typical dielectric permittivity for tissues of high-water-content such as muscle and most organs, and tissues of low-water-content, which include bone and fat. Clearly, the reflection of RF and microwaves from planar tissue into air is smaller for low-water-content tissue compared to that of high-water-content tissue. Reflections are smaller for higher microwave frequencies than for lower ones, and it ranges from roughly 90% to 15%. Conversely, the coupling of RF and microwaves from air into planar tissue is greater for low-water-content tissue compared to that of high-water-content tissue. It is greater for higher microwave frequencies than for lower ones and ranges from about 15% to 90%.

**TABLE 5.2**
**Depth of Penetration of Microwaves in Biological Tissues as a Function of Frequency**

| | Tissue Type | | | | |
|---|---|---|---|---|---|
| | Saline | Blood | Muscle (Skin) | Fat (Bone) | Lung |
| Frequency MHz | Depth of Penetration (cm) | | | | |
| 433 | 2.8 | 3.7 | 3.0 | 4.7 | 16.3 |
| 915 | 2.5 | 3.0 | 2.5 | 4.5 | 12.8 |
| 2450 | 1.3 | 1.9 | 1.7 | 2.3 | 7.9 |
| 5800 | 0.7 | 0.7 | 0.8 | 0.7 | 4.7 |
| 10,000 | 0.2 | 0.3 | 0.3 | 0.3 | 2.5 |

**TABLE 5.3**
**Propagation Characteristics of Plane Waves in Low- and High-Water-Content Biological Tissues at 37°C**

| Frequency (MHz) | Dielectric Constant | | Conductivity (S/m) | | Reflection Coefficient | | Skin Depth (cm) | | Transmission Coefficient | |
|---|---|---|---|---|---|---|---|---|---|---|
| $H_2O$ Content | High | Low | High | Low | High | Low | High | Low | High | Low |
| 27 | 113 | 20 | 0.61 | 0.03 | 0.86 | 0.44 | 14 | 77 | 0.14 | 0.56 |
| 40 | 97 | 15 | 0.69 | 0.03 | 0.83 | 0.38 | 11 | 59 | 0.17 | 0.62 |
| 100 | 72 | 7.5 | 0.89 | 0.05 | 0.78 | 0.26 | 27 | 106 | 0.22 | 0.74 |
| 433 | 53 | 5.6 | 1.43 | 0.08 | 0.64 | 0.18 | 3.6 | 183 | 0.36 | 0.82 |
| 915 | 51 | 5.6 | 1.60 | 0.10 | 0.60 | 0.17 | 2.5 | 13 | 0.40 | 0.83 |
| 2450 | 47 | 5.5 | 2.21 | 0.16 | 0.37 | 0.16 | 1.7 | 8.1 | 0.43 | 0.84 |
| 5800 | 43 | 5.1 | 4.73 | 0.26 | 0.36 | 0.15 | 0.8 | 4.7 | 0.44 | 0.85 |
| 10,000 | 40 | 4.5 | 10.3 | 0.44 | 0.55 | 0.13 | 0.3 | 2.6 | 0.45 | 0.87 |

### 5.2.1 Angle of Incidence and Polarization

Microwave radiation of general or unspecified polarization may be decomposed into its orthogonal linearly polarized components whose electric or magnetic field parallels the interface (see Chapter 3, Eqs 3.67 and 3.68). These components can be treated separately and combined afterward. Figures 5.3 and 5.4 illustrate the magnitude and phase of the reflection coefficients of representative tissue interfaces at a temperature of 37°C for 2450 MHz microwave exposures. The figures clearly show the difference between E and H polarization. E polarization, also called perpendicular polarization and H polarization, often referred to as parallel polarization, are defined in Chapter 3. For E polarization, there is only a slight variation in magnitude and phase of the reflection coefficient with incidence angle. For H polarization, however, there is a pronounced dependence on the incidence angle. The reflection coefficient reaches a minimum magnitude and has a phase angle of 90° at Brewster's angle (see Chapter 3, Eq. 3.72). Thus, the H-polarized wave is totally transmitted into the muscle medium at Brewster's angle.

## 5.3 MULTIPLE TISSUE LAYERS

In a layered tissue structure with different dielectric permittivity, the reflection and transmission characteristics become more complicated. Multiple reflections can occur between the skin and subcutaneous tissue boundaries, with a resulting modification of the reflection and transmission coefficients (see Chapter 3, Eqs 3.68 and 3.69). In general, the transmitted wave combines with the reflected to form standing waves in each layer. The standing-wave phenomenon becomes especially pronounced if the thickness of each layer is less than the penetration depth for that tissue. The peaks of the standing waves can result in greater coupling of RF and microwave energy into the tissue layer. The standing-wave phenomenon also becomes especially

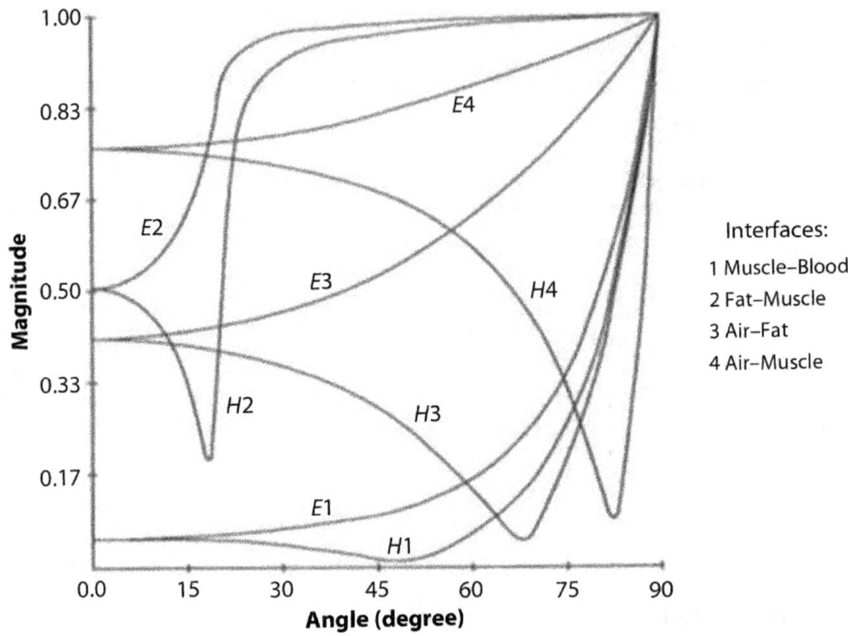


**FIGURE 5.3** Magnitude of reflection coefficients for E and H polarized microwaves at 2450 MHz with a plane wavefront.

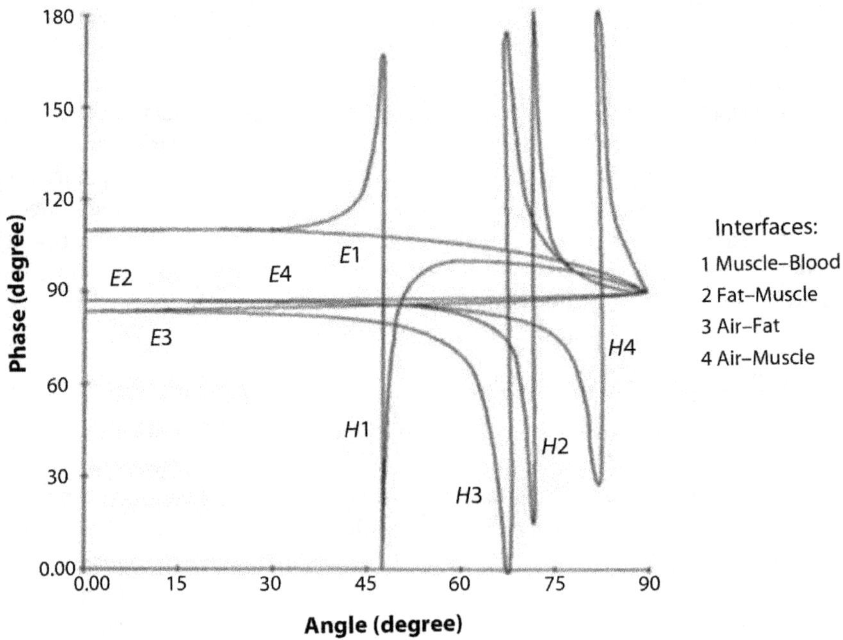


**FIGURE 5.4** Phase of reflection coefficients for E and H polarized 2450 MHz microwaves with a plane wavefront.

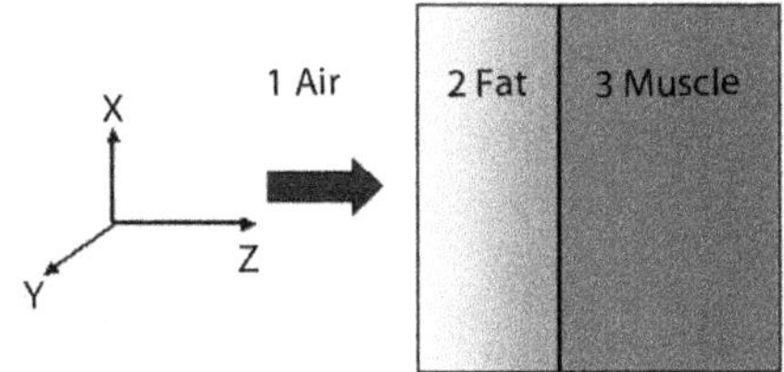


**FIGURE 5.5** Plane wave in air impinging on a composite fat-muscle layer.

pronounced if the thickness of each layer is greater than the penetration depth for that tissue and is approximately one-half wavelength or longer at the RF and microwave frequency. This dependence of standing-wave oscillation peaks on layer thickness is a manifestation of layer resonance, which can enhance power transmission and energy absorption.

For the layered tissue model depicted in Figure 5.5, the electric field strength in the fat layer is given by

$$E_f = F_l E_0 \left[ e^{-(\alpha_2 + j\beta_2)z} + \Gamma_{32} e^{(\alpha_2 + j\beta_2)z} \right] \tag{5.4}$$

and the electric field in the underlying muscular tissue is given by

$$E_m = F_t E_0 e^{-(\alpha_3 + j\beta_3)z} \tag{5.5}$$

where $\alpha_2$, $\beta_2$, and $\alpha_3$, $\beta_3$ are the attenuation and propagation coefficients in fat and muscle, respectively. The layer function $F_l$ and the transmission function $F_t$ are given by

$$F_l = \frac{T_{12}}{e^{(\alpha_2 + j\beta_2)l} + \Gamma_{21} \Gamma_{32} e^{-(\alpha_2 + j\beta_2)l}} \tag{5.6}$$

$$F_t = \frac{T_{12} T_{23}}{e^{(\alpha_2 + j\beta_2)l} + \Gamma_{21} \Gamma_{32} e^{-(\alpha_2 + j\beta_2)l}} \tag{5.7}$$

where $T_{12}$ and $T_{23}$ are the transmission coefficients at the air–fat and fat–muscle boundaries, respectively. $\Gamma_{21}$ and $\Gamma_{32}$ denote the reflection coefficients at the respective boundaries, and l is the thickness of the fat layer. The power deposition or attenuation in a given layer can be obtained from equations given in Chapter 3.

Computed results of SAR distribution or attenuation and absorption in fat–muscle layers for four different frequencies are given in Figure 5.6. The values are normalized to the SAR in muscle at the fat–muscle boundary. Note the absorbed energy is much lower in fat than in muscle. However, the reflection from the fat–muscle boundary produces a standing wave in fat. The standing-wave maximum at a quarter wavelength from the boundary becomes bigger in fat, and the penetration into muscle becomes less as the frequency increases. It is important to note that for fat tissues less than 3-cm thick, the corresponding values can be simply obtained by deleting portions of the curves to the left of the actual fat thickness displayed. The SARs will remain as shown for smaller fat thicknesses. Thus, the distribution of the

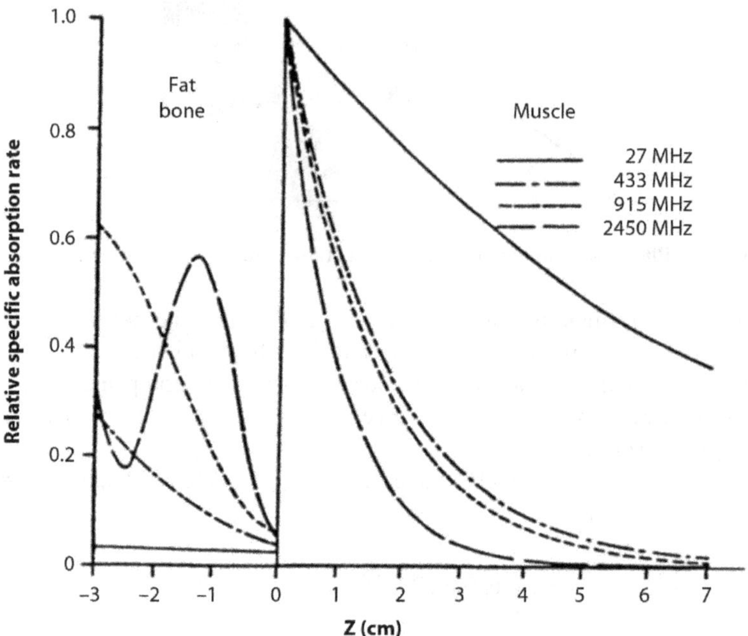


**FIGURE 5.6** Relative specific absorption rate in planar fat-muscle layers.

relative SAR corresponding to a 1 cm thick fat layer would be the same as shown in the figure for fat and muscle.

The microwave energy deposited in models composed of three planar layers of skin, fat, and muscle may be analyzed in a similar manner, except the distribution of absorbed energy becomes more complex [Lin, 2000]. Multiple reflections could occur between tissue interfaces. The reflected component will combine with the transmitted component to form standing waves in each tissue layer. The standing wave effect becomes especially pronounced if the thickness of each layer is longer than the skin depth for that tissue, namely, one-quarter wavelength or longer. This phenomenon is a manifestation of layer resonance. Some examples of the dependence of peak SAR on the thickness of the fat layer in a planar tissue model of skin–fat–muscle layers at different frequencies are shown in Figure 5.7. The skin thickness is 2 mm, and the incident power density is 10 $W/m^2$. It is interesting to note that for fat layers up to 3 cm thick, the peak SAR is higher in the skin tissue for each of the frequencies studied.

It is important to note that the multiple reflections from discontinuities of the dielectric permittivity of various tissue layers can cause multipath signals to be present at the receiver. These multipath backscattered signals from the same target can arrive at the receiver via a different propagation path. The presence of multipath reflections along with the direct reflection can produce distortion in the received signal and give rise to incorrect interpretation of the target's characteristics. Thus, signal processing techniques may be required to separate the direct reflection from the multipath backscatter.

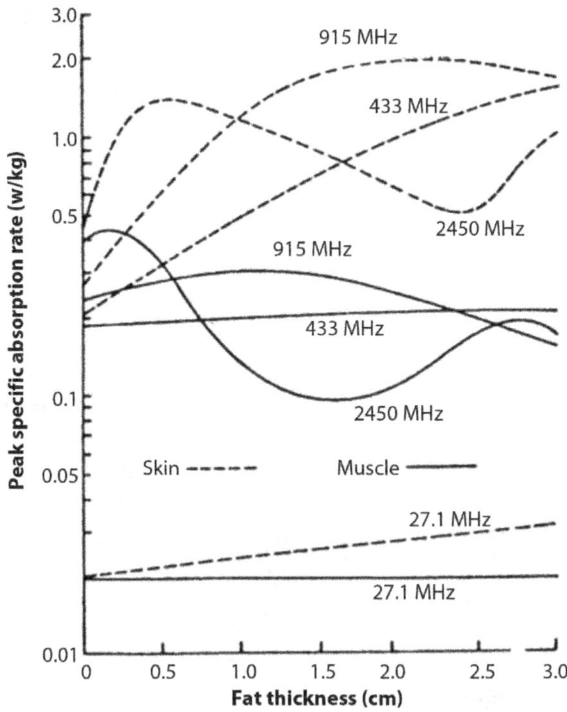


**FIGURE 5.7** The peak specific absorption rate as a function of fat-layer thickness in a planar layered tissue model of skin-fat-muscle at different frequencies. The skin thickness is 2 mm, and the incident power density is 10 W/m$^2$.

## 5.4 ANATOMIC PHANTOM MODELS

Although depth of penetration and reflection and transmission characteristics in planar tissue models provide considerable insights into coupling and distribution of RF and microwave energy, biological structures are complex in form and exhibit substantial curvature that can affect microwave energy reflection, transmission, and distribution. These complexities place limitations on the analytical calculations of reflected and transmitted microwave energy for bodies of various shapes with complex permittivity.

Many models of the human body have been developed with millimeter and in some cases, sub-millimeter resolutions as better or more realistic representations of the complex geometry and structural organization of the human body [Christ et al., 2010; FDA, 2017; Findlay et al., 2005; Li et al., 2015; Nagaoka and Watanabe, 2009; Nagaoka et al., 2004; Uusitupa et al., 2010; Wu et al., 2011]. Some of the models have been applied to compute RF and microwave reflection, transmission, absorption, and distribution both in and outside the human body. The models include constructions using small-volume cubic cells or cell meshes, and anatomically based models generated from X-ray computerized tomography (CT) and magnetic resonance imaging (MRI) data. One of the earliest and most frequently used high-resolution, three-dimensional (3-D) human models come from the "Visible Human (VH) Project" of the National Library of Medicine [Ackerman, 1998], representing an adult human male and female. The VH data sets for both the male and female include photographic images obtained through the cryosectioning of human cadavers and digital images acquired through CT and MRI of cadavers. The male data set, the first to be constructed (released in 1994), consists of 1871 digital axial images obtained at 1.0 mm intervals with a pixel resolution of 1 mm, while the female data set contains 5189 digital axial images (released in 1995) and was achieved with a finer spatial grid of 0.33 mm.

While these digital data sets represent a unique tool to explore human anatomy, their direct use for computational RF and microwave investigations is limited by the fact that the image data set cannot be directly used as an input for a numerical electromagnetic computational algorithm or tool, but must be converted to a so-called "segmented" version by segmentation of the original image sets [Mason et al., 2000]. A segmented model is a model where every pixel, usually called a "voxel," does not contain information about the color (like in digital images), but rather a label that is uniquely assigned to a given tissue. In such a way, it is possible to know which tissue fills each of the model voxels and, hence, assigns the correct complex permittivity values to be used in numerical computations and simulations.

A computer simulation of the reflection, scattering, and absorption characteristics of an anatomically realistic numerical head model using a Finite Integration Technique (FIT) tool and microstrip antenna showed a nominal –15 to –20 dB (10% to 18%) reflection from the head model [Mobashsher et al., 2016]. These numbers are comparable to those obtained for prolate spheroidal bodies discussed in Section 5.7, but are lower than the 50% expected for plane-wave reflections from planar tissue surfaces. Typically, the reflection coefficients vary with anatomy and size of the head model. Figure 5.8 illustrates the normalized electric field amplitudes in and outside the horizontal section of a phantom head model exposed to 1 GHz microwave radiation. It is seen that the electric field is the highest between the antenna and the forehead. The transmitted electric field amplitude varies as it progresses into the head structure, with different tissue types at different distances. Note that different locations inside the head model showed differences in the electric field patterns due to the heterogeneous tissue dielectric properties. The variation reveals how the field attenuates inside the head, which would have implications of signal detection capability in a fading propagation channel.

### 5.4.1 SAR in Anatomical Models

Aside from the influence of transmitted and reflected field variations on signal detection, SAR analysis is often performed to evaluate the safety of exposure to RF and microwaves on humans [Christ et al., 2010; Dimbelow et al., 1997; 2002; 2007; Findley et al., 2005; 2006; Lin and Wang, 2005; Piuzzi et al., 2011; Wang et al., 2006; 2008; 2008]. Thus, anatomically realistic human body models have been used to examine whole-body and partial-body (head or head-and-shoulder) exposure to RF and microwave radiation from various sources. It involves solving Maxwell's equations in the differential form (Chapter 3) using the computational algorithm based

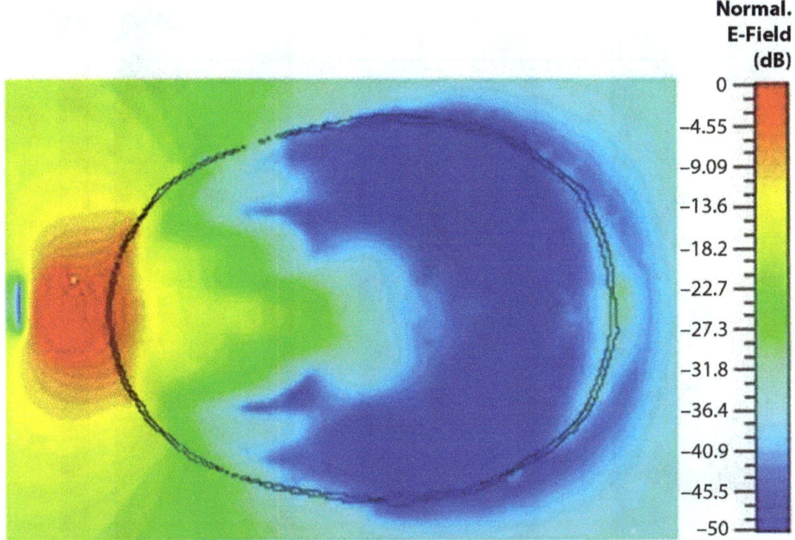


**FIGURE 5.8** Normalized amplitudes in and outside the horizontal section of a phantom head model exposed to microwave radiation. (From Mobashsher et al., 2016.)

on the numerical method of the finite-difference time-domain (FDTD) technique [Kunz and Luebbers, 1993; Yee, 1966].

Examples of computed SAR distributions for an anatomical model of a human body exposed to plane-wave sources of microwaves are shown in Figures 5.9. The whole-body anatomical Duke human model is comprised of 110 × 58 × 360 cell elements with 1 mm spatial resolution and 78 different types of tissue. The dielectric permittivity properties for the 78 different tissues were taken from Gabriel and Gabriel [1996] and Gabriel et al. [1996a,b]. The incident plane wave's electric vector is aligned along the long axis and propagates from the front to back of the body. Figure 5.9 presents SAR distributions in the central coronal section of the anatomical Duke human body model [see FDA, 2017] for plane-wave exposures at three microwave frequencies: 700, 1800, and 2700 MHz [Cavagnaro and Lin, 2019]. Shown are computed values, normalized to 1 W/kg (at 0 dB). These results indicate a highly nonuniform SAR distribution inside the body at all three frequencies, although SAR distribution at 700 MHz is considerably more uniform than at 2700 MHz, where higher SAR values are seen in more superficial tissues, including the head region. As expected, the higher the microwave frequency, the shallower the penetration depth of the microwaves. Note that the higher frequency SARs in the center of this coronal section of the body and head are negligible in comparison to the skin and subcutaneous tissues. Thus, there is a relatively strong concentration of microwave power deposition close to the body and head surface at higher microwave frequencies. However, SARs are much more uniformly distributed among all tissues in the arms and legs, mainly because of their narrower cross sections.

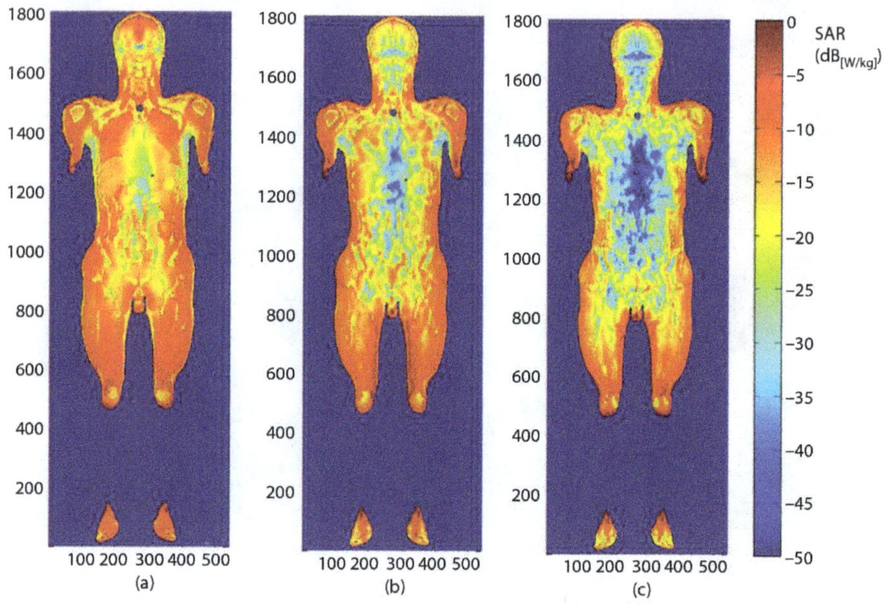


**FIGURE 5.9** Plane wave specific absorption rate distribution in the central coronal section of a human body model at three microwave frequencies: (a) 700 MHz; (b) 1800 MHz; (c) 2700 MHz normalized to 1 W/kg (0 dB).

## 5.5 FREQUENCY DEPENDENCE AND RESONANCE ABSORPTION

As seen earlier in the chapter, SAR distribution in the same anatomical human can vary with microwave frequency. It is instructive to further study the phenomenon via canonical models such as the spherical body to gain insights into their fundamental interactions [Lin and Bernardi, 2007; Lin and Gandhi, 1996; Lin and Wang, 2005]. The relative absorption coefficients for a 14 cm diameter homogeneous sphere of brain-and-muscle equivalent materials exposed to a plane wave are shown in Figure 5.10 as a function of the sphere's size-to-wavelength ratio (ka) at frequencies from 100 MHz to 10 GHz [Lin, 2018, 2020, 2021]. The absorbed energy varies widely with sphere size and frequency. In general, both for brain and muscle tissues, absorption increases rapidly with increasing radius and frequency, and is then followed by some wavelength-dependent geometrical resonant behavior.

However, as shall be shown next, with increasing frequency, microwave energy is absorbed in a decreasingly smaller volume of mass because of the shortened penetration depth. The peaks of these resonant oscillations are related to the maxima in the SAR distributions inside the tissue model. For ($ka = 2\pi a/\lambda_0$) <0.4, where a is the sphere radius and $\lambda_0$ is the wavelength in vacuum or free space, SAR peaks do not occur inside the sphere. However, for some combinations of exposure frequency and radius (0.4 <ka <2.0), peak absorption will occur, which is an example of geometric resonance phenomenon. For larger tissue spheres, the maximum absorption appears at the anterior portion (first exposed surface) of the tissue sphere, and the diminished penetration depth at the surface becomes a dominating factor for exposures at

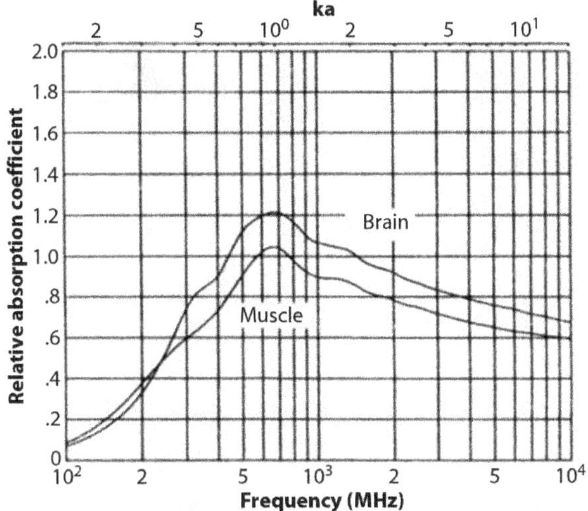


**FIGURE 5.10** Frequency and size dependence of absorption in a 14-cm diameter spherical model of the human brain and muscle equivalent materials from 100 MHz to 10 GHz.

frequencies in this range. Furthermore, the planar model discussed previously may be applied to obtain a theoretical estimation of absorbed energy distribution in this case.

For a plane wave linearly polarized in the x direction and propagating along the positive z direction, the SAR distributions through the center of the brain sphere along the coordinate axes calculated from analytical formulations for a homogeneous spherical model of the human adult (9 cm radius) brain exposed to 915 MHz plane waves is shown in Figure 5.11. Note the location of a peak SAR near the center

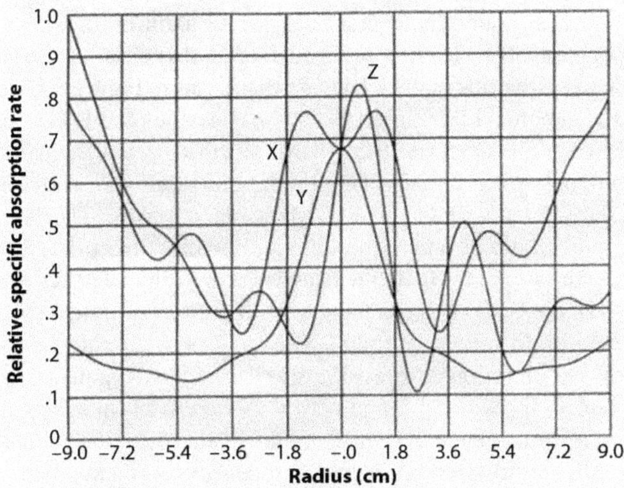


**FIGURE 5.11** Specific absorption rate distribution in a homogeneous spherical brain model (18 cm diameter) exposed to a 915 MHz plane wave. The direction of microwave propagation is along the z axis.

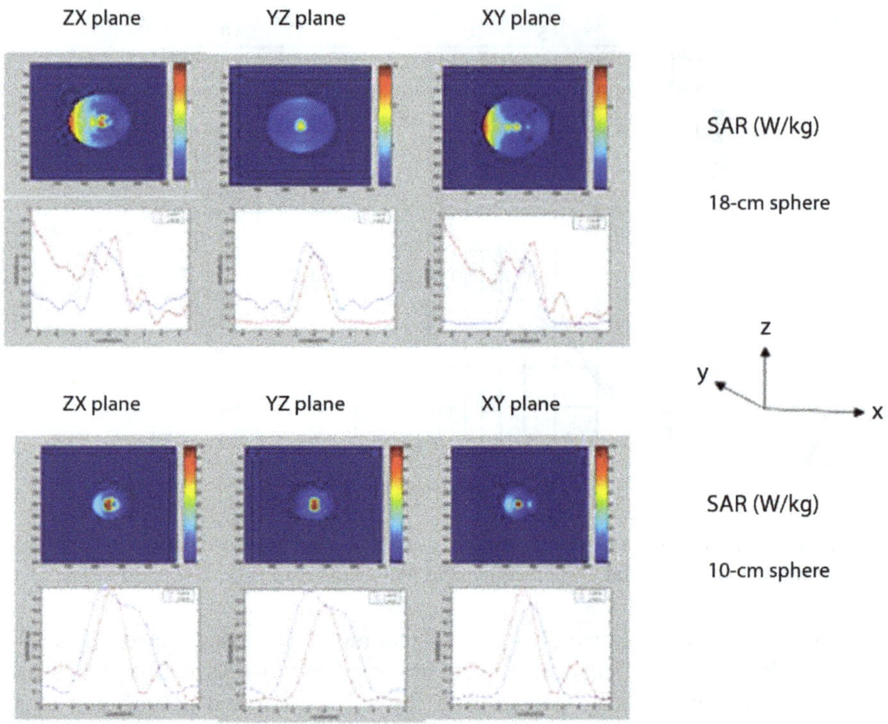


**FIGURE 5.12** Specific absorption rate characteristics in 2-D displaying microwave absorption in the canonical brain models exposed to 915 MHz plane waves propagating along the x direction. Note symmetry in the transverse dimension.

of the brain sphere, although the center peak for an adult brain is about 20% down from peak absorption at the leading brain surface in this case.

SAR patterns in two dimensions (2-D) are displayed in Figure 5.12 for microwave absorption in the canonical brain models. These examples of FDTD-computed SAR distributions through the center of the sphere over the three principal cross sections are for homogeneous spherical models of the human adult (18 cm diameter) or child (10 cm diameter) brains exposed to 915 MHz plane waves. The line graphs give the SAR distributions through the center along the axial directions. The plane-wave microwave exposure impinges from the negative x direction. The results for the adult head at 915 MHz are in good agreement with the analytic calculations. As noted, for an adult-sized brain sphere, the peak SAR moves to an anterior location in the incident microwave direction. However, a small peak SAR appears near the center of an adult brain. Both exposed human child and adult brain spheres exhibit clear peak absorption near the center and inside of the head. Note that the location of peak SAR for the smaller child-sized brain sphere appears prominently near the center for 915 MHz microwaves. This result reveals the fact that for microwave exposure, the same plane-wave source can produce very different SAR distributions inside different sized human body models.

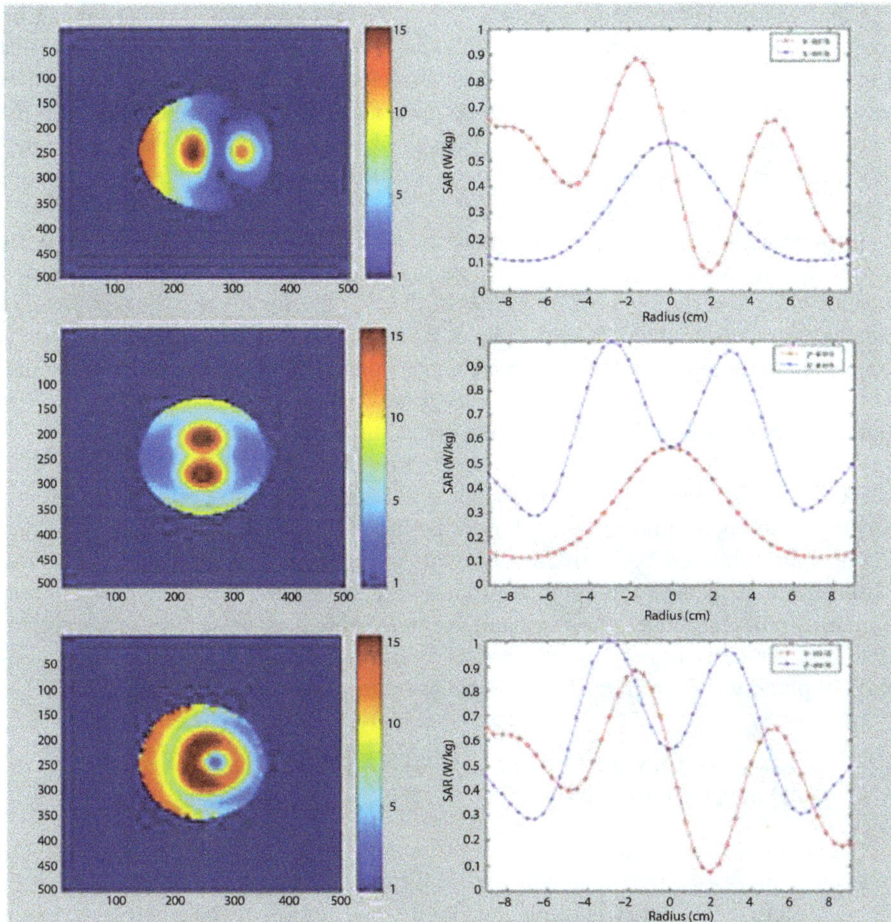


**FIGURE 5.13** Specific absorption rate distributions inside a 9-cm radius adult brain sphere exposed to a 400 MHz plane wave. The three rows represent XY, ZX, and YZ plane patterns, respectively. The corresponding line distributions are along the direction of propagation (red) and transverse (blue) to the direction of propagation shown on the right. The direction of wave propagation is along the X axis.

A 2-D display of microwave absorption in a 9 cm radius homogeneous brain sphere for a 400 MHz plane wave is shown in Figure 5.13. Note that the left-side 2-D graphs and right-side line graphs of the model show equal magnitudes in the transverse planes because of symmetry of the brain model and uniform transverse fields of the incident microwave. Also, the SAR distributions have different peaks deep inside the brain sphere and the local peaks may be several times greater due to exponential or penetration losses in planar homogeneous models. The enhancement is the result of the refraction of incident plane waves into the brain sphere by the curved tissue surface and a geometrical resonance phenomenon in the form of standing waves. Although SAR in the shadow region is lower compared with the front surface, it can still be substantial.

Clearly, microwaves can overcome exponential losses and produce enhanced coupling at a greater depth in bodies with curved surfaces. Typically, if the largest dimension of the body is comparable to the wavelength of the impinging microwave, energy deposition and distribution will be influenced by the surface curvature of the whole or partial body part and tissue composition. In particular, the ratio of geometric dimension and wavelength or the factor ka affects the extent and characteristics of microwave energy coupling.

In general, standing-wave SAR patterns with multiple peaks and valleys are observed. The peak absorption may be several times greater than the average, and the enhanced absorptions near the center of these brain models may be significantly greater than that expected from the planar tissue models. The increased absorptions are due to a combination of the high dielectric constant and curvature of the model, which produces a strong focusing of energy toward the interior of the sphere that more than compensates for transmission losses through the tissue.

The coupling of RF plane waves into more complex models of the body such as the human head structure, where a spherical core of brain is surrounded by five concentric shells of other tissues, shows that the effect of skin, fat, skull, dura, and cerebrospinal fluid on SAR distribution is to increase SAR in the skin [Lin, 1976]. Absorptions in fat and the skull are the lowest among the tissue layers [Lin and Gandhi, 1996]. Moreover, the peak and average SARs may be several times greater than for homogeneous models. The enhancement is apparently due to resonant coupling of plane-wave RF into the brain sphere by the outer tissue layers.

## 5.6 ORIENTATION AND POLARIZATION EFFECTS FOR ELONGATED BODIES

For nonplanar, elongated bodies such as human or animal bodies, or a prolate spheroidal model where the height-to-width ratio is larger than 1, the coupling of RF and microwave energy is influenced by the orientation of the electric field vector (i.e., polarization) with respect to the body. The three principal polarizations of the impinging plane wave to be distinguished are: E polarization, in which the electric vector is parallel to the long axis of the body; H polarization, in which the magnetic vector is parallel to the long axis of the body; and K polarization, in which neither the electric nor magnetic vector is parallel to the long axis of the body. For K polarization, the plane wave impinges along the long axis of the body. The frequency at which the highest (resonant) absorption occurs is a function of both polarization and the exposed subject's geometry. In general, the shorter the subject, the higher the resonance frequency, and vice versa. E polarization couples microwave energy more efficiently to the body in a plane-wave field for frequencies up to and slightly above the resonance region, where the body dimension and wavelength are roughly equal.

For RF frequencies well below resonance, such that the ratio of long-body dimension (L) to free-space wavelength ($\lambda_o$) is less than 0.2, the average SAR is characterized by a $f^2$ dependence. SAR goes through the resonance region in which $0.2 < L/\lambda_o < 1.0$. Specifically, the SAR rapidly increases to a maximum near $L/\lambda_o = 0.4$ and then falls off as 1/f. At frequencies for which $L/\lambda_o > 1.0$, the whole-body absorption decreases slightly, but approaches asymptotically to about one-half of the incident power is transmitted into biological body; thus, about the same amount is reflected since it is proportional to the value of (1 – power reflection coefficient). Resonance absorptions are not nearly as well defined for H polarization as for E polarization. The average SAR for H polarization gradually reaches a plateau throughout the RF spectrum [Lin and Bernardi, 2007].

## 5.7 SCATTERING COEFFICIENT FOR PROLATE SPHEROIDAL BODIES

As mentioned, human and animal bodies generally are complex in form and exhibit variations in curvatures that can modify microwave reflection and transmission. The wave propagation characteristics can depend critically on the polarization and orientation of the incident wave with respect to the body and the ratio of body size to wavelength. These complications place severe limitations on reflection and transmission determinations, especially for bodies of arbitrary shape and complex permittivity. The issue may be approached by choosing a prolate spheroidal tissue model to serve as a prototype that can be used to estimate the scattering characteristics in related cases.

The scattering coefficient, defined as the ratio of scattered energy to incident energy for a 14 cm long homogeneous prolate spheroid with a major-to-minor axis (A/B) ratio of 1.5 is shown in Figures 5.14 and 5.15 for 915 and 2450 MHz

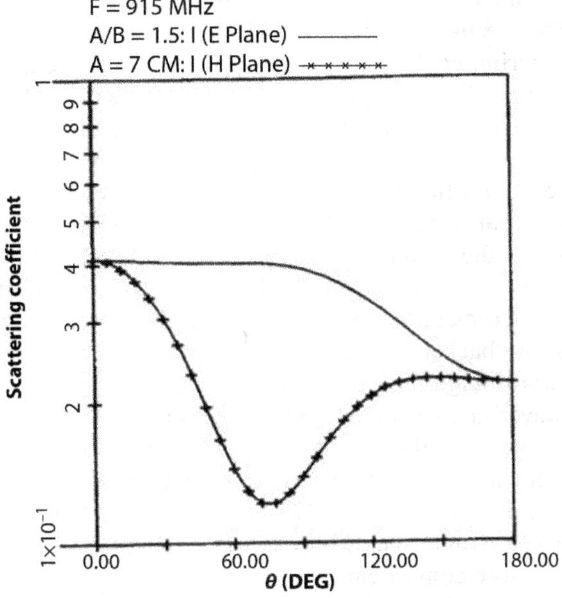


**FIGURE 5.14** The scattering coefficient for a 14-cm long homogeneous prolate spheroidal tissue model with a major-to-minor axis ration of 1.5 exposed to a 915 MHz plane wave.

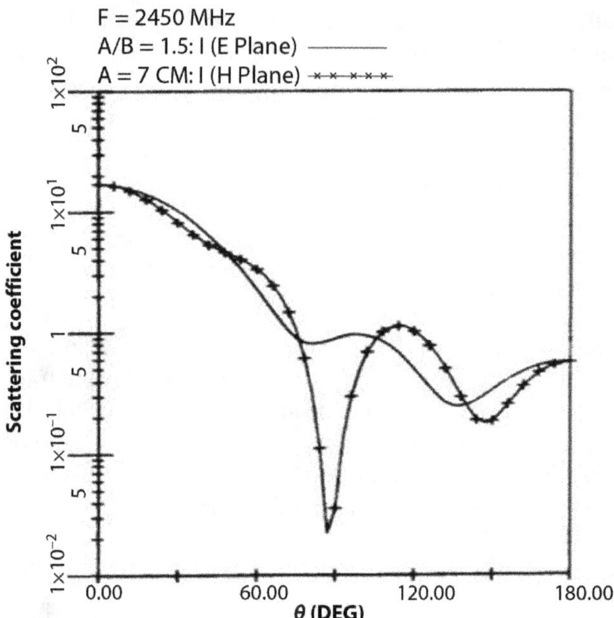


**FIGURE 5.15** The scattering coefficient for a 14-cm long homogeneous prolate spheroidal tissue model with a major-to-minor axis ration of 1.5 irradiated by 2450 MHz microwaves.

plane waves incident from air. Dielectric constants of 35 or 32 and conductivity of 0.73 or 1.32 S/m are used for 915 and 2450 MHz, respectively [Lin, 1986]. It is seen that the scattering coefficients in the E-plane (plane parallel to the electric field vector) and in the H-plane (plane parallel to the magnetic field vector) differ from each other except for the forward- (0°) and backscattered (180°) components. The scattered energy varies widely with the angle of observation, especially in the H-plane. The reason that the scattering coefficient for 915 MHz is smoother and fluctuates less than for 2450 MHz is because the 14 cm spheroid represents a smaller fraction of the wavelength at 915 MHz than at 2450 MHz. In general, the smaller the ratio of body size to wavelength, the more uniform the variation of the scattering coefficient as a function of the observation angle. It is significant to note that the backscattered (reflected) microwave energy at 915 MHz is on the same order of magnitude as the forward scatter component, and the backscattered microwaves at 2450 MHz are less than one-tenth of the forward scatter component — a level near those obtained for a human head model described in Section 5.4. Nonetheless, this finding suggests that while transmission measurement may be more efficient at 2450 MHz, both reflection and transmission measurements should be equally applicable to 915 MHz. Also, measurement in the E-plane is usually more convenient.

Thus far, the propagation phenomenon has been described in terms of plane waves impinging on parallel layers of tissues and simple volumes isolated in free space. In many practical situations, however, interaction can occur in the near field rather than the far field where plane waves dominate. Furthermore, they may involve applicators or antennas that are comparable in dimensions to the wavelength. This combination, along with the fact that most biological targets consist of complex surfaces of irregular shape, as evidenced by the anatomical models, make the propagation characteristics complex to describe with accuracy or precision. However, from a signal processing perspective, it is an approachable challenge.

Because of the fundamental nature of plane-wave interaction, the understanding obtained serves a useful purpose when used with proper precautions. So, to be used effectively, they must be supplemented by further detailed information on the nature of the problem. For example, the data given in Table 5.3 show that microwave energy at 433 MHz can penetrate three times as deep into the tissues as energy at 5800 MHz. This implied advantage of lower frequencies is somewhat misleading because as the frequency is decreased, the wavelength, antenna, and applicator size become proportionally larger until it is no longer possible to direct the wave to a desired biological target with reasonable applicator dimensions. If the applicator is not increased in size as the frequency is lowered, the radiated energy will rapidly diverge and be scattered by the target; only a small fraction of the available energy will penetrate into tissue.

## 5.8 DOPPLER EFFECT FROM TARGET MOTION

When microwaves are scattered from a biological target moving relative to the transmitter and receiver, the received signal undergoes an apparent frequency change, called the Doppler shift. Using the scheme illustrated in Figure 5.16, a relation can be obtained [Gill, 1965; Lin, 1986, 1989] between the Doppler frequency change $f_d$ and the target velocity $\boldsymbol{u}$ as

$$f_d = -\frac{1}{2\pi}(\boldsymbol{k}_r - \boldsymbol{k}_t) \cdot \boldsymbol{u} \tag{5.8}$$

where $\boldsymbol{k}_t$ and $\boldsymbol{k}_r$ are propagation vectors associated with the transmitter and receiver, respectively.

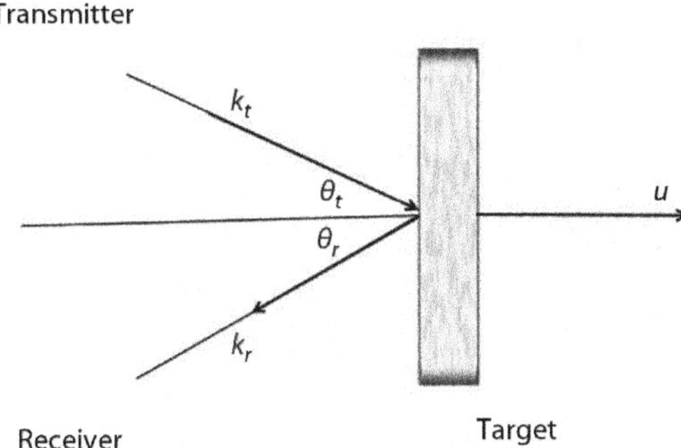


**FIGURE 5.16** Scattering of a plane wave by a moving biological target with velocity, $u$.

If the receiving and transmitting antennas are in close proximity of each other or are the same, i.e., $\boldsymbol{k}_r = -\boldsymbol{k}_t$, Eq. (5.8) then reduces to

$$f_d = \frac{1}{2\pi}(\boldsymbol{k}_t \cdot \boldsymbol{u}) = -\frac{1}{2\pi}(\boldsymbol{k}_r \cdot \boldsymbol{u}) = -2f\left(\frac{u}{v}\right)\cos\theta \tag{5.9}$$

where $f$ is the source frequency, $v$ is the velocity of microwave, and $\theta$ is the angle between the target velocity vector $\boldsymbol{u}$ and the direction of wave propagation. It is seen from Eq. (5.8) that $f_d$ is directly proportional to the target velocity $u$ and takes on the largest value when $\theta = 0$ or 180° such that

$$f_d = \pm 2f\left(\frac{u}{v}\right) \tag{5.10}$$

where the plus and minus signs account for movements toward and away from the transmitter, respectively.

In noninvasive sensing of physiological changes, various parts of the target may fill all or an appreciable portion of the incident microwave beam, the target velocity can vary over the beam so that the Doppler component will consist of a spectrum of frequencies. For example, during contraction, the heart is known to rotate anteriorly by about 4°. Considering the situation depicted in Figure 5.17, where a rotation imparts an angular velocity $\omega_r$ of the target about its center of gravity, two fixed points on the target, a distance $z$ apart, will have a relative radial velocity toward the transmitter of

$$\Delta u = u_1 - u_2 = (\omega_r z)\cos\theta_r \tag{5.11}$$

Hence, from Eq. (5.11), the difference in Doppler frequencies between these two points is

$$\Delta f_d = 2f\left(\frac{\Delta u}{v}\right) = 2f\frac{(\omega_r z)\cos\theta_r}{v} \tag{5.12}$$

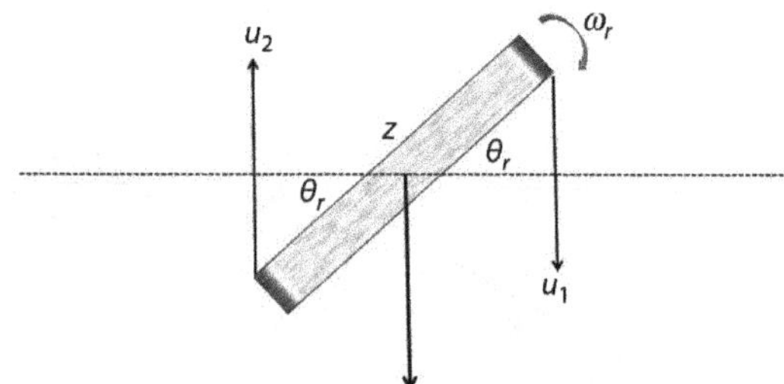


**FIGURE 5.17** Effect of target rotation on reflected microwave signal.

Thus, the Doppler spectrum will be proportional to the angular velocity of the target and the gross aspect of the target. In a Doppler system, the spectrum will be detected as the frequency shifts relative to the transmitter frequency. This is usually accomplished through mixing the backscattered wave with the transmitted wave and then measuring the difference in frequency by using a digital counter or by passing the demodulated signal through a set of bandpass filters.

When multiplying Eq. (5.10) by $2\pi$ and integrating over time, while neglecting the constant term, the instantaneous phase variation $\phi(t)$ corresponding to the distance $x(t)$ traveled by the target becomes

$$\phi(t) = 2\pi \int f_d\,(t)\,dt = 4\pi f\left[\frac{x(t)}{v}\right] \tag{5.13}$$

This is the Doppler phase shift, which is proportional to target displacement $x(t)$. Doppler frequency is proportional to target velocity. If the demodulated waveform is fed through a low-pass filter, the output $g(t)$ will be a signal that varies with time and target motion such that

$$g(t) = G\ sin\ \phi(t) = G\ sin\left\{4\pi f\left[\frac{x(t)}{v}\right]\right\} \tag{5.14}$$

where $G$ is the signal amplitude associated with the reflected wave. Since the instantaneous displacement of the target involved is small compared to the wavelength in tissue or air for microwave frequencies of most interest, an approximate relation for $g(t)$ is obtained as

$$g(t) = G\left\{4\pi f\left[\frac{x(t)}{v}\right]\right\} = 4\pi G\left[\frac{x(t)}{\lambda}\right] \tag{5.15}$$

for $f\lambda = v$. Therefore, the displacement of the target is directly proportional to the output of the filter under these conditions, and it is linearly related to the biological target's displacement. Moreover, the signal strength will be stronger for microwaves with shorter wavelengths for a given target displacement.

## 5.9 RANGE AND VELOCITY RESOLUTION

The Doppler frequency shift provides a direct measure of relative motion or velocity. There are other related considerations that have relevance in microwave noninvasive sensing of physiological changes. The signal filtration schemes alluded to previously offer a simple technique to help detect the Doppler signal under the continuous wave (CW) operation domain. However, the CW Doppler approach does not provide target range information and is sensitive to motions from all ranges. An alternative is to employ a train of narrow pulses transmitted at a rate lower than the expected Doppler frequency component. This approach is called range gating or pulse Doppler.

Resolution defines the ability of a sensing system to differentiate two closely spaced targets. This ability depends partially on the signal processing scheme employed. In the case of range, resolution is achieved mainly through proper selection of the bandwidth of the transmitted waveform. It has been found that two targets can be resolved in range quite simply if they are separated by at least by 0.8 of a pulse width [Skolnik, 1980]. Similarly, two targets can be resolved in angle if they are separated by at least 0.8 of a beam width [Skolnik, 1975]. When several targets with different velocities are present, the received signal is a composition of the corresponding number of Doppler-shifted signals. To adequately separate multiple targets in motion, it will be necessary to apply the signal for a sufficient duration. In general, the longer the duration of the signal and the higher the microwave frequency, the more accurate the measurement. Thus, resolution in Doppler signal depends on the signal duration. It is possible to isolate multiple targets using either high-range resolution or a narrow-band Doppler filter. However, large signal-to-noise ratios (SNR) are necessary if good resolution is desired. A general rule suggests that the SNR must be greater than 20 dB to obtain satisfactory results.

The pulse Doppler technique combines the range discrimination ability of the system with the frequency discrimination of CW systems by using a coherent pulse train, i.e., a train of pulses that are samples of a single unmodulated sine wave. When the pulse train is reflected by a moving target, the signal is Doppler-frequency shifted in proportion to the target velocity. In the presence of multiple targets with different velocities, the reflected signal is a superposition of a corresponding number of pulse trains, each with its own Doppler shift. A range gate is used to select only those pulses reflected from the target. A narrow-band filter following the range gate passes only the frequencies corresponding to a particular Doppler component, thus, blocking all those pulse trains that pass the range gate but do not have the proper Doppler shift. The pulse Doppler technique offers the capability of measuring range and velocity unambiguously over a predetermined plane of the ambiguity domain in the presence of multiple targets, albeit at the expense of considerably more system complexity.

Instead of a tonal signal or a train of pulses, other waveforms such as pulsed CW radars (PCW), frequency-modulated CW (FMCW), stepped-frequency CW (SFCW), and ultra-wide-band (UWB) radar sensors have been introduced to overcome the limitations of CW Doppler radars. Further discussion on use of FMCW and UWB radars for vital-sign monitoring are presented in Chapter 6, Section 6.2.3 and other chapters that follow.

## REFERENCES

Ackerman, M. J., 1998. The visible human project. Proc. IEEE, 86:504

Cavagnaro, M., Lin, J. C., 2019. Importance of exposure duration and metrics on correlation between RF energy absorption and temperature increase in a human model. IEEE Trans. Biomed. Eng., 66(8):2253–2258

Chou, C. K., Bassen, H., Osepchuk, J., Balzano, Q., Peterson, R., Meltz, M., Cleveland, R., Lin, J. C., Heynick, L., 1996. Radio frequency electromagnetic exposure: Tutorial review on experimental dosimetry. Bioelectromagnetics, 17:195–208

Christ, A., Kainz, W., Hahn, E. G., Honegger-Zefferer, K., Neufeld, M., Rascher, E., Janka, W., Bautz, R., Chen, W., Kiefer, J., Schmitt, B., Hollenbach, P., Shen, H. P., Oberle, J., Szczerba, M., Kam, D., Guag, A., Kuster, N., 2010. The Virtual Family—development of surface-based anatomical models of two adults and two children for dosimetric simulations. Phys. Med. Biol., 55:23–38

Dimbylow, P. J., 1997. FDTD calculations of the whole-body averaged SAR in an anatomically realistic voxel model of the human body from 1 MHz to 1 GHz. Phys. Med. Biol., 42:479–490

Dimbylow, P. J., 2002. Fine Resolution calculations of SAR in the human body for frequencies up to 3 GHz, Phys. Med. Biol., 47:2835

Dimbylow, P. J., 2007. SAR in the mother and foetus for RF plane wave irradiation. Phys. Med. Biol., 52:3791–3802

FDA, 2017. Virtual Family data set https://www.fda.gov/about-fda/cdrh-offices/virtual-family, U.S. Food and Drug Administration

Findlay, R. P., Dimbylow, P. J., 2005. Effects of posture on FDTD calculations of specific absorption rate in a voxel model of the human body. Phys. Med. Biol., 50:3825–3835

Findlay, R. P., Dimbylow, P. J., 2006. FDTD calculations of specific energy absorption rate in a seated voxel model of the human body from 10 MHz to 3 GHz. Phys. Med. Biol., 51:2339–2352

Gill, T. P., 1965. Doppler Effect. London: Logo Press

Guido, K., Kiourti, A., 2020. Wireless wearables and implants: A dosimetry review. Bioelectromagnetics, 41:3–20

Kunz, K. S., Luebbers, R. J., 1993. The Finite-Difference Time-Domain Method for Electromagnetics. Boca Raton, Florida: CRC Press

Laakso, I., Uusitupa, T., Ilvonen, S., 2010. Comparison of SAR calculation algorithms for the finite-difference time-domain method. Phys. Med. Biol., 55:421–431

Li, C., Chen, Z., Yang, L., Lv, B., Liu, J., Varsier, N., Hadjem, A., Wiart, J., Xie, Y., Ma, L., Wu, T., 2015. Generation of infant anatomical models for evaluating the electromagnetic fields exposure. Bioelectromagnetics 36:10–26

Lin, J. C., 1976. Interaction of two cross-polarized electromagnetic waves with mammalian cranial structures. IEEE Trans. Biomed. Eng., 23:371–375

Lin, J. C., 1986. Microwave propagation in biological dielectrics with application to cardiopulmonary interrogation. In: Larsen, L. E., Jacobi, J. H., Eds., Medical Applications of Microwave Imaging (pp. 47–58), New York: IEEE Press

Lin, J. C., 1989. Microwave noninvasive sensing of physiological signatures. In: Lin, J. C., Ed., Electromagnetic Interaction with Biological Systems (pp. 3–25), New York: Plenum

Lin, J. C., 2000. Mechanisms of field coupling into biological systems at ELF and RF frequencies. Advances in Electromagnetic Fields in Living Systems (Vol. 3, pp. 1–38), New York: Kluwer/Plenum

Lin, J. C., 2007. Dosimetric comparison between different possible quantities for limiting exposure in the RF band: Rationale for the basic one and implications for guidelines. Health Phys., 92(6):547–453

Lin, J. C., 2018. Computational methods for predicting electromagnetic fields and temperature increase in biological bodies. Bioengineering and Biophysical Aspects of Electromagnetic Fields (4th ed, pp. 299–397, Chapter 9), CRC Press

Lin, J. C., 2021. Auditroy Effect of Microwave Radiation (Chapter 5), Switzerland: Springer

Lin, J. C., Bernardi, P., 2007. Computer methods for predicting field intensity and temperature change. In: Barnes, F., Greenebaum, B., Eds., Handbook of Biological Effects of Electromagnetic Fields (pp. 293–380), Chapter 10, Boca Raton, FL: CRC Press

Lin, J. C., Gandhi, O. P., 1996. Computer methods for predicting field intensity. In: Polk, C., Postow, E., Eds., Handbook of Biological Effects of Electromagnetic Fields (pp. 337–402), CRC Press

Lin, J. C., Wang, Z. W., 2005. SAR and temperature distributions in canonical head models exposed to near- and far-field electromagnetic radiation at different frequencies. Electromagn. Biol. Med., 24(3):405–421

Mason, A. P., Hurt, W. D., Walters, T. J., D'Andrea, J. A., Gajšek, P., Ryan, K. L., Nelson, D. A., Smith, K. I., Ziriax, J. M., 2000. Effects of frequency, permittivity, and voxel size on predicted specific absorption rate values in biological tissue during electromagnetic-field exposure. IEEE Trans. Microw. Theory Tech., 48:2050

Mobashsher, A. T., Bialkowski, K. S., Abbosh, A. M., Crozier, S., 2016. Design and experimental evaluation of a non-invasive microwave head imaging system for intracranial haemorrhage detection. PLoS ONE, 11(4): e0152351. doi: 10.1371/journal.pone.0152351

Nagaoka, T., Watanabe, S., 2009. Voxel-based variable posture models of human anatomy. Proc. IEEE, 97:2015–2025

Nagaoka, T., Watanabe, S., Sakurai, K., Kunieda, E., Watanabe, T., 2004. Development of realistic high-resolution whole-body voxel models of Japanese adult male and female of average height and weight and application of models to radio-frequency electromagnetic-field dosimetry. Phys. Med. Biol., 49:1–15

NCRP, 1981. Radio Frequency Electromagnetic Fields: Properties, Quantities, Units, Biophysical Interactions, and Measurements, Rpt 67, Bethesda, MD: NCRP

Piuzzi, E., Bernardi, P., Cavagnaro, M., Pisa, S., Lin, J. C., 2011. Analysis of adult and child exposure to uniform plane waves at mobile communication systems frequencies (900 MHz – 3 GHz). IEEE Trans. Electromagn. Compat., 53:38–47

Skolnik, M. I., 1975. Comments on the angular resolution of radar. Proc. IEEE, 63(9):1354–1355

Skolnik, M. I., 1980. Introduction to Radar Systems, 2nd ed, McGraw Hill

Uusitupa, T., Laakso, I., Ilvonen, S., Nikoskinen, K., 2010. SAR variation study from 300 to 5000 MHz for 15 voxel models including different postures. Phys. Med. Biol., 55:1157–1176

Wang, J., Fujiwara, O., Kodera, S., Watanabe, S., 2006. FDTD calculation of whole-body average SAR in adult and child models for frequencies from 30 MHz to 3 GHz. Phys. Med. Biol., 51:4119–4127

Wang, Z. W., Lin, J. C., Mao, W. H., Liu, W. Z., Smith, M. B., Collins, C. M., 2007. SAR and temperature: Simulations and comparison to regulatory limits for MRI. J. Magn. Resona. Imag., 26(2):437–441

Wang, Z. W., Lin, J. C., Vaughan, J. T., Collins, C. M., 2008. On consideration of physiological response in numerical models of temperature during MRI of the human head. J. Magn. Resona. Imag. 28(5):1303–1308

Wu, T., Tan, L., Shao, Q., Zhang, C., Zhao, C., Li, Y., Conil, E., Hadjem, A., Wiart, J., Lu, L., Wang, N., Xie, Y., Zhang, S., 2011. Chinese adult anatomical models and the application in evaluation of wideband RF EMF exposure. Phys. Med. Biol., 56:2075–2089

Yee, K. S., 1966. Numerical solutions of initial boundary value problems involving Maxwell's equations in isotropic media. IEEE Trans. Ant. Propag., 14:302–307

# 6 System Analysis and Signal Processing

In microwave sensing of physiological signatures and changes, a framework is established where the physiological events are transformed by electronic systems into electrical signals. The events may be bodily motion and fluctuation, organ function and behavior, tissue feature and reaction, or surface and volume change in health and disease. The signals that mimic the response of one or more physiological events with their unique attributes are amenable to computer processing and mathematical analysis as well as probing via electronic systems and software algorithms.

The purpose of this chapter is to define the essential mathematical relationships and describe the applicable mathematical tools that are useful in analyzing microwave sensing systems and physiological signals as a linear process. The goal is to explain the various fundamental concepts and to facilitate physical insight into the microwave sensing system's operation and the behavior of physiological signals and signatures. Another objective is to assist readers in gaining an understanding of the techniques used for analysis and processing of linear systems and biomedical signals. It will begin with fundamental concepts, but confine the descriptions to the most pertinent topics rather than a comprehensive discussion of the processing and analysis of biological signals. Applicable and more sophisticated methods in signal processing are highlighted alongside subsequent chapters that discuss specific areas of noninvasive physiological sensing applications.

## 6.1 SIGNALS AND SYSTEMS

Signals and systems are integral parts of sensing methodologies. It is the signal that makes the system take necessary actions for accomplishing its chosen purpose. The input signal or excitation to a system is a force to which the system can respond in some appropriate fashion. In a microwave radar sensing system, this force is a microwave signal. The output is the response of the system to the input in the form of a modulated microwave signal. In this case, the signals are all functions of time. They may be simple and well known, such as a sinusoid or pulse, or may be complicated and largely unknown functions of time, such as heartbeat variability or the vital-sign waveforms of people in a crowded room. It is important to note that, generally, signals can be representable mathematically for analysis and processing.

### 6.1.1 Linear Systems

Like many electronic systems and physical phenomena, the signals described in mathematical expressions behave in such a way that the response to a single input acting individually, or inputs acting simultaneously, is equal to the sum of the responses

DOI: 10.1201/9781003315223-6

that each of the inputs would produce individually. For example, in a microwave radar system, if the signal from the source antenna is doubled, the received signal will double. These types of behavior are linear phenomena, and the system is referred to as a linear system.

A process or system is linear, mathematically, if it fulfills the following conditions, where $a$ is a constant, and $f(t)$ and $g(t)$ represent the source and receiver signals, excitation and response, or input and output signals. For

$$af(t) = ag(t), \quad \text{Scaling preservation} \tag{6.1}$$

and

$$f_1(t) + f_2(t) = g_1(t) + g_2(t), \quad \text{Superposition or Additivity} \tag{6.2}$$

Combining the two conditions, then

$$a\left[f_1(t) + f_2(t)\right] = a\left[g_1(t) + g_2(t)\right] \tag{6.3}$$

where $f_1(t)$, $f_2(t)$ and $g_1(t)$, $g_2(t)$ are two separate inputs and outputs of the system. Thus, Eq. (6.3) becomes the criteria for linearity. The methods and procedures for treating linear signals and systems provide a powerful set of tools for analyzing physiological events and their temporal change patterns.

### 6.1.2 Orthogonal Signals

An appropriate way to represent complex signals is to use a linear combination of a set of elementary time functions. The practice is convenient in working with linear systems. It decomposes a complicated input into a number of more simple inputs to find the response of the system to each of these elementary functions and to superimpose the individual response to obtain the total response. These elementary functions are selected because they have certain desirable properties, often referred to as orthogonality. A set of such functions is orthogonal if each member is orthogonal (or at right angles to each other) to every other member of the set. The functions are called basis functions. For example, the well-known sinusoidal time functions in exponential or trigonometric form

$$e^{\pm j(\omega_0 t)} = cos\ (\omega_0 t) \pm jsin\ (\omega_0 t), \tag{6.4}$$

are orthogonal over its period. In this case, the sinusoidal functions may serve as basis functions.

Here, a signal representation using orthogonal functions is discussed first in general, and the operation is illustrated using sinusoidal functions in the next section. A basis function $f(t)$ is orthogonal to $h(t)$ if

$$\int_{t_1}^{t_2} f(t)h^*(t)dt = 0, \quad over\ (t_1, t_2) \tag{6.5}$$

where $h^*(t)$ is the complex conjugate of $h(t)$.

A set of elementary time functions $g_n(t)$ is orthogonal over the time interval $(t_1, t_2)$ if

$$\int_{t_2}^{t_1} g_j(t) g_k^*(t) dt = 0, \quad for\ j \neq k \tag{6.6}$$

where $g_k^*(t)$ is the complex conjugate of $g_k(t)$. A generalized time function *x(t)* may be represented by a set of basis functions $g_n(t)$ such that

$$x(t) = \sum_{n=1}^{N} c_n g_n(t), \quad N \to \infty \tag{6.7}$$

or

$$x(t) \approx \sum_{n=1}^{N} c_n g_n(t), \quad N < \infty \tag{6.8}$$

where $c_n$ are constant coefficients. Since $g_n(t)$ is orthogonal,

$$\int_{t_2}^{t_1} x(t) g_7^*(t) dt = c_1 \int_{t_1}^{t_2} g_1(t) g_7^*(t) dt + \cdots + c_7 \int_{t_1}^{t_2} \left| g_7^2(t) \right| dt + \cdots + c_n \int_{t_1}^{t_2} g_N(t) g_7^*(t) dt \tag{6.9}$$

becomes

$$\int_{t_1}^{t_2} x(t) g_7^*(t) dt = c_7 \int_{t_1}^{t_2} \left| g_7^2(t) \right| dt \tag{6.10}$$

Then,

$$c_7 = \frac{\int_{t_1}^{t_2} x(t) g_7^*(t) dt}{\int_{t_1}^{t_2} \left| g_7^2(t) \right| dt} \tag{6.11}$$

In general, the coefficients $c_n$ are given by

$$c_n = \frac{\int_{t_1}^{t_2} x(t) g_n^*(t) dt}{\int_{t_1}^{t_2} \left| g_n^2(t) \right| dt} \tag{6.12}$$

and $c_n$ may be viewed as a projection of *x(t)* on $g_n(t)$.

The best-known orthogonal basis function is the set of sinusoidal functions. The resulting decomposition equation is known as the Fourier series representation. The familiar sinusoidal functions are popular basis functions because they remain sinusoidal after various mathematical operations. The addition and subtraction of two sinusoids of the same frequency is still a sinusoid, and the differentiation or integration of a sinusoid is still a sinusoid. Over the interval of any period, $T = \frac{1}{f_0}$ of the periodic signal $g(t)$ where $f_0$ is the fundamental frequency of the sinusoidal functions

$$\int_{t_0}^{t_0+T} g_m(t)\, g_n^*(t)\, dt = 0,\ m \neq n \tag{6.13}$$

## 6.2 FOURIER SERIES REPRESENTATION OF SIGNALS

The signal representation by the Fourier series uses the sinusoidal functions as basis functions. The complex exponential form is chosen for this discussion for reasons previously mentioned. The resulting series can be converted into trigonometric (sine and cosine) series, if needed, by the familiar relation given in Eq. (6.4). The specific equations for conversions are given in a later section.

The requirements of the signal *f(t)* being single-valued has a finite number of maxima and minima within $(t_1, t_2)$, and the existence of Dirichlet conditions need to be fulfilled so that

$$\int_{t_1}^{t_2} |f(t)|\, dt = \int_{a}^{a+T} |f(t)|\, dt < \infty \tag{6.14}$$

A condition any physical signal will satisfy.

To illustrate, the exponential form of the sinusoidal function is used as the basis function

$$e^{jn\omega_0 t}, \qquad n = 0, \pm 1, \pm 2, \pm 3, \ldots, \pm \infty \tag{6.15}$$

where the angular frequency is

$$\omega_0 = \frac{2\pi}{T} \tag{6.16}$$

The Fourier series representation of a time domain signal $f(t)$, according to Eq. (6.7), is given by

$$f(t) = \sum_{n=-\infty}^{\infty} D_n e^{jn\omega_0 t}, \quad \omega_0 = 2\pi f_0 = 2\pi\left(\frac{1}{T}\right) \tag{6.17}$$

where

$$D_n = \frac{1}{T}\int_{t_1}^{t_1+T} f(t)\, e^{-jn\omega_0 t}\, dt \tag{6.18}$$

In this case, the calculations begin with multiplication of Eq. (6.17) by the complex conjugate, $e^{-jm\omega_0 t}$, and exchanging the integration and summation operations by invoking the properties of linearity to obtain

$$\int_{t_1}^{t_1+T} f(t)e^{-jm\omega_0 t}dt = \int_{t_1}^{t_1+T}\sum_{-\infty}^{\infty} D_n e^{jn\omega_0 t}e^{-jm\omega_0 t}dt \tag{6.19}$$

$$= \sum_{n=-\infty}^{\infty} D_n \int_{t_1}^{t_1+T} e^{jn\omega_0 t}e^{-jm\omega_0 t}dt \tag{6.20}$$

Since $e^{\pm jm\omega_0 t}$, $e^{\pm jn\omega_0 t}$ are orthogonal functions, such that

$$\int_{t_1}^{t_1+T} e^{jn\omega_0 t}e^{-jm\omega_0 t}dt = \begin{cases} T, & m = n \\ 0, & m \neq n \end{cases}$$

Therefore, Eq. (6.18) results as given

$$D_n = \frac{1}{T}\int_{t_1}^{t_1+T} f(t)e^{-jn\omega_0 t}dt \tag{6.21}$$

Note that the results shown in Eq. (6.21) are in frequency domain and the coefficients $D_n$ are given in terms of fundamental frequency $\omega_0$.

### 6.2.1 Example of Fourier Series Representation of Signals

This example details the process of finding the Fourier series representation for the periodic sequence of rectangular pulses shown in Figure 6.1, using exponential basis functions.

The rectangular pulse in the periodic signal is defined as

$$\begin{aligned} f(t) &= \text{A}, \quad 0 < t < t_0 \\ &= 0, \quad t_0 < t < T \end{aligned} \tag{6.22}$$

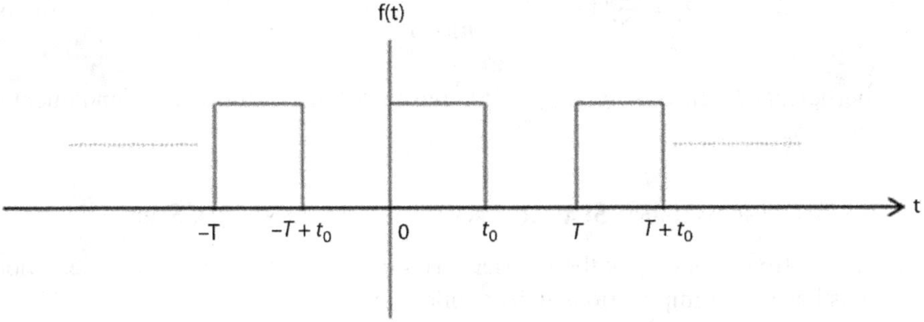


**FIGURE 6.1** A periodic sequence of rectangular $t_0$ wide pulses with a period of T.

The formal representation of the exponential Fourier series is

$$f(t) = \sum_{-\infty}^{\infty} D_n e^{jn\omega_0 t} \tag{6.23}$$

The coefficients are found as

$$D_n = \frac{1}{T}\int_0^{t_0} A e^{-jn\omega_0 t}\,dt = \frac{A}{T}\left[\frac{1-e^{-jn\omega_0 t_0}}{jn\omega_0}\right]$$

$$= \frac{A}{T} e^{-\frac{jn\omega_0 t_0}{2}}\left[\frac{e^{\frac{jn\omega_0 t_0}{2}} - e^{-\frac{jn\omega_0 t_0}{2}}}{jn\omega_0}\right]$$

$$= \frac{2A}{T} e^{-\frac{jn\omega_0 t_0}{2}}\left(\frac{1}{n\omega_0}\right)\left(\frac{1}{2j}\right)\left(e^{\frac{jn\omega_0 t_0}{2}} - e^{-\frac{jn\omega_0 t_0}{2}}\right)$$

$$= \frac{2A}{T} e^{-\frac{jn\omega_0 t_0}{2}}\left(\frac{1}{n\omega_0}\right)\sin\left(\frac{n\omega_0 t_0}{2}\right)$$

after conversion to sine functions using Euler's Identity.

$$\sin x = \left(\frac{1}{2j}\right)\left(e^{jx} - e^{-jx}\right) \tag{6.24}$$

Hence, the coefficients in Eq. (6.23) $D_n$ expressed in fundamental frequency $\omega_0$ are

$$D_n = \frac{At_0}{T} e^{-\frac{jn\omega_0 t_0}{2}}\left(\frac{1}{n\omega_0 t_0/2}\right)\sin\left(\frac{n\omega_0 t_0}{2}\right) \tag{6.25}$$

For $\omega_0 = \frac{2\pi}{T}$, the coefficients $D_n$ can be written as

$$D_n = \frac{At_0}{T}\left[e^{-n\pi t_0/T}\left(\frac{1}{n\pi t_0/T}\right)\sin\left(\frac{n\pi t_0}{T}\right)\right] \tag{6.26}$$

The coefficients $D_n$ in Eqs. (6.23), (6.25), and (6.26) are expressed in fundamental frequency $\omega_0$.

### 6.2.2 Time Shifting and Scaling Properties of the Fourier Series

The time-shifting property of the Fourier series decomposition or the representation of signals has useful implications in its application.

The **time-shifting** property reveals that shifting a signal by $t_o$ changes the spectrum or phase distribution (the exponential factor $e^{-jn\omega_0 t}$) by $\omega_0 t_0$, that is, a linear phase shift in its spectrum. However, the amplitude spectrum does not change its distribution or spectrum. The process is shown next.

For

$$f(t)=\sum_{n=-\infty}^{\infty}a_n e^{jn\omega_0 t},\quad a_n=\frac{1}{T}\int_T f(t)e^{-jn\omega_0 t}dt \tag{6.27}$$

and a time shifting $(t-t_0)$ such that

$$g(t)=f(t-t_0)=\sum_{n=-\infty}^{\infty}b_n e^{jn\omega_0 t} \tag{6.28}$$

$$b_n=\frac{1}{T}\int_T g(t)e^{-jn\omega_0 t}dt=\frac{1}{T}\int_T f(t-t_0)e^{-jn\omega_0 t}dt$$

$$=e^{-jn\omega_0 t_0}\frac{1}{T}\int_T f(t')e^{-jn\omega_0 t'}dt'$$

By letting

$$t'=t-t_0;\ dt'=dt$$

and rewriting

$$b_n=e^{-jn\omega_0 t_0}a_n$$

$$g(t)=\sum_{n=-\infty}^{\infty}e^{-jn\omega_0 t_0}\left[a_n\right]e^{jn\omega_0 t} \tag{6.29}$$

Thus, shifting a signal in time by $t_o$ changes by a factor of $e^{-jn\omega_0 t_0}$, or an equivalent linear phase shift of $n\omega_0 t_0$.

The **time-scaling** property indicates that in the time compression of a signal by a factor of $k$, the frequency varies faster, resulting in its spectral expansion by a factor of $k$ varying more slowly. Likewise, time expansion of the signal results in its spectral compression. If a signal expanded in time, then the frequency of its Fourier components are lowered, implying that its frequency spectrum is compressed.

## 6.3 THE IMPULSE FUNCTION AS A SIGNAL

The impulse function is one of the most important functions in the study of systems and signals (Figure 6.2). It is defined as,

$$\delta(t)=\begin{cases}\to\infty, & t=0\\ 0, & t\neq 0\end{cases} \tag{6.30}$$

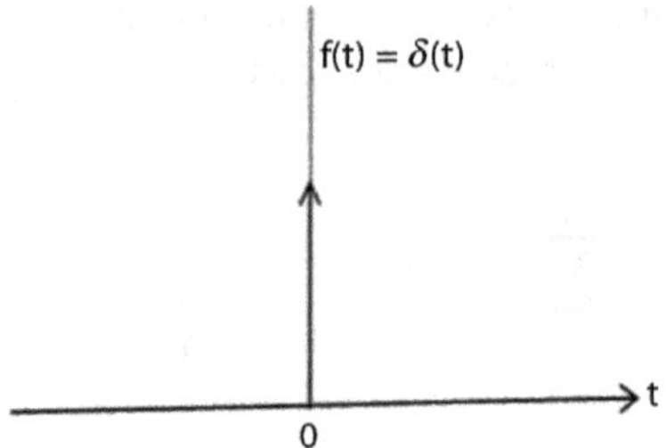


**FIGURE 6.2** The impulse function.

and

$$\int_{-\infty}^{\infty} \delta(t)dt = 1 \tag{6.31}$$

So, $\delta(t) = 0$ is equal to zero everywhere except at $t = 0$, where it is defined as infinite but with a unit area. Thus, it is often called the unit impulse. The importance and usefulness of the unit impulse function becomes evident from the following operations when it is multiplied by another function $f(t)$, known to be continuous at $t = 0$. Since $\delta(t)$ exists only at $t = 0$, and the value of $f(t)$ at $t = 0$ is f(0), we have

$$f(t)\delta(t) = f(0)\delta(t) \tag{6.32}$$

Similarly, if $\delta(t)$ is shifted or delayed in time to $t - T$ for $\delta(t - T)$, then

$$f(t)\delta(t-T) = f(T)\delta(t-T) \tag{6.33}$$

provided $f(t)$ is continuous at $t = T$.

### 6.3.1 Fourier Series for an Impulse Train

The Fourier series for an impulse train (Figure 6.3) is given by

$$f(t) = \delta(t) = \sum_{n=-\infty}^{\infty} D_n e^{jn\omega_0 t}, \; \omega_0 = \frac{2\pi}{T}$$

with

$$D_n = \frac{1}{T} \int_{-\frac{T}{2}}^{\frac{T}{2}} \delta(t) e^{-jn\omega_0 t} dt = \frac{1}{T}.$$

The value of $D_n$ is shown in Figure 6.4, which is also a representation of the spectrum associated with the Fourier series for an impulse train. It can be seen that

$$\delta(t) = \frac{1}{T} \sum_{-\infty}^{\infty} e^{jn\omega_0 t}, \; \omega_0 = \frac{2\pi}{T} \tag{6.34}$$

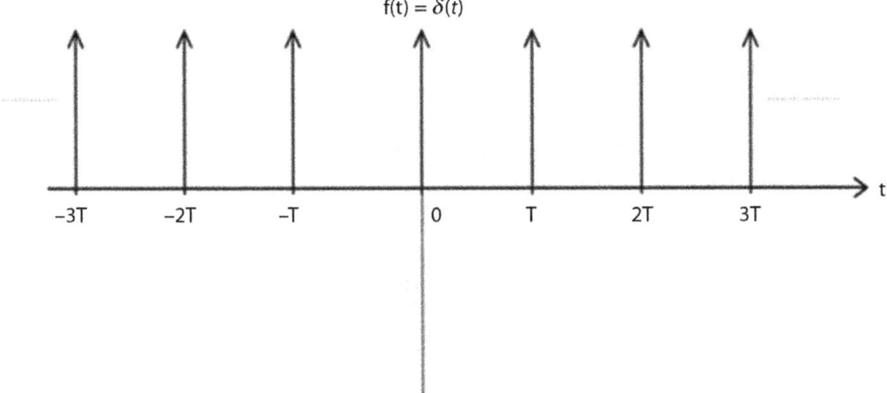


**FIGURE 6.3** An impulse train, $f(t) = \delta(t)$ with a period, $T$.

### 6.3.2 Sifting or Sampling Property of the Unit $\delta(t)$ Function

For any function $f(t)$ continuous at $(t_0)$, the sampling or sifting property provides,

$$\int_{-\infty}^{\infty} f(t)\delta(t-t_0)dt = f(t_0) \tag{6.35}$$

This is a very useful property, and it demonstrates an important property of the unit impulse function, δ(t) from Eqs. (6.31) and (6.32) that,

$$\int_{-\infty}^{\infty} f(t)\delta(t)dt = f(0)\int_{-\infty}^{\infty}\delta(t)dt = f(0) \tag{6.36}$$

since $\int_{-\infty}^{\infty}\delta(t)dt = 1$. Also, it follows from Eq. (6.33) that,

$$\int_{-\infty}^{\infty} f(t)\delta(t-T)dt = f(T) \tag{6.37}$$

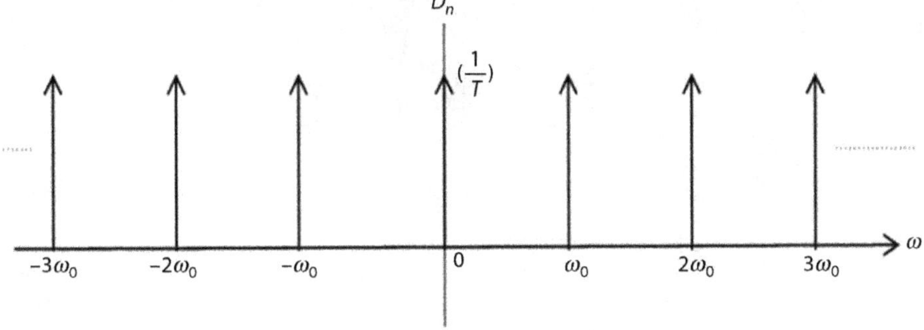


**FIGURE 6.4** The spectrum of Fourier series for an impulse train.

where $f(t)$ is continuous at $t = T$. This is another statement of the sampling or sifting property of the unit impulse function. Therefore, the area under the curve, $f(t)\delta(t-T)$ is the value of $f(t=T)$.

## 6.4 MULTIPLICATION PROPERTY OF FOURIER SERIES

The Fourier series representation of two signals $f(t)$ and $g(t)$ are given as

$$f(t)=\sum_{n} a_n e^{jn\omega_0 t}, \quad g(t)=\sum_{m} b_m e^{jm\omega_0 t} \tag{6.38}$$

The product of these two signals $y(t)$ is given by

$$y(t)=f(t)g(t)=\sum_{k} c_k e^{jk\omega_0 t} \tag{6.39}$$

and

$$c_k=\frac{1}{T}\int_{T} y(t)e^{-jk\omega_0 t}dt=\frac{1}{T}\int_{T} f(t)g(t)e^{-jk\omega_0 t}dt$$

$$=\frac{1}{T}\int_{T}\sum_{n} a_n e^{jn\omega_0 t}\sum_{m} b_m e^{jm\omega_0 t}e^{-jk\omega_0 t}dt$$

$$=\frac{1}{T}\int_{T}\sum_{n}\sum_{m} e^{j(n+m)\omega_0 t}e^{-jk\omega_0 t}dt\left[a_n b_m\right]$$

Rearranging and from linearity

$$=\frac{1}{T}\sum_{n}\sum_{m} a_n b_m\int_{T} e^{j[(n+m)-k]\omega_0 t}dt$$

and for $\delta[\{k-(n+m)\}\omega_0]=\frac{1}{T}\int_T e^{j[(n+m)-k]\omega_0 t}dt$,

$$c_k=\sum_{n}\sum_{m} a_n b_m\delta\left[\{k-(n+m)\}\right]\omega_0$$

$$=\sum_{n} a_n b_{k-n} \tag{6.40}$$

after noting the identities:

$$k-n-m=0, \quad m=k-n, \quad \delta(\omega)=\delta(\omega)e^{j\omega t}$$

## 6.5 IMPULSE RESPONSE OF A LINEAR SYSTEM

A linear system shown in block diagram form in Figure 6.5 can be represented by a linear operator $L$, such that the output $g(t)$ in response to an input $f(t)$ is given by

$$g(t) = L\left[f(t)\right] \tag{6.41}$$

Using the sifting property Eq. (6.35)

$$g(t) = L\left[\int_{-\infty}^{\infty} f(t')\delta(t'-t)dt'\right] \tag{6.42}$$

From linearity, Eq. (6.42) can be rewritten as,

$$g(t) = \int_{-\infty}^{\infty} f(t')L\left[\delta(t'-t)\right]dt' \tag{6.43}$$

where the impulse response, $h(t)$ can be recognized as given by,

$$L\left[\delta(t'-t)\right] = h(t) \tag{6.44}$$

Thus, Eq. (6.42) may be expressed in terms of $h(t)$, such that

$$g(t) = \int_{-\infty}^{\infty} f(t')h(t'-t)dt' \tag{6.45}$$

The impulse response $h(t)$ from a linear system is typically straightforward to obtain.

Eq. (6.45) is a superposition integral. It shows that the output $g(t)$ is a linear superposition of input $f(t)$ for all values of $(t)$. Specifically, the output $g(t)$ is a result of convolution of the input $f(t)$ with the impulse response of the linear system $h(t)$. Therefore, once the impulse response is known for a sensing system, one can find the output to any input excitation by way of a convolution integral.

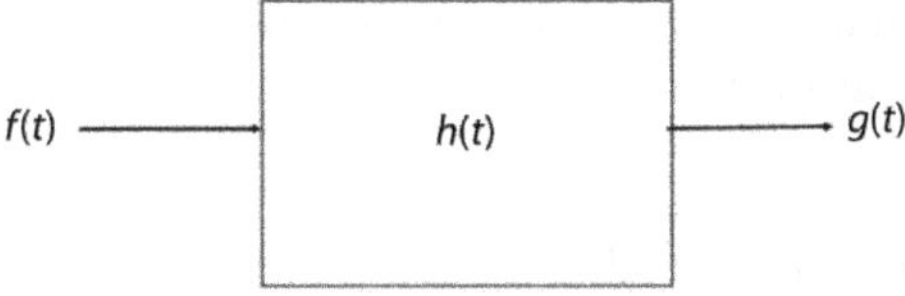


**FIGURE 6.5** The input $f(t)$ and output $g(t)$ of a linear system $h(t)$ in block diagram form.

## 6.6 FOURIER TRANSFORMS

The concept of Fourier decomposition of periodic signals may be extended to aperiodic signals through a process called Fourier transform. In this case, an aperiodic time-domain signal is represented by a continuum of complex exponential functions in the frequency domain. The Fourier-transformed signals provide a direct measure of the frequency content and bandwidth of the time domain signal. Fourier transform technique can greatly facilitate or even simplify the analysis of signals and systems by operating in the frequency domain.

The required and sufficient mathematical conditions on $f(t)$ for its Fourier transform to exist are:

1. $f(t)$ is sectionally continuous and has a finite number of finite discontinuities in any finite time interval.
2. $f(t)$ is absolutely integrable over time $t$,

$$i.e., \int_{-\infty}^{\infty} |f(t)| < \infty. \tag{6.46}$$

The Fourier transform $F(\omega)$ is defined by the Fourier integral

$$F(\omega) = \mathcal{F}[f(t)] = \int_{-\infty}^{\infty} f(t) e^{-j\omega t} \, dt \tag{6.47}$$

where $\mathcal{F}[f(t)]$ designates the Fourier transform operation on $f(t)$. An inverse Fourier transform operation is applied to recover the time domain signal as defined by

$$f(t) = \mathcal{F}^{-1}[\omega] = \frac{1}{2\pi} \int_{-\infty}^{\infty} F(\omega) e^{j\omega t} \, d\omega \tag{6.48}$$

where $\omega$ is the angular or radian frequency. The functions $f(t)$ and $F(\omega)$ in Eqs. (6.46) and (6.47) are called Fourier transform pairs. The same information is contained in the Fourier transform pairs. In practice, a Fourier transform pair exists for any physically generated signals.

### 6.6.1 Fourier Transform Properties and Relations

Several Fourier transform operations occurring more frequently in signal and systems analysis have established operations both in time and frequency domains. The more commonly encountered properties and relationships are described to further the utility of Fourier transform operations.

#### Linearity

If $A$ and $B$ are constants, then

$$\mathcal{F}[Af(t) + Bg(t)] = A\mathcal{F}[f(t)] + B\mathcal{F}[g(t)] \tag{6.49}$$

The transforms of the weighted sum of two functions are the weighted sum of their individual transforms.

### Translation

$$\mathcal{F}\left[f(t-t_0)\right]=F(\omega)e^{j(\omega t_0)} \tag{6.50}$$

The translation of a function in the time domain introduces a linear phase shift in the frequency domain. For example, a delay in the time domain corresponds to the introduction of a phase shift in the frequency domain that varies linearly with frequency.

### Reciprocal translation

$$\mathcal{F}\left[f(t)e^{-j(\omega_0 t)}\right]=F(\omega+\omega_0) \tag{6.51}$$

Conversely, a translation in the frequency domain introduces a linear phase shift in the time domain.

### Magnification or scale change

$$\mathcal{F}\left[f(at)\right]=\frac{1}{|a|}F\left(\frac{\omega}{a}\right) \tag{6.52}$$

The expansion in time domain results in a proportionate contraction in the frequency domain along with a change in the amplitude of the spectrum by a constant scaling factor.

### Symmetry about time origin

Any time function can be considered as being made of an even and an odd part, with the evenness and oddness being determined relative to the time origin. Thus,

a. If $f(t)$ is real, i.e. $f^*(t)=f(t)$ (6.53)

then

$$F^*(-\omega)=F(\omega) \tag{6.54}$$

$$F^*(\omega)=F(-\omega) \tag{6.55}$$

b. $f(t)$ is real and even,
then

$$f(t)=f^*(t)=f^*(-t) \tag{6.56}$$

$$F(\omega)=F^*(-\omega)=F^*(\omega) \tag{6.57}$$

c. $f(t)$ is real, but odd,
then

$$f(t)=f^*(t)=-f(-t) \tag{6.58}$$

$$F(\omega)=-F(-\omega)=F^*(-\omega) \tag{6.59}$$

These relations are useful in determining time functions from their spectra and vice versa.

**Separable function**
If a function $f(t,t')$ is separable such that

$$f(t,t')=f(t)f(t') \tag{6.60}$$

then

$$\mathcal{F}\left[f(t,t')\right]=\mathcal{F}\left[f(t)f(t')\right]=F(\omega,\omega') \tag{6.61}$$

and

$$\mathcal{F}\left[f(t,t')\right]=F(\omega)F(\omega')=F(\omega,\omega') \tag{6.62}$$

These simple relationships can facilitate evaluation of Fourier transforms.

**Time differentiation**

$$\mathcal{F}\left[\frac{d^n}{dt^n}f(t)\right]=(j\omega)^n F(\omega) \tag{6.63}$$

Differentiation in the time domain leads to multiplication by $j\omega$ in the frequency domain, indicating a process that tends to emphasize the higher frequency components.

**Time integration**

$$\mathcal{F}\left[\int_{-\infty}^{t} f(t)dt\right]=\frac{1}{j\omega}F(\omega)+\pi\, F(0)\delta(\omega) \tag{6.64}$$

Integration in the time domain results in enhancement of the lower frequencies in the frequency domain.

**Convolution**
If

$$\mathcal{F}\left[f(t)\right]=F(\omega)$$

$$\mathcal{F}\left[g(t)\right]=G(\omega)$$

the Fourier transform of the convolution integral of the two functions $f(t)$ *and* $g(t)$ is given by

$$\mathcal{F}\left\{\int_{-\infty}^{\infty} f(t)g(t'-t)dt\right\} = F(\omega)G(\omega) \tag{6.65}$$

or

$$\mathcal{F}\left[f(t) * g(t)\right] = F(\omega)G(\omega) \tag{6.66}$$

where * denotes convolution operation between $f(t)$ *and* $g(t)$. Thus, the convolution of two functions in time domain is equivalent to simply multiplying their spectra in the frequency domain. This relationship is fundamental in signal and system analysis because the output of the system is the result of convolution of the input with the impulse response of the linear system. The results shown in Eqs. (6.65) and (6.66) suggest that the output is obtained simply through multiplication of the spectra of the input signal and impulse response of the system in the frequency domain. In this process, it converts the convolution operation from complex calculus to elementary algebraic manipulation.

Closely related to convolution is the process of correlation. In general, correlation gives the expected or mean value of the product between two signals or functions.

## Autocorrelation

If two functions describe the same process, the autocorrelation function is defined as

$$R(t) = \int_{-\infty}^{\infty} f(t)f^{*}(t'+t)dt \tag{6.67}$$

where $f^{*}(t)$ is the complex conjugate of $f(t)$, and

$$\mathcal{F}\left[R(t)\right] = \mathcal{F}\left[\int_{-\infty}^{\infty} f(t)f^{*}(t'+t)dt\right] = \left|F(\omega)\right|^{2} \tag{6.68}$$

Let ** denote correlation operation, then

$$\mathcal{F}\left[R(t)\right] = \mathcal{F}\left[f(t) ** f^{*}(t)\right] = \left|F(\omega)\right|^{2} \tag{6.69}$$

Conversely,

$$\mathcal{F}^{-1}\left[\left|F(\omega)\right|^{2}\right] = R(t) \tag{6.70}$$

The autocorrelation $R(t)$ can be thought of as a measure of similarity of the signal $f(t)$ and the signal $f(t'+t)$. Note that the largest autocorrelation function value always occurs at $t' = 0$.

**Cross correlation**

The cross correlation between two functions $f(t)$ and $g(t)$ is defined by

$$\int_{-\infty}^{\infty} f(t)g^*(t'+t)dt \tag{6.71}$$

Then

$$\mathcal{F}\left[\int_{-\infty}^{\infty} f(t)g^*(t'+t)dt\right] = F(\omega)G^*(\omega) \tag{6.72}$$

or

$$\mathcal{F}\left[f(t)**g^*(t)\right] = F(\omega)G^*(\omega) \tag{6.73}$$

The cross correlation provides a measure of how much two functions depend on one another. Indeed, the specific cross correlation between system input and output takes on a very important physical meaning and significance in system analysis. For example, if $f(t)$ is the transmitted microwave signal and $g(t)$ is the reflected (received) signal from a biological target, a strong cross correlation for some value of $(t')$ will signify not only the presence of a target but also define a relative time shift of the reflected signal $g(t)$ with respect to the transmitted signal, $f(t)$. For a known speed of microwave propagation, the time shift will produce a measure of the distance (range) of the target from the transmitting source.

## 6.7 SYMMETRY OF FOURIER TRANSFORMS

The equations defining direct (Eq. 6.46) and inverse (Eq. 6.47) Fourier transform operations are very similar, suggesting a close relationship between the transform of a function in $t$ and the inverse transform of that same function in $\omega$. Thus, if

$$\mathcal{F}\left[f(t)\right] = F(\omega) \tag{6.74}$$

then

$$F(t) = \mathcal{F}^{-1}\left[f(-\omega)\right] = 2\pi\, f(-\omega) \tag{6.75}$$

These properties can be used to gain further insights into corresponding time and frequency representation of signals and systems. As an example, consider the time function for a transform that is constant over a specified frequency band and zero elsewhere, as shown in Figure 6.6. The transform is a rectangular pulse of width $t_0$

(a)

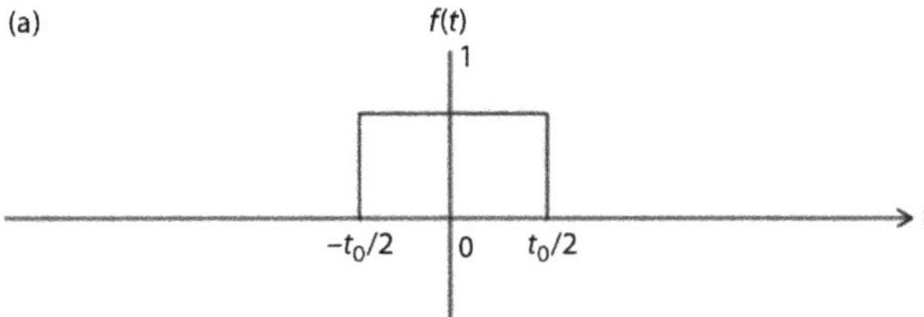


(b)

(c)

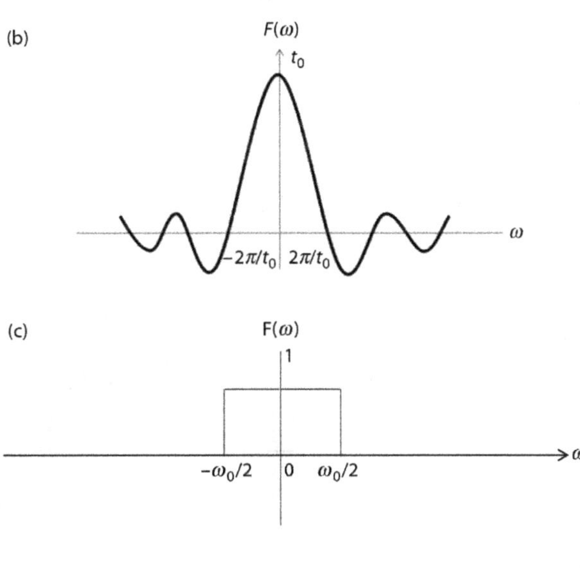


(d)

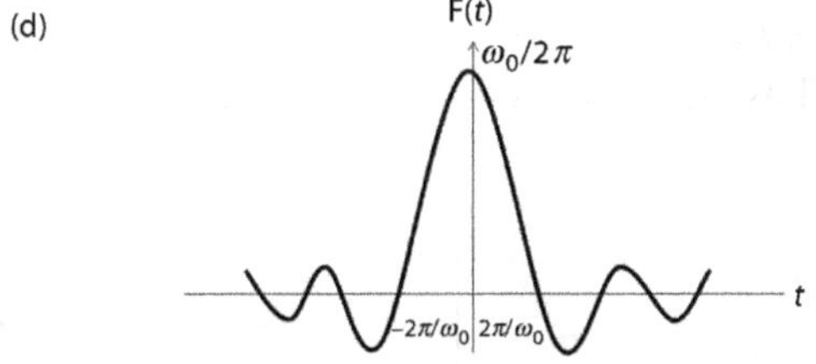


**FIGURE 6.6** An illustration of the symmetry of Fourier transform pairs: (a) rect (t), (b) Fourier transform of rect (t), spectrum with constant over a specific frequency band and zero elsewhere, and (d) time function or inverse transform of (c).

and unit *or* $2\pi$ amplitude, as the case may be (see Table 6.1). The phase function is assumed to be zero. The Fourier transform of rect (t) is given by

$$\mathcal{F}[f(t)] = \mathcal{F}\left[rect(t) = \begin{cases} 1, |t| \le \frac{1}{2}t_0 \\ 0, \textit{otherwise} \end{cases}\right] = t_0 sinc\left(\frac{\omega t_0}{2}\right) = t_0 \frac{\sin\left(\frac{\omega t_0}{2}\right)}{\left(\frac{\omega t_0}{2}\right)} = F(\omega) \tag{6.76}$$

**TABLE 6.1**
**Fourier Transform Pairs of Common and Specialized Functions**

| Time Function | Fourier Transform |
|---|---|
| $\delta(t)$ | $1$ |
| $1$ | $2\pi\delta(\omega)$ |
| $\sin\omega_0 t$ | $j\pi\lfloor\delta(\omega+\omega_0)-\delta(\omega-\omega_0)\rfloor$ |
| $\cos\omega_0 t$ | $\pi\lfloor\delta(\omega+\omega_0)+\delta(\omega-\omega_0)\rfloor$ |
| $e^{j\omega_0 t}$ | $2\pi\delta(\omega-\omega_0)$ |
| $rect(t)=\begin{cases}1, & \lvert t\rvert\le\frac{1}{2}t_0\\ 0, & otherwise\end{cases}$ | $t_0 sinc\left(\frac{\omega t_0}{2}\right)=t_0\frac{\sin\left(\frac{\omega t_0}{2}\right)}{\left(\frac{\omega t_0}{2}\right)}$ |
| $\wedge(t)=\begin{cases}1-\frac{2\lvert t\rvert}{t_0}, & \lvert t\rvert<\frac{t_0}{2}\\ 0, & otherwise\end{cases}$ | $\frac{t_0}{2}sinc^2\left(\frac{\omega t_0}{4}\right)$ |
| $circ(t)=\begin{cases}1, & t\le 1\\ 0, & otherwise\end{cases}$ | $\frac{2\pi}{\omega}J_1(\omega)$, Bessels function |
| $Gaussian=a^2e^{-a^2t^2}$ | $e^{-\frac{\omega^2}{a^2}}$ |

The corresponding inverse transform can be found directly from Eq. (6.75). In this case, $F(\omega)$ is the same as $F(t)$ with t replaced by $\omega$, and $f(-\omega)$ is the same as $f(t)$ with $t$ replaced by $-\omega$. Thus, the symmetry property produces

$$F(t)=t_0 sinc\left(\frac{tt_0}{2}\right)=\left[t_0\frac{\sin\left(\frac{tt_0}{2}\right)}{\left(\frac{tt_0}{2}\right)}\right]=\mathcal{F}^{-1}\left[rect(-\omega)\right]=2\pi\ f(\omega) \tag{6.77}$$

Note the use of $rect(-t)=rect(t)$ because $rect(t)$ is an even function. Figure 6.6 shows graphically the symmetry property for this pair. Note that the impulse response depicted clearly shows that this is not a physically realizable system because the input occurs prior to the application of the input. One way to approximate the ideal filter response is to employ a system having a response in the form of Figure 6.6, but delayed in time. The greater the delay, the more nearly the shape of Figure 6.6 can be reproduced by a physically realizable filter. The effect of the delay in the frequency domain is to produce a phase shift that varies linearly with frequency.

## 6.8 SYSTEM TRANSFER FUNCTION

A general linear system is shown schematically in Figure 6.5. The output $g(t)$ is given by the convolution of the input signal $f(t)$ and the impulse response $h(t)$ of the time-invariant linear system.

$$g(t) = \int_{-\infty}^{\infty} f(t)h(t'-t)dt' \tag{6.78}$$

The Fourier transform of the convolution integral according to Eq. (6.65) yields

$$G(\omega) = F(\omega)H(\omega) \tag{6.79}$$

where $G(\omega)$ is the Fourier transform of output $g(t)$ given by the product of two Fourier transforms (see Figure 6.7) $F(\omega)$ and $H(\omega)$of input $f(t)$, and impulse response of the system $h(t)$. Eq. (6.75) can be rearranged in the form of a ratio

$$H(\omega) = \frac{G(\omega)}{F(\omega)} \tag{6.80}$$

The function $H(\omega)$ is called a system transfer function and it can be provided by the Fourier transform of impulse response of the system $h(t)$. It is a mathematical model obtained by the solution of the equations representing the system. In general, $H(\omega)$has finite amplitude and phase variations. The concept of the system transfer function is valuable in the analysis of systems and the use of it often simplifies the computation of system response.

## 6.9 SAMPLING OF CONTINUOUS SIGNALS

So far, the discussions have been concerned only with signals that are continuous functions of time. These are signals that are explicitly defined for every instant in time. In signal analysis and processing, it is useful and convenient to represent continuous signals as sampled signals. In this case, a sampled signal is derived from a continuous signal by obtaining its values at a set of equally spaced time intervals. Intuitively, one would expect to obtain a more accurate representation if the sampled values were taken at more closely spaced time intervals, and that an exact description would require that the instants between samples approach zero. However, it can be shown that for band-limited signals, an exact description of the continuous signal can be obtained from samples taken with nonzero sampling intervals. A band-limited signal is one for which the Fourier transform is identically zero everywhere,

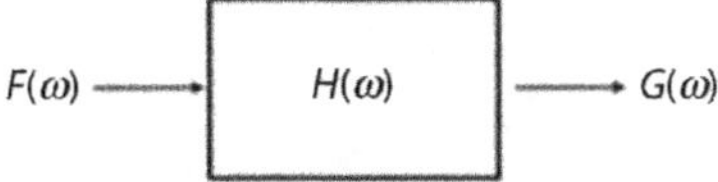


**FIGURE 6.7** The system transfer function for a generalized linear system.

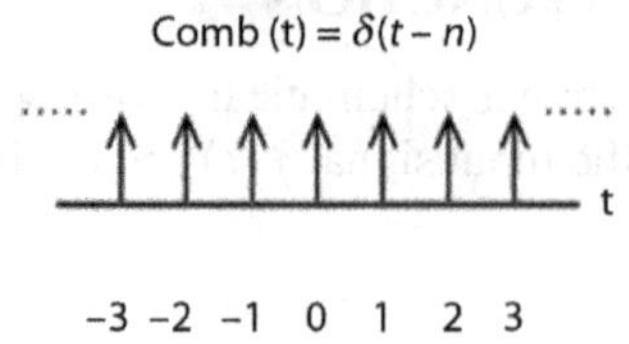

Comb (t) = δ(t − n)

−3 −2 −1 0 1 2 3 t

**FIGURE 6.8** An impulse train: comb function.

except for a finite range of frequencies. In practice, there is always some range of frequencies outside of which the spectral amplitude is negligibly small, so that it can be assumed as zero. The **sampling theorem** provides the conditions under which sampled values completely define a continuous function.

Let

$$f_c(t) = comb(t) \tag{6.81}$$

If this comb function (Figure 6.8) is used to sample a band-limited signal $f(t)$, then the resultant sampled signal is the product of these two functions:

$$f_s(t) = f(t)f_c(t) = f(t)[comb(t)] \tag{6.82}$$

The Fourier transform of a comb function is another comb function such that

$$\mathcal{F}[comb(t)] = comb(\omega) \tag{6.83}$$

For $\delta$ function separated by $t_0$,

$$f_s(t) = f(t)f_c(t) = f(t)\left[comb\left(\frac{t}{t_0}\right)\right] \tag{6.84}$$

This is the resultant sampled signal. The spectrum of the sampled signal is given by

$$F_s(\omega) = F(\omega) * comb(\omega) \tag{6.85}$$

where

$$\mathcal{F}\left[comb\left(\frac{t}{t_0}\right)\right] = t_0 comb(t_0\omega) \tag{6.86}$$

and

$$t_0 comb(t_0\omega) = \sum_{n=-\infty}^{\infty} \delta\left(\omega - \frac{n}{t_0}\right) \tag{6.87}$$

Therefore,

$$F_s(\omega) = \sum_{n=-\infty}^{\infty} F\left(\omega - \frac{n}{t_0}\right) \tag{6.88}$$

$F_s(\omega)$ is a summation of shifted replicas of $F(\omega)$. Since $f(t)$ is band limited,

Then
$$F(\omega)=0, \; for \; |\omega|>\omega_{max} \tag{6.89}$$

The replicas of $F(\omega)$ will not overlap if the frequency,

$$\frac{1}{t_0}=2\omega_{max} \tag{6.90}$$

Thus, if the sampling rate ($\frac{1}{t_0}$) is at least twice the maximum frequency of the signal, $F(\omega)$ will not overlap according to Eq. (6.90), which is known as the Nyquist criterion.

A single replica of $F(\omega)$ can be isolated through a low-pass filtration operation with the transfer function

$$H(\omega)=rect(t_0\omega) \tag{6.91}$$

The output spectrum

$$G(\omega)=F_s(\omega)H(\omega)=\frac{F(\omega)}{t_0} \tag{6.92}$$

which gives the original image by inverse Fourier transformation,

$$\mathcal{F}^{-1}\{F(\omega)=t_0\;G(\omega)\}=f(t) \tag{6.93}$$

or

$$\begin{aligned} g(t) &= f(t)\left[comb\left(\frac{t}{t_0}\right)\right]*h(t) \\ &= t_0\sum_{n=-\infty}^{\infty} f(nt_0)\delta(t-nt_0)*\left(\frac{1}{t_0}\right)sinc\left(\frac{t}{t_0}\right) \end{aligned} \tag{6.94}$$

and

$$g(t)=\sum_{n=-\infty}^{\infty} f(nt_0)sinc\left[\frac{1}{t_0}(t-nt_0)\right] \tag{6.95}$$

Therefore,

$$f(t)=g(t) \tag{6.96}$$

The sampling relation provides an exact procedure for reconstructing any band-limited signal from its values at a discrete set of sampling points.

In summary, according to the sampling theorem, a signal whose spectrum is band limited to $\omega_{max}$ can be reconstructed exactly from samples taken uniformly at a rate greater than $\omega_{max}$, or more precisely, at a minimum rate of 2 $\omega_{max}$.

### 6.9.1 Aliasing from Undersampling

Aliasing occurs when an inadequate number of samples are taken from a continuous signal. This can happen in principle because all time functions are of finite duration, are not band limited, and potentially can possess infinite bandwidth. Thus, regardless of the sampling rate, it would fall short of that required by the Nyquist criterion. The lost frequency tail would show as a frequency component lower than the one-half of the sampling frequency and folded into the reconstructed spectrum. The folded components reappear, aliased, as lower-frequency distortion. In general, aliasing may be reduced by the use of antialiasing filters with a sharp high-frequency cutoff (a low-pass filter) prior to any sampling operation. However, in practice, real signals are always band limited; aliasing distortion typically occurs due to undersampling. For example, if $f_s(t) = 100$ Hz for a continuous-time physical signal with an upper-frequency limit of 120 Hz, aliasing distortion will occur. A physical signal with a frequency of 20 Hz, when sampled at the 100-Hz rate is indistinguishable from a signal with a frequency of 120 Hz, when sampled at the same rate. The signal reconstruction process uses frequencies within the band of $f_s(t)/6$. The reconstructed signal will have a 20 Hz lower frequency component, corresponding to $f(t) - f_s(t) = 120 - 100 = 20$ Hz folded signal, appearing as an aliasing distortion.

### 6.9.2 Quantization of Sampled Signals

Sampling of continuous functions enables digitization of continuous-time signals by a discrete sequence of numbers, which leads to the topic of digital signal processing. The quantization of sampled values of signals allows processing discrete sequences of numbers equivalent to processing continuous-time signals, if not more efficiently. A continuous function as an analog signal can assume an infinite number of minute amplitudes over a continuous range of values. An analog signal is converted to a digital signal (for example by using A-to-D converter hardware) via sampling and digitization. The amplitude of digital signals can take on only a finite number of assigned values. The binary digital signal is commonly used where the signal can have only two values (0 or 1). In this case, the binary digit is called a bit by combining and contracting the two words.

The most popular is the natural binary in fractional binary form

$$N = a_1 2^{-1} + a_2 2^{-2} + a_3 2^{-3} + \cdots + a_n 2^{-n} \tag{6.97}$$

where $a_n = 0 \; or \; 1$, and n is the resolution level. For example, the analog number 0.625 may be represented by $n = 4$ (1010) as a number with 4-bit resolution

$$0.625 = 1 \times 2^{-1} + 0 \times 2^{-2} + 1 \times 2^{-3} + 0 \times 2^{-4} \tag{6.98}$$

Analog output is quantized to digital values of $2^n$ binary states; each state will have an analog value $D$ of

$$D = \frac{\textit{Full Scale Range}}{2^n} \tag{6.99}$$

For this example, $n = 4$; $2^n = 2^4$, and there are 16 states with 4-bit resolution.

The uncertainty introduced by the process of quantization of an analog signal, the quantization error, can be as large as $\pm D/6$. It is a source of noise infused into the signal with zero mean but a root mean square value of $\frac{D}{\sqrt{12}}$ for this example. This noise cannot be eliminated but can be reduced by using higher levels of resolution. Specifically, the signal-to-noise ratio (SNR) is given by

$$SNR = \frac{2^n D}{\left(\frac{D}{\sqrt{12}}\right)} = 2^{n+1}\sqrt{3} \tag{6.100}$$

or, in the relative scales,

$$SNR(dB) = 20\log\left[\frac{2^n D}{\left(\frac{D}{\sqrt{12}}\right)}\right] = 6.02n + 10.8 \tag{6.101}$$

Accordingly, the SNR can be increased by 6.02 dB for each additional bit of resolution.

## 6.10 OPTIMAL DETECTION USING MATCHED FILTER

Matched filters are a class of filters that are exceedingly important and powerful tools in signal analysis and processing. They are linear systems with impulse responses that are tuned to the input signal to produce the maximum output signal. The purpose of this discussion is to introduce the basic ideas.

An application in which matched filters have played a pivotal role is radar systems. The fundamental notion of radar is that a microwave pulse transmitted at a target is reflected by the target and will return to the sender a signal with a delay proportional to the distance to the target. Ideally, the received signal will simply be a scaled and shifted version of the original transmitted signal. Thus, the operation of a simple radar system is based on using a matched filter with transmitted waveform and noting the time at which the output of the system reaches its maximum value. In practice, it is a problem of signal detection in the presence of additive noise.

Let the input to the filter be a signal $s(t)$ plus noise $n(t)$

$$f(t) = s(t) + n(t),\ s(t) \text{ is a known function} \tag{6.102}$$

The output of filter $g(t)$ is given by the convolution of the input signal $f(t)$ with the impulse response of the filter $h(t)$

$$g(t) = f(t) * h(t) \tag{6.103}$$

The filter is to produce a spike response when a signal is present at arbitrary time $t = t_1$. Thus, the design criteria for the filter is to maximize the SNR at time $t = t_1$, such that

$$Max\ [SNR] = \frac{\left[s(t_1) * h(t_1)\right]^2}{\sigma_n^2} \tag{6.104}$$

where the numerator is proportional to signal power and the denominator is the mean squared noise power of the output,

$$\sigma_n^2 = \overline{\left[n(t_1) * h(t_1)\right]^2} \tag{6.105}$$

The noise from filters and most system components of interest such as amplifiers and transducers is assumed to follow a Gaussian probability density function, and $\sigma_n^2$ represents the variance of the Gaussian with zero mean.

For stationary noise, $\sigma_n^2$ can be expressed in frequency domain as

$$\sigma_n^2 = \int_{-\infty}^{\infty} N^2(\omega)\left|H(\omega)\right|^2 d\omega \tag{6.106}$$

and $\sigma_n^2$ can be expressed in frequency domain for white noise as

$$\sigma_n^2 = N^2(\omega)\int_{-\infty}^{\infty} \left|H(\omega)\right|^2 d\omega \tag{6.107}$$

and

$$\left[s(t_1) * h(t_1)\right]^2 = \left|\int_{-\infty}^{\infty} S(\omega)H(\omega)e^{j\omega t_1} d\omega\right|^2 \tag{6.108}$$

Therefore,

$$SNR = \frac{\left|\int_{-\infty}^{\infty} S(\omega)H(\omega)e^{j\omega t_1} d\omega\right|^2}{N^2(\omega)\int_{-\infty}^{\infty} \left|H(\omega)\right|^2 d\omega} \tag{6.109}$$

Normalizing the top and bottom by total signal power $\int_{-\infty}^{\infty} |S(\omega)|^2\, d\omega$ and noise power spectrum $N^2(\omega)$

$$SNR = \frac{\left|\int_{-\infty}^{\infty} S(\omega)H(\omega)e^{j\omega t_1} d\omega\right|^2}{\left[\int_{-\infty}^{\infty} \left|S(\omega)\right|^2 d\omega\right]\left[\int_{-\infty}^{\infty} \left|H(\omega)\right|^2 d\omega\right]} \tag{6.110}$$

The objective is to maximize the SNR of Eq. (6.110). From the Schwarz inequality,

$$\frac{\left|\int_{-\infty}^{\infty} f(x)g(x)dx\right|^2}{\left[\int_{-\infty}^{\infty} |f(x)|^2 dx\right]\left[\int_{-\infty}^{\infty} |g(x)|^2 dx\right]} \le 1 \quad (6.111)$$

which holds only if $f(x)$ is proportional to $g^*(x)$. Let $f = H$, $g = \mathcal{S}e^{j\omega t_1}$, and for Max [SNR]

$$H(\omega) = A\mathcal{S}^*(\omega)e^{-j\omega t_1} \quad (6.112)$$

where $e^{-j\omega t_1}$ represents a phase shift. Thus, the inverse Fourier transform of the system transfer function $\mathcal{F}^{-1}[H(\omega)]$ of Eq. (6.107) yields an impulse response for the matched filter

$$h(t) = As(t_1 - t) \quad (6.113)$$

Therefore, the matched filter is given by $h(t)$, a shifted and time-reversed replica of the input signal for optimal detection. For $t_1 = 0$ (no time delay), the output is given by

$$g(t) = f(t) * h(t) = \int_{-\infty}^{\infty} f(t')h(t' - t)dt' \quad (6.114)$$

Or upon substitution of Eq. (6.108),

$$g(t) = A\int_{-\infty}^{\infty} f(t')s(t' + t)dt' \quad (6.115)$$

which is recognized as a correlation process,

$$g(t) = A[f(t) ** s(t)] \quad (6.116)$$

Thus, matched-filter detection is equivalent to correlating the input with the signal of interest in detecting.

## 6.11 CASCADED LINEAR SYSTEMS AND FILTERS

The concept of representing a system using a single block diagram with input and output may be extended to represent more complex systems of several blocks with appropriate interconnections. Figure 6.9 shows two cascaded systems in a time domain with impulse responses of $h_1(t)$ and $h_2(t)$, and the usual input and output given by $f(t)$ and $g(t)$, respectively. The corresponding system transfer functions in the frequency domain can be obtained by Fourier transform.

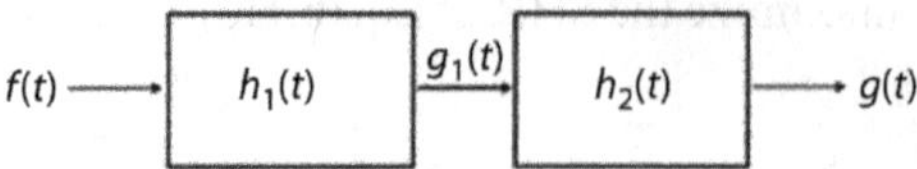


**FIGURE 6.9** Block diagram representation of two cascaded systems in time domain.

Let

$$H_1(\omega) = \mathcal{F}\left[h_1(t)\right]$$

$$H_2(\omega) = \mathcal{F}\left[h_2(t)\right]$$

$$F(\omega) = \mathcal{F}\left[f(t)\right]$$

$$G_1(\omega) = \mathcal{F}\left[g_1(t)\right]$$

$$G(\omega) = \mathcal{F}\left[g(t)\right]$$

Then,

$$G_1(\omega) = F(\omega)H_1(\omega) \tag{6.117}$$

Since $g_1(t)$ is the input signal to $h_2$,

$$G(\omega) = F(\omega)H_1(\omega)H_2(\omega) \tag{6.118}$$

$$G(\omega) = F(\omega)H(\omega) \tag{6.119}$$

where

$$H(\omega) = H_1(\omega)H_2(\omega) \tag{6.120}$$

is a system transfer function obtained by the product of the individual transfer functions of a cascaded system. The concept of finding a single transfer function that represents a complete system composed of several system blocks is an important one in system analysis. The ease in combining transfer functions in the frequency domain is an advantage that can often avoid many algebraic manipulations. A simple example is given here using an inverse filter.

An **inverse filter** can be used to restore degradation introduced into signals. For exact compensation, the requirement is such that

$$g(t) = f(t) \tag{6.121}$$

This can be satisfied if the cascaded system's impulse response is a $\delta(t)$ function, so that the system transfer function takes the form of

$$H(\omega) = H_1(\omega)H_2(\omega) = 1 \tag{6.122}$$

To achieve the requirement, an inverse filter $H_2(\omega)$ needs to be an exact inverse of $H_1(\omega)$,

$$H_2(\omega) = \frac{1}{H_1(\omega)} \tag{6.123}$$

With an impulse response given by

$$h_2(t) = \mathcal{F}^{-1}\left\{\frac{1}{H_1(\omega)}\right\} = \frac{1}{2\pi}\int_{-\infty}^{\infty}\left(\frac{1}{H_1(\omega)}\right)e^{[j(\omega t)]}d\omega \tag{6.124}$$

Unfortunately, the $H_1(\omega)$ in physical systems have frequency bands over which $H_1(\omega) \to 0$. While mathematically exact, this inverse filter is not physically realizable. As indicated in the upcoming discussion, with some minor modification, it can become realizable with an ideal low-pass-inverse filter.

### 6.11.1 An Ideal Low-Pass Inverse Filter

Consider a continuous-time impulse response is in the form of a train of rectangular pulses whose width is $t_o$ and period is T. The system transfer function in Figure 6.10 is specified as

$$H(\omega) = 2\pi\frac{t_0}{T}\sum_{n=-\infty}^{\infty}\frac{\sin\frac{\pi n t_0}{T}}{\frac{\pi n t_0}{T}}\delta\left(\omega - \frac{2\pi n}{T}\right) \tag{6.125}$$

with the output $F_2$ given by

$$F_2 = F(\omega)H(\omega) \tag{6.126}$$

Moving $F(\omega)$ inside the summation to form a product with $\delta(\omega - \frac{2\pi n}{T})$ to obtain $F(\omega - \frac{2\pi n}{T})$,

$$F_2 = F(\omega)\left\{2\pi\frac{t_0}{T}\sum\frac{\sin\frac{\pi n t_0}{T}}{\frac{\pi n t_0}{T}}\delta\left(\omega - \frac{2\pi n}{T}\right)\right\} \tag{6.127}$$

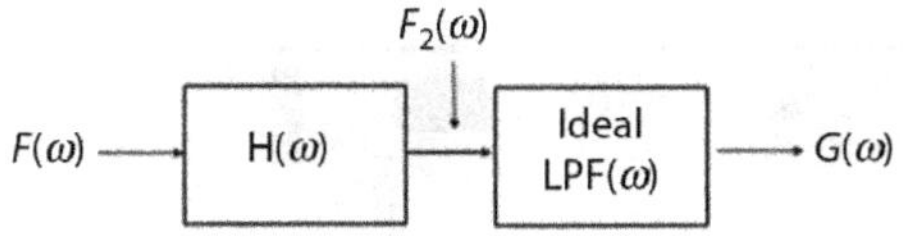

**FIGURE 6.10** Block diagram for a cascaded system with an ideal low-pass inverse filter.

or

$$F_2 = 2\pi \frac{t_0}{\mathrm{T}} \sum sinc \frac{\pi n t_0}{\mathrm{T}} F\left(\omega - \frac{2\pi n}{\mathrm{T}}\right) \tag{6.128}$$

By setting $n = 0$, a single replica of $F_2(\omega)$ can be isolated through an low-pass filter (LPF) operation with the transfer function, so that

$$G(\omega) = F_2(\omega)[LPF] \tag{6.129}$$

Then

$$G(\omega) = F_2 = 2\pi \frac{t_0}{\mathrm{T}} F(\omega) \tag{6.130}$$

Thus, the original signal can be recovered from degradation by passing the received image through an ideal LPF having a gain $\frac{\mathrm{T}}{t_0}$.

### 6.11.2 A Realistic Inverse Filter

Suppose the sensing system has a Gaussian blur whose impulse response is represented by

$$h_1(t) = e^{-a^2 t^2} \tag{6.131}$$

as shown in Figure 6.11. The Fourier transform is found as

$$\mathcal{F}\{h_1(t)\} = H_1(\omega) = \frac{\sqrt{\pi}}{a} e^{-\frac{\omega^2}{4a^2}} \tag{6.132}$$

and its frequency spectrum is displayed in Figure 6.12.

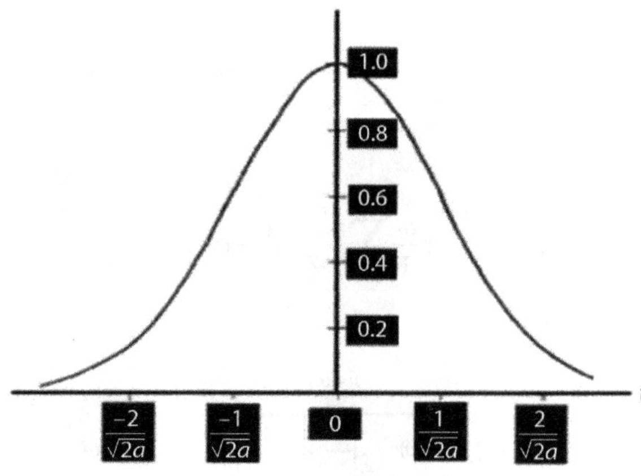


**FIGURE 6.11** Normalized Gaussian impulse response function where $1/\sqrt{2}a$ is half-pulse width.

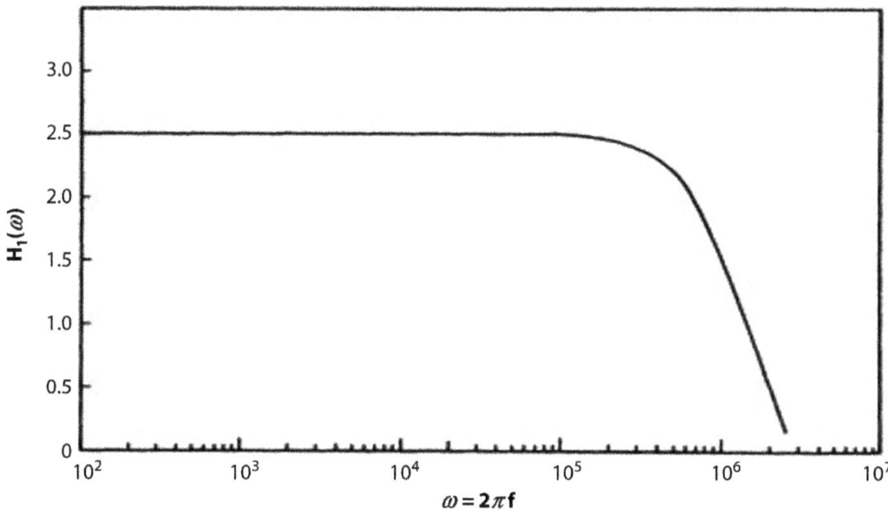


**FIGURE 6.12** System transfer function (spectral distribution) of a Gaussian pulse with a half-pulse width, $1/\sqrt{2}a = 1\mu s$.

The inverse filter to compensate for this distortion is given by

$$H_2(\omega) = \frac{1}{H_1(\omega)} = \frac{a}{\sqrt{\pi}} e^{+\frac{\omega^2}{4a^2}} \tag{6.133}$$

Since this exact inverse filter cannot be realized because $\omega \longrightarrow \infty$, let $\omega_{max}$ be the cutoff, such that

$$H_2(\omega) = \begin{cases} \dfrac{a}{\sqrt{\pi}} e^{+\frac{\omega^2}{4a^2}} & |\omega| \le \omega_{max} \\ 0 & otherwise \end{cases} \tag{6.134}$$

which is shown in Figure 6.13. Then

$$H(\omega) = H_1(\omega) H_2(\omega) = \begin{cases} 1, & |\omega| \le \omega_{max} \\ 0, & otherwise \end{cases} \tag{6.135}$$

and is recognized as an ideal LPF with $\omega_{max}$ being the cutoff. Accordingly,

$$G(\omega) = F(\omega) H(\omega) = F(\omega) \tag{6.136}$$

Once an appropriate $\omega_{max}$ is selected, the impulse response $h_2(t)$ needed to realize the Gaussian inverse filter can be specified by Fourier inversion. For the spectrum shown in Figure 6.13, a realistic choice could be $10^6$ for $\omega_{max}$. In practical systems, there is noise that does not have predictable response and may be high for

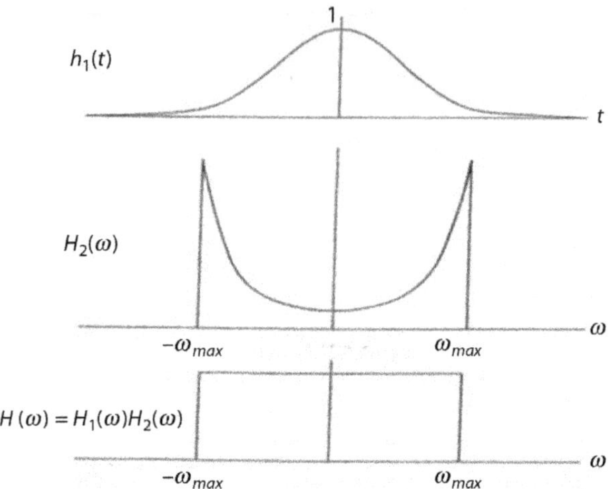


**FIGURE 6.13** An inverse filter, $H_2(\omega)$ with $\omega_{\max}$ cutoff to realize an ideal low-pass inverse filter, $H(\omega) = H_1(\omega)\, H_2(\omega)$ with $\omega_{\max}$ cutoff.

all frequencies, especially for $\omega_{max} \to \infty$, which could lead to a greater probability of noise content and limit the useful range of the inverse filter.

### 6.11.3 Distortionless Filter and System

The medium, space, or system between a source and receiver is called a channel. The channel is often the principal source of distortion for signal transmission. A system that allows a signal to pass without distortion requires the output waveform to be a replica of the input waveform within a constant factor. Also, if a system's output has a time delay but retains the input waveform, it is considered distortionless. Thus, for a distortionless system, the output *g(t)* is the same as the input *f(t)*

$$g(t) = f(t) \tag{6.137}$$

The linear system can be expressed in the frequency domain as

$$G(\omega) = F(\omega)H(\omega) \tag{6.138}$$

where $H(\omega)$ represents the system's transfer function, which can be expressed in terms of an amplitude response $A(\omega)$ and a phase response $e^{j\phi(\omega)}$, such that

$$H(\omega) = A(\omega)e^{j\phi(\omega)} \tag{6.139}$$

and

$$G(\omega) = F(\omega)\; A(\omega)e^{j\phi(\omega)} \tag{6.140}$$

This shows that the conditions of a distortionless system are for the amplitude response to be a constant and the phase response to vary as a linear function of $\omega$, as illustrated in Figure 6.14.

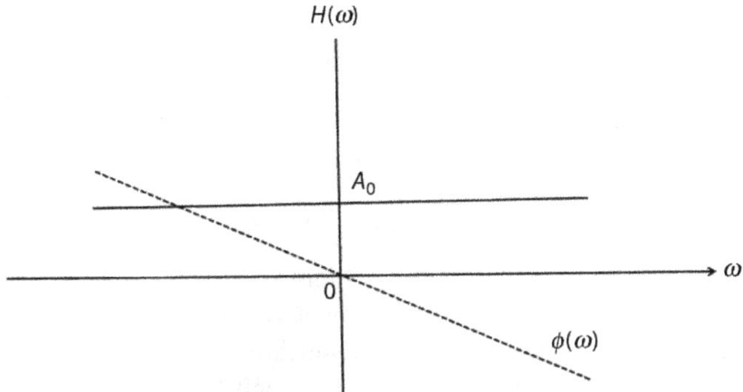


**FIGURE 6.14** Amplitude and phase response of $A_0\, e^{(-j(\omega t_0))}$ of a distortionless system.

The impulse response can be determined by an inverse Fourier transform operation on Eq. (6.135) according to

$$g(t) = \frac{1}{2\pi} \int_{-\infty}^{\infty} F(\omega)\left[A(\omega)e^{j\phi(\omega)}\right]e^{j\omega t}\, d\omega \tag{6.141}$$

Or

$$g(t) = \frac{1}{2\pi} \int_{-\infty}^{\infty} F(\omega)A(\omega)\left[e^{j\phi(\omega)}e^{j\omega t}\right]d\omega \tag{6.142}$$

Again, for *g(t)* to have the same shape as *f(t)*, the requirements are the amplitude response must be a constant alongside a linear phase shift in the frequency domain.

Let $A_0$ be a constant and $t_0$ be a fixed time delay, such that

$$A(\omega)e^{j\phi(\omega)} = A_0 e^{-j(\omega t_0)} \tag{6.143}$$

then

$$g(t) = \frac{1}{2\pi} A_0 \int_{-\infty}^{\infty} F(\omega)e^{j\omega(t-t_0)}\, d\omega \tag{6.144}$$

which is recognized simply as

$$g(t - t_0) = \frac{1}{2\pi} A_0 \int_{-\infty}^{\infty} F(\omega)e^{j\omega(t-t_0)}\, d\omega \tag{6.145}$$

or

$$g(t - t_0) = A_0 f(t - t_0) \tag{6.146}$$

Thus, the delayed output retains the waveform undistorted with respect to the input waveform. As mentioned earlier, the concept of time delay and linear phase shift in the frequency domain can also facilitate the analysis and implementation of physically realizable ideal filters.

### 6.11.4 Ideal High-Pass and Band-Pass Filters

Time invariant linear systems are typically applied to model physical systems and can be used to represent the ideal behavior that a system is expected to exhibit. Ideal filters allow distortionless transmission of a certain band of frequencies and block all other frequencies. A system that eliminates high-frequency signals and allows the low-frequency components to pass through unaltered is called a low-pass filter. The low-pass filter has been analyzed and its uses have been described previously. Figures 6.15 and 6.16 illustrate the ideal high-pass and band-pass filter characteristics. Specifically, a system that suppresses the low-frequency components and passes the high frequencies ($>\omega_m$) unaltered is called a high-pass filter (Figure 6.15). The band-pass filter allows only frequencies above and below certain ranges to pass and suppresses all other frequency components.

The system transfer function for the band-pass filter shown in Figure 6.16 is

$$H(\omega) = A_0 e^{-j(\omega t_0)} \begin{cases} 1, & \omega_0 - \omega_m \leq |\omega| \leq \omega_0 + \omega_m \\ 0, & otherwise \end{cases} \tag{6.147}$$

The corresponding impulse response can be found by an inverse Fourier transform operation and takes the form of

$$h(t) = \frac{2A_0}{\pi}\omega_m \frac{\sin(\omega_m t)}{\omega_m t} \cos\omega_0 t = \frac{2A_0}{\pi}\omega_m \mathrm{sinc}(\omega_m t)\cos\omega_0 t \tag{6.148}$$

where $\omega_0$ is the center frequency of the pass band and $2\omega_m$ is its band width centered around $\omega_0$. A band-pass filter with a varying center frequency and bandwidth can serve as the basis of spectrum analyzers, using, for example, a bank of fixed-frequency band-pass filters under the control of a computer. Alternatively, the

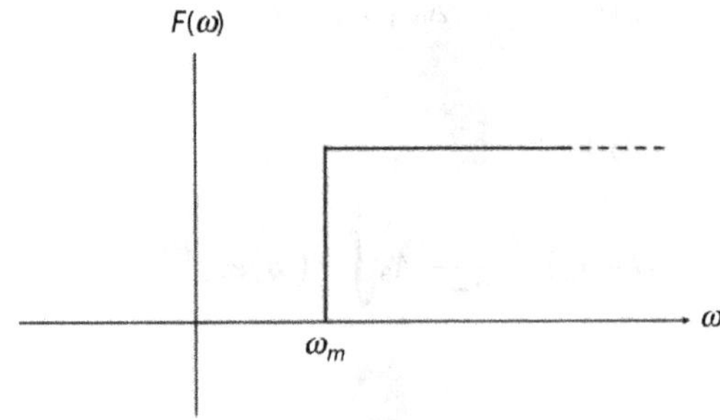


**FIGURE 6.15** Ideal high-pass filter characteristics.

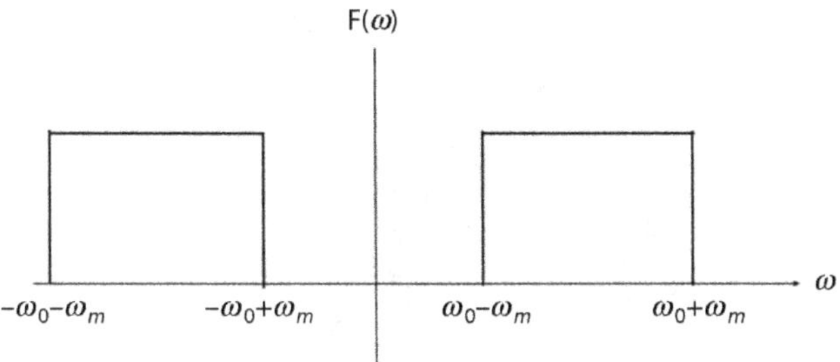


**FIGURE 6.16** The system transfer function for an ideal band-pass filter.

variation of a tuned capacitor circuit can sample the waveform and perform the spectrum analysis by a computer. In either situation, the spectral resolution improves as the bandwidth becomes narrower.

### 6.11.5 A Practical Realizable Filter

While ideal filters are conceptually useful, the sharp corners of ideal filter behavior displayed in Figures 6.15 and 6.16 are impossible to physically implement. Typically, a practical band-pass filter with 0.1 Hz high-pass and 10 Hz low-pass characteristics would be suitable to remove any DC offset and avoid aliasing for use with cardiopulmonary and vital-sign sensing [Droitcour et al., 2004]. The fundamental frequency of respiration is usually below 0.4 Hz, while the heart rate is usually above 1 Hz. A physically realizable band-pass filter with a 12th-order elliptic infinite impulse response (IIR) that passes 0.9–9 Hz but blocks frequencies below 0.8 Hz is shown in Figure 6.17 for heartbeats.

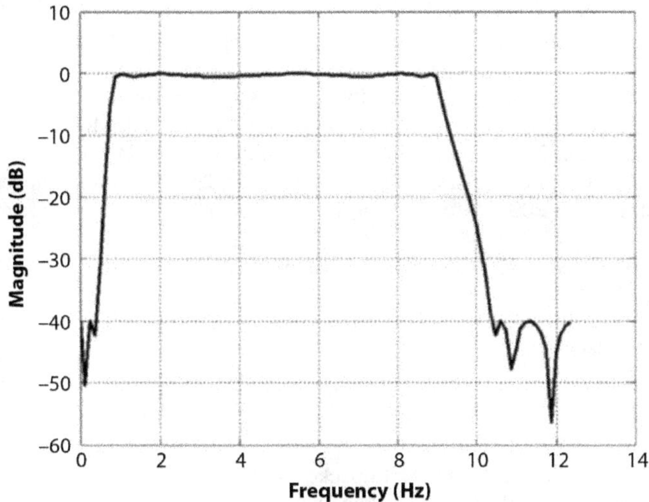


**FIGURE 6.17** Frequency response of a 12th-order elliptic infinite impulse response filter to separate the heart signal from a signal that includes both heart and respiration information.

## 6.12 ADVANCED SIGNAL CONDITIONING AND PROCESSING METHODS

Many of the fundamental theories, techniques, and algorithms discussed in this chapter aided investigations on the microwave sensing of physiological signals in a wide range of applications. It is noteworthy that a variety of implementations of advanced methods in signal processing were applied to specific cases of microwave noninvasive physiological sensing applications and developments. They have provided insights, improved results, rendered clearer understanding of how the signals behave, and enhanced the signal's detectability. The advanced methods include automated clutter cancellation, active Capone beamforming, feature extraction, independent component analysis, principal component analysis, generalized eigenvalue decomposition, frequency estimation algorithm, parametric spectral estimation, wavelet transform and packet decomposition, characteristic stability index classification, multiple signal classification, estimation of signal parameters via rational invariance techniques, independent component analysis, joint approximation diagonalization of eigenmatrices, artificial intelligence, and machine learning, among others. Likewise, there are many innovative decision-making algorithms for extracting signals of interest or suppressing undesired signals such as directionally constrained minimization of power, blind source separation, direction of arrival, maximum-likelihood method, multiple-signal classification, phased and adaptive array processing, sequential Monte Carlo filtering, and ensemble Kalman filtering. Brief descriptions of some of the advanced methods in signal processing and various algorithms for signal extraction are included in later chapters, alongside discussions on specific areas of noninvasive physiological sensing applications. They provide specific examples, demonstrating how they were applied and found suitable, appropriate, and helpful during research and development in noninvasive biomedical sensing and monitoring.

## GENERAL REFERENCES

Bracewell, R. N., 2000. The Fourier Transform and its Applications, 3rd ed, McGraw Hill
Carlson, A. B., Crilly, P. B., 2009. Communication Systems, 5th ed, McGraw Hill
Haykin, S., Moher, M., 2005. Modern Wireless Communications, Pearson Prentice Hall
Lathi, B. P., 2021. Signal Processing and Linear Systems, 2nd ed, Oxford University Press
Lee, E. A., Varaiya, P., 2003. Structure and Interpretation of Signals and Systems, Addison Wesley
McClellan, J. H., Schafer, R. W., Yoder, M. A., 1998. DSP First: A Multimedia Approach, Prentice Hall
Oppenheim, A. V., Willsky, A. S., 1997. Signals and Systems, 2nd ed, Prentice Hall
Stoica, P., Moses, R. L., 2005. Spectral Analysis of Signals, vol. 1, Prentice Hall

## REFERENCE CITED

Droitcour, A. D., Boric-Lubecke, O., Lubecke, V. M., Lin, J., Kovacs, G. T. A., 2004. Range correlation and I/Q performance benefits in single chip silicon Doppler radars for noncontact cardiopulmonary monitoring. IEEE Trans. Microw. Theory Techn., 52(3):838–848

# 7 Vital Sign Sensing
## *Heartbeat and Respiration*

A group of three clinical measurements is commonly taken to indicate the general state of physical health of a person. These fundamental components of clinical care, known as vital signs, are the heart and respiratory rates alongside body temperature. While blood pressure is not considered a vital sign, it is often measured along with the vital signs. Hence, they are often referred to as a group of the four most important clinical vital-sign measurements to be measured consistently and recorded accurately. They are also the essential parameters in identifying clinical deterioration in the hospital. For example, physiological abnormalities could develop up to 24 hours after major surgery, if changes in vital signs and blood pressure are not monitored or interpreted properly. Thus, vital-sign monitoring has an important role in healthcare delivery and its potential in alerting significant adverse consequences cannot be overstated. These considerations can be extended to include vital-sign monitoring of patients with critical burns and neonatal monitoring in premature babies when direct contact with the subject is either impossible or undesirable. The noncontact approaches can help to overcome some of the inability and sensitivity due to electrodes or sensors that must be attached or strapped onto patients for proper recording.

Beyond the hospital doors, vital-sign detection and monitoring have potential applications in search and rescue missions of victims of natural disasters. They may render critically needed support in searching for survivors after earthquakes, building collapses, avalanches, or human-caused disasters such as hazardous environments due to chemical spills, nuclear contamination, or fire [ Lin, 1986, 1989, 1992, 1999, 2004, 2006; Rozzell and Lin 1987]. They are also used in home and elderly healthcare and safety-alert monitoring circumstances [Li et al., 2013].

Remote measurement and noncontact detection of vital signs (heart and respiration rates) are particularly useful when direct contact with the subject is either impractical or unsuitable. Remote noncontact microwave detection of vital signs has been measured at distances of a few centimeters to tens of meters [Chan and Lin 1985, 1987; Chen et al., 1986, 2000; Lin 1975, 1993; Lin et al., 1977, 1979; Popovic et al., 1984; Seals et al., 1983, 1987; Sharpe et al.,1986; Stuchly et al. 1980]. Microwaves can penetrate light, dry, or thick clothing and physical barriers, and do not require any coupling agent t]be applied on the skin. Thus, noninvasive microwave sensing of heart and respiratory rates provides a platform for inconspicuous, yet continuous physiological monitoring.

This chapter provides a description of the characteristics of the principal biological structures and physiological targets of interest in cardiopulmonary monitoring and interrogation — the heart and lungs in the thoracic cavity. It presents discussions on results of experimental measurements and monitoring procedures as examples of the types of instrumentation and techniques that are useful in microwave

DOI: 10.1201/9781003315223-7

cardiopulmonary interrogation and vital-sign monitoring, including abnormal breathing conditions in infants and the elderly as well as the infirm.

## 7.1 ORGANS IN THE THORAX

The biological targets of primary interest to cardiopulmonary interrogation are the heart and the lungs in the thoracic cavity. Both organs exhibit characteristic dimensional and functional changes in health and in disease. Therefore, they may be particularly useful in microwave interrogation. However, the cardiovascular and respiratory systems are complex; a detailed description of their anatomy and physiology is beyond the scope of this chapter. In this section, we shall briefly describe some of the structure, physiology, and dynamics involved in cardiopulmonary functions. The guiding principle is to start with a brief introduction to the specific topics and relevant background information on anatomical structure and physiology. The aim is to facilitate understanding of the measurements and differences in various tissue and organ system functions.

### 7.1.1 The Heart and Coronary Vessels

The heart is a muscular organ located in the chest cavity. In humans, it is divided longitudinally into left and right halves, each consisting of two chambers, an atrium, and a ventricle (Figure 7.1). The chambers on each side of the heart are connected to each other, but the left chambers do not communicate directly with those on the right. Between the chambers in each half of the heart are valves that open to permit blood to flow from atrium to ventricle (the tricuspid valve between the right atrium and ventricle and the mitral valve between the left atrium and left ventricle) but not vice versa. There are also valves at the entrances of pulmonary artery (pulmonary valve between the right ventricle and the pulmonary artery) and aorta (the aortic valve between the left ventricle and the aorta), which permit blood to flow into

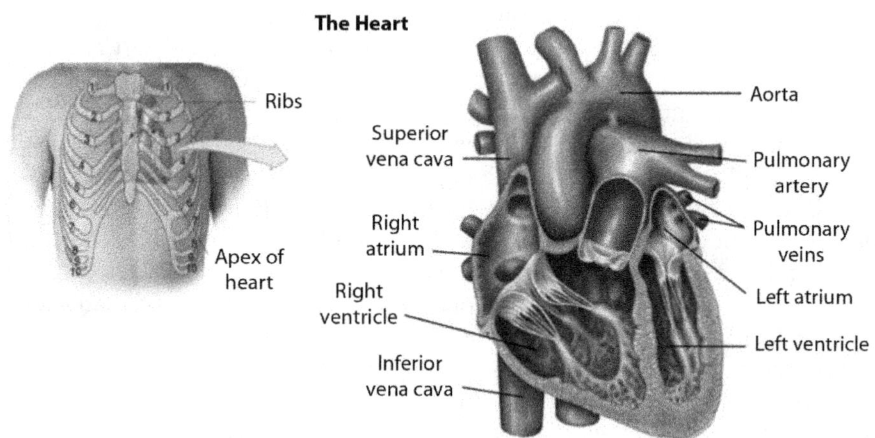


**FIGURE 7.1** Anatomic structure of the human heart and its position in the thorax.

these arteries but close, immediately preventing the reflux of blood in the opposite direction [Silverthorn, 2016; Vander et al., 1990].

Normally, blood flows from superior or inferior vena cava to the right atrium, right ventricle, pulmonary arteries, left atrium, left ventricle, and the aorta. This orderly flow of blood through the various parts of the heart is accomplished by the active contraction of the cardiac muscle, which is triggered by a coordinated process of depolarization of the muscle membrane.

The movements of the heart in the chest cavity, and the intrinsic volume-pressure changes in the heart chambers also produce displacements or motions of the chest wall. As the wave of cardiac electric excitation traverses the Purkinje system over the endocardial surface of the ventricles, the trabeculae carneae and capillary muscle begin to contract. With the onset of this contraction, the internal length of the heart decreases as the mitral valve is pulled toward the ventricular cavity.

Simultaneously, there is no expansion of the circumference of the ventricular wall. The intracavitary pressure is generated and the circumference continues to increase in size until the movement of aortic valve opening. This coincides with the maximal outward displacement of the chest produced by the heart. During the blood ejection phase, the circumference diminishes and the ventricular pressure continues to decrease until the atrium begins to fill. This causes the inward displacement of the chest wall. These movements correspond to physiological changes that occur during the cardiac cycle. Contraction of the heart muscle sets in motion the precordium overlying the apex.

The heart's mass varies with height and skeletal structure. It averages from 250 to 300 g in females and 300 to 350 g in males. The normal thickness of the free wall of the right ventricle is 0.3–0.5 cm and that of the left ventricle is 1.3–1.5 cm [Cotran et al., 1994]. It is interesting to note that during contraction, the heart shortens by approximately 75% and rotates by about 4° [Brower and Meester, 1979].

There are five great blood vessels entering and leaving the heart: the superior and inferior vena cava, the pulmonary artery, the pulmonary vein, and the aorta (Figure 7.1). The superior vena cava and inferior vena cava are large veins that carry blood to the heart. They return deoxygenated blood from circulation in the body and empty it into the right atrium. The pulmonary artery carries blood to the lungs for oxygenation. The pulmonary veins carry oxygenated blood from the lungs and empty it into the left atrium and ventricle. The aorta carries oxygenated blood to the body.

### 7.1.2 The Lungs

Anatomically, there are two lungs — the left and right, each divided into several lobes. Together with the heart, great vessels, trachea, esophagus, bronchus, and ribs, the lungs completely fill the chest cavity (Figure 7.2). The lungs consist of air-containing tubes, blood vessels, and connective tissues. The smallest tubes end in tiny air sacs, the alveoli, which are the sites of gas exchange within the lungs. The lungs, however, lack muscle and are, therefore, passive elastic containers with no inherent ability to change their volume. Lung expansion is accomplished by action of the diaphragm (the tissue that separates the chest and abdominal cavities) and muscles that move the ribs. Accordingly, respiratory changes are also associated with movement of the abdominal cavity.

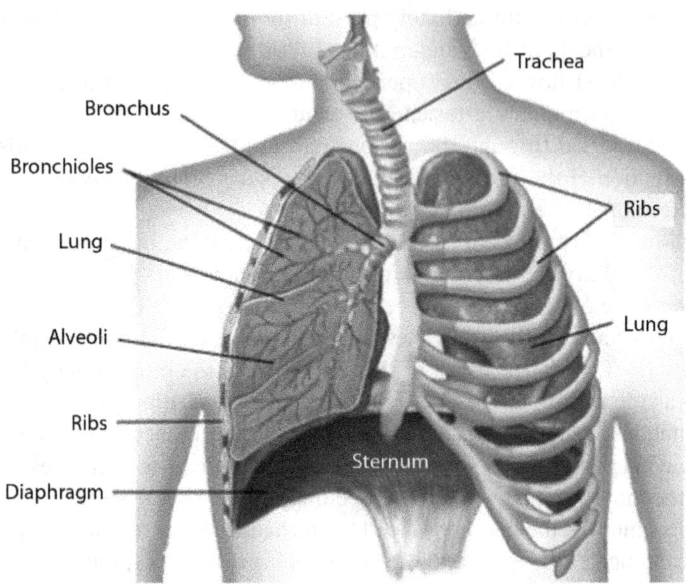


**FIGURE 7.2** The lungs within the human chest and rib cage.

The lungs can be expanded and contracted by elevation and depression of the ribs to increase and decrease the anteroposterior diameter of the chest cavity from 1 mm to as much as 5 mm. During expiration, the ribs slant downward, thus allowing the sternum to fall backward toward the spinal column. During inspiration, the rib cage is elevated. The ribs project directly forward so that the sternum moves forward away from the spine. The anteroposterior thickness of the chest can be 20% greater during maximum inspiration than during expiration.

The normal pulmonary capillary pressure is only 10–15 mm Hg. This, in combination with osmotic gradients and alveolar surface tension, allows the alveoli to remain dry, a feature essential for normal gas exchange. However, if the pulmonary capillary pressure increases greatly, because of pulmonary venous hypertension (e.g., with left ventricular failure), or because of direct increases in capillary permeability, fluid may accumulate in the interstitial spaces or in the alveoli. Pulmonary edema with intra-alveolar components prevents gas exchange across the alveolar wall.

The determination of respiratory system functions is important both for diagnostic and therapeutic medicine. A deviation of respiration rate of 4 per min (beat/min) from the normal range could indicate an impending medical emergency such as cardiac arrest due to cerebral hypoxia. A persistent abnormal respiration rate (<6 or >24 per min) is a predictor of imminent death.

## 7.2 MEASUREMENT OF RESPIRATION

### 7.2.1 Respiratory Parameters

Measurement of respiratory air flow, volume, and efficiency of gas transfer from the alveoli in the lungs to the blood provide valuable diagnostic information. Continuous monitoring of respiration activities in recovery rooms and for patients with impending or existing respiratory failure is also essential to assess the function of the vital respiratory organs. In addition, during the first days of life, premature and low-birth-weight infants often have apneic spells that may require continuous monitoring.

The rate of breathing is the simplest test of respiratory function and, clinically, it is mostly done by inspecting the color of skin and mucous membranes, or through simple counting. However, it is both time consuming and demanding on the part of healthcare personnel, and it does not lend to situations where continuous monitoring is required. Therefore, there is a need for a reliable means to continuously measure and monitor respiratory activity.

A variety of techniques have been developed over the years for measurement and extraction of respiration and cardiovascular information from chest displacement to movement-related signals; none of them is completely satisfactory. Among these are strain gages, resistance pneumogram, and impedance pneumography. Strain gauges and resistance pneumograms measure changes in the length of the chest. Body movements cause artifacts, which are dimensional changes unrelated to lung volume changes. The impedance pneumogram is reliable and has been extensively used especially as an apnea monitor for prematurely born infants. During the inspiration, the lung tissue fills with air and becomes more resistive. Electrodes are placed on the chest wall of patients. Detection cannot be made without direct contact with the patient. These systems have considerable differences in sensitivity that may result from applying electrodes and sensors directly on the skin with varying contact pressures.

### 7.2.2 Microwave Measurement of Respiration

Microwave sensing is predicated on its ability to measure the displacement of a moving biological target and to detect its velocity (see Chapter 5, Section 5.8) as well as to sense time-dependent permittivity changes from outside the body (see Chapter 5, Sections 5.2 and 5.3). A microwave technique to remotely monitor the respiratory movement of humans and animals (cats, rats, and rabbits) using a continuous wave (CW) Doppler system was first reported in the 1970s [Lin, 1975; Lin and Salinger, 1975]. In this case, low-power microwave energy at 10 GHz was directed by a standard gain horn toward the subject. The microwave energy reflected from the chest is compared to the transmitted signal to give a measure of the respiratory movements. The noncontact or remote sensing technique is based on the backscattering of microwave radiation. A beam of microwave radiation is directed toward the upper torso of the subject, the reflection from the chest is mixed with the transmitted energy, and the resultant signal is displayed to provide respiratory information. The method is convenient, simple, noninvasive, and does not require any contact or sensor attachment to the subject; in fact, the subject may be fully clothed or covered with fur, as the case may be.

Microwave energy as shown in Figure 7.3 is derived from an X-band sweep oscillator, which has a maximum output of 10 mW. In this experiment, the output frequency of the source was adjusted to 10 GHz, and the incident power density was projected to be in the milliwatt per square meter (mW/m$^2$) range. The forward signal was passed through a variable attenuator and a 20 dB directional coupler before

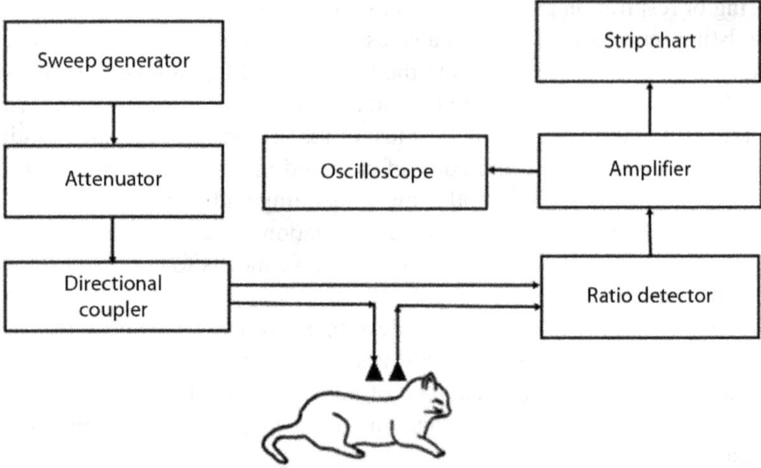


**FIGURE 7.3** Block diagram of a continuous wave microwave radar sensor for respiration. Note that received microwave signal is mixed or compared with a portion of the transmitted microwave serving as a reference signal at the same frequency, the result is a baseband signal. The scheme is called homodyne detection.

being radiated through a rectangular horn antenna. Upon incidence on the subject, the microwave signal was modulated both in amplitude and in phase by the moving chest wall. The scattered energy modulated by the respiratory movements was detected by a crystal detector mounted on a receiving horn antenna. This signal was led to the ratio meter where the amplitude was compared with a portion of the forward signal detected by a similar crystal attached to the directional coupler. The ratio meter calculated the instantaneous ratio between the scattered and the reference signals. The output of the ratio meter is a voltage whose frequency corresponds to the rate of respiration. The outputs from the microwave respiration monitor were capacitively coupled to an oscilloscope and recorded using a strip-chart recorder.

Note that the output voltage whose frequency corresponds to the rate of respiration through the equation for an amplitude modulated signal, either as

$$v(t) = A + Bsin(\omega_r t) \tag{7.1a}$$

or

$$v(t) = A + Bcos(\omega_r t) \tag{7.1b}$$

where $A$ and $B$ are constants and $\omega_r = 2\pi f_r$ and $f_r$ is the frequency of the moving chest wall.

The microwave measured respiratory activity was compared with the results from a thermistor-based hot-wire anemometer air-flow transducer. The outputs from the microwave respiration monitor and the hot-wire anemometer pulmonary function analyzer were capacitively coupled to a dual trace oscilloscope and recorded using a dual channel strip-chart recorder.

In one series of experiments, a 5.1 kg albino rabbit was confined to a cardboard box but not anesthetized. The air-flow transducer was attached to the inlet of a plastic mask, which was placed over the rabbit's head. The distance between the horn antenna and the rabbit was approximately 30 cm. The receiving horn may be located either right next to the transmitting horn or at an angle but was always aimed at the chest of the rabbit. A typical strip-chart recording is shown in Figure 7.2. Notice that the hot-wire anemometer recording is related to the absolute value of respiratory flow. Therefore, its variations are at twice the rate of respiration.

The results obtained using the experimental setup for a seated human subject breathing deliberately at approximately 51 times per minute is shown in Figure 7.5. The distance between the subject and the antenna was 30 cm. The upper traces in these figures are for microwave measurement and the middle curves are the air flow measurements. The bottom curves are time markers at 1-second intervals.

It can be seen from Figures 7.4 and 7.5 that the continuous microwave technique can provide reliable measurements of the respiratory rate. The comparisons between microwave and anemometer measurements also indicate that it may be possible to use microwaves to assess respiratory volume. (The output voltage of the hot-wire anemometer flow meter corresponds to 0.1 volt/liter/min). In fact, Moskalenko [1960] has suggested the use of changes of microwave reflectance and transmittance as a measure of physiologically significant parameters such as circulatory and respiratory volume changes. More details on the topic will be described in Chapter 8.

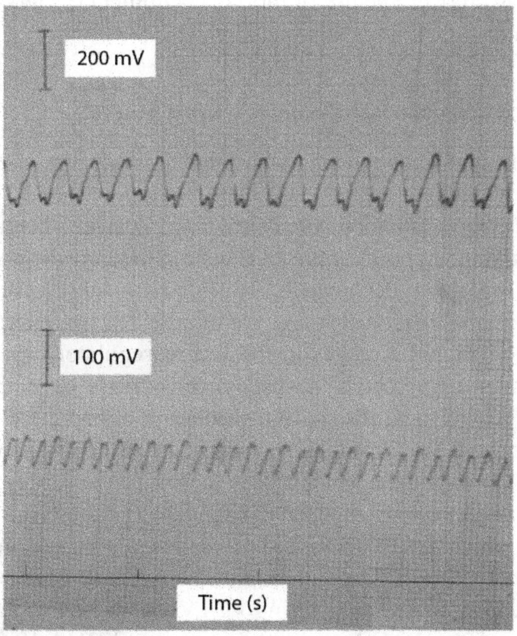


**FIGURE 7.4** Measurements of respiratory movement of an intact (unanesthetized) rabbit: upper tracing for microwave sensing; lower tracing for anemometer.

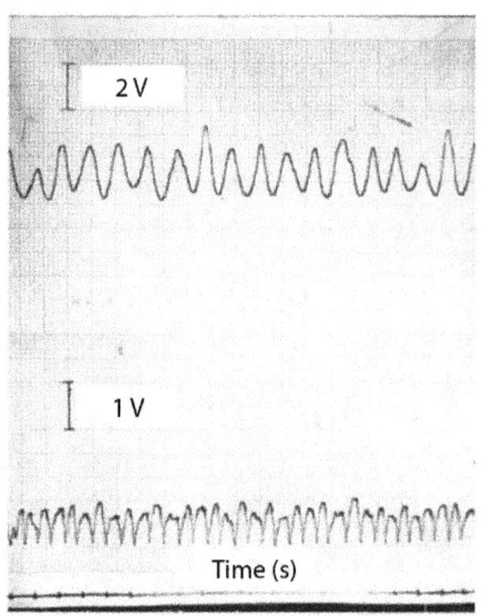


**FIGURE 7.5** Respiratory measurement from a human subject: upper tracing for microwave; lower tracing for anemometer.

The microwave sensing method has several advantages over more conventional techniques because it does not require any direct contact with the subject. Problems such as skin irritation, restriction of breathing, and loose electrode connections are easily eliminated. Moreover, the use of ratio measurement renders the stability of the microwave oscillator less of an issue or challenge.

### 7.2.3 Respiratory Sensing of Animal Under Stress

Humans, mammals, and birds are warm-blooded animals or homeotherms, and they thrive in a relatively narrow range of body temperatures around 37–38°C. The main regulators of the thermoregulatory system are in the head and central nervous system (CNS). The CNS and the hypothalamus of the brain mediate the classic physiological responses to heat sensation. Perturbations to this relatively constant body temperature may lead to thermal discomfort and are manifested by general stress responses characterized by functional changes in the thermoregulatory systems of the body. When the hypothalamus perceives an excessive increase in temperature, the CNS often reacts by effecting heat dissipation through a cooperative behavior between two different processes. For example, in cats, heart and respiratory rates are modified in response. The augmented blood flow increases the supply of warm blood to the lungs, and panting increases the heat exchange with the environment and accelerates heat loss from the lungs to help maintain a constant body temperature.

A continuous record of a Doppler microwave-sensed respiratory history of an anesthetized cat (alpha chloralose, 55 mg/kg I.V.) subjected to selective heating of the head is shown in Figure 7.6 [Lin, 1989; Lin et al., 1973]. A 10 GHz standard gain horn antenna, as shown in Figure 7.3, is directed toward the thorax of the animal at 2 m. The record shows that the microwave sensor was able to register instantaneous

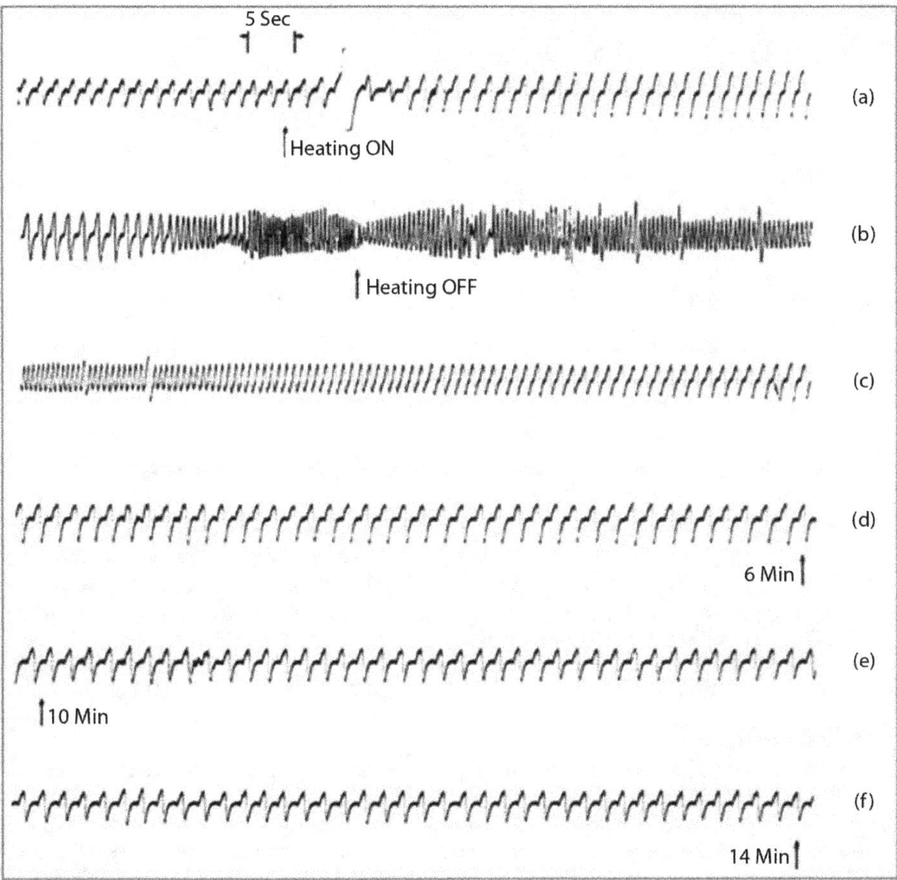


**FIGURE 7.6** A continuous wave microwave sensor monitored respiratory record (uninterrupted from a-f) of a cat subjected to a brief period of selective heating of the head (see heating on and off arrows).

changes in respiration. The respiration rate increases simultaneously with brain heating. Also, a period of hyperventilation is followed by an intense tachypnea. The rapid panting gradually stabilized and ended about 14 minutes after the secession of brain heating, returning to normal breathing. The Doppler sensor-recorded respiratory dynamics in the live cats clearly highlights the role of physiological thermoregulation and the behavioral effects in laboratory animals in response to localized brain heating without any physical contact with the animal.

### 7.2.4 Contactless Microwave Apnea Monitor

During the first days of life, premature and low-birth-weight infants often exhibit apneic spells. Although the connection is neither clear nor simple, prolonged apneic periods during sleep have been identified in crib-death or sudden infant death syndrome (SIDS). Continuous monitoring of respiratory activities is helpful because stimuli sufficient to wake the infant are usually strong enough to re-establish breathing.

A variety of motion signals are generated by an awakened infant; however, such signals should not be a problem since this is presumably not the high-risk period. During sleep when apneic periods are identified, the dominant chest motion is respiratory in origin and can be equated with the rate of breathing.

A remote contactless microwave sensor based on CW radar was reported for an apnea monitor [Lin et al., 1977]. It follows the basic CW radar architecture shown in Chapter 1, Figure 1.3. The device consists of an active sensing head and a signal-processing unit. It uses Doppler microwaves to sense infant respiratory movement (Figure 7.7). The sensor is a low-power (3 mW) microwave circuit module (MCM – GEC 2070M) Doppler transceiver that combines transmitting and receiving functions. The operating frequency is 10.5 GHz and the maximum power density is less than 0.1 W/m$^2$ at 30 cm from a subject. Microwaves from a 3 × 3 cm horn antenna are scattered by the chest of the subject. The backscattered microwaves with their Doppler-shifted frequency (see Chapter 5) are mixed with a portion of the transmitted signal by the bulk-effect diode inside the microwave circuit module.

The resultant Doppler signal is amplified by a pair of cascaded band-pass amplifiers, each having a gain of 25 from 0.08–14 Hz. It is then buffered by a transistor and converted to digital signals, which are used for detection. The sensitivity is about 0.1 mm at the lower end of the frequency response region. An analog output is provided for display, recording, and/or for listening through a loudspeaker. A 30-second delay timer is used to turn on visual and audible alarms if no signal is detected within the specified periods. Note that both the upper frequency limit of the band-pass amplifiers and the time delay interval were selected in testing the device with laboratory animals. These variables can be changed as appropriate, for example, by changing the value of a capacitor. (In fact, changing the settings of frequency limits for the band-pass filter using different capacitances would provide a device for heart-rate monitoring.)

The performance of the Doppler microwave apnea monitor was tested with 3.5 kg cats and 2.5 kg rabbits. Anesthesia was induced in the cat with intravenous thiamylal sodium at a dose of 17.5 mg/kg of body mass until effect to allow tracheal

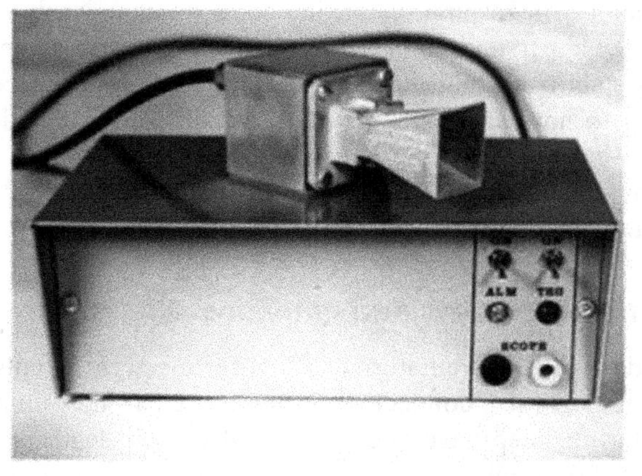


**FIGURE 7.7** A contactless microwave apnea monitor.

intubation and was maintained with methoxyflurane using a non-rebreathing system on a gas anesthetic machine. In the rabbit, anesthesia was induced with intramuscular ketamine hydrochloride at dose of 60 mg/kg body mass followed by sodium pentobarbital I.V. at 30 mg/kg of body mass to effect. The rabbit was intubated by means of a tracheostomy and ventilated as needed with a bag. After induction of anesthesia, the animal was placed in an incubator in lateral recumbency.

Respiratory difficulty, such as prolonged apnea, is known to follow a period of hyperventilation. In these experiments, the Doppler microwave sensor front end was mounted on the top of an incubator. Artificial hyperventilation was induced by inflation of the animal's lungs with room air from a pump. Figure 7.8 shows the Doppler microwave apnea detector-recorded instantaneous changes in respiration, including artificially induced apnea following hyperventilation and return to normal breathing. Both the audio and visible alarms were triggered whenever an apnea lasted 30 seconds or longer.

These findings indicate that microwave sensing of respiration is viable as a remote noncontact apnea sensor. The Doppler microwave device can register instantaneous respiratory activity and changes. The advantages of the device include contactless application, which eliminates such problems as loose electrode connections, skin irritation, and restriction of breathing functions. The remote-sensing feature allows monitoring without the subject becoming conscious of the procedure. In addition, movements in the immediate vicinity of the incubator did not interfere with the operation of the microwave detector. One limitation of the simpler single-channel device is the associated dead spot with the nulls of the standing wave pattern resulting from the backscattered microwave. This difficulty is resolvable by use of a quadrature detection scheme, which splits the received signal into two orthogonal channels, as prescribed in Eq. (7.1), so that the signal provided by one channel is stronger than the other and vice versa [Lin, 1989].

There have been many radio frequency (RF) and microwave devices and systems introduced for continuously monitoring apnea and respiration, including some commercial products since the 1970s However, none of them is completely satisfactory [Liu et al., 2019; Villarroel et al., 2014]. Indeed, to date, more than one high profile company has attempted to commercialize microwave radar technology to track and monitor for signs of sleep apnea. It is noteworthy that infants with delicate skin would benefit most from noncontact monitoring by avoidance of adhesive electrodes. While there have been investigations under clinical settings in recent years, studies

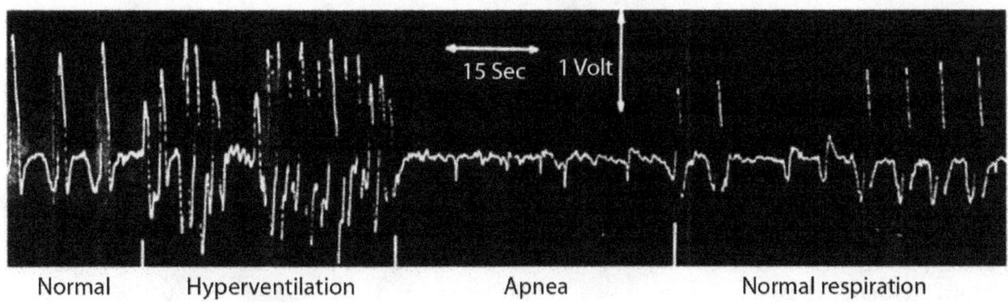


**FIGURE 7.8** A microwave apnea detector recorded respiratory activity of an anesthetized cat showing apneic episode and recovery.

on infants in the neonatal intensive care units are still limited [Al-Naji et al., 2017, Beltrão et al. 2022, Khanam et al., 2021]

### 7.2.5 Other Developments in Microwave Respiratory Monitoring

Respiratory-rate measurement has been introduced to a range of early detection systems in recognition of its potential in early detection of a patient's decline in health [Subbe et al., 2003]. Furthermore, while the respiration rate is acknowledged clinically as an early indicator of serious events, its determination has been commonly recorded by manual methods. Research has indicated that determination by manual counting could be inaccurate [Edmonds et al., 2002; Lim et al., 2002; Lovett et al., 2005]. In addition to the infant apnea monitor discussed previously, a need for reliable assessment of potential sleep apnea-hypopnea syndrome (SAHS) has been identified among the adult population. SAHS is a multifactorial disease characterized by recurrent hypopnea or respiratory interruption during sleep, which causes intermittent hypoxemia (an abnormally low concentration of oxygen in the blood), hypercapnia (excessive carbon dioxide in the bloodstream), and sleep disturbances.

Respiration rate is a very important physiological parameter that is not well monitored in a range of healthcare settings [McBride et al., 2005]. Since the pioneering investigations in 1970s and 1980s, many microwave methods have been proposed and studied for automated and continuous monitoring of respiration rate. However, they are mostly at the experimental feasibility or prototype stage [Liu et al., 2019; Zakrzewski et al., 2015]. In recent years, substantial interest and resources have been devoted to improving Doppler microwave sensing to achieve a noninvasive, convenient, unobtrusive, accurate, continuous, and automatic measurement systems, including noncontact and remote respiratory activity monitoring [Hong et al., 2018, 2019]. The Doppler radar sensor's ability to record different types of breathing patterns was further investigated in which results from Doppler radar were compared with conventional respiration belt measurements correlation coefficients between 90 and 98% (see Table 7.1) [Lee et al., 2014].

**TABLE 7.1**
**Doppler Radar Compared to Conventional Respiration Belt Measurements Associated with Different Respiratory Disorders**

| Type of Breathing | Mean Square Error (MSE) | Correlation Coefficient |
|---|---|---|
| Ataxic | 0.0038 | 0.9465 |
| Biot | 0.0063 | 0.9762 |
| Central sleep apnea | 0.0121 | 0.9427 |
| Cheyne-Stokes | 0.0094 | 0.9376 |
| Cheyne-Stokes variant | 0.0089 | 0.9650 |
| Dysrhythmic breathing | 0.0236 | 0.9355 |
| Normal breathing | 0.0461 | 0.9198 |
| Kussmaul breathing | 0.0764 | 0.9006 |

Over the years, the potential of noninvasive sensing has attracted a great deal of interest for a wide variety of applications. The potential and interest have prompted the development of many bench-top prototypes and system-concept verifications. Advances in the past decade have come in the form of low profile and flexible antennas, new front-end architectures, baseband signal processing schemes, pattern recognition, software implementation, and system-level integrations. These developments have helped to improve detection accuracy and robustness. In the case of wireless respiratory sensing, the efforts also incorporated preliminary trials under a clinical environment for sleep research and apnea detection. Some salient examples of the efforts are presented in the following sections.

## 7.3 MICROWAVE RESPIRATORY SENSOR ON A CHIP

The noncontact Doppler radar apnea monitoring device shown in Figure 7.7 was small for the time. The CW radar transceiver employed conventional architectures with typical AC and DC coupling schemes [Lin et al., 1977]. It was fabricated with lumped circuit elements and bulky waveguide components. Nonetheless, it was able to render proper phase demodulation — a noninvasive contactless CW Doppler radar was able to accurately sense and monitor respiration motions from human participants and animal subjects. Developments in wireless technologies have made it feasible to integrate such a microwave radar on a single chip for the first time [Droitcour et al., 2004].

### 7.3.1 Doppler Radar Apnea Monitoring on a Single Chip

The single-chip sensor is compact and lightweight and, importantly, the miniaturized circuitry consumes less power. A direct-conversion microwave Doppler-radar transceiver was fully integrated using 0.25 $\mu$m silicon CMOS and BiCMOS technologies [Droitcour et al., 2002, 2003, 2004, 2009]. Also, the miniaturization and low power consumption can potentially render smaller apnea detectors that are less expensive to produce. It was envisioned that the single-chip microwave Doppler radar sensor could potentially be used in home monitoring for sleep apnea detection both for infants and adults. Furthermore, the development ushered in low-cost compact modern radar systems capable of being integrated in sensor networks and delivering high-accuracy measurements.

Another significant design improvement is the inclusion of a quadrature scheme for detection mentioned earlier, which could enhance detection sensitivity and mitigate against the detection ambiguity due to the nulls in microwave propagation associated with backscattering in single-channel devices [Lin, 1989]. A functional block diagram of the 2.4 GHz ISM band single-chip quadrature radar transceiver is shown in Figure 7.9 [Droitcour et al., 2004]. It follows the basic Doppler-radar architecture shown in Chapter 1, Figures 1.3 and 7.3. The chip uses two identical receiver channels to provide quadrature outputs to avoid the phase-demodulation null points. The $RF_{out}$ and LO signals from the voltage-controlled oscillator (VCO) are split without using a balun. The LO is amplified with a low-noise amplifier (LNA) and is then split with a resistor–capacitor–capacitor–resistor (RCCR) circuit into two quadrature

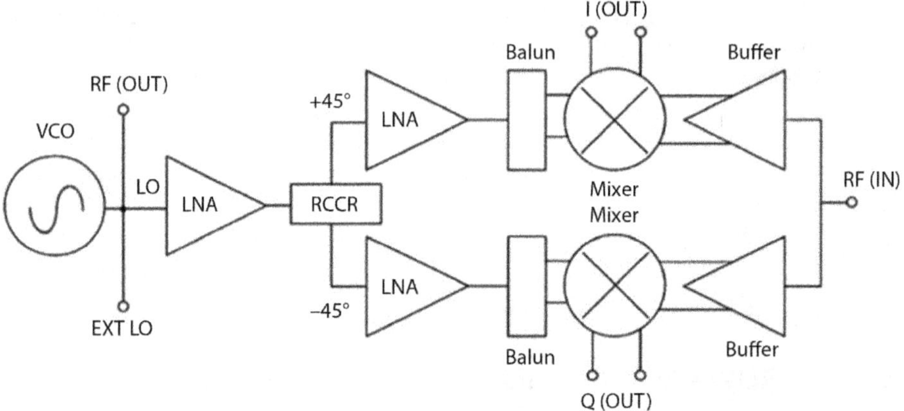


**FIGURE 7.9** Functional block diagram of a single-chip quadrature radar transceiver.

LO signals for the in-phase (I) and quadrature (Q) receiver channels. Another LNA amplifies each of these signals to provide isolation between the LOs of I and Q, and a passive LC balun transforms each single-ended LO into the differential LO required by the double-balanced mixer. A commercially available 2.4 GHz ISM-band patch antenna (Antenna Specialists ASPPT2988) with 60° × 80° beamwidth was used at the front end. The RF input is split in two for the I and Q channels, and active baluns provide differential RF signals to feed the mixer. The baseband $I_{out}$ and $Q_{out}$ channel outputs are filtered, and the respiration rate is then extracted.

The chip was implemented with 0.25 $\mu$m silicon CMOS and BiCMOS technologies in a 48-pin package. Figure 7.10 presents a photograph of the chip [Droitcour

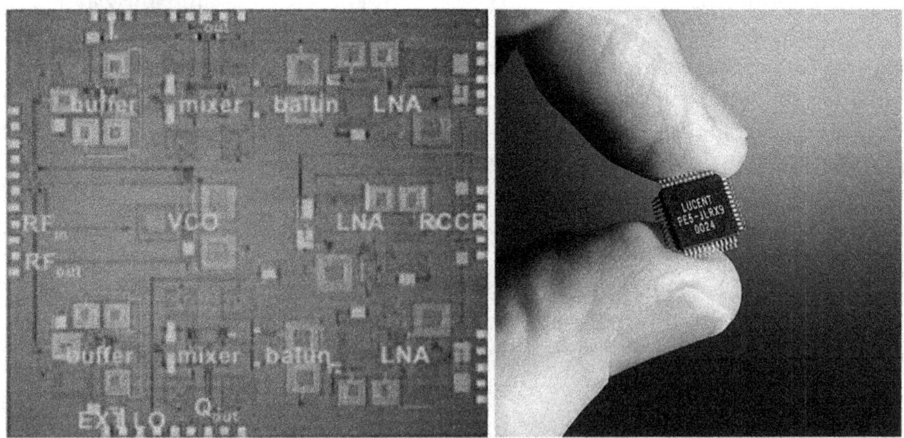


**FIGURE 7.10** Architecture and photograph of single chip quadrature Doppler radar transceiver for noncontact physiological sensing. (Courtesy of Jenshan Lin, University of Florida and Bell Laboratories.)

et al., 2003]. The chip is 4.0 × 4.2 $mm^2$ and it is reported to consume 180 mW of DC power and deliver 2 mW output power. Note that in addition to the 2.4 GHz quadrature CMOS chips, 1.6 GHz single-channel BiCMOS chips and 1.6 GHz single-channel CMOS chips with similar power output were investigated. Some experimental measurements with the 1.6 and 2.4 GHz ISM-band quadrature single-chip radar sensors can be found in Figures 7.45 and 7.46.

### 7.3.2 System-on-Chip Ultrawide-band Pulse Radar for Measuring Respiration Rate

An ultrawide-band (UWB) system-on-chip (SoC) radar sensor for contactless respiratory rate monitoring was implemented in 90 nm CMOS technology [Zito et al., 2011]. As a new class of devices, UWB systems have a 7.5 GHz-wide bandwidth in the frequency range from 3.1 to 10.6 GHz. In principle, UWB radar transceivers have lower circuit complexity compared to CW radars because they do not involve frequency conversions, which leads to lower power consumption for longer battery life [Baldi et al., 2014; Bernardi et al., 2014; Boryssenko et al., 2007]. A system diagram of the UWB pulse radar sensor is shown in Figure 7.11. The pulse generator (PG) transmits short pulses (see Figure 7.12 for a 350 ps-wide pulse) toward the subject at a set pulse repetition frequency ($f_{PR}$). The microwaves reflected by the target are captured by the RX antenna, amplified by the LNA, and multiplied and integrated (correlated) with a delayed replica of the transmitted pulses generated on-chip by the shaper circuit. The signal at the output of the multiplier with information on body movement is integrated to increase the signal-to-noise ratio (SNR) and isolated using a low-pass filter. Figure 7.13 shows the output for three different relative delays between the input pulses $V_P$ and $V_Q$.

The operating principle of the UWB radar sensor is based on the delay generator (DG) to provide a delay equal to the entire time-of-travel (round trip) of the transmitted and received pulses. If the target is not moving (stationary target), the local replica and the amplified echo are aligned and the multiplier provides the same output pulse with $f_{PR}$, as shown in Figure 7.11(b), Case A. Therefore, the signal at the output of the integrator is nearly constant, as shown in Figure 7.11(c). Note that the integrator will provide a constant output voltage regardless of the relative shift $\Delta$ between the local replica and amplified echo, for any other constant, $\Delta$. If the target is moving, the movement causes a time-varying $\Delta$ between the local replica and the echo amplified by the LNA. Therefore, the multiplier provides an output pulse that may be positive, negative, or zero, depending on the $\Delta$ caused by the time-varying distance between radar and target and due to the target movements around its motionless position.

The UWB radar sensor operates in two operating modes: ranging mode (RM) and tracking mode (TM). During RM, the 5-bit programmable monotonic DG provides a variable delay to span the range of interest and identify the target (see Figure 7.11[a]). During RM, the radar sensor identifies the presence of a target and the time of travel. When a target is detected, the radar switches to TM, in which the DG provides a fixed delay (the time of travel identified in RM) to monitor a

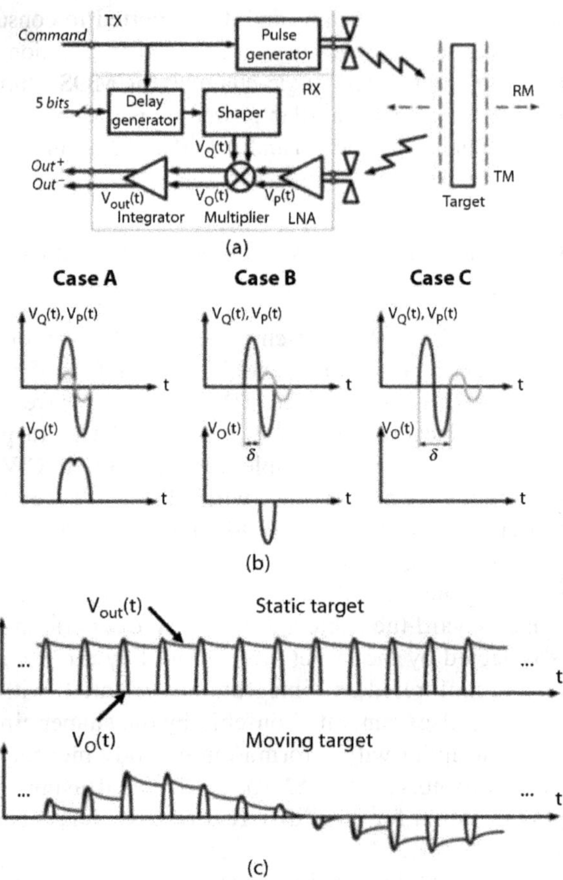


**FIGURE 7.11** System diagram of SoC UWB pulse radar (a). The dashed lines around the target indicate the range spanned by the radar in ranging (RM) and tracking (TM) modes. Representation of the pulses at the input and output of the multiplier for three different cases of relative shift between the input pulses (b). Representation of the input and output voltages of the integrator for stationary and moving targets (c).

fixed range gate (see Figure 7.11[a]). Therefore, the output voltage is directly proportional to the chest movement in case of respiratory rate monitoring. Figure 7.14 shows the radar test chip die and package. The overall power consumption is 73.2 mW including bias. The SoC radar packaged in QFN32 was mounted on a test-board with TX and RX antennas having a 2.3 dBi gain at 3.5 GHz for the 2.8 to 5.4 GHz frequency band of interest. In experimental test setup, the UWB radar detected longitudinal target movements with 2 cm displacements at distances up to 70 cm.

The experimental results from female and male human participants are illustrated in Figures 7.15 and 7.16. In Figure 7.15, a female subject is seated in front of

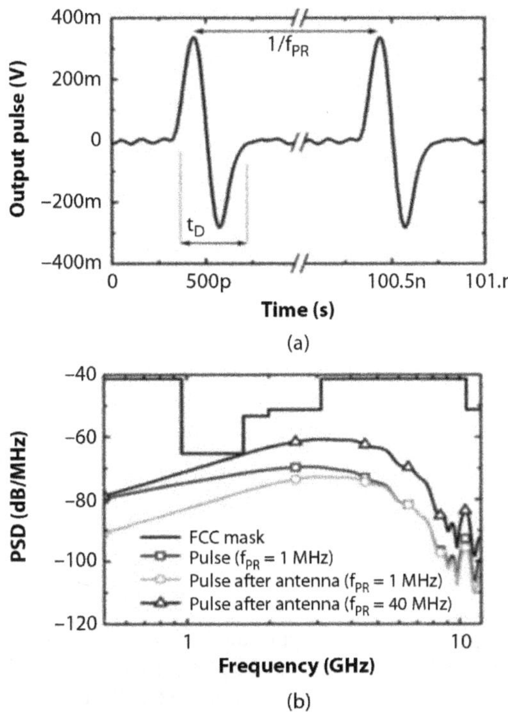


**FIGURE 7.12** Output from PG of the SoC radar: (a) Ultrawide-band (UWB) pulses with 350 ps duration; (b) The power spectral density (PSD) of pulse measured before and after antenna filtering and FCC UWB masking.

the radar sensor at 30 cm. The UWB radar detected a respiratory rate of 0.3 Hz. The maximum chest displacement during respiration was about 0.7 cm. Similarly, Figure 7.16 shows the measurement during an experiment in which the subject with normal breathing was instructed to voluntarily stop breathing before resuming normal breathing. It is seen that the UWB radar sensor was able to track the entire episode of the respiration maneuver. In this case, the maximum chest displacement during respiration was about 1 cm and the radar detected a respiration rate of 0.4 Hz. These results suggest that UWB radar could be useful in contactless sleep apnea monitoring applications.

### 7.3.3 Radar Measurement of Respiration During Cancer Radiotherapy

Accurate respiratory gating is crucial in motion-adaptive cancer radiotherapy to ensure proper dose delivery and minimize radiation damage to normal tissue. In many anatomic sites (e.g., lung and liver), tumors can move substantially (2–3 cm) with respiration. Respiratory gating limits ionizing radiation exposure to a portion of the breathing cycle when the tumor is in a predefined gating window. Conventional

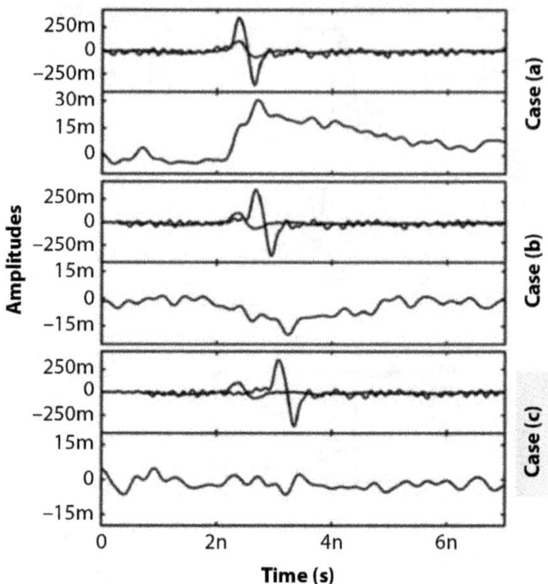


**FIGURE 7.13** Input (upper trace) and output (lower trace) signals of the multiplier measured for three cases: (a) monocycle input pulses without relative delay (i.e., time alignment), (b) a relative delay of half of the time duration, and (c) relative delay equal to the time duration.

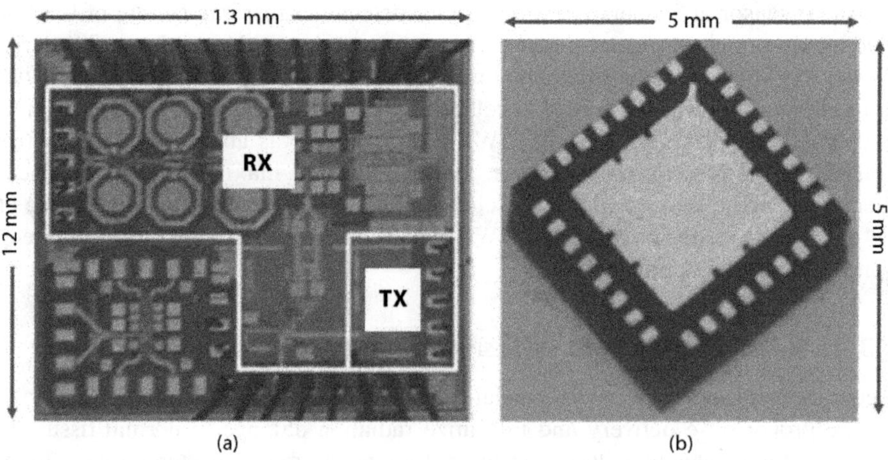


**FIGURE 7.14** System on chip ultrawide-band pulse radar. Micrograph of the radar chip (a). The die size is 1.5 × 1.3 mm (including the multiplier as stand-alone device). Radar testchip packaged in a leadless package (bottom view) with exposed ground pad (size 5 × 5 mm) (b).

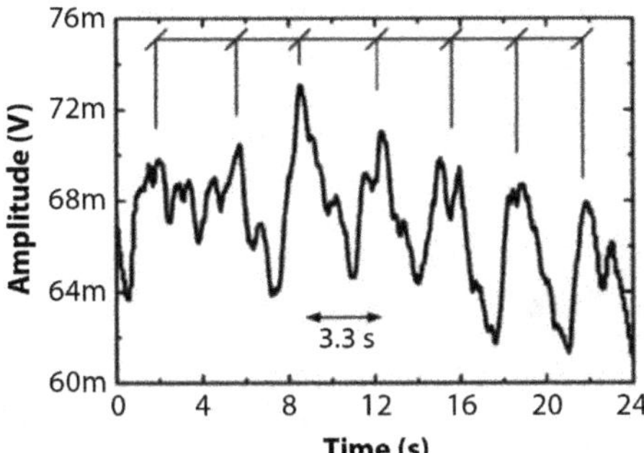


**FIGURE 7.15** Respiration record of a seated female detected with ultrawide-band radar sensor at 30 cm in front of chest. The measured output voltage in TM mode (fPR at 40 MHz) is expressed in mV and shows a respiratory rate about 0.3 Hz.

methods for respiration measurement are incompatible because they are either invasive, such as fiducial markers, or do not have sufficient accuracy [Jiang, 2007]. In addition, measurement of respiratory signals based on conventional approaches often requires the physical device to be in contact with the patient, which often causes unwanted patient discomfort-related motion during the radiation therapy session. Furthermore, for the treatment to be effective, the tumor's location must be known with a high degree of precision and in real time. To address these issues, a DC-coupled CW radar sensor was developed to provide a noninvasive contactless method for respiration measurement [Gu et al., 2012].

The scenario for a radar-respiration-gated motion-adaptive radiotherapy system in operation is shown in Figure 7.17 (inset [c] shows the 2.4 GHz miniature microwave radar sensor). Radiotherapy involves two major steps: treatment planning and the treatment session, which delivers the ionizing radiation dose to the patient. Treatment planning is a virtual process that designs the patient treatment using the patient model built at the simulation stage. At the simulation stage, the patient and tumor geometrical information is collected through computed tomography (CT)

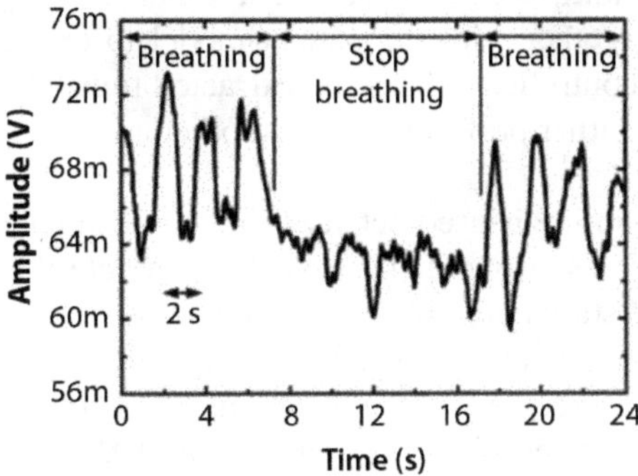


**FIGURE 7.16** Output voltage (mV) showing respiratory record of a male subject from before and after voluntarily holding his breath at 25 cm from the radar.

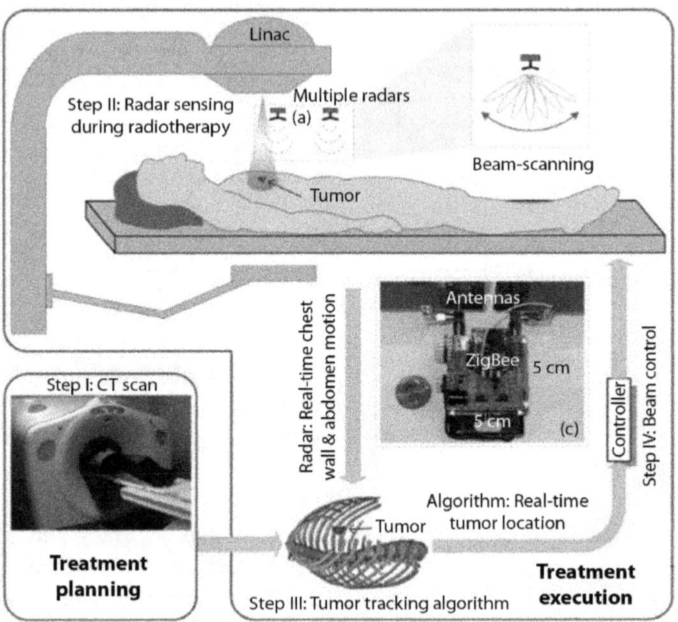


**FIGURE 7.17** Motion-adaptive radiotherapy based on radar respiration sensing. The process includes two steps: treatment planning and treatment execution sessions. Insets: (a) multiple radars, (b) beam-scanning radar, and (c) the 2.4-GHz miniature radar sensor (see quarter coin for size comparison). (Courtesy of Changzhi Li, Texas Tech University.)

scan and then a 3-D patient model is built for the target tumor and organs at risk. During the radiotherapy session, a medical linear accelerator (LINAC) would work with two radar sensors that dynamically monitor the chest wall and abdomen to provide real-time motion information. The LINAC could also be integrated with a radar sensor with beam-scanning capability, as shown in inset (b) of Figure 7.17, which would make it possible to use one radar sensor to simultaneously measure the breathing motions at multiple body locations. A tumor-tracking algorithm combines motion information together with the patient model to extract the tumor location in real-time. Then, a controller utilizes the extracted tumor location information to control the LINAC to either perform gated radiotherapy or steer the radiation beam to track the tumor.

Commonly, AC coupling is used between the RF front end and baseband circuit in CW radar respiration-sensing applications to eliminate the undesired DC offset due to reflections from stationary objects near the body. However, respiration motion is dominated by low-frequency and even DC components and it tends to pause at the end of expiration. To overcome the complications this phenomenon presents in respiration-gating, the radar sensor incorporates a smart DC-coupled adaptive tuning architecture that includes RF coarse-tuning and baseband fine-tuning (Figure 7.18). The RF coarse tuning adds a portion of the transmitted signal to the receiver signal to cancel most of the clutter reflection. To further calibrate the remaining undesired DC

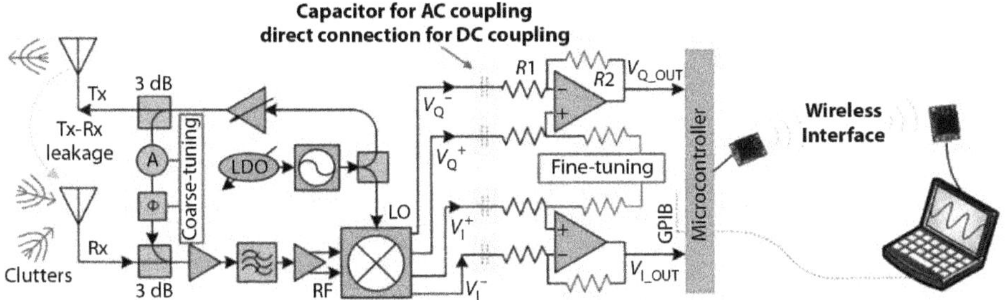


**FIGURE 7.18** Block diagram of DC-coupled radar sensor system with RF coarse-tuning and baseband fine-tuning architectures. ZigBee protocols are used to transmit data and receive commands wirelessly. (Courtesy of Changzhi Li, Texas Tech University.)

offset, the baseband fine-tuning adaptively adjusts an amplifier bias to the desired level that allows both high gain amplification and maximum dynamic range at the baseband stage.

The smart radar sensor was validated with a LINAC in a clinical setting. The radar sensor and an on-board, real-time position management (RPM) system were used to measure the same motion in a phantom on the treatment platform with the radiation treatment beam turned on. The measurement demonstrated a submillimeter accuracy as measured using phantom motion (Table 7.2). Also, the smart radar sensor was set up for measurement with a human participant who laid on the treatment platform. The subject was coached to dynamically adjust breathing to generate a reproducible respiration signal to place the end of expiration (EOE) position within the shaded area (Figure 7.19). The accurate measurement provided by the DC-coupled and RF-tuned radar sensor allows the coaching reference data domain to be chosen near the position of end of inspiration (EOI). With the radar-measured accurate respiration pattern shown, gating signals could be easily obtained.

**TABLE 7.2**
**Accuracy of Radar Measurement for Various Motion Amplitudes**

| Amplitude (mm) | Period (s) | RMS Error (mm) |
|---|---|---|
| 20 | 4 | 0.202 |
| | 5 | 0.209 |
| | 6 | 0.211 |
| 10 | 4 | 0.176 |
| | 5 | 0.175 |
| | 6 | 0.179 |
| 5 | 4 | 0.103 |
| | 5 | 0.091 |
| | 6 | 0.115 |

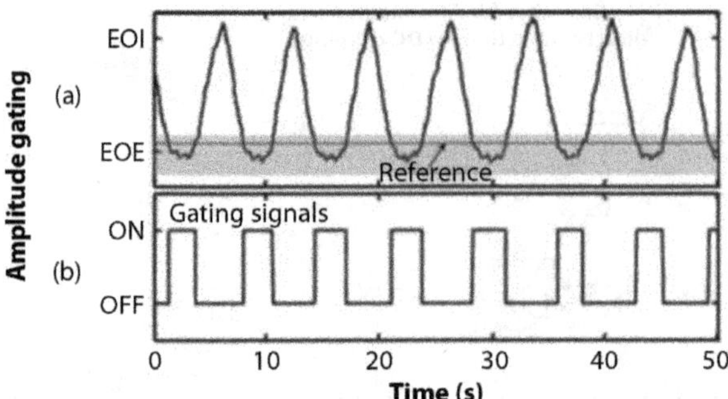


**FIGURE 7.19** DC-coupled sensor measured respiratory signal of a human participant: (a) Radar measured respiration signal; (b) Generated gating signal. The shaded area indicates the coach reference data domain, and the line represents the reference for gating.

## 7.4 CONTINUOUS RESPIRATORY MONITORING WITH FREQUENCY-MODULATED CW RADAR

The microwave signal returned from a target consists of backscattering due to target movement and reflections of stationary objects within its field of propagation. AC coupling is commonly used between the RF front end and baseband circuit in CW Doppler radar respiration sensing applications, for example, to eliminate undesirable DC offset due to reflections from stationary objects near the body. A related limitation of Doppler CW radars comes from their inability to discriminate between reflections from multiple targets to provide absolute range or their vulnerability to stationary objects and the motions of unwanted targets, which manifest as radar clutter (see Chapter 5).

As mentioned in Chapter 5, Section 5.9, instead of a tonal signal used in the CW Doppler radar, other waveforms such as pulsed CW radars (PCW), frequency-modulated CW (FMCW), stepped-frequency CW (SFCW), and ultrawide-band (UWB) radar sensors have been introduced to overcome the limitations of CW Doppler radars [Skolnik, 1980; Wang et al., 2014; Rabbani and Ghafouri-Shiraz, 2016; Muñoz -Ferreras et al., 2017]. In all the cases, the objective is to capitalize on the large bandwidth of device architecture aided by sophisticated signal processing schemes to achieve better range resolution. In pulse Doppler radars, the transmitter's CW RF signal is multiplied with a rectangular pulse signal at a pulse repetition frequency (PRF). The receiver downconverts the target-reflected signal using the original CW signal. Therefore, the receiver output spectrum is shifted from DC to an intermediate frequency (IF) that is equal to the PRF, for example, 100 Hz. This single-channel pulse Doppler low-IF radar architecture overcomes a limitation of conventional quadrature radars, quadrature channel imbalance [Mostafanezhad and Boric-Lubecke, 2014]. An example of respiratory-rate monitoring with FMCW radar is discussed in this section, and discussions on use of UWB radars follow in subsequent sections.

### 7.4.1 FMCW Radar Sensor

The functional schematics of FMCW radar sensors are essentially the same as those depicted in Chapter 1, Figure 1.3 or Figure 7.3 for CW Doppler radar, except for the modulation impressed on the microwave source. In CW Doppler radar, a simple tone or a sample of a single sine wave is used to modulate the sinusoidal source of microwaves. In FMCW radar, other waveforms such as a train of periodic sawtooth waveforms with rising frequency modulates the microwave source. Figure 7.20 illustrates the conventional sawtooth waveform for FMCW radar [Peng et al., 2017; Skolnik, 1980]. The instantaneous bandwidth is given by $B = f_2 - f_1$, the period $T$, and the carrier frequency is designated by $f_c$. The ramps may be generated through modulation of the microwave source with a linear periodic voltage. Therefore, the transmitted signal is represented by a frequency modulated sine wave,

$$x(t) = sin\left\{2\pi t\left(f_c + \left[\frac{Bt}{2T}\right]\right)\right\} \tag{7.1}$$

The microwave signal travels to a distance $R$, and the total two-way time it takes the reflected signal to travel back to the receiver at speed $v$ is

$$t_d = \frac{2}{v}R(t) \tag{7.2}$$

The microwave signal received back at the receiving antenna is identical to the transmitted signal, but delayed in time by $t_d$, such that

$$y(t) = sin\left\{2\pi(t - t_d)\left(f_c + \left[\frac{B(t - t_d)}{2T}\right]\right)\right\} \tag{7.3}$$

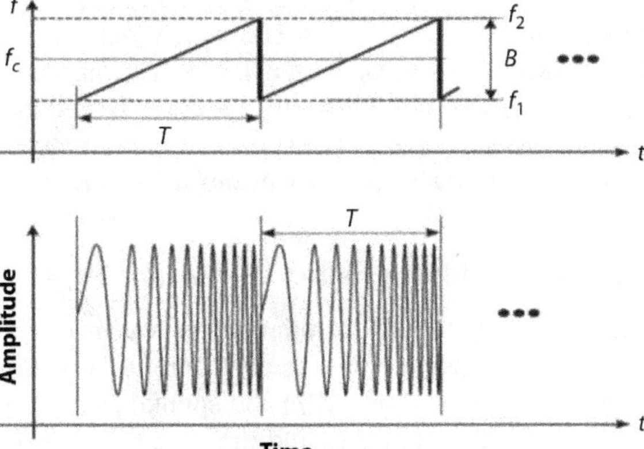


**FIGURE 7.20** Transmitted waveform of a sawtooth frequency-modulated continuous wave (FMCW) radar: Ramp frequency modulation versus time (upper) and instantaneous amplitude variation with time (lower).

Following correlation of $y(t)$ with $x(t)$ over $T$, and passing the result through a low-pass filter, the output signal $z(t)$ is proportional in frequency to target range $R(t)$ and takes the form, after substituting Eq. (7.2),

$$z(t) = sin\left[4\pi\left(\frac{f_c}{v}R(t)\right) + 4\pi\left(\left(\frac{B}{T}\right)\left(\frac{t}{v}\right)R(t)\right)\right] \tag{7.4}$$

where the frequency of the baseband beat signal

$$f_b = 2\left(\frac{B}{T}\left(\frac{1}{v}\right)R(t)\right) \tag{7.5}$$

is proportional to the distance to the target. The phase component in Eq. (7.4),

$$\phi(t) = 4\pi\left(\frac{f_c}{v}R(t)\right) \tag{7.6}$$

provides an expression for the target range extraction,

$$R(t) = \left(\frac{v}{4\pi f_c}\phi(t)\right) \tag{7.7}$$

Furthermore, FMCW has a range resolution that varies with the modulation bandwidth B, such that

$$\Delta R = \frac{v}{2B} \tag{7.8}$$

Figure 7.21 shows a prototype ramp based FMCW radar with two patch array antennas [Wang et al., 2014]. For a microwave carrier frequency $f_c$ = 5.8 GHz, the ramp modulation bandwidth $B$ = 160 MHz, which yields a range resolution of $\Delta R = 0.94$ m and the sampling period of $T = 2$ ms, which is long enough to sample the breathing pattern shown in Figure 7.22. In this case, the seated human subject was at 1.5 m from the radar and stayed quiet while breathing normally. Displacements in the chest wall associated with the respiratory events are clearly identifiable.

### 7.4.2 Preclinical Study Using a Prototype FMCW Sensor

In a preclinical study, a prototype FMCW radar sensor was investigated to determine whether the noninvasive contactless radar system can reliably measure respiration in patients during mechanical ventilation (MV) and spontaneous breathing [van Loon et al., 2016]. Specifically, the preclinical study involved adult patients who underwent elective laparoscopic prostatectomy or hysterectomy and were monitored after surgery during recovery. Nursing and medical staff were blinded to the study's measurement with FMCW radar. The prototype radar sensor operated at a frequency of 9.5 GHz with a radiated power of 14 mW. The FMCW radar sensor (a small box-sized

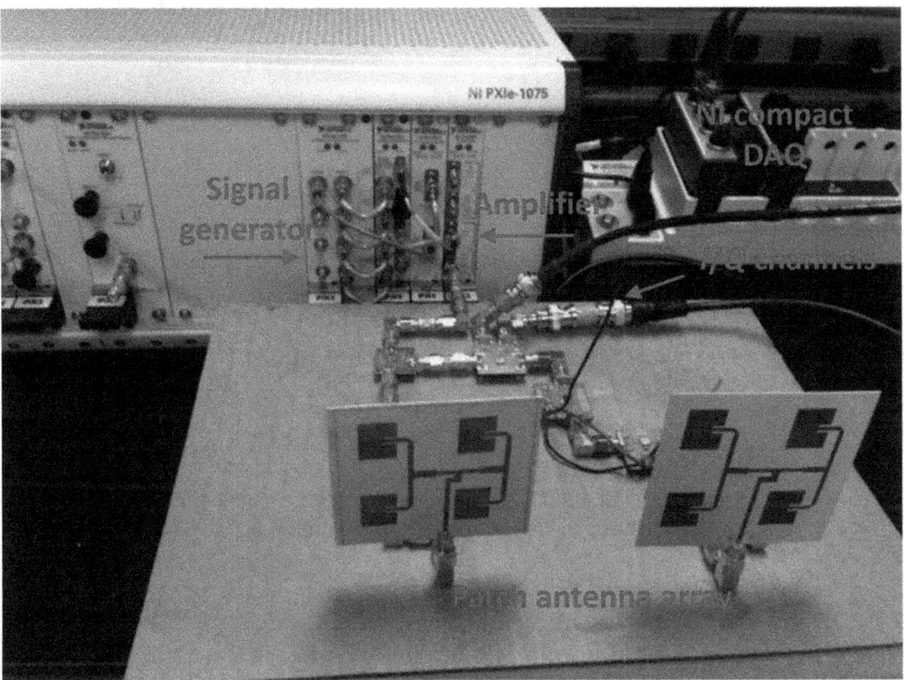


**FIGURE 7.21** Photograph of prototype quadrature frequency-modulated continuous wave radar showing signal generator and patch array antennas with low-noise amplifier (LNA), data acquisition (DAQ ), and local oscillator (LO). (Courtesy of Changzhi Li, Texas Tech University.)

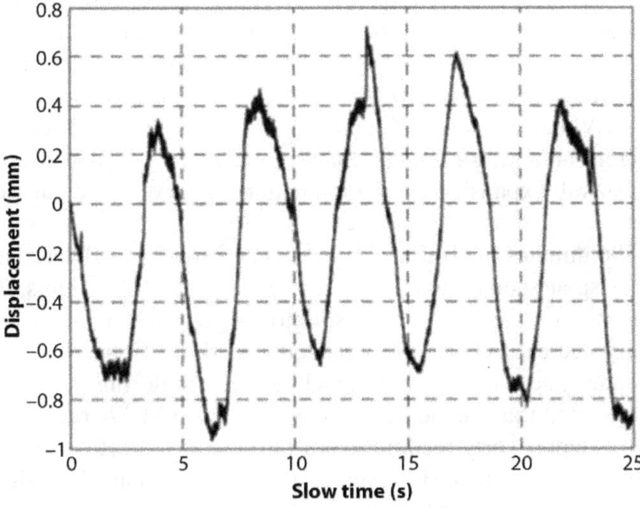


**FIGURE 7.22** Human respiration pattern showing chest-wall displacement obtained using a 5.8 GHz frequency-modulated continuous wave radar sensor.

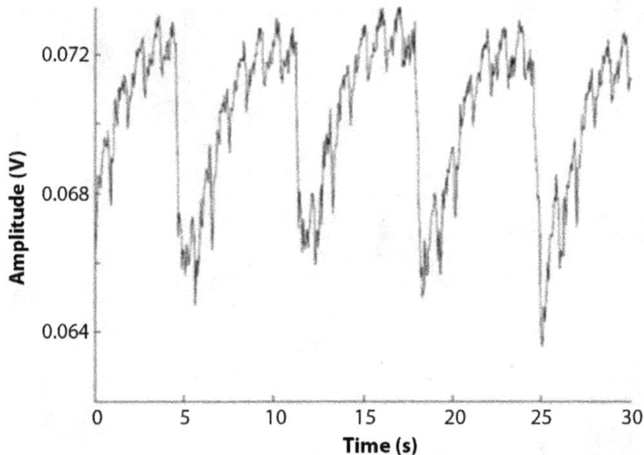


**FIGURE 7.23** Frequency-modulated continuous wave radar-detected patient breathing patterns with superimposed heartbeats during mechanical ventilation.

7.5 × 10 cm) was mounted to the ceiling above the patient's bed. Its output signals were recorded simultaneously with those from the reference standard. During MV, the reference standard was the pneumotachograph ventilator, which has an accuracy of ±1 breath/min. During spontaneous breathing, the reference standard was a capnograph, which has an accuracy of ±1 breath/min in the range 4–20 breaths/min. A capnograph measures the partial pressure of carbon dioxide ($CO_2$) in exhaled breath. A simple nonrespiratory movement artifact removal algorithm was used to eliminate movement artifacts bias.

Figure 7.23 illustrates FMCW radar detected patient breathing patterns. Although this study focused on detection of respiration during mechanical ventilation, it is seen that a heartbeat signal is superimposed on the respiration pattern, demonstrating the FMCW radar sensor is also capable of detecting heart rate noninvasively. An example of FMCW radar-monitored spontaneous breathing is depicted in Figure 7.24 showing different breathing patterns. Each inspiratory cycle is characterized by a first peak (chest-wall expansion during inhalation), followed by a curved peak (during exhalation).

A total of 796 minutes of observation time during mechanical ventilation and 521 minutes during spontaneous breathing were examined in 8 patients. The FMCW radar was able to accurately measure respiratory rate in MV patients (within 95%), but the accuracy decreased during spontaneous breathing. Considering the ability of the FMCW radar system to accurately track respiration during mechanical ventilation, it was suggested that the noninvasive contactless FMCW radar technique has the potential to support early recognition of physiological decline in spontaneously breathing patients in hospitals. However, further optimization of the signal processing algorithms is needed to enable tracking of respiration rate trend of spontaneously breathing postoperative patients recovering from general anesthesia on a minute-to-minute basis.

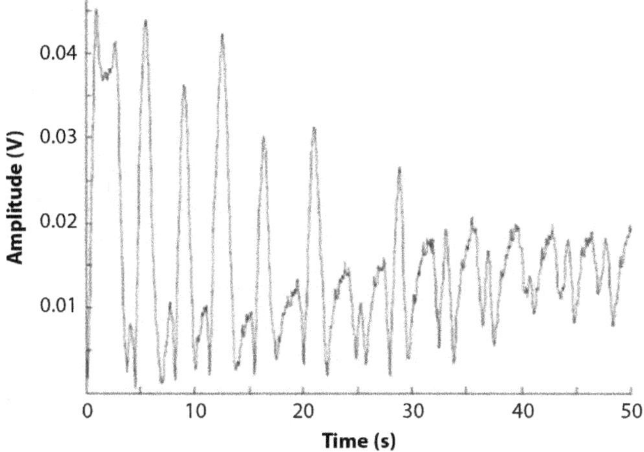


**FIGURE 7.24** Frequency-modulated continuous wave radar monitored spontaneous breathing with different breathing patterns. Each inspiratory cycle is characterized by a first peak (chest-wall expansion during inhalation) followed by a curved peak (during exhalation).

Note that the use of a ceiling-mounted microwave (1215 MHz) radar antenna for noncontact monitoring of respiratory activities was reported earlier in a nursing care setting [Uenoyama et al., 2006]. It involved 8 healthy and 8 elderly participants in bed with soft coverings. Respiration rates measured correlated well with rates measured using conventional sensors ($r = 0.97$, $P < 0.001$ for healthy participants; $r = 0.98$, $P < 0.0001$ for elderly participants). It was suggested that ceiling-mounted microwave radars could monitor subtle changes in respiration rate, with the possibility of monitoring respiratory rate increases caused by disorders such as pneumonia.

Also, sleep apnea-hypopnea syndrome (SAHS) is being recognized as a potential cause or significant contributor to such chronic medical conditions as hypertension, heart failure, and diabetes. Early diagnosis of disease can positively impact treatment outcome and efficacy. Description of continuous noninvasive contactless microwave Doppler radar respiratory monitoring as a diagnostic tool for SAHS in sleep medicine can be found in Chapter 11, where the topic of microwave sensing in sleep research and medicine alongside recent advances will be discussed.

## 7.5 HEARTBEAT SENSING AND MICROWAVE CARDIOGRAPHY

Displacements and vibrations on the chest wall manifest events generated by the beating heart inside the chest. These mechanical events are measurable using Doppler microwave and related radar techniques. Like the cardiac electrical events recorded in electrocardiography (ECG), the motions can be recorded to provide an index for assessing cardiac performance. The principle of operation is based on detection of the changes in the backscattered microwaves caused by the movement of the chest wall in response to ventricular contraction [Byrne et al., 1986; Chan and Lin, 1985, 1987; Lin et al., 1979]. The microwave-sensed pulsatile response gives the same heart rate recorded simultaneously by the ECG and phonocardiography (PCG). A significant difference is that contactless microwave radar measurement eliminates direct contact with the skin, and it does not require attaching electrodes or any other device on the body surface for it to function.

Biomechanical events can be measured using the techniques known as apexcardiography (ACG) or seismocardiography (SCG). ACG is a direct method for sensing and recording of the precordial movements. It represents the left-ventricular movement caused by low-frequency displacements of the precordium overlying the apex of the heart [Benchimol and Dimond 1963] and it is correlated with the hemodynamic events within the left ventricle [Denef et al., 1973; Tavel et al., 1965; Voigt and Friesinger, 1970; Willems et al., 1971, 1979]. The complex ACG tracings are reported to reveal changes in left ventricular volume, compliance, position, and intracardiac pressures as well [Voigt and Friesinger, 1970]. In conventional systems used to record ACG, either a linear displacement or velocity gradient microphone is used to sense and convert the mechanical movement and vibration into electrical signals. It is necessary to strap or tape the microphone to the patient's chest. These approaches have been found to be unreliable since a tremendous variation in sensitivity results from differing pressures applied to the skin through the microphone.

Similarly, a conventional SCG is acquired with an accelerometer placed near the xiphoid process on the lower sternum or midsternum over the apex of the heart (see Figure 7.25) [Bozhenko, 1961; Sørensen et al., 2018]. SCG is typically recorded by attaching an accelerometer directly to the skin. Thus, both ACG and SCG recordings have considerable variations in sensitivity that could result from applying the microphone or accelerometer on the skin with different contact pressures. The ACG and SCG recordings may be combined with ECG data to derive an index for a global assessment of cardiac health and performance.

A contactless noninvasive Doppler microwave cardiography technique was developed to detect changes in the reflected microwaves caused by precordial displacements of the chest wall and the vibrations in response to ventricular contraction (Figure 7.26). The remote-sensing approach alleviates any change in sensitivity, discomfort, intrusion, or obstruction caused by attaching sensors to the chest. The

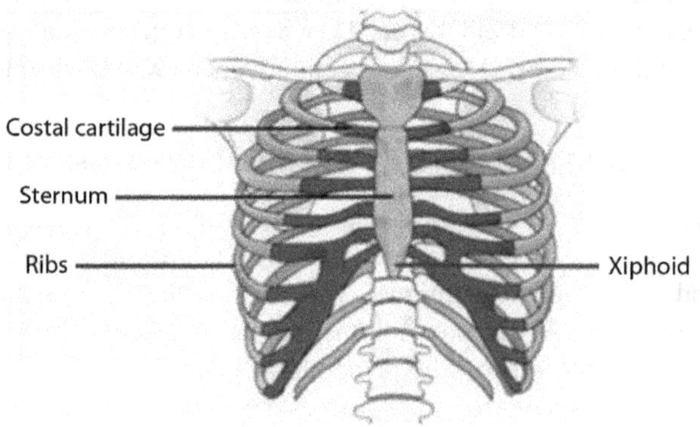


**FIGURE 7.25** The sternum, xiphoid, and thoracic cage.

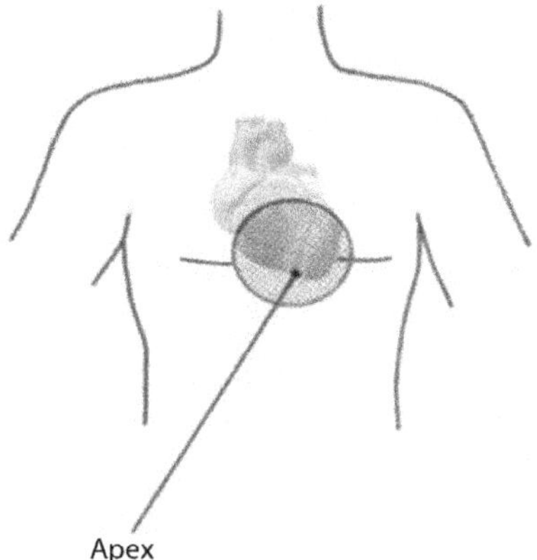


**FIGURE 7.26** Antenna located over the apex of the heart for microwave apexcardiography.

microwave technique was named microwave apexcardiography (MACG), recognizing that microwave ACG involves detecting variations in the microwave signal reflected using an antenna positioned over the apex of the heart [Lin et al., 1979]. Figure 7.27 gives an illustration of ECG, ACG, and MACG recordings. MACG is related to the hemodynamic events within the left ventricle and matches up with the conventional SCG recording. Also, the salient features of MACG measurement echo the simultaneously recorded ECG. The MACG signal is deterministic and noninvasive, however, in contrast to ECG, ACG, and SCG sensors, MACG measurements do not require attachment of the radar sensor to the chest. The MACG fiducial points are associated with characteristic events during the cardiac cycle. Noninvasive Doppler

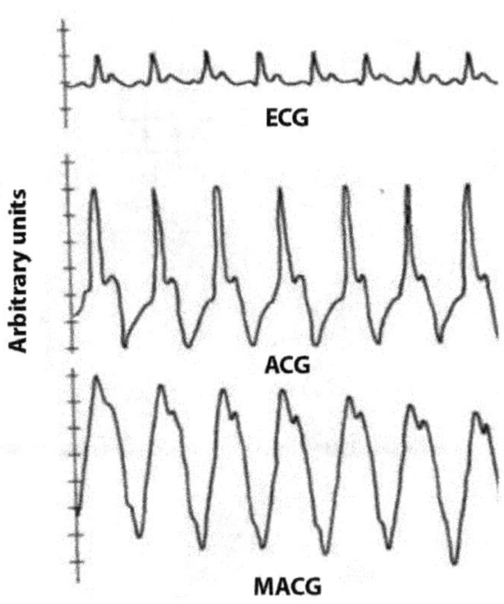


**FIGURE 7.27** Illustration of electrocardiography (ECG), apexcardiography (ACG), and microwave apexcardiography (MACG) recordings in arbitrary units.

microwave radar sensors can successfully and reproducibly measure cardiovascular signal waveforms of diagnostic quality [Papp et al., 1987]. Thus, MACG may be useful as a noninvasive measuring technique of cardiac performance and its condition of health. MACG or microwave cardiography can be advantageous because it relies on wireless remote noncontact sensing.

### 7.5.1 Measurement of MACG

The measurement of MACG involves detecting the amplitude or phase variation in the microwave signal reflected using an antenna located over the apex of the heart. A schematic diagram of the Doppler microwave system is shown in Figure 7.28 [Lin et al., 1979]. Microwave energy is derived from a signal generator. The incident power is fed through a 20 dB directional coupler and emitted by way of an antenna (coaxial applicator) operating at 2450 MHz [Lin et al., 1982]. The reflected microwave signal is modulated both in amplitude and in phase by the moving chest wall. Using the forward signal as a reference, the amplitude and phase of the reflected signal are measured as a function of precordial displacement over the apex of the heart, with a vector voltmeter. The output voltage corresponding to either the amplitude or the phase variation is presented on a multichannel chart recorder.

For the experimental results shown in Figure 7.29, the human subject was lying on a table in the supine position. The coaxial applicator held by a stand was located over the apex of the heart with a spatial separation of 3 cm between the applicator surface and chest wall. The amplitude and phase changes depend closely on the applicator location. It is important that the applicator is placed directly over the apex. The figure shows the microwave-sensed pulsatile ACG (the more sensitive phase variation in this case) for a healthy young male who held his breath throughout the

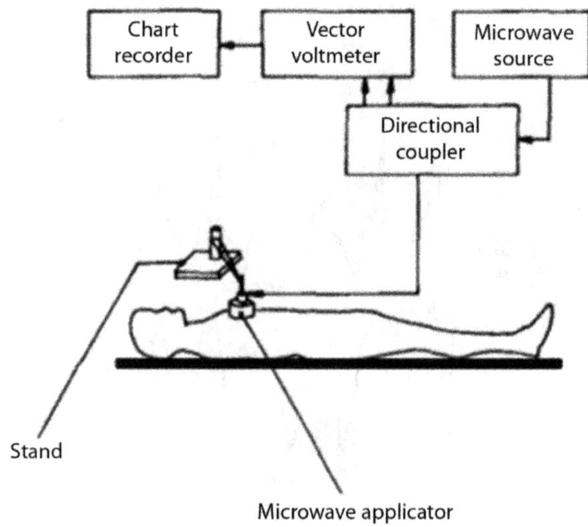


**FIGURE 7.28** Experimental diagram for microwave cardiography - noncontact microwave measurement of precordial movements using homodyne detection.

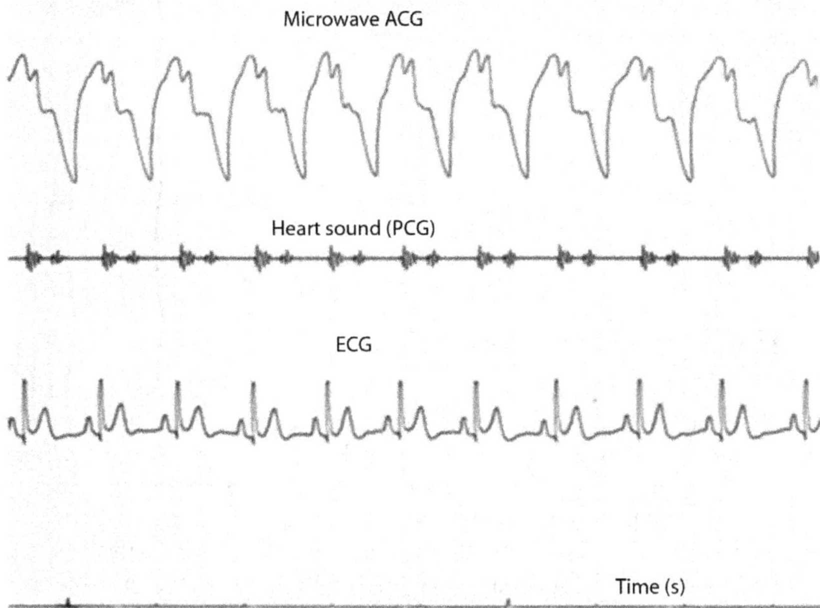


**FIGURE 7.29** Microwave pulsatile microwave apexcardiography (MACG) for a healthy young male along with electrocardiography (ECG) and phonocardiography (PCG) tracings. Note the same heart rate is recorded by the ECG, PCG, and MACG.

measurement. The ECG and PCG (heart sound) tracings for the same subject are recorded simultaneously. It is seen that the same heart rate is provided by the ECG, PCG, and pulsatile MACG.

The salient features of microwave-sensed ventricular movement in a healthy young male who held his breath throughout the measurement is shown in Figure 7.30

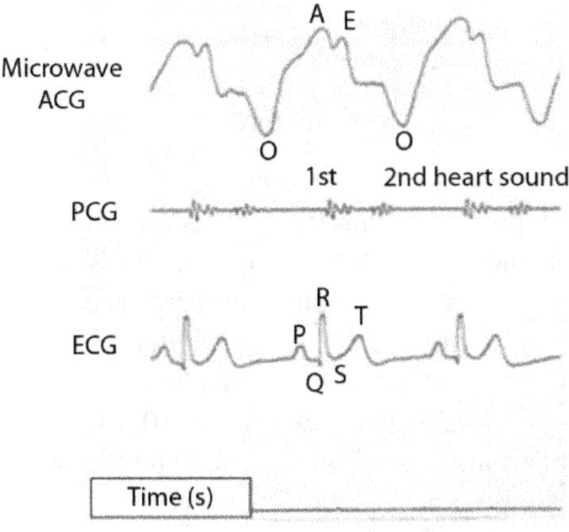


**FIGURE 7.30** Salient features (landmarks) of microwave-measured ventricular movement in a healthy young male.

alongside the simultaneously recorded ECG and PCG. It is seen that toward the end of systole, a rapid rising wave occurs due to ventricular filling, which is completed by atrial contraction occurring between the P-wave and QRS complex in ECG. A rapid downward deflection represents maximal ventricular ejection following a period of isometric contraction, just after the QRS complex. The ventricular movement reaches a plateau at the level of midsystole, and it is then followed by another downward deflection, which coincides with the aortic valve opening and completes the cardiac cycle. The noninvasive microwave method, therefore, may be used to delineate fine details of the hemodynamic movements associated with ventricular contraction.

## 7.6 VITAL SIGN MEASUREMENTS

The heartbeat and respiratory rate alongside temperature and blood pressure are a group of the four most important clinical vital-sign measurements taken to indicate the general state of physical health of a person. The results discussed in Sections 7.2 and 7.5 for Doppler microwave-measured respiratory rate and heartbeat, respectively, reveal individually their efficiency for assessing the status of the body's vital functions. Furthermore, the noncontact and remote operational capability suggest potential applications of vital-sign detection beyond patient health assessment to include fitness sensing, neonatal monitoring, and burn management under normal conditions, to wider use in emergency situations where direct contact with the subject is either impossible or undesirable. The scenarios span rescue campaigns necessitated by disasters like fire, chemical or nuclear accidents, and natural catastrophes such as earthquakes or building collapses [Chan and Lin, 1985, 1987; Chen et al., 1986, 2000; Lin, 1986, 1989, 1992, 1999, 2004; Popovic et al., 1984]. Several contactless and remote Doppler microwave vital-sign monitors for detection of heart and respiration rates have been investigated using microwaves from 400 MHz to 60 GHz. Indeed, research and development have expanded to involve many other types of microwave radar technologies. The description will begin with the fundamental results and contributions, and progress to discussions on both recent advances in applications and technological innovations concerning microwave remote contactless vital sign detection and monitoring.

### 7.6.1 A Portable Contactless Vital-Sign Monitor

A portable protype microprocessor-based noninvasive contactless cardiopulmonary rate monitor was developed for use in situations where direct contact with the subject is either impossible or undesirable [Chan and Lin, 1985, 1987; Popovic et al., 1984]. It uses Doppler microwaves to detect chest movement at few centimeters to tens of meters from the subject. Information on the frequency and regularity of the heartbeat and respiration rates is extracted from the chest movement.

The front end is comprised of a low-power (10.5 GHz, 5–10 mW) microwave transceiver and a X-band antenna (Figure 7.31). The transceiver consists of a tuned CW Gunn diode oscillator and a Schottky barrier mixer diode, assembled into a compact waveguide package. The horn antenna directs microwaves from the Gunn diode toward the moving chest. The total output power from the transceiver is about

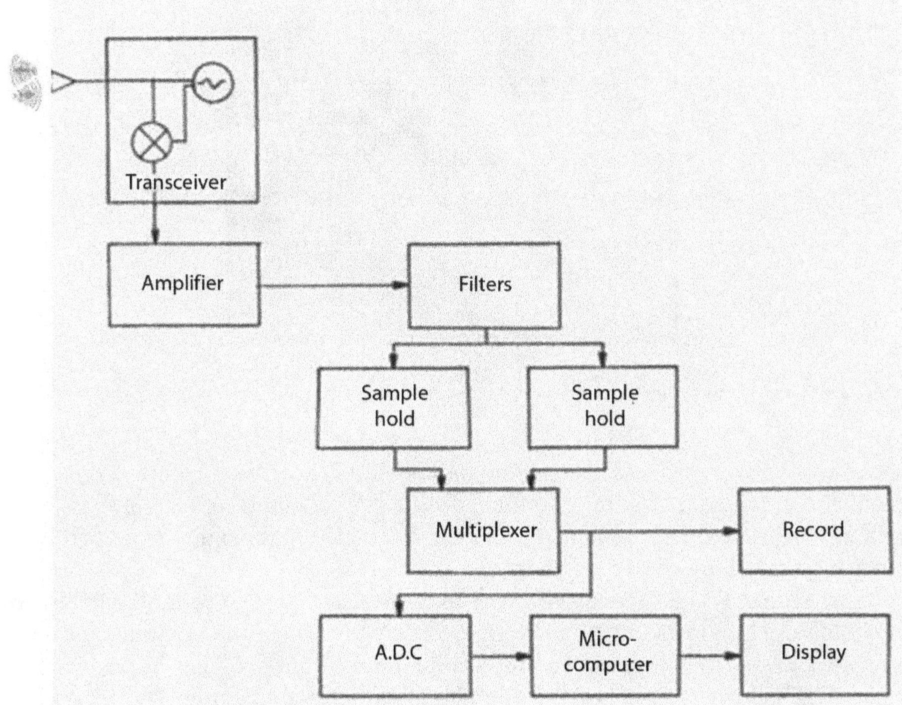


**FIGURE 7.31** Functional diagram of a portable contactless vital sign monitor.

10 mW for a power density of less than 1 mW/m$^2$. The mixer diode combines the backscattered signal with the transmitted microwave as a reference via homodyne detection to produce the Doppler shift frequency component. The output from the transceiver is proportional to the displacement of the chest-wall movement associated with expansion and contraction of the heart and lungs.

The microwave wavelength dictates the spatial resolution of the microwave monitor. The depth of microwave penetration determines the target or source of motion detection, whether it is from the surface or at depth. In this case, the wavelength in air is 2.8 cm and the depth of penetration is about 0.3 cm in skin and muscle. These characteristics allow the monitor to detect chest-surface motion with millimeter (mm) spatial resolution.

As can be seen from the transceiver's output shown in Figure 7.32, the heart signal is typically superimposed on breathing as an artifact. The output from the transceiver mixer is fed into an analog signal processing circuit to maximize dynamic range through amplification, while filtering separates the heart and respiration signals. A multiplexer presents either the heart signal or the breathing signal to an analog-to-digital converter for conversion to digital form. The circuits include a combination of filters. The band-pass filter with a high frequency cutoff at 3.3 Hz removes the high-frequency noise and sets the upper limit of the heartbeat signal, and a low-frequency cutoff at 0.03 Hz to filter out the DC component of the transceiver output and limits

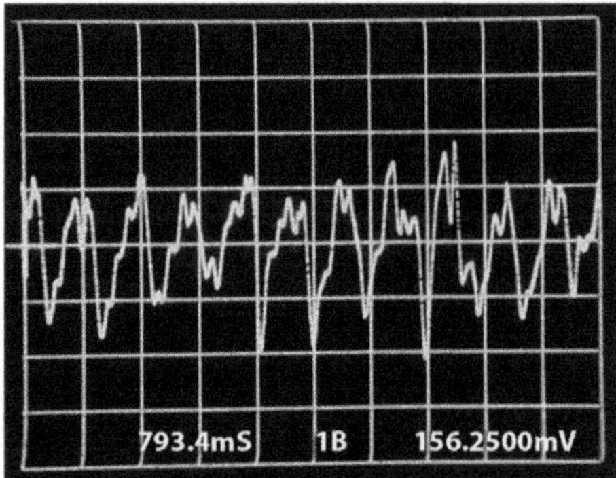


**FIGURE 7.32** Transceiver output signal sensed from human chest.

the lowest breathing rate detectable by the monitor. These filters are followed by a parallel combination of a low-pass filter with a 0.5 Hz cutoff and a high-pass filter with a 0.6 Hz cutoff to separate the higher frequency heart signal from the lower frequency breathing signal.

Approximately 12 seconds of heart and 48 seconds of breathing signals are taken at sampling rates of 80 and 10 Hz, respectively. The same software algorithm was used to detect both heart and respiration rates (discussed later in the chapter). Figure 7.33 shows typical heart and breathing waveforms recorded from a healthy young adult. As expected, the two signals have clearly distinguishable characters. The breathing signal resembles a typical sinusoidal signal. The heart signal, while periodic, exhibits the usual complex characteristics.

The performance of the vital-sign (heart rate and respiration) monitor was tested both on rats and human subjects. The anesthetized rats (500 g, sodium pentobarbital, 40 mg/kg IP) breathed regularly and produced minimal motion artifacts. The maximum counting error of the monitor was less than 3% out of 17 readings. A scatter graph for the monitor measured and visually identified breathing rates taken from an oscilloscope is shown in Figure 7.34. The calculated correlation coefficient is 0.99 in this case, showing excellent agreement.

The vital sign monitor's performance was also tested on humans in standing or supine positions. A comparison of monitor-detected and visually counted heart and

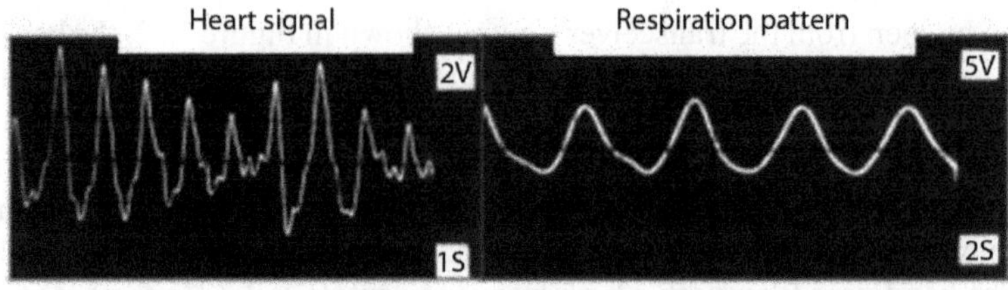


**FIGURE 7.33** Typical heart and breathing waveforms recorded by the portable contactless vital sign monitor from a healthy young adult.

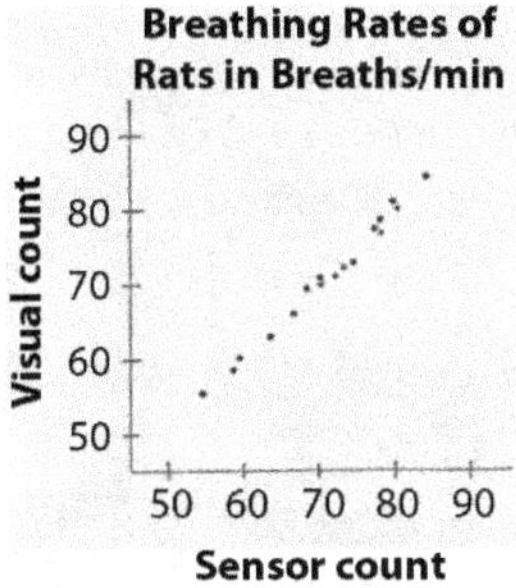


**FIGURE 7.34** Scatter plot of measured and visually identified breathing rates of rats.

respiration rates is given in Table 7.3. The maximum errors between the sensor and visual determinations are 7% and 9%, respectively, with 0.98 and 0.99 calculated correlation coefficients. Scatter graphs for the monitor measured and visually identified heart and respiration rates for human subjects are shown in Figure 7.35. Thus, results obtained both from animals and humans showed excellent agreement with visual determinations. Clearly, noninvasive contactless and microprocessor-based microwave vital sign monitors can provide a reliable system for measuring the vital heart and respiration rates.

Through the 1980s, computers had been used mainly to process and enhance the detected microwaves to facilitate signal analysis and cardiopulmonary rate extraction. The approaches involved a considerable amount of manual treatment in addition to that done by the computer. Aside from microprocessor control, the monitor provided a pattern recognition algorithm to enable machine or automatic extraction of cardiopulmonary rates through software processing of the chest movement signal detected by Doppler microwave radar [Chan and Lin, 1987]. A single algorithm was used to process and analyze both heart and breathing signals, whose shapes are very different from each other, as shown in Figure 7.33. In comparison, the respiration signal resembles a sinusoidal waveform.

#### 7.6.1.1 Pattern Recognition Algorithm

A graphical representation of the logical steps in the pattern recognition is depicted in Figure 7.36. Specifically, they involve: 1) Locate all the maxima for the whole length of data, 2) Set the noise threshold, 3) Locate the minimum point from each

**TABLE 7.3**
**Statistics of Microwave Sensor and Visual Determination of Heart and Respiration Rates of Adult Human Subjects (11 Readings for Each Parameter)**

| Vital Signs | Maximum Error (%) | Mean Error (%) | Correlation Coefficient |
|---|---|---|---|
| Heart rate | 7.0 | 2.1 | 0.98 |
| Respiration rate | 9.0 | 3.1 | 0.99 |

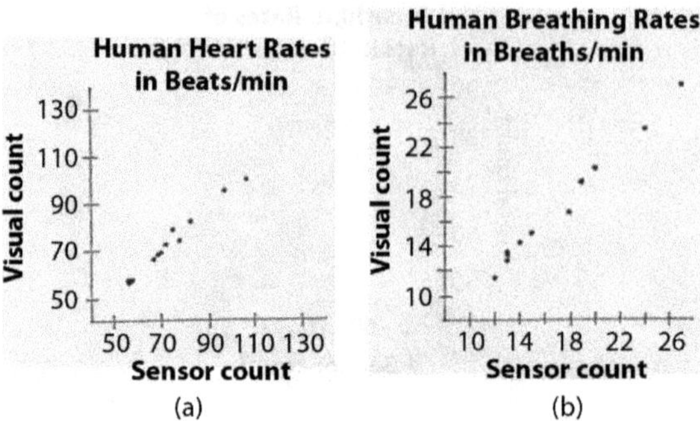


**FIGURE 7.35** Scatter graphs of the vital-sign monitor displaying measured and visually identified heart (a) and respiration rates (b) for human subjects.

remaining maxima and if it is below a set point, it is defined as the foot (F) of the cycle, and 4) The first maximum from the foot is the peak (P) of the waveform cycle [Chan and Lin, 1987].

The first attempt to locate the peak of each cycle is made by performing a slope test for every point in one cycle. Points at which the signal changes from upslope to

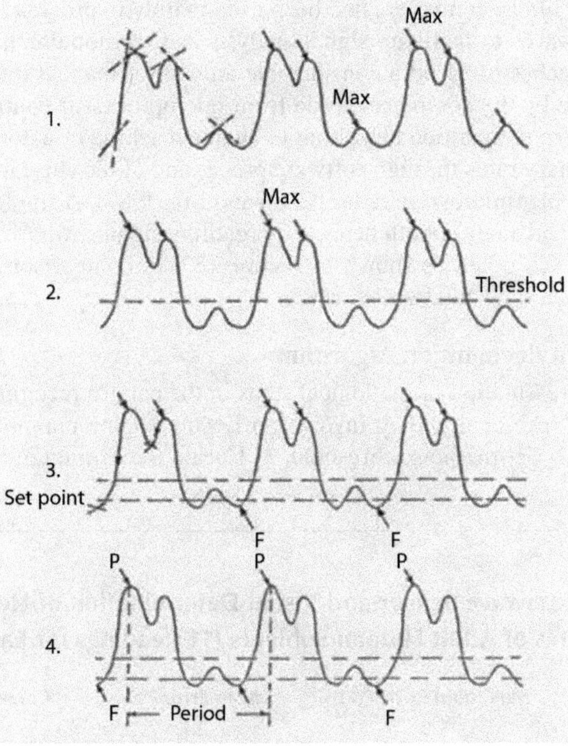


**FIGURE 7.36** Summary of basic steps in the pattern recognition software algorithm.

downslope are the local maxima. To improve the dynamic range of the system, the peak voltage of the signal is adjusted to a value higher than one volt. Local maxima less than 0.5V are mainly due to noise and motion artifacts. They do not contribute significantly to the cardiopulmonary rate determination. Therefore, a threshold of 0.5V is set to eliminate them.

The next step is to identify the foot of each cycle. This is accomplished by proceeding back from the remaining local maxima to a point where the slope becomes negative. This minimum point is the foot, or beginning, of the cycle if its amplitude is less than a set point (zero is used for this program). The first maximum point from the foot is defined as the peak of the cycle (either the systolic peak or the peak of inspiration). Each succeeding cycle is analyzed as described previously. The peaks located by the pattern recognition programs are used in the waveform analysis described later in this chapter.

#### 7.6.1.2 Waveform Analysis

The time difference between two succeeding peaks is calculated first. A median of all the periods calculated is used as a reference point to delete those values that are too large or too small. An average is calculated from those that remain. For comparison, analog forms of the chest-movement signals are displayed on a storage oscilloscope and the rates are counted from visually identified points on these records. Scatter diagrams of the values calculated from the computer-identified points against those obtained from the visually identified points are plotted both for heart rates and respiratory rates, and the correlation coefficients are computed (see Figures 7.31 and 7.32, and Table 7.3).

### 7.6.2 Remote Noncontact Vital-Sign Sensing

The advantages and potential applications of microwaves for remote noncontact detection of such vital signs as heartbeat and respiration rate were expanded to rescue-related operations beyond healthcare or controlled environments. The microwave radar approach has been explored for conditions under which direct contact with the subject is either difficult or unsuitable, such as fire, chemical accidents, and natural disasters or emergencies such as earthquakes or collapsed buildings [Lin, 1989, 1992; Sharpe et al., 1986]. Some of the most important considerations include robust designs that minimized various noise sources and achieved high sensitivity with low levels of radiated power.

#### 7.6.2.1 Remote Detection of Heartbeat and Respiration

A Doppler microwave system was demonstrated that can detect heartbeat and respiration rates of human subjects lying on the ground at 30 m or more, or behind a 15 cm thick cinder block wall [Chen et al., 1986]. A schematic diagram of the X-band system is shown in Figure 7.37. A phase-locked oscillator at 10 GHz produced a stable output of 20 mW. The output was amplified by a low-noise microwave amplifier to a power level of about 200 mW and was fed through a directional coupler, a variable attenuator, a circulator, and then to a horn antenna. The directional coupler branched out to provide a reference signal for clutter cancellation and for the mixer.

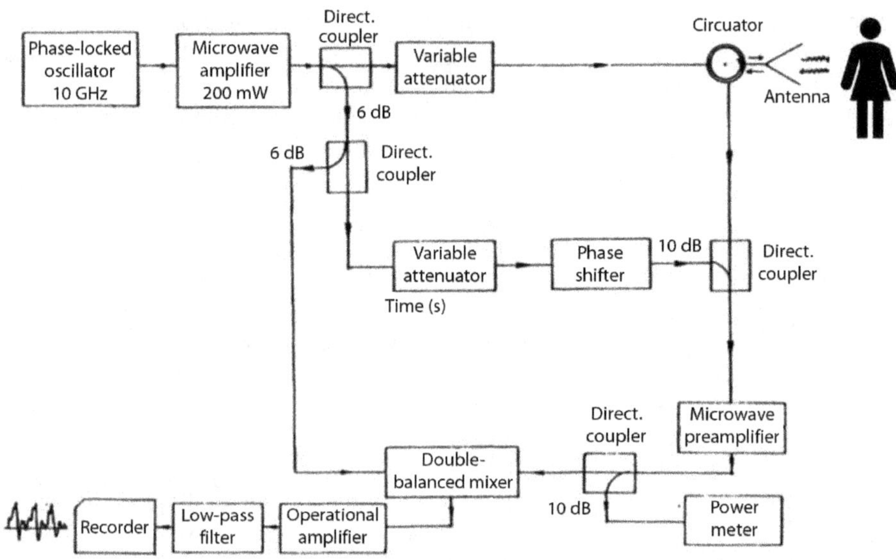


**FIGURE 7.37** Schematic diagram of the remote heart and respiration rate detection system.

The horn antenna radiated a microwave beam of about 15° beamwidth aimed at the human subjects lying on the ground. The signal received by the antenna consisted of clutters and signals backscattered from the bodies. The clutter signal was cancelled by one of the reference signals, the amplitude and phase of which were adjusted by using a variable attenuator and a phase shifter in a directional coupler. After clutter cancellation, the output of the directional coupler contained mainly the backscattered signal from the bodies, modulated by breathing and the heartbeat. It was then amplified by a low-noise microwave preamplifier and mixed with another reference signal in a double-balanced mixer, which produced the low-frequency signals resulting from breathing and heartbeat motions. The output from the mixer was amplified using an operational amplifier and passed through a low-pass filter with a 4 Hz cutoff for recording.

Figure 7.38 presents the microwave radar system-detected heartbeat and respiration rate of a subject seated 2 m from and behind a 15 cm thick cinder block wall [Chen et al., 1986]. Figure 7.39 shows the measured heart signal of a human subject lying on the ground in a supine position and holding his breath. The subject at 30 m had the body aligned perpendicular to the 10 GHz microwave beam. As expected, the performance is affected by distances of separation both between the microwave antenna and the targeted subject as well as subject's location from the walls. It is noteworthy that the effect of clothing over the sensitivity of the system was found to be insignificant for up to four layers of thick jackets. While the report suggests that the device's sensitivity was found to be the same in all three cases investigated, — circular, linear-vertical, and linear-horizontal polarization were employed — the remarks on lack of any effect of linear polarizations likely was related to how the investigation was conducted. Polarization dependence is well-recognized and is the motivation for

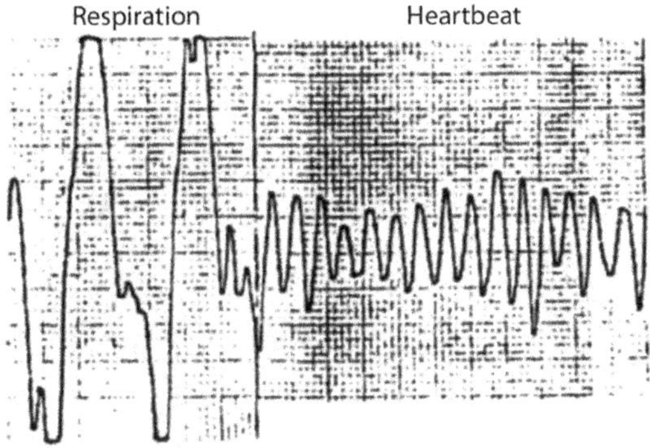


**FIGURE 7.38** Microwave sensing of heartbeat and respiration from a human subject sitting at 2 m from and behind a 15 cm thick cinder block wall.

the important quadrature detection scheme due to null points in linear polarization measurements. In fact, circular polarization is another approach to mitigate detection deficiencies resulting from the polarization related effect. Nonetheless, similar systems may find utility in a variety of search-and-rescue-related operations where direct physical contact with the subject is impractical or not possible. However, the operation of the system was found to be vulnerable if a large time-varying clutter such as that produced by moving objects or trees and bushes. Aside from the more directive and higher gain antennas, other signal processing schemes including adaptive noise cancellation may be applied to help resolve the limitations.

#### 7.6.2.2 Microwave Life-Detection Systems

Later, more sensitive microwave life-detection systems were constructed that can be used to locate human subjects buried under earthquake rubble or hidden behind various material barriers [Chen et al., 2000]. The lower and more deeply penetrating frequencies in the L or S band range were used to construct two new systems: one operating at 450 MHz and the other at 1150 MHz. Similar to the system described

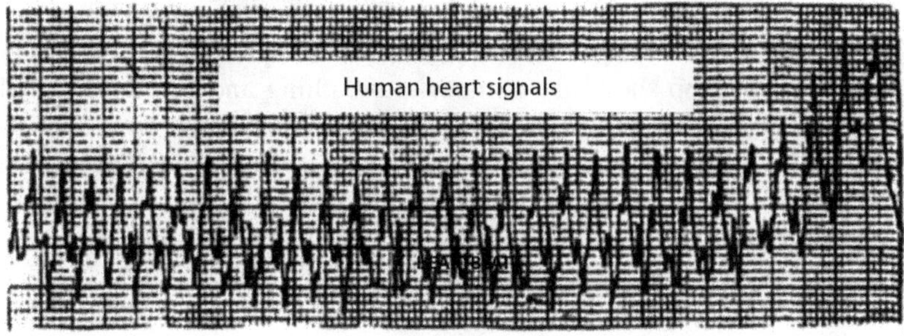


**FIGURE 7.39** Heart signals of a human subject lying on the ground at 30 m measured with a 10 GHz microwave Doppler radar beam.

previously, each of the new systems has advantages and disadvantages depending on the nature of the rubble and ruins under investigation. The basic system architectures of the 450 MHz and 1150 MHz microwave life-detection systems are like those shown in Figures 7.26, 7.28, and 7.34 and are based on the same microwave propagation principles. It was found that the 450 MHz microwave has difficulty penetrating layers of reinforced concrete slabs with imbedded metallic wire of 4 in (~10 cm) spacing. However, the 1150 MHz microwave can pass through rubble with layers of reinforced concrete slabs with metallic wire mesh more easily than that of 450 MHz microwaves. Nonetheless, 450 MHz can penetrate deeper into rubble without metallic wire mesh than that of 1150 MHz microwaves.

A schematic diagram of the system structure of the 1150 MHz microwave system is illustrated in Figure 7.40. The more sophisticated microwave life-detection system has four major modules: 1) a microwave circuit system that generates, amplifies, and distributes microwave signals to various microwave components, 2) a microprocessor-controlled clutter cancellation module [Chuang et al., 1991] that creates an optimal signal to cancel the clutter from the rubble and the background, 3) a dual-antenna system that consists of two separate antennas energized sequentially, and 4) a laptop computer that controls the microprocessors, monitors, and displays the output signal.

The major departures from or improvement to the system shown in Figure 7.37 include a phase-locked oscillator that generates a stable microwave at 1150 MHz with an output power of 400 mW (25.6 dBm). The system has two separate antennas, one more directive than the other. They are electronically switched at a frequency of 100 Hz, and the outputs are combined to reduce the background clutter noise and to provide the most reliable sampled signal from the objects simultaneously. The function of the digitally controlled phase-shifters, especially the one installed in front of the local reference signal port of the double-balanced mixer is to control the phase of the local reference signal for increasing system sensitivity.

The performance of constructed systems operating at 450 or 1150 MHz was tested for detection of breathing and heartbeat signals of human subjects through obstacles such as earthquake rubble or layers of building materials as thick as 10 ft (~3 m). A human subject was lying down in the space at the bottom of the rubble. As shown in Figure 7.41, the breathing and heartbeat signals can be extracted from human subject buried under earthquake rubble, and a subject hidden behind construction barriers can be located with the 450 MHz system. Fast Fourier transform (FFT) of the time-domain signal shows the frequency components of the microwave sensor-detected signal. The graph on top shows the composite breathing and heartbeat signal. The FFT results show that the time-domain breathing signal has a dominant peak at 0.3 Hz and a heartbeat signal of 1.36 Hz (the second largest peak). The third largest peak at 0.6 Hz is the second harmonic of the breathing signal. Similarly, experimental results were obtained with the 1150 MHz system using simulated rubble on detection of breathing and heartbeat signals of human subjects.

The systems were tested in a field test using a realistically simulated earthquake rubble environment [Chen et al. 2000]. Figure 7.42 presents the results of a test conducted with a reflector antenna and a human subject. In this case, the microwaves had to penetrate six layers of reinforced concrete slabs and two double-T beam structures

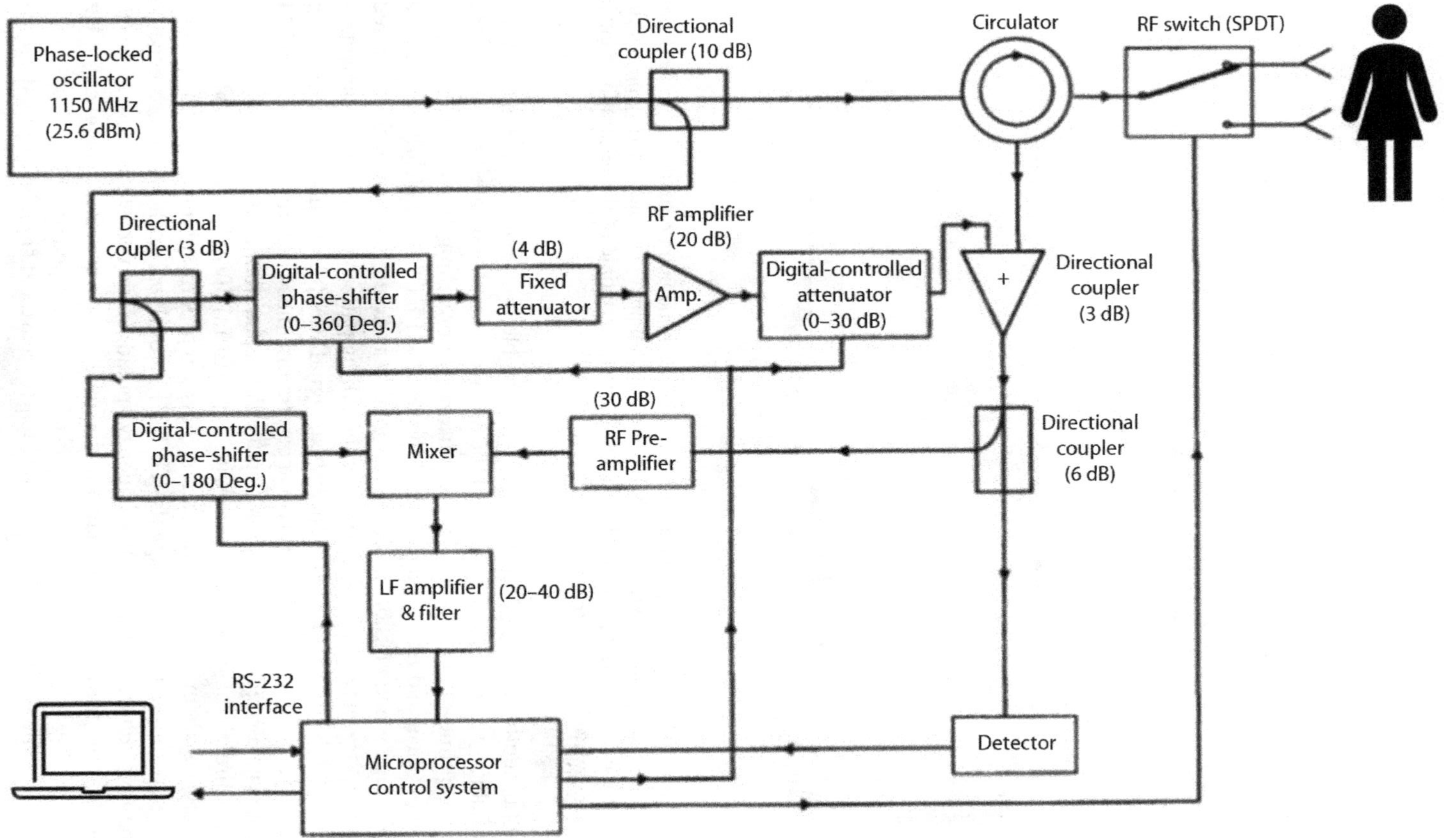


**FIGURE 7.40** Schematic diagram of a 1150-MHz microwave life-detection system.

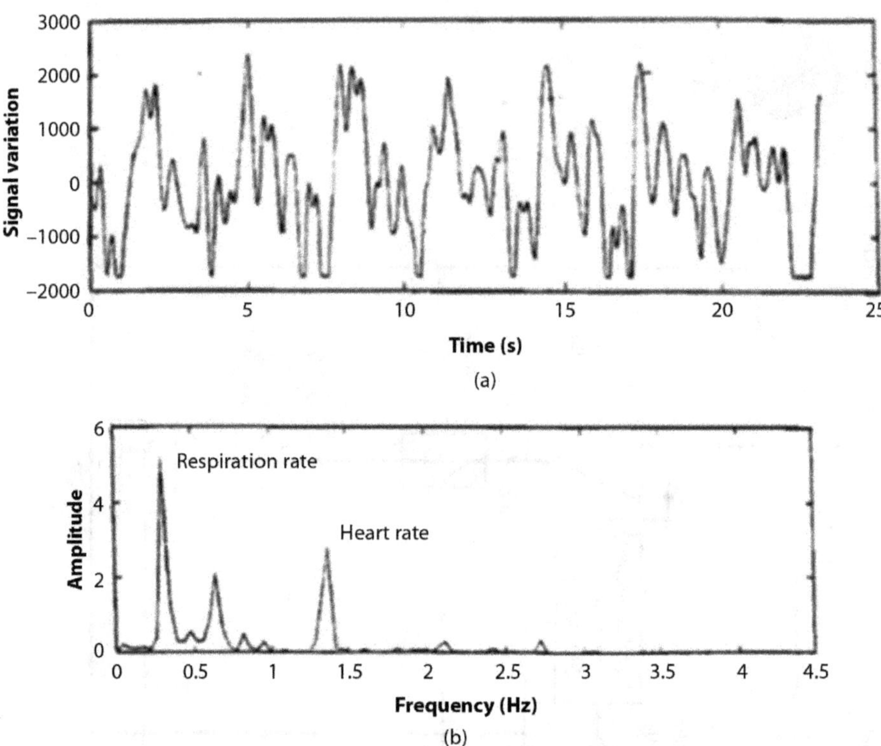


**FIGURE 7.41** Heartbeat and respiration signals of a female human subject recorded from the top of simulated rubble with a 450 MHz reflector antenna. The subject is lying within a cavity in the rubble. The peak at 0.6 Hz is the second harmonic of the respiration signal. (a) Temporal waveform, (b) frequency spectrum.

for a total depth of 9 ft (~2.74 m). The dense rubble between the antenna and the human subject reduced the amplitude of the received signal compared with simulated rubble. The time-domain signal shows a distinctive breathing signal and a complex mixture of noise and heartbeat signal. However, the FFT results clearly indicated a breathing signal and possibly a heartbeat signal. It is noted that two peaks appeared near 0.2–0.3 Hz may be due to the uneven breathing pattern of the human subject.

The system's ability to detect a heartbeat signal was further demonstrated using two sets of signals received from two separate antennas (Figure 7.43). Figure 7.44 depicts the measured heartbeat signals created by a phantom heart model placed 7 ft (~2.13 m) directly below the antennas with 3 ft (0.91 m) of rubble with metallic wire mesh between them. The time-domain signals from both antennas A and B show the noise corrupted heartbeat signals. Their FFT results also show the presence of a strong noise clutter with a wide frequency spread. However, when these two sets of signals were cross correlated, a distinctive peak of the heartbeat signal at 0.8 Hz is seen with drastically reduced noise levels. The second peak at 1.6 Hz suggests a second harmonic of the heartbeat signal. Clearly, heartbeat signals may be detected by cross correlation.

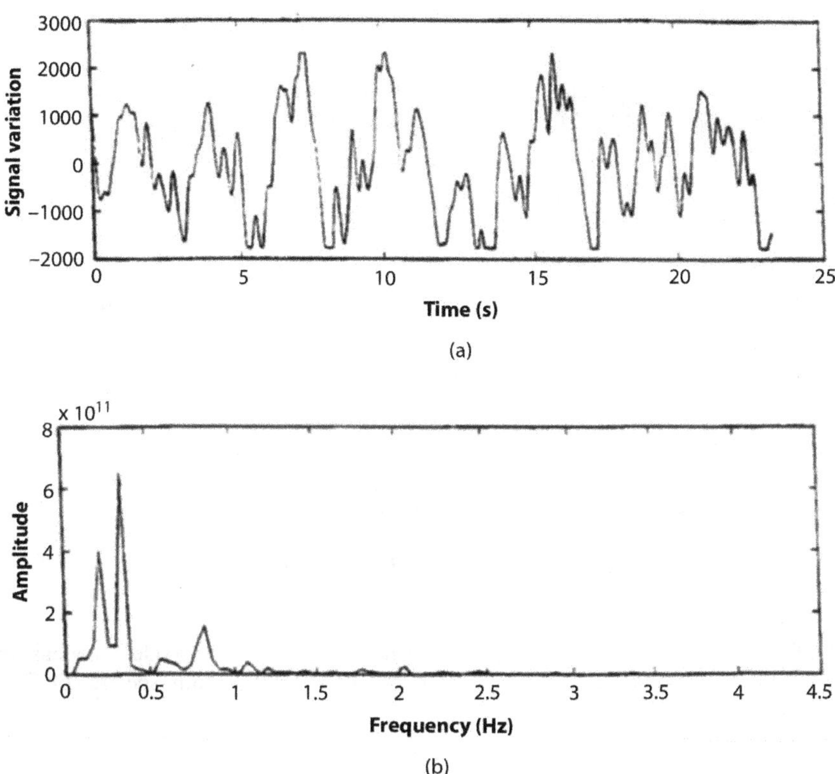


**FIGURE 7.42** Breathing and heartbeat signals recorded from a human subject lying beneath 9 ft (~2.74 m) of rubble by a 450 MHz life-detection system. (a) Temporal waveform, (b) frequency spectrum.

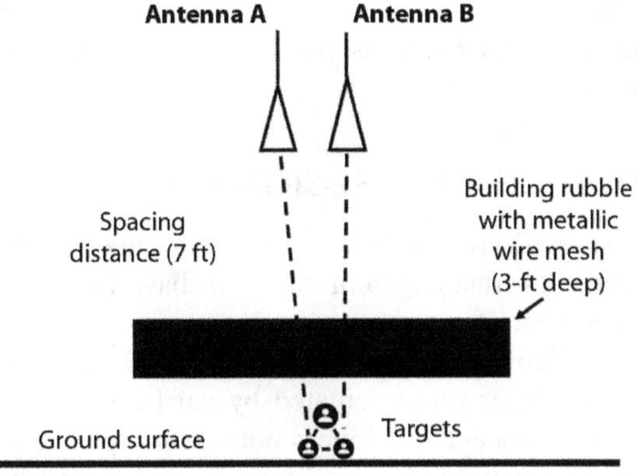


**FIGURE 7.43** Sensing of heartbeat signals by two side-by-side antennas in a 1150 MHz life-detection system. Simulation of human subjects or a phantom heart model under 3 ft of wire-mesh rubble.

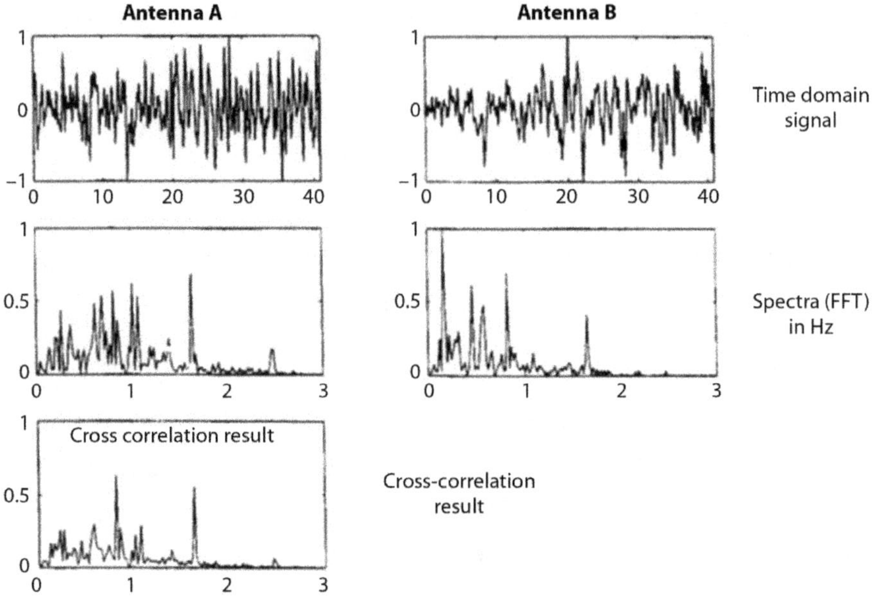


**FIGURE 7.44** Phantom heartbeat signals sensed by two side-by-side antennas in a 1150 MHz life-detection system. Results are displayed as time-domain, spectra (FFT), and cross correlations.

The performance of the 1150 MHz system is similar to that of the 450 MHz system. The major difference is that microwaves at 1150 MHz can penetrate through rubble consisting of layers of reinforced concrete slabs with imbedded metallic wire mesh of 4 in (~10 cm) spacing, better than microwaves at 450 MHz. Thus, the 1150 MHz system should be more effective in detecting the breathing and heartbeat signals of trapped victims under collapsed reinforced concrete and masonry structures than the 450 MHz system. In comparison, the 450 MHz system may be more effective in searching for trapped victims under rubble that does not have fine metallic wire mesh imbedded.

## 7.7 RECENT ADVANCES IN VITAL-SIGN SENSING

The investigations discussed previously on microwave remote noncontact detection and monitoring of vital signs that began in the 1970s have found applications in and out of hospital environments for infant and adult apnea monitoring, detection of abnormal breathing conditions, respiration monitoring of patients after surgery, and the search for survivors under rubble created by earthquakes or following structural collapses. Thus, the concept of wireless noncontact sensing of vital signs was not only successfully demonstrated but well recognized by the turn of the century. Microwave sensing techniques are noninvasive, contactless, unobtrusive, convenient, and can be used for continuous long-term monitoring with minimal intrusion and without pain or stress. Since 2000, the research efforts have been moving the technology toward development of smarter devices with lower power, lighter weight, smaller form factor, better accuracy, expanding to wider application domains [Li et al., 2013, 2021, Kim & Jeong 2020; Muñoz-Ferreras et al., 2017; Walsh et al., 2014]. Indeed, aside from humans, the research was extended to animals beyond benchtop feasibility testing in veterinary laboratories where it has been used to monitor vital signs from animals with varying sizes and skin surfaces, including birds, fish, hamsters, tortoises, mice, cats, rabbits, dogs, cows, and even sea elephants [Hui and Kan, 2018, 2019; Wang et al., 2020; Zhou et al., 2020].

This section discusses recent advances in remote microwave noninvasive vital-sign sensing. The discussions include integrated radar chipsets, bench-top prototypes, and portable system implementations from concept verification to technology validations under clinical environments. It will provide details of a variety of architectures and different technologies such as CW Doppler, FMCW, and UWB radars.

### 7.7.1 Chip Scale Radar Sensors

The concept of a microwave radar on a single chip by circuit miniaturization and integration was successfully brought about in the form of a direct-conversion quadrature Doppler-radar transceiver for vital sign detection and monitoring [Droitcour et al., 2004, 2009]. The chip was implemented with 0.25 $\mu$m silicon CMOS. and BiCMOS technologies in a 48-pin package. The functional block diagram is found in Figure 7.9. Figure 7.10 presents a photograph of the chip. Other details are given in Section 7.3.1 on functions of each of the circuit modules. In addition to the 2.4 GHz quadrature radar chips, a 1.6 GHz single-channel chip with similar power output was also investigated in this study.

Some experimental measurements with the 1.6 and 2.4 GHz band quadrature single-chip radar sensors are shown in Figures 7.45 and 7.46. The performance of the single-chip radar sensors in detecting heart rate and respiration involved a fully clothed human subject seated 50 cm from the antenna, facing the antenna, and breathing normally. A piezo-electric finger-pressure pulse transducer was used during the measurements to provide a reference signal for heart activity. The baseband output was filtered with 0.1 Hz high-pass and 10 Hz low-pass filters with a 12 dB/decade slope, and a total gain of 33 dB were used to remove DC offset and avoid aliasing. Although the high-pass analog filter reduces the amplitude of the respiration signal, the respiration rate can still be extracted since the respiration signal amplitude is significantly larger than that of the heart signal. The resulting waveforms were digitized with a digital oscilloscope. The digitized signals were processed to determine the heart and respiration rates over time. The heart-rate accuracy was calculated as the percentage of the measurement interval. The heart rate measured using the single-chip Doppler radar was within 1 beat per min of the rate measured with the finger pulse reference.

The signals were digitally filtered with a 12th-order elliptic IIR bandpass filter, which passed 0.9–9 Hz, blocking frequencies below 0.8 Hz (See Chapter 6, Figure 6.17). The signals were windowed and then autocorrelated, and an FFT of the autocorrelated signal was calculated. The heart rate was extracted from the frequency where the FFT had its maximum. Respiration rates were obtained using a similar method, without digital filtering. However, it is noted that the unfiltered

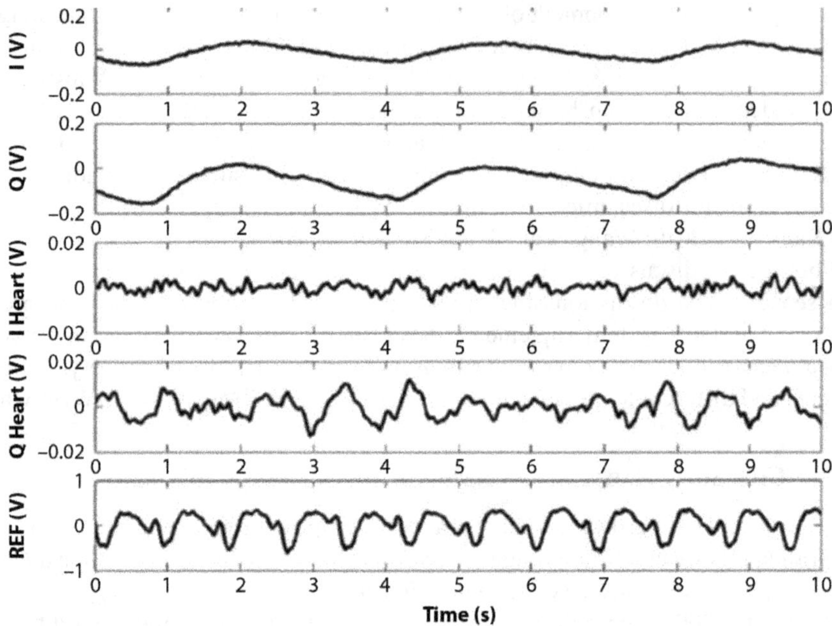


**FIGURE 7.45** Heart and respiration activity measured with the 2.4 GHz quadrature radar chip. The analog filtered I and Q outputs, which contain both heart and respiration information, are shown at the top, followed by the digitally filtered I and Q signals, with only heart information. Neither the I nor Q output is at the maximum sensitivity point or at the null point. They have similar amplitudes and accuracies. The I output is within 1 beat per min of the reference 82% of the time, and the Q output is correct 81% of the time.

analog signals contain both heart and respiration information, with the heart signal superimposed on the slower but stronger respiration signal.

The data collected using the 2.4 GHz quadrature transceiver are shown in Figure 7.45, where neither in phase (I) or quadrature (Q) outputs are in quadrature maximum or at null point for sensitivity. The analog filtered I and Q outputs, which contain both heart and respiration signals, are shown at the top. The heart information is superimposed on the slower but stronger respiration signal. The radar sensor provided a heart rate of 70 beats per min, which is within one beat per min of the rate measured with the pulse reference for 82% and 81% of the measurement intervals, respectively. The respiration rate is 18 breaths per min.

Results from the 1.6 GHz BiCMOS radar chip are shown in Figure 7.46. The analog filtered I and Q outputs, which contain both heart and respiration signals, are shown at the top. The heart is seen as a modulation on the slower but stronger respiration signal. After digital filtering, the heart signal from the BiCMOS chip was within 1 beat per min of the pulse reference 100% of the time, while the raw signal after digital filtering agreed with the pulse reference 92% of the time. In contrast, these measurements were made near the optimum phase-demodulation point. For comparison with measurements made with the 2.4 GHz chip at nonoptimal

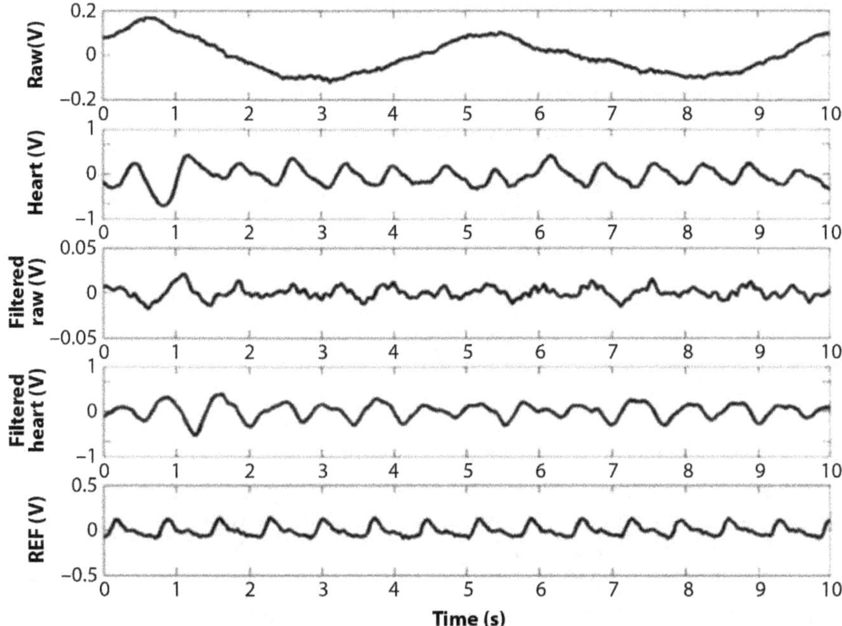


**FIGURE 7.46** Heart and respiration activity measured with the 1.6 GHz BiCMOS chip. The top trace is the analog-filtered raw signal, and the second is the analog-filtered heart signal. The third and fourth traces are the raw and heart signals, respectively, after digital filtering. The bottom trace is the pulse reference. The filtered heart signal was within one beat per minute of the reference 100% of the time, while the filtered raw signal agreed 92% of the time.

phase-demodulation points, the 1.6 GHz BiCMOS chip has about 12 dB lower phase noise than the 2.4 GHz CMOS chip. Thus, using the BiCMOS chip, it is possible to obtain a clearer signal and to achieve a higher accuracy than with the CMOS chip. Nevertheless, it should be noted that while the work demonstrated the feasibility of RF integration of on-chip Doppler radar for vital sign sensing, external bias circuits, filters, and baseband amplifiers are still required for the detectors to function.

The front end of the microwave architecture plays an important role in maximizing the sensitivity, extending the detection range, and rejecting interferences, apart from directivity of the antenna, as demonstrated in this integrated single chip radar sensor. Various front-end architectures have been explored in prototype bench-mark projects. In addition to the quadrature homodyne exemplified above, double-sideband architectures [Li et al., 2008; Ma et al., 2018], low intermediate-frequency (IF) and direct IF sampling [Ma et al., 2018; Mostafanezhad and Boric-Lubecke, 2014] and self and mutual injection locking were recently investigated [Li et al., 2009, Tang et al. 2017 Wang et al., 2011, 2020a,b]. Discussions on the design and performance of some of these front-end architecture implementations on integrated chips are given below.

Several radar-on-chip for noncontact vital sign sensing have been explored since completion of the previously discussed effort. For example, a fully integrated 5 GHz double-sideband radar chip was demonstrated using 0.18 $\mu$m CMOS process

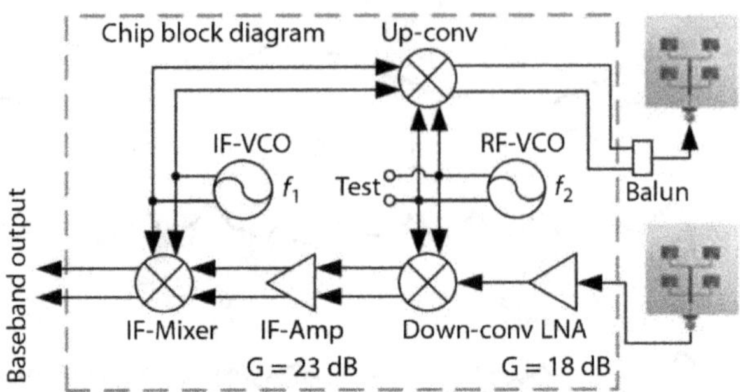


**FIGURE 7.47** Schematic diagram of the 5 GHz radar transceiver with interfaces for input/output antennas. (Courtesy of Changzhi Li, Texas Tech University.)

[Li et al., 2008]. Double-sideband transmission for noncontact vital-sign sensing was demonstrated previously using a bench-top prototype system [Xiao et al., 2007]. However, the 5 GHz integrated CMOS double-sideband radar sensor chip uses a differential architecture (Figure 7.47), which can effectively reduce local oscillator leakage. The chip radar has more than a 1 GHz tuning range, which empowers the advantage of avoiding the null detection point by its wide frequency tuning range. It has successfully detected heartbeat and respiration from subjects seated at 0.5 and 2 m away, facing the antenna. Figure 7.48(a) shows the radar chip designed with a double-sideband architecture and fabricated with 0.18 $\mu$m process. The CMOS radar-on-chip integrates all the RF building blocks so that the output of the transmitter can be directly transmitted to a target and the output from the receiver is directly transferred to and processed by the on-chip baseband circuitry.

The design of a high-sensitivity noncontact vital-sign radar chip sensor was accomplished by appropriately choosing the baseband bandwidth and flicker noise corner [Li et al., 2010]. Figure 7.48(b) shows a 1.1 × 1.2 mm$^2$ direct-conversion Doppler radar integrated on a single CMOS chip implemented using a 0.13 $\mu$m process. The chip is software configurable to set the operation point and detection range for optimal performance. All the analog functions shown in Figure 7.49 are integrated on-chip so that the output can be digitally sampled for signal processing.

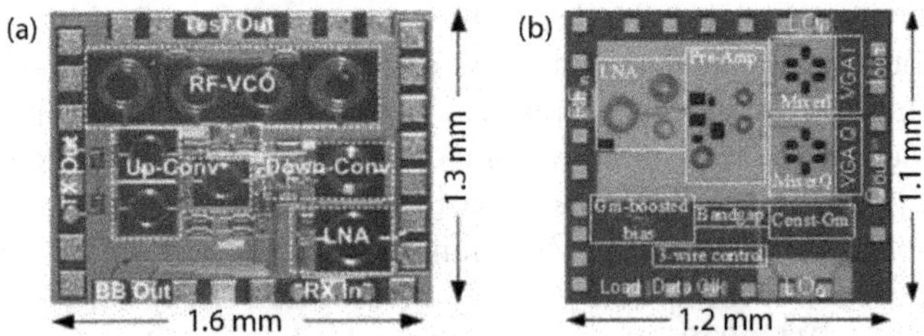


**FIGURE 7.48** Photomicrograph of integrated chip sensors: (a) a double sideband vital-sign detection radar fabricated in 0.18 $\mu$m CMOS process (Li et al., 2008) and (b) a direct conversion radar fabricated in 0.13 $\mu$m CMOS process. (Courtesy of Changzhi Li, Texas Tech University.)

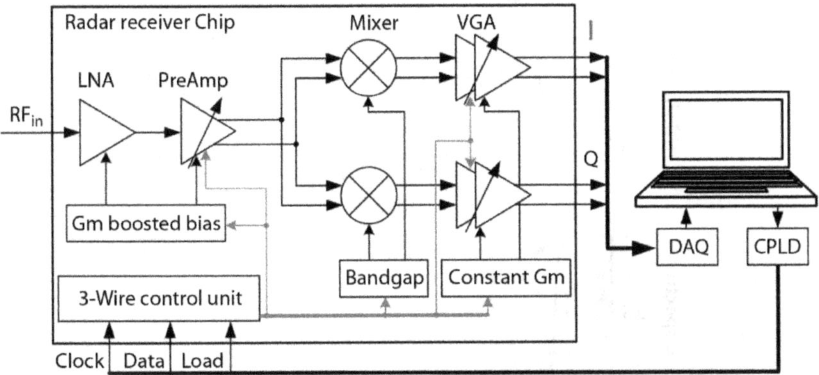


**FIGURE 7.49** Schematic block diagram of the software-configurable 5.8 GHz quadrature continuous wave radar-on-chip sensor. (Courtesy of Changzhi Li, Texas Tech University.)

The 5.8 GHz CW radar chip has a homodyne quadrature architecture with two output channels. A clutter cancellation mechanism was also implemented in the SoC. The paper showed that although in general a CMOS receiver chip has a high noise figure around the signal of interest due to flicker noise, it is possible to design a high-sensitivity noncontact vital-sign detection chip with a reduced total noise level for real-time vital-sign monitoring.

Performance of the CMOS chip CW radar system was experimentally tested in a laboratory environment with a 2 × 2 patch antenna arrays to transmit and receive 5.8 GHz microwaves with power supplied by a 1.5 V battery. Figure 7.50 shows an example of the vital-sign signals detected from the back of a seated human subject.

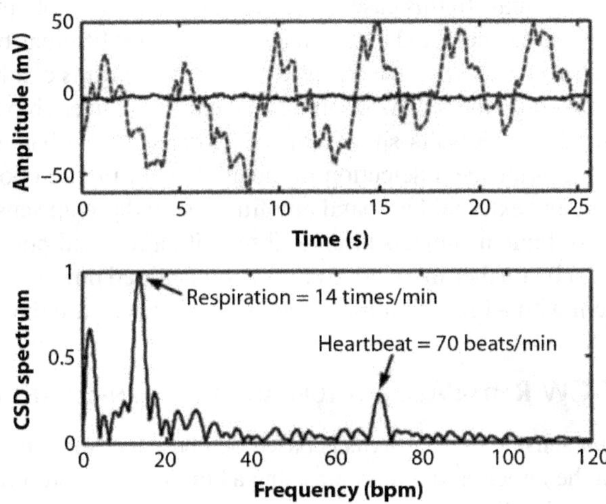


**FIGURE 7.50** Radar-on-chip output signal detected from the back of a human subject: Waveforms of I (dashed line) and Q (solid line) channels (top) and frequency spectrum of demodulated (CSD) signal (bottom).

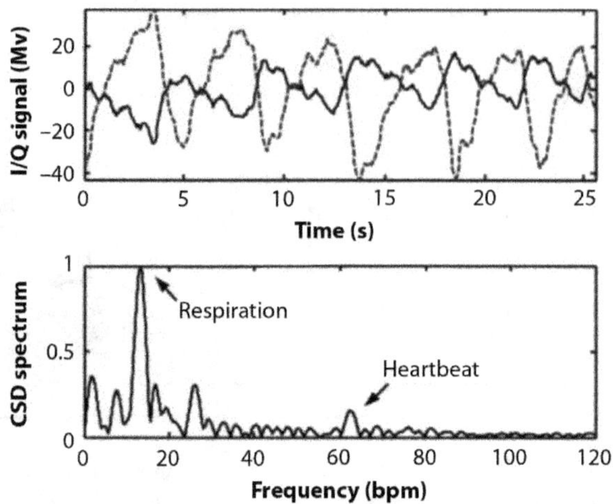


**FIGURE 7.51** CMOS radar-on-chip sensor output signal detected from the front of a human subject at 1.5 m: Waveforms of I (dashed line) and Q (solid line) channels (top) and frequency spectrum of demodulated (CSD) signal (bottom).

Note the clean time-domain heart and respiration signals. In this case, the detection was performed at a distance position where one channel is near the optimal detection point, while the other channel is close to the null detection point. The respiration and heartbeat signals identified from the spectrum, show a respiration rate of 14 times/min and a heartbeat rate of 70 beats/min.

Figure 7.51 gives an example of vital sign detection by using the CMOS radar-on-chip sensor. It shows the output signal obtained from in front of a human subject seated at 1.5 m from the antennas. In this case, the detection position is not optimized. Thus, amplitude waveforms of the I and Q channels are slightly different but are equally clean. It is interesting to observe that the time-domain waveforms exhibited less noise than those determined by the 5 GHz double-sideband transceiver chip described previously [Li et al., 2008]. Results show that the fabricated chip has a sensitivity of greater than 100 dBm for ideal detection in the absence of random body movement. Moreover, without any external baseband amplifier, the radar chip sensor was able to detect vital signs of human subjects at up to 3 m, with a reduced power budget. The detection range can be further increased if higher transmitted power or a data acquisition (DAQ) system with a higher sampling rate is used to increase the SNR.

### 7.7.2 Low-IF CW Radar Architecture and Injection-Locked Oscillators

Doppler CW radar sensing of vital signs is based on phase modulation of the backscattered signal from the target tissue interface using a homodyne receiver architecture. Its advantages include simplicity and accuracy due to range correlation and guaranteed cancellation of phase noise, but it has its limitations. Doppler CW radar sensing is susceptible to various inherent and other noise sources within its detection environment. A heterodyne architecture is one way to resolve the issue of noise, especially the low-frequency noise for vital sign detection. Also, the frequency-tuning method and quadrature detection scheme described previously can be used to circumvent the distance ambiguity associated with the null point problem of a homodyne receiver. In what follows, a coherent low-IF architecture is described that preserves the range correlation benefits of the homodyne system, while minimizing the baseband flicker noise. It will be followed by discussions on self-injection-locked oscillator as an alternative means to enhance the SNR and overcome the null point limitation of a single-channel system.

In a coherent low-IF system, the same microwave source is used to create a down-conversion LO that is correlated in phase noise to that of the transmitted signal, allowing it to take advantage of the range correlation to provide a system with higher precision [Gu et al., 2010; Mostafanezhad and Boric-Lubecke, 2014]. The low-IF system has a heterodyne architecture with an IF low enough to be digitized directly. It requires only one receiver chain for full phase recovery, resulting in simpler architecture and lower DC power consumption, but it requires a considerably faster sampling rate, which results in a large amount of data for signal processing. Nonetheless, DC coupling associated with data loss and channel imbalance issues is eliminated. A schematic diagram of the coherent low-IF system is given in Figure 7.52. It can be seen from signal flow that the low-IF component is generated locally within the system by single-sideband (SSB) modulation of the same LO that generated the transmit signal. This assures that the two signals are coherent.

The reported performance demonstrated with a human subject showed that using the coherent low-IF system improved the SNR for the combined fundamental and harmonics of the heart signal by 17 dB [Mostafanezhad and Boric-Lubecke, 2014]. The SNR for just the fundamental frequency of the heart signal is also increased by 7 dB compared to homodyne detection. This effectively lowers the required transmit power by a minimum of 7 dB, or for the same transmit power, it extends the radar range by 50%. Heart rate accuracy better than 1 beats/min was achieved at 2.95 m with a transmit power of 10 mW.

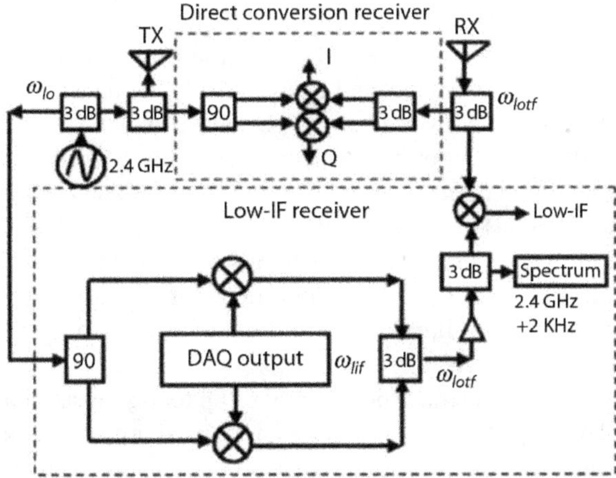


**FIGURE 7.52** Schematic diagram of coherent low-IF system showing signal flow.

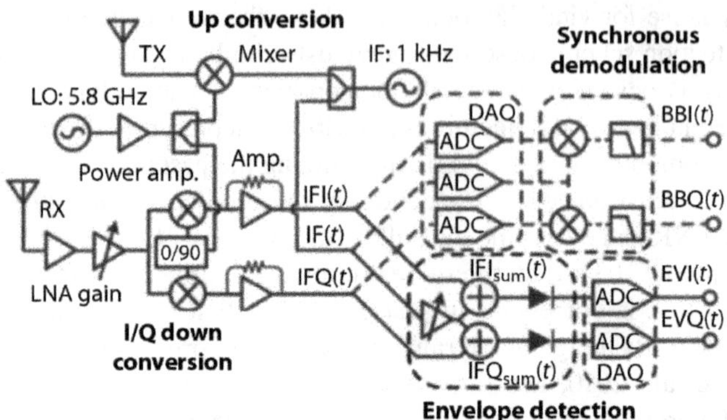


**FIGURE 7.53** Schematic diagram of a 5.8 GHz double-sideband low-IF continuous wave radar system with both envelope detection (ED) and synchronous demodulation (SD) demonstrated at the output.

To simplify the architecture of a low-IF system and reduce the high sampling-rate (ADC) requirements, an envelope detection (ED) algorithm for a double-sideband low-IF CW radar was proposed [Ma et al., 2018]. Specifically, the ED is realized in hardware rather than software. In this way, the low-frequency envelopes at I and Q outputs can be sampled by a very low sampling frequency such as 20 Hz. In this case, the ADC requirement is reduced significantly to a level similar to homodyne detection, while a better SNR is achieved by adopting a low-IF architecture.

The architecture of the double sideband low-IF CW radar is depicted in Figure 7.53, where the same local oscillator (LO) and IF sources are shared by the transmitter (TX) and the receiver (RX) for motion detection. In the TX chain, the low-frequency IF is up-converted with a double-sideband mixer. Thus, the output spectrum contains the lower sideband $f_L = LO - IF$, the upper sideband $f_U = LO + IF$, and the leaked LO signal. After reflected from a moving target, both the double-sideband signal and the leaked LO signal are modulated with the phase information produced by target movement. In the RX chain, the backscattered double-sideband CW signal is down-converted into I and Q channels by a quadrature mixer, whereas the reflected LO signal is converted to a DC offset, which can be eliminated by AC coupling. For the coherent or synchronous detection (SD) section, IFI(t), IFQ(t), and IF(t) are sampled simultaneously with a sampling rate of 20 kHz. In the digital domain, BBI(t) and BBQ(t) are first generated by down-converting IFI(t) and IFQ(t) with the IF carrier. The signal is filtered by a low-pass filter with a 10 Hz cutoff frequency. For the ED section, the envelope detector is realized with a switching diode. RC filters are used to filter out the DC offsets from $IFI_{sum}(t)$ and $IFQ_{sum}(t)$ at the output of the envelope detector.

A bench-top prototype and the experimental setup for test measurements are shown in Figure. 7.54. The 5.8 GHz low-IF radar system used a pair of 2 × 2 patch antennas for transmitting and receiving microwave signals. In an experiment designed to test the prototype's ability to measure vital signs, a human subject was seated 1 m in front of the antennas. Figure 7.55a and b shows the ED and SD data from a 20-second

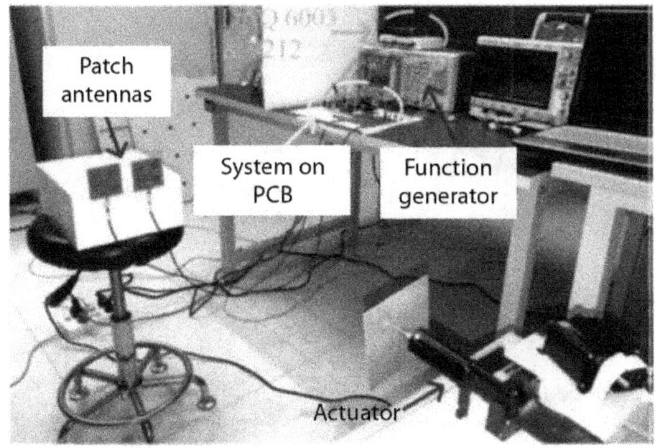


**FIGURE 7.54** Experimental setup for motion measurements using the 5.8 GHz low-IF radar system with a pair of 2 × 2 patch antennas for microwave transmission and reception. The human subject would be in the position of actuator and metal plate shown. (Courtesy of Lianming Li, Southeast University.)

recording. It is seen that the time-domain waveforms from the ED and SD approaches have the same amplitudes, indicating that the two methods can achieve the same results. Also, the power spectrum yielded a respiration rate of 19 breaths/min and a heartbeat of 91 beats/min. Thus, with substantially relaxed ADC requirements, the ED method can achieve the same SNR performances as that of the SD method. For performance during longer monitoring periods, Figure 7.56 shows the results of

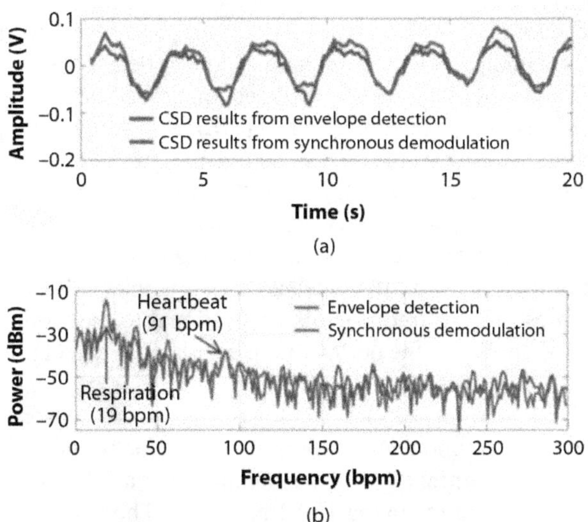


**FIGURE 7.55** Comparison between the envelop detection and synchronous demodulation methods for vital sign detection. The 20-s waveform (a-top) and corresponding power spectrum under normal (freely) breathing conditions (b-bottom).

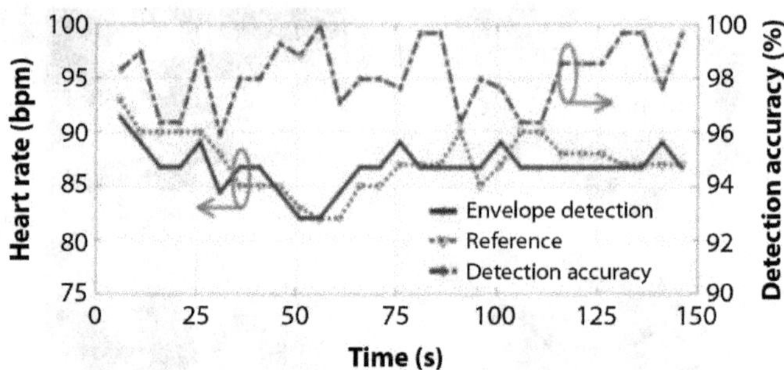


**FIGURE 7.56** Prolonged human vital-sign (heartbeat) monitoring by envelope detection (ED) method. The total detection interval is 140 s. Detected vital-sign (heartbeat) results are the same as the reference pulse rate. The detection accuracy is better than 96%.

vital-sign variations observed over a 140-second session. A 10-second window is adopted for the FFT and a 5-second incremental step size is used for data update. For reference, the real-time heartbeat rate was recorded by a finger pulse monitor. Only results from the proposed ED method are shown. The detected heartbeat is in good agreement with the reference for a detection accuracy better than 96%.

### 7.7.3 Injection-Locked Oscillator Architectures

Doppler radars using self and mutual injection-locking architectures have been investigated extensively for vital-sign detection and physiological sensing [Wang et al., 2020a,b]. Some of the advantages of injection-locking systems include clutter noise and random body motion cancellation, increased SNR for better sensitivity, reduced system complexity, and potentially longer detection range for the same power budget [Wang et al., 2010, 2011]. This section describes various approaches to microwave sensors using self-injection locked (SIL) oscillator and frequency demodulator system architecture for detection of vital signs. In a SIL architecture, a part of the output from the receiver, which is modulated by the target motion is injected back into the microwave transmitter source oscillator (VCO), to bring the VCO into a self-injection-locking state. Thus, instead of mixing the received microwave signal with the output of the oscillator, the received signal is injected into the VCO oscillator. The shift in oscillation frequency is proportional to the motion. A frequency demodulator can be applied at the output of the oscillator to detect the Doppler effect associated with the target motion.

A schematic diagram of the conventional SIL radar sensor is depicted in Figure 7.57. The main components of the CW SIL radar include an SIL oscillator (SILO), an IQ delay discriminator which is composed of a delay line and IQ mixers, and transmitting (TX) and receiving (RX) antennas. The SILO is the only active component in some cases. The RX antenna in the SIL radar is connected to the SILO's injection port and the injection signal $S_{inj}(t)$ is used to bring the oscillator into SIL state. No LNA is required for near-field or short-range applications (see Figure 7.58), in contrast to CW Doppler radars.

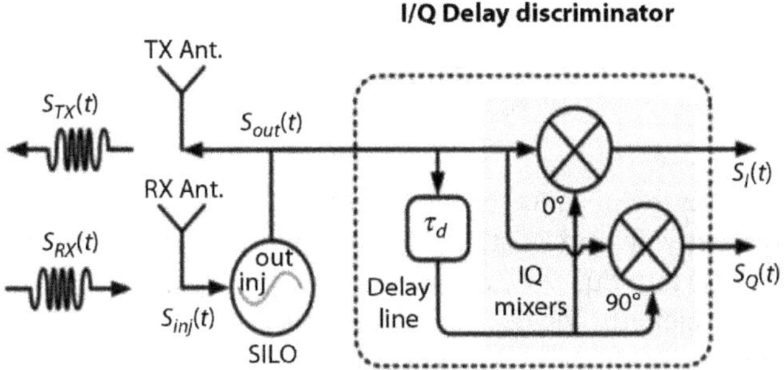


**FIGURE 7.57** Schematic diagram of a self-injection-locked oscillator (SILO) radar system.

For a constant free-running signal $S_{osc}(t)$ of the SILO with a constant amplitude of $E_{osc}$ and a constant frequency of $\omega_{osc}$, the injection signal $S_{inj}(t)$ has a constant amplitude of $E_{inj}$. When the SILO is operating in the SIL state, $\omega_{out}(t)$ can be obtained as [see Horng, 2013; Wang et al., 2010]:

$$\omega_{out}(t) = \omega_{osc} - \omega_{LR}\ sin\ \phi(t) \tag{7.9}$$

The locking range $\omega_{LR}$ is given by

$$\omega_{LR} = \left(\frac{\omega_{osc}E_{inj}}{2QE_{osc}}\right), \tag{7.10}$$

where Q is the quality factor of the SILO's resonant tank circuit. The phase difference $\phi(t)$ from $S_{inj}$ (t) to $S_{osc}$ (t) is the sum of the phase delay $\phi_{inj}$ and the Doppler phase modulation $\phi_m(t)$ introduced in the SIL path, such that

$$\phi(t) = \phi_{inj} + \phi_m = \frac{2\omega_{osc}}{v}\left[R + x(t)\right] \tag{7.11}$$

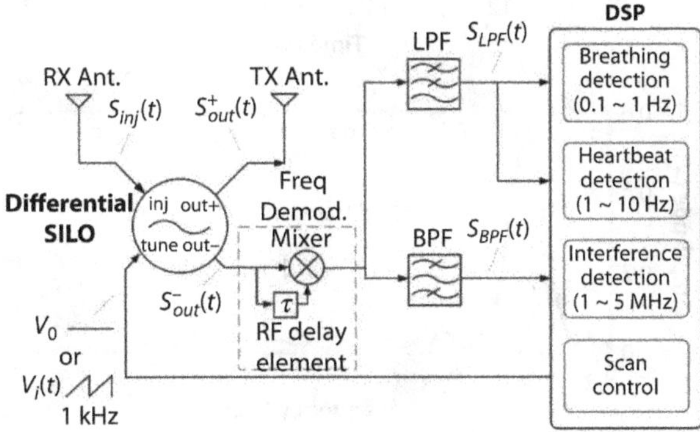


**FIGURE 7.58** Schematic diagram of an SIL radar sensor developed for vital-sign measurement using an ISM band. It includes annotated specifications of key system components.

and

$$\phi_m = \left( \frac{2\omega_{osc}}{v} x(t) \right) \tag{7.12}$$

where $R$ and $x(t)$ are the distance to the target and the instantaneous displacement of the target, respectively, and $v$ is the speed of microwave propagation. Substituting Eqs. (7.10) and (7.11) into Eq. (7.9), with the assumption that $x(t)$ is much smaller than the free-space wavelength, yields the frequency-demodulated mixer output signa $S_{out}(t)$, following appropriate approximation, as

$$S_{out}(t) = \left( \frac{\omega_{osc}^2 \tau_d \, E_{inj}}{Qv \, E_{osc}} \right) \cos\left[ \left( \frac{2\omega_{osc}}{v} R \right) x(t) \right] \tag{7.13}$$

where $\tau_d$ is the two-way propagation time delay. The phase component in Eq. (7.13) is clearly a linear function of the time-varying displacement $x(t)$ between the SIL radar sensor and the target. Thus, the SILO's output frequency will change with the relative motion between the target and the radar antenna. It is significant to note from Eq. (7.13) that the output signal from the SIL radar is proportional to the square of the microwave source frequency $\omega_{osc}$, suggesting that a doubling of the source frequency will increase (quadruple) the SIL radar output signal's strength by four-fold.

For the vital-sign detection experiment shown in Figures 7.59 and 7.60, a human subject was seated 1 m away from a prototype SIL radar sensor depicted in

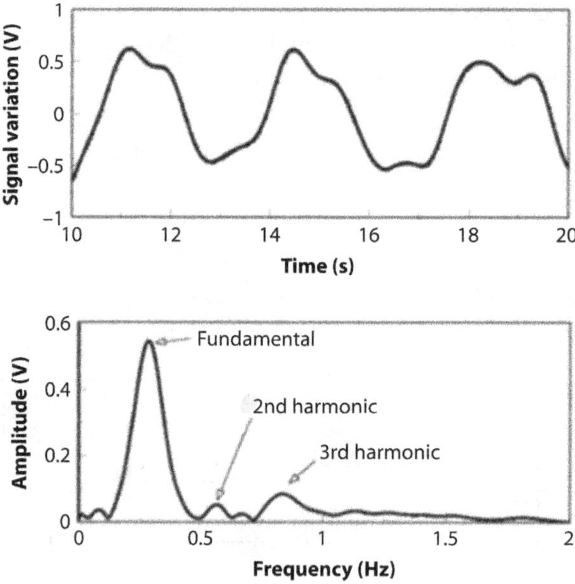


**FIGURE 7.59** Vital signs detected using ISM band SIL radar: Breathing waveform (top) and frequency spectrum showing a rate of 17 beats/min (below).

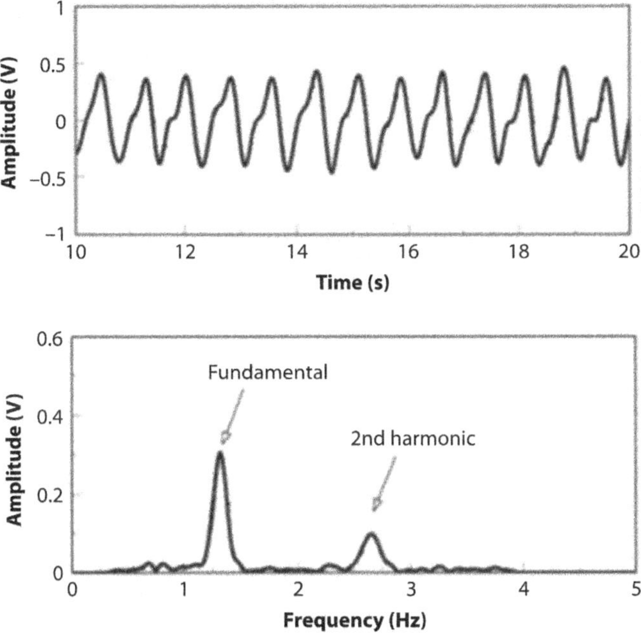


**FIGURE 7.60** Heartbeat detected using an ISM SIL radar sensor: (a) Heartbeat waveform and (b) Frequency spectrum indicating a heartbeat of 79 beats/min.

Figure 7.61, for ISM band operation. The frequency-demodulated output signal was first sent through a low-pass filter. The respiration and heartbeat information are then extracted by applying digital filters with the following passbands: 0.1–1 Hz for respiration and 1–10 Hz for heartbeat. A breathing rate of 17 per min and a heartbeat of 79 beats/min are identified. The sensitivity of SIL radar detection is exemplified by clarity of the signals.

A special feature of the SIL sensor architecture is that the system SNRs are proportional to the fourth power of source frequency. Since the received power, in general, decreases with the square of sensing distance, doubling the operating frequency should increase the SNR by a factor of four (see Eq. 7.13). This phenomenon is validated experimentally for the SIL sensor by detecting heart signals at different frequencies and distances between the SIL radar and the subject as illustrated in Figures 7.58–7.60. In these figures, the VCO in the SIL sensor system was operating in the single-frequency mode and the selected output frequencies are at 1.8, 2.4, and 3.6 GHz. The distances of separation between SIL sensor and subject are 0.5, 1, 2, and 4 m.

Figure 7.62 depicts the heart signal detection results at 2.4 GHz. It is seen that the amplitude of the output waveform is reduced by roughly half (50%) as the sensing distance doubles. Note that digital processing of the results at 4 m was not able to provide an accurate measure of the heartbeat rate, and thus suggesting a maximum sensing distance is 2 m for the SIL sensor operating at 2.4 GHz. In a similar fashion,

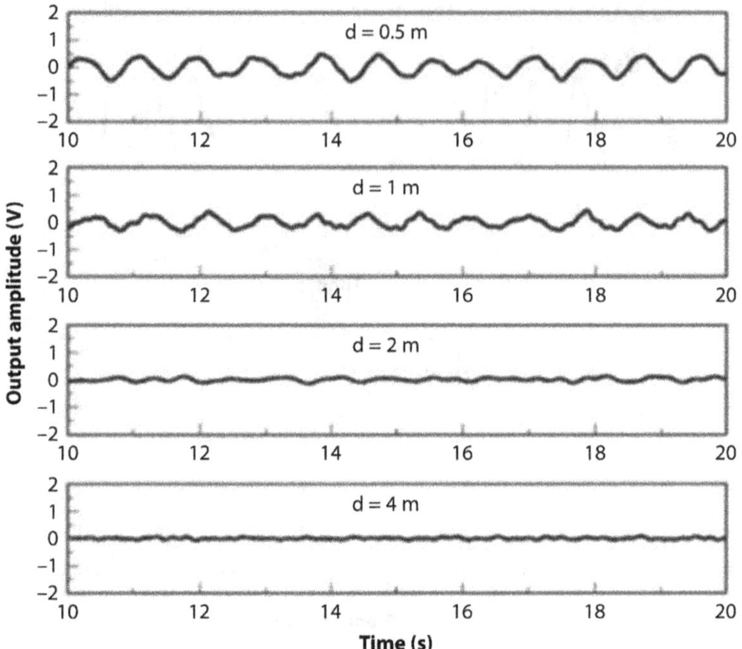


**FIGURE 7.61** Heart signal detection results at different distances between the subject and SIL sensor operating at 1.8 GHz.

Figures 7.61 and 7.63 give the heartbeat detection results at 1.8 and 3.6 GHz, respectively. Using the same criterion for assessing the detectability of heartbeat rates, the maximum distance for accurate sensing is 1 and 4 m, respectively, for these SIL sensors operating at 1.8 and 3.6 GHz and at an output power level of 1 mW. This result is consistent with expected SIL sensor performance of increasing the sensing distance four-fold by doubling the operating frequency. A further advantage of the SIL architecture is seen by allowing the VCO to sweep its output frequency, which helps to resolve the null detection point problem (see Figure 7.64). It also enables the SIL sensor to minimize external RF interference and stationary clutters.

The SIL radar sensors are gaining increasing attention for applications in noninvasive contactless vital-sign monitoring. During the past decade, various prototype systems have been developed to investigate some of the useful features of SIL radar for potential healthcare sensing applications. The proof-of-concept studies, whether on bench-top setups or using commercially available components on PCB circuits, have mostly been successful in demonstrating expected performances. While several chips for noncontact vital sign detection have been implemented, the prototype SIL radar sensors as a development opportunity with potential for SoC realization remains [Wang et al., 2020a]. It should be mentioned that aside from system architectures based on the conventional designs without a LNA, many of the more recent prototypes have incorporated LNA [Wu et al., 2013], and quadrature detection

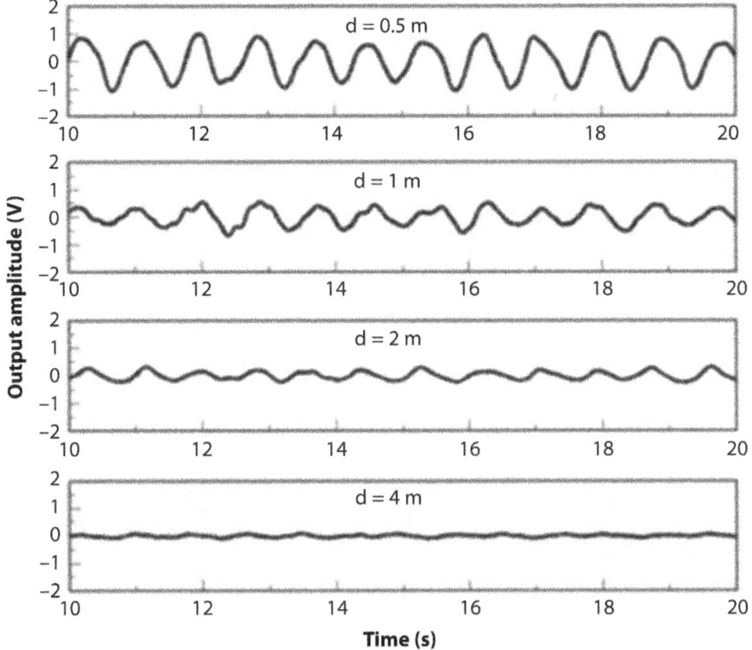


**FIGURE 7.62** Heart signal detection results at different distances between the subject and SIL sensor operating at 2.4 GHz.

schemes are appearing on some SIL radar architectures [Wang et al., 2019], especially for nonsmall-signal application scenarios. Nonetheless, the SIL radar sensor's advantages of high detector sensitivity, low system complexity, and less vulnerability to clutter noise remain as major attractions. The discussions that follow provide additional examples of applications of SIL radar, current advances, and associated technological innovations.

#### 7.7.3.1 Active-Integrated-Antenna SIL Sensors

An SIL radar sensor with active integrated antenna (AIA) and differentiator-based envelope detector was reported for vital-sign detection from the chest wall [Tseng et al., 2018]. The AIA sensor is designed for 5.6 GHz operation in proximity of the chest. A schematic diagram of the self-oscillating AIA based on the feedback-loop oscillator configuration is given in Figure 7.65(a) and (c) along with a photograph of the prototype sensor's circuitry (Figure 7.65[b]). In this configuration, the circular patch antenna, aside from transmitting microwaves, acts as a frequency-selective element for stabilizing the oscillator. The backscattered signal from the target is injected into and locks the AIA oscillator, and simultaneously introduces a variation in magnitude and a shift in frequency of the oscillator. The output signal is a frequency-modulated carrier with an amplitude-varying envelope. To extract the vital signs from the modulated signal, an envelope detector is integrated with a microwave

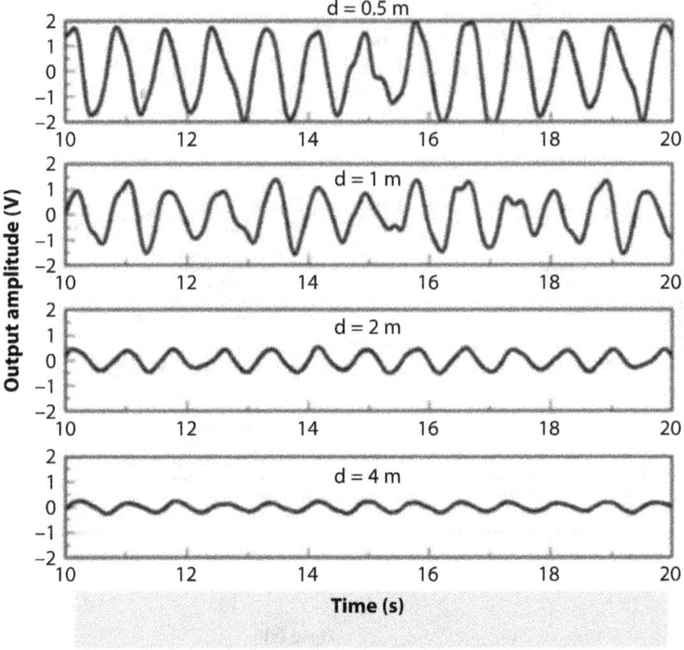


**FIGURE 7.63** Heart signal detection results at different distances between the subject and SIL sensor operating at 3.6 GHz.

differentiator to form a differentiator-based envelope detector in demodulating the output signal of the AIA.

For the cardiopulmonary rate measurement test setup, the AIA sensor was arranged in front of the left side of the chest of a human subject seated at 1.5–2 cm without contact with the chest wall. The measured time-domain waveform is shown in Figure 7.66(a). Except for subtracting the 2.5 V DC voltage level of the baseband

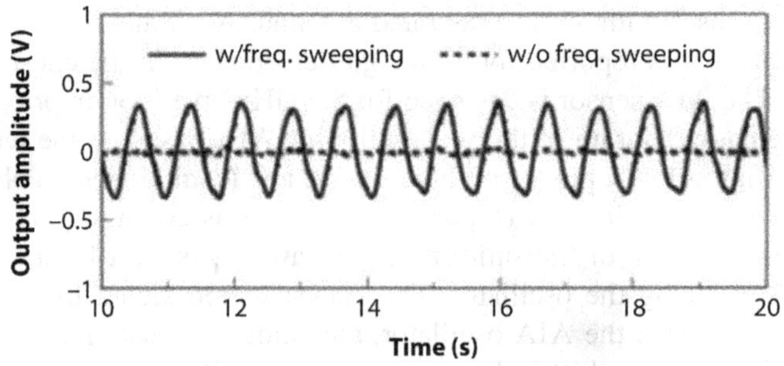


**FIGURE 7.64** Heart signal detection using an SIL sensor at a continuous wave Doppler radar "null" point showing heart-signal detection with frequency sweeping compared to that without.

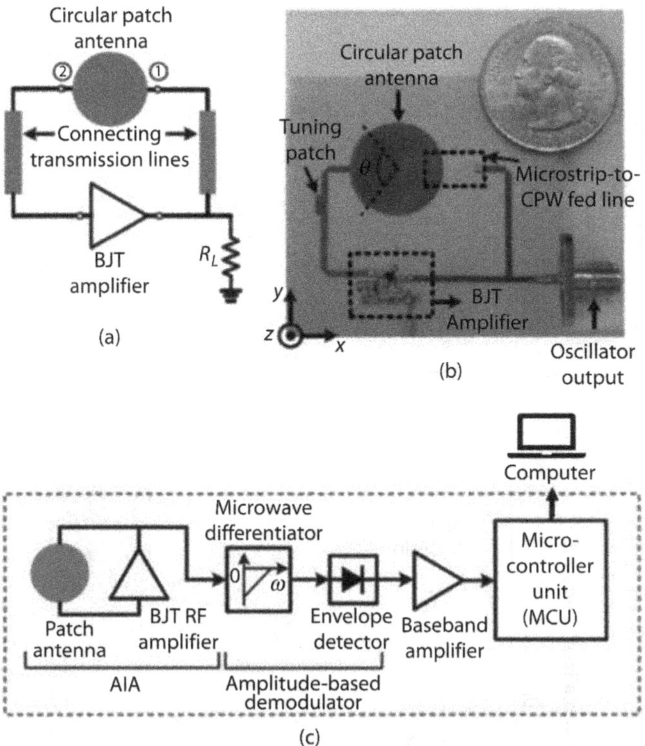


**FIGURE 7.65** SIL AIA radar sensor: (a) Circuit diagram of self-oscillating AIA sensor, (b) Photograph of AIA, and (c) Schematic diagram showing differentiator-based envelop detector. (Courtesy of Chao-Hsiung Tseng, National Taiwan University of Science and Technology.)

amplifier, signal processing procedures are applied on the raw data acquired by the DAQ module. As can be seen, the amplitude of the waveform is about 2 V, and this time-domain signal can be easily acquired by a low-cost microcontroller with a 10-bit ADC functionality. The time-domain waveform is converted to the frequency-domain spectrum via FFT, as shown in Figure 7.66(b). The two clear spectrum peaks show measured respiration and heartbeat rates of 20.8 and 79.2 beat/min, respectively. For reference and to demonstrate effectiveness of the AIA SIL sensor, a finger pulse oximeter was used to measure the heartbeat for comparison. The measured heartbeat by the AIA SIL sensor agrees closely with that acquired by the finger pulse oximeter, as illustrated in the inset of Figure 7.66(b). These results suggest that in addition to the AIA SIL's simple architecture, some advantages may be derived from the frequency-scalable nature of the demodulator architecture.

#### 7.7.3.2 Modulated SIL Radar for Remote Vital-Sign Detection

The introduction of frequency modulation into conventional SIL radar yielded a design architecture that supports remote ranging and tracking capabilities by allowing the system's operation to switch between CW and FMCW modes [Wang et al.,

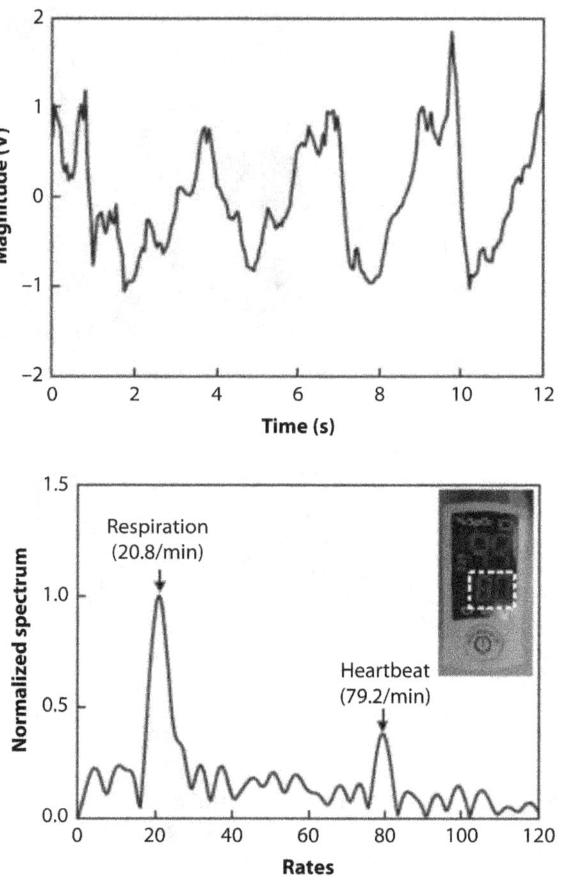


**FIGURE 7.66** SIL AIA sensor measurement of a cardiopulmonary signal: (a) Time-domain results of cardiopulmonary detection and (b) Spectrum showing respiration and heartbeat rates. Inset: Reference pulse rate from finger.

2013, 2020b]. The schematic and timing diagram of a prototype modulated SIL system is shown in Figure 7.67. When the tuning voltage $V_t(t)$ and scanning voltage $V_s(t)$ are ramp and constant, respectively, the radar operates in FMCW mode. In CW mode, $V_t(t)$ remains a constant and the ramp signal of $V_s(t)$ enters the phase shifter to scan the beam direction and detect the Doppler shifts at various azimuths. A sum-difference pattern detection technique is applied to track the azimuth of individual subjects. It has been shown that the modulated SIL radar architecture's remote ranging and tracking capabilities can allow the SIL radar signal to go through walls to track subjects based on detection of their cardiopulmonary signatures.

In the experiment shown in Figure 7.68(a), two subjects are seated (2–5 m) behind a 180 × 200 × 3 cm$^3$ wooden office partition wall and surrounded by various items that generate clutter signals. The SIL oscillator frequency was 2.4 GHz in CW mode. It was swept from 2.4 to 2.7 GHz in FMCW mode. The azimuth tracking angle was scanned from 55° to 125°. As shown in Figure 7.68(b), the reconstructed SIL image

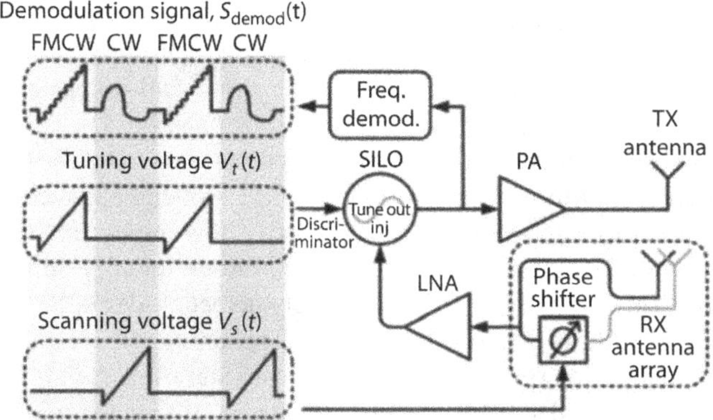


**FIGURE 7.67** Schematic and timing diagram of the frequency modulated SIL radar architecture.

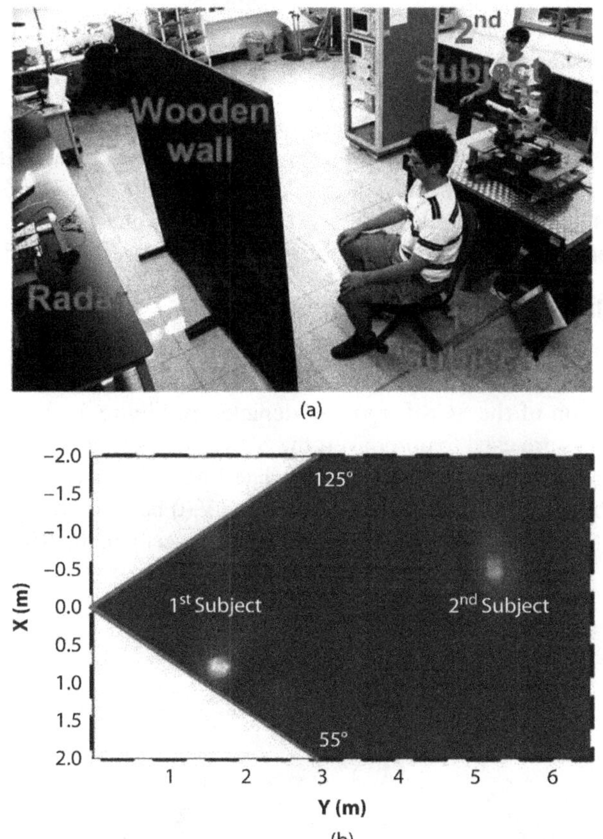


**FIGURE 7.68** Experimental arrangement for remote SIL radar detection of location and cardiopulmonary signatures: (a) Photograph of two subjects seated 2–5 m behind a wooden partition wall and (b) Reconstructed image of subject locations. (Courtesy of T.S. Jason Horng, National Sun Yat-Sen University.)

clearly shows the location of two subjects. The tint and brightness of the two image blobs change with time as functions of the subjects' cardiopulmonary signatures, especially respiration, which can cause greater chest wall displacements than the heartbeat.

It is noted that modulated SIL radar for remote detection for the experiment shown in Figure 7.68 with subjects seated behind a wooden partition wall has been referred to as "see-through-wall (STW SIL) radar" [Wang et al., 2013]. The ranging and tracking capabilities along with the cardiopulmonary sensing feature to enable the SIL to see through walls and remotely detect hidden subjects clearly offer advantages for search and rescue operations. The unique accomplishment in this case is the demonstration of remote sensing of vital signs and ranging using the SIL radar system at modest distances, which is the topic of discussion in the following section for a related SIL radar.

The ability for microwaves to penetrate walls constructed of low-loss, low dielectric constant materials is considerable. The dielectric constants are 2–5 for Plexiglas, window glass, dry wood, plastics, etc. (see Chapter 4). Theoretical and experimental studies suggest that minimal perturbation by walls constructed with dielectric or equivalent materials occurs if its broadside orientation is normal to the direction of microwave propagation. The backscattering is less than 10% in most cases [Lin et al., 1977; Lin and Wu, 1976]. The microwave transmission coefficients for planar surfaces are as large as 60% to 80% and the transmitted microwave signals can pass through with little distortion. Indeed, similar rationales have led to CW microwave Doppler radars being applied in detecting vital signs of human and animal victims buried under bricks or building rubble during disaster relief (see Section 7.7.2).

### 7.7.3.3 Single-Conversion SIL Radar

The single-conversion SIL (SCSIL) hybrid mode radar architecture is a variation of the modulated SIL radar for remote sensing of vital signs [Wang et al., 2020a,b]. The schematic diagram of the SCSIL radar is depicted in Figure 7.69. In this case, frequency converters are used to up-convert the SILO's output signal and down-convert the received signal to establish a SIL loop. The FMCW and CW mode operations are accomplished by switching the tuning voltage $V_t(t)$ between ramp and DC waveforms. Unlike the modulation SIL radar previously described, the SILO in the SCSIL radar operates at a fixed free-running frequency to minimize bandwidth limitations

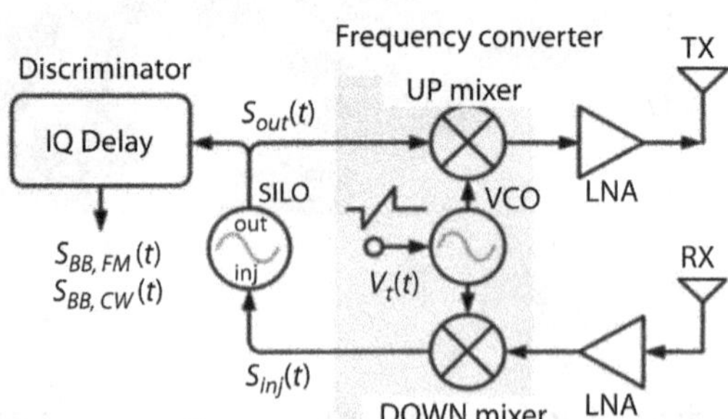


**FIGURE 7.69** Schematic diagram of single-conversion SIL (SCSIL) hybrid mode radar sensor.

and potential instability issues. With coherent sampling, the output signals of the IQ delay discriminator, $S_{BB,FM(t)}$ and $S_{BB,CW(t)}$ are used to extract the range and Doppler information. Each tone's phase is ideally proportional to the propagation delay in the SIL path, and this proportionality as a frequency-phase relationship may be compromised if the distance between neighboring subjects is less than the range resolution of the FMCW radar. The specific condition of this architecture can predetermine the frequency range in which the resolution issue arises.

The popular signal processing algorithms such as MUSIC (multiple signal classification) and ESPRIT (estimation of signal parameters via rational invariance technique) are not suitable for application to an SIL radar because of its specific mechanism of noise shaping. A novel frequency estimation algorithm (FEA) for super-resolution analysis was proposed [Wang et al., 2020b]. FEA assumes that the input signal is a combination of multiple sine wave signals and uses FFT and Newton's method to evaluate the frequency and amplitude of each component with an iterative method. The process is repeated until the residual-to-input energy ratio is less than the threshold (approximately 10%).

The experimental arrangement of the SCSIL radar system for remote monitoring of vital signs of two seated subjects is shown in Figure 7.70. The center frequency of the radar is 5.8 GHz; the bandwidth is 150 MHz and, therefore, the theoretically estimated range resolution is 1 m. Subject A is at a radial distance of 1.9 m with an azimuth angle of 90° while subject B is at a radial distance of 2.5 m and an azimuth angle of 95°. The two subjects are close to each other, and the body of subject A partially occludes subject B. Measured range and spectrum results are shown in Figure 7.71(a) and (b). The black and gray lines with circles represent the output spectra of the baseband signals obtained by conventional FFT and the proposed FEA, respectively. It is seen that FEA can overcome the resolution issue caused by insufficient modulation bandwidth in FMCW mode and sensing time in CW mode, and the signal reflected from subject B

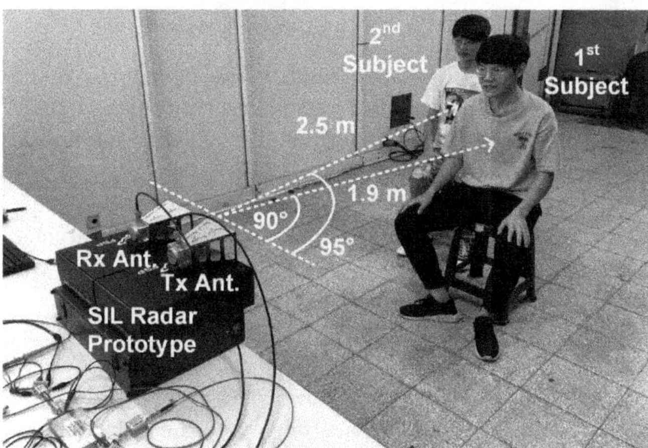


**FIGURE 7.70** Experimental arrangement for remote single-conversion SIL (SCSIL) radar detection and sensing of the vital signs of two seated subjects. (Courtesy of Fu-Kang Wang, National Sun Yat-Sen University.)

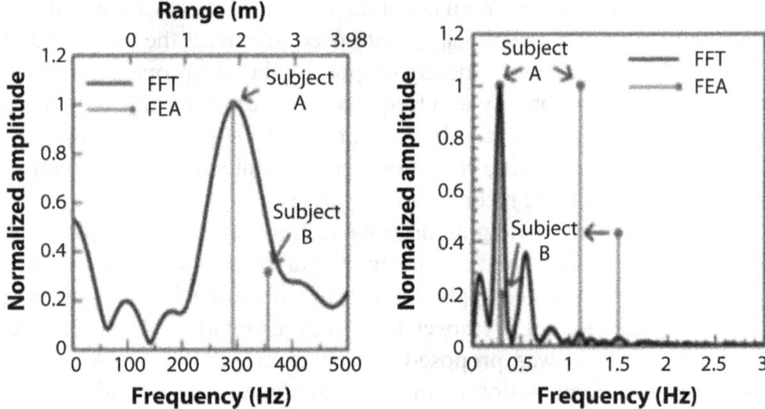


**FIGURE 7.71** Experimental results obtained using fast Fourier transform (FFT) and frequency estimation algorithms (FEA). The black and gray lines with circular symbols represent the output spectra of the baseband signals: (a) Range detection and (b) Vital-sign detection.

is almost completely blocked by subject A, with reduced amplitude. Nonetheless, Figure 7.71 shows that vital signs of multiple subjects can be identified from the tone's amplitude. The estimated range error is 5 cm. With a measurement time of 20 seconds, the errors of respiration and heart rates are 2 breaths and 3 beats per min, respectively. Therefore, although the amplitude-based method for identifying multiple subjects is successfully demonstrated with various radial distances, the issue of accuracy remains. Further research is essential to develop algorithms for range-Doppler mapping including two-dimensional FEA, to enhance accurate range and vital sign detection of multiple subjects at the same time and place.

### 7.7.4 High Sensitivity CW Doppler CMOS Radar Chips

The advancements discussed indicate significant development of microwave radar sensors for contactless and remote vital-sign monitoring for humans. The hardware has been demonstrated from bench-top prototype systems to radar-on-chip or SoC architectures. Various detection schemes have been tested to improve range, reduce effective phase noise, or improve phase-modulation sensitivity. A seminal advantage of the microwave radar technique and technology is the human target's sizable radar cross section (RCS) or its relatively large detectable target areas with microwave noncontact detection from remote locations compared to most alternative technologies. Nonetheless, the advantages and disadvantages of various systems are continuously being assessed.

A logical factor from the free-space wavelength perspective, or perhaps apparent tactic in realizing high-detection sensitivity, is to use radar sensors with higher operating frequency, which simply translates to wavelength-based better spatial resolution of target displacement or movements. As mentioned in Chapter 1, while it would be valuable, there may not be an optimal frequency for remote noncontact sensing. Instead, the effectiveness may be dependent on specific application in target space and accessible frequency source. Nevertheless, the use of higher frequency millimeter wave (mmW) bands for better receiver sensitivity are being explored. Furthermore, at the mmW frequencies, a chip-size radar detector could be implemented in CMOS architecture. It is worthy of note that higher sensitivity may potentially elicit more pronounced noise sources to interfere with vital-sign detection, including the presence of higher harmonics of vital sign signals. Furthermore, there are concerns that the high spatial resolution of mmW frequencies might not be most suited for remote contactless sensing of the vital signs of humans because the short wavelength might be too sensitive for the relatively large chest displacements associated with respiratory activity.

#### 7.7.4.1 CW Doppler mmW Radar Sensors

The first reported experimental study of a contactless 60 GHz mmW vital-sign detection system was performed by using V-band mmW waveguide components on a laboratory bench [Chuang et al., 2012]. Figure 7.72(a) shows a photograph of the 60 GHz prototype system. The V-band waveguide components shown includes a mmW signal source, PA, circulator, horn antenna, variable phase shifter, variable attenuator, LNA, and a mixer. A clutter canceller is implemented in the system with an attenuator and phase shifter. The clutter canceller performs the cancellation for the transmitted power leakage to the receiver and background reflection clutter to enhance the detecting sensitivity of the vital signals. Noncontact vital-signal measurements were taken from a human subject at 1–2 m. The transmitting power is 8 dBm and the horn antenna gain is 25 dBi. The time- and frequency-domain results indicated clear heartbeat signals during 20-second sessions. However, the robustness of respiration detection is limited. In this case, the large difference between heartbeat and respiration amplitudes and complex phase modulation significantly increases the signal detection difficulty in the presence of a strong respiratory signal. The prototype system has led to the development and implementation of a 60 GHz CMOS chip design [Kuo et al., 2016], based on direct-conversion Doppler radar sensor architecture with a clutter canceller for single-antenna contactless vital-sign detection in humans (see Section 7.7.4.3 for additional discussions).

#### 7.7.4.2 CMOS Flip-Chip-Integrated Radar at 60 GHz

This section discusses the first flip-chip-packaged and fully integrated 60 Hz Doppler radar in 90 nm CMOS for contactless vital sign detection. The compact 60 GHz core (0.73 mm) provides a 36 dB peak down-conversion gain and transmits 1 mW of power at 55 GHz [Kao et al., 2013]. A quadrature circuit at the intermediate frequency stage of the heterodyne receiver safeguards effective signal detection by eliminating the null detection point issue. A system block diagram is shown in Figure 7.73, including the CMOS transceiver chip, patch antennas for TX and RX, and metal trace on the laminate (zoom-in area) designed for flip-chip integration, without a high-power amplifier.

A quadrature receiver is required to eliminate the well-known null detection points. I/Q separation is realized at the IF stage of the heterodyne receiver instead of a direct-conversion design, which minimizes the loss, mismatch, and power consumption of 60 GHz I/Q separation and distribution. Because the phase noise is

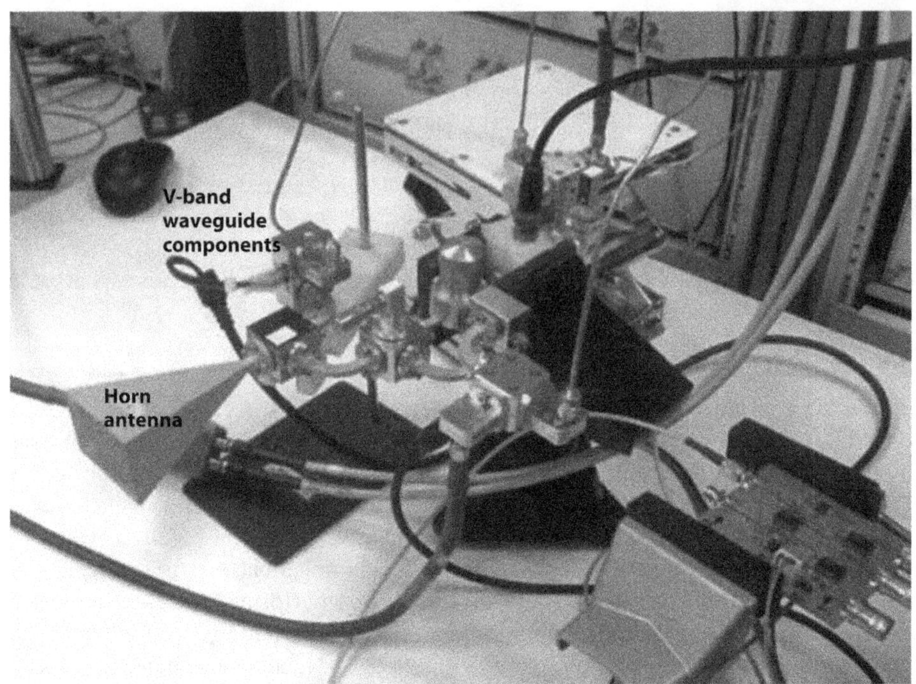


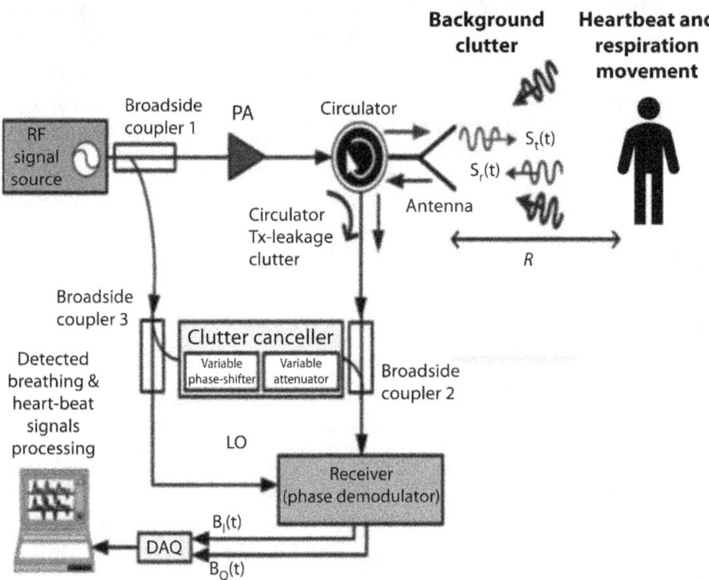


**FIGURE 7.72** Photograph (a) and schematic diagram (b) of a 60 GHz prototype vital-sign measurement system setup using V-band waveguide components. (Courtesy of Tzuen-Hsi Huang, National Cheng Kung University.)

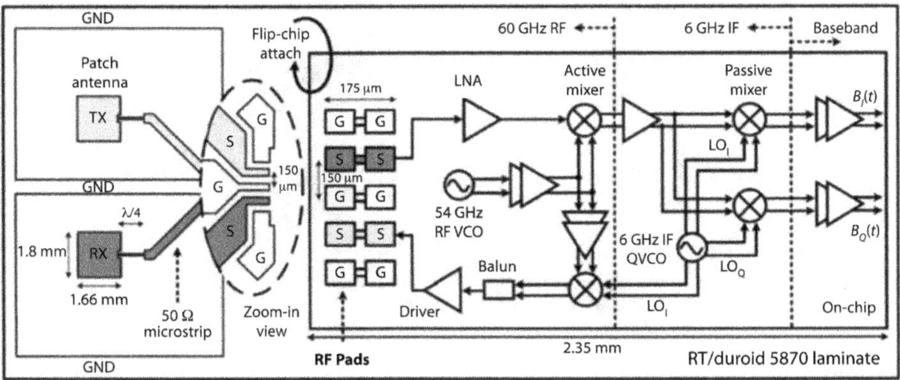


**FIGURE 7.73** System block diagram illustrating CMOS Doppler radar, flip-chip integration, TX and RX PCB patch antennas, 60 GHz RF section, 6 GHz IF, and baseband I/Q outputs. The overall dimensions are 31.3 × 45 mm.

significantly reduced by range correlation effect, a compact free-running quadrature ring VCO is used for IF to drive two passive mixers with large transistor size. The large passive mixers are used to minimize low flicker noise, which is not cancelled through range correlation. The wide tunable IF provided by the ring VCO is used to compensate the possible RF drift due to mmW uncertainty and to improve the system robustness. Also, the IF frequency chosen about a decade away from the LO (54 GHz) makes the LO feed-through more effectively attenuated by the output tank of the RF mixer. A photomicrograph of the 60 GHz CMOS radar chip is shown in Figure 7.74. The final system configuration used in human experiments is shown in Figure 7.75, where the lightweight PCB was pasted to an upright piece of cardboard facing the target. The photograph shows the flipped chip, TX and RX patch antennas, and DC bias wires.

The compact 60 GHz CMOS Doppler radar sensor chip system has successfully demonstrated detection of heartbeat at 0.3 m at first pass from human chest. The experimental results showed that for heartbeat detection, random body movement often results in the transition between optimal and null detection points every

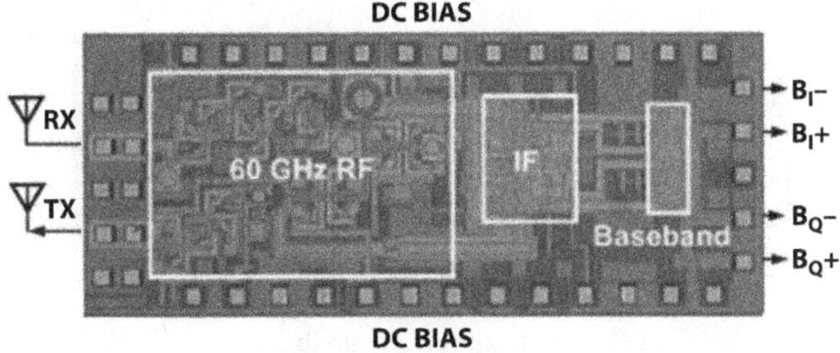


**FIGURE 7.74** Photomicrograph of the 60 GHz CMOS radar chip. (Courtesy of Jenshan Lin, University of Florida.)

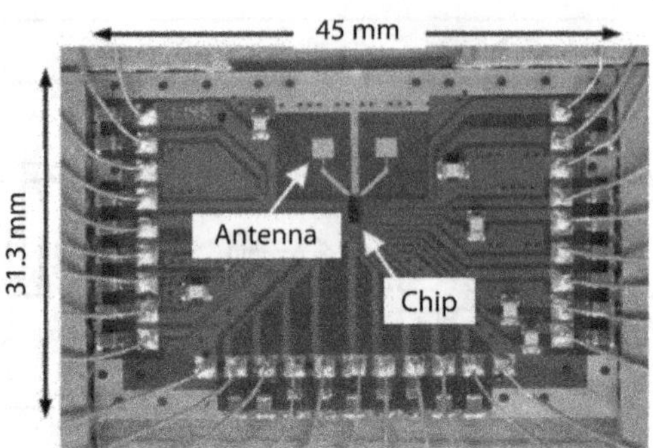


**FIGURE 7.75** Final system photograph including the flipped chip, TX and RX patch antennas, and DC bias wires. (Courtesy of Jenshan Lin, University of Florida.)

$\lambda/8$ (~0.6 mm) in chest displacement variations. The quadrature scheme can ensure robust detection. When the movement is comparable to or greater than $\lambda$, the modulated phase, $4\pi\ x(t)/\lambda$ travels through multiples of $2\pi$, and the detector output is no longer monotonic during inhale and exhale cycles. This shows up in the spectrum as harmonics and intermodulation, which can seriously degrade the detection accuracy. Figure 7.76 gives the detection results of two different displacements, when the respiration rate is 15 breath/min at 0.3 m. Figure 7.76(b) shows a possible respiration peak at 15 breath/min; however, the presence of other large peaks makes the

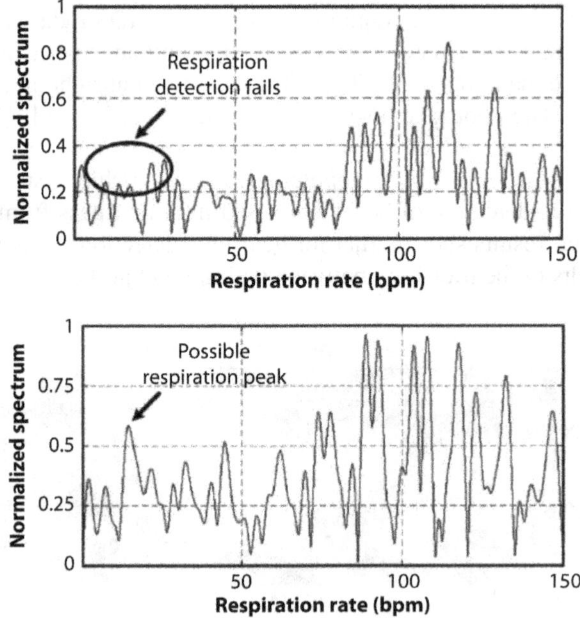


**FIGURE 7.76** Spectrum of respiration signal detection from two different displacements: (a) No prominent respiration peak and (b) possible respiration peak at 15 breath/min.

detection unreliable. In other cases, shown in Figure 7.76(a), as the displacement changes, the main respiration peak can be swamped, and respiration rate detection completely fails.

Because the same distorted signals do not appear in I and Q channels simultaneously, an algorithm was developed to preserve the undistorted portion of the waveform and recover the distorted portion to solve the detection problem when target displacement is comparable to or greater than $\lambda$. In Figure 7.77(a), the algorithm was applied to the I and Q baseband outputs of Figure 7.76(a), and the respiration rate was recovered from both I and Q channels. The recovered spectrum in Figure 7.77(b) shows a correct respiration peak at 15.11 breath/min. Nevertheless, the complexity and robustness remain as challenges and need a dedicated algorithm to extract a correct vital sign, which suggests room for further improvement when the movement is comparable to or greater than $\lambda$ adopted for the radar system. The use of a shorter wavelength can achieve higher sensitivity compared with previous work performed at a longer wavelength, but there are tradeoffs to be considered.

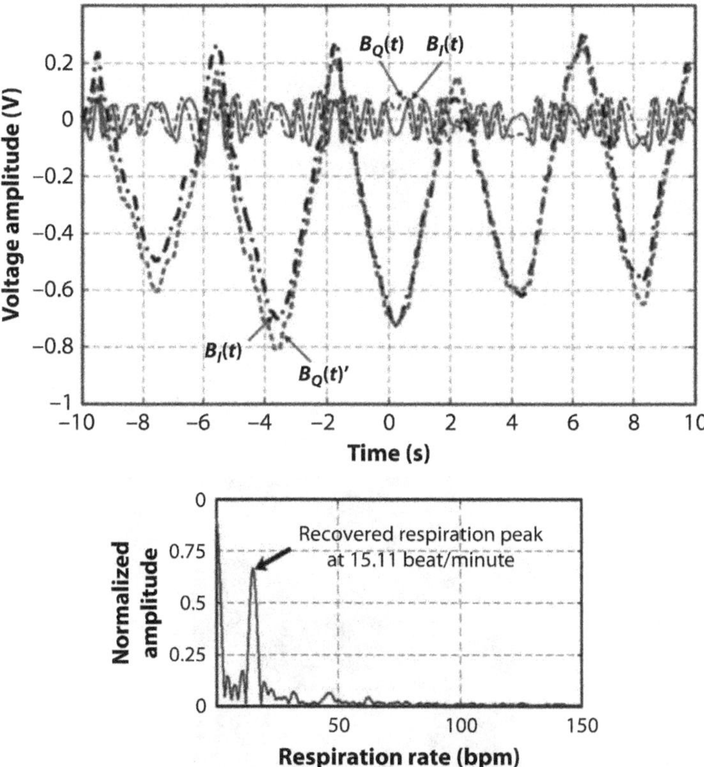


**FIGURE 7.77** 60 GHz CMOS radar chip detected respiration signals: (a) I and Q outputs before recovery algorithm is applied and I and Q outputs after recovery algorithm is applied and (b) spectrum of recovered respiration peak from I and Q outputs for the signal shown in Figure 7.76(a).

#### 7.7.4.3 CMOS Integrated Direct-Conversion Doppler Chip Radar

Section 7.7.4.1 described a research project aimed at reducing the modulator noise, increasing detection sensitivity, and extending the vital-sign sensing range using 60 GHz mmW. Further development in this effort has manifested in a fully integrated 60 GHz CMOS direct-conversion Doppler radar RF sensor (Figure 7.78 for photomicrograph) with a clutter canceller for single-antenna contactless human vital-sign detection [Kuo et al., 2016]. A high isolation quasi-circulator (QC) is designed to reduce the transmitter's (TX) power leakage to the receiver (RX). The clutter canceller performs cancellation for the TX leakage power from the QC and the stationary backscattered clutter to enhance the detection sensitivity of weak vital-sign signals. The integration of the 60 GHz sensor consists of the VCO, divided-by-2 frequency divider (FD), power amplifier (PA), QC, clutter canceller consisting of variable-gain amplifier (VGA) and 360 phase shifter (PS), LNA, in-phase (I)/quadrature-phase (Q) subharmonic mixer, and three couplers. The mmW vital-sign Doppler radar sensor chip is fabricated in 90 nm CMOS technology with a chip size of 2 × 2 mm, including the test pads and metal dummy, and consumes 217 mW of power. A schematic diagram of the 60 GHz CMOS direct-conversion Doppler radar sensor with clutter canceller circuits for single-antenna contactless human vital sign detection is depicted in Figure 7.79. The inset figure to the right illustrates the principle of clutter cancellation.

The principle of clutter cancellation can be described as follows. The TX leakage from QC may be expressed as,

$$A_{Leak}\cos(\omega t+\theta_{Leak}) \tag{7.14}$$

and the stationary background clutter as,

$$A_c\cos(\omega t+\theta_c) \tag{7.15}$$

The sum of these two signals is the equivalent signal (see inset of Figure 7.76),

$$V_{eq}(t)= A_{Leak}\cos(\omega t+\theta_{Leak})+ A_c\cos(\omega t+\theta_c) \tag{7.16}$$

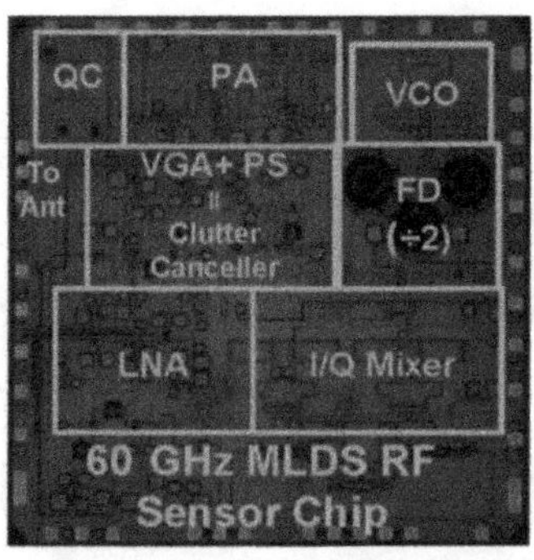


**FIGURE 7.78** Photomicrograph of 60 GHz CMOS direct-conversion Doppler radar chip (size 2 × 2 mm). (Courtesy of Huey-Ru Chuang and Tzuen-Hsi Huang, National Cheng Kung University.)

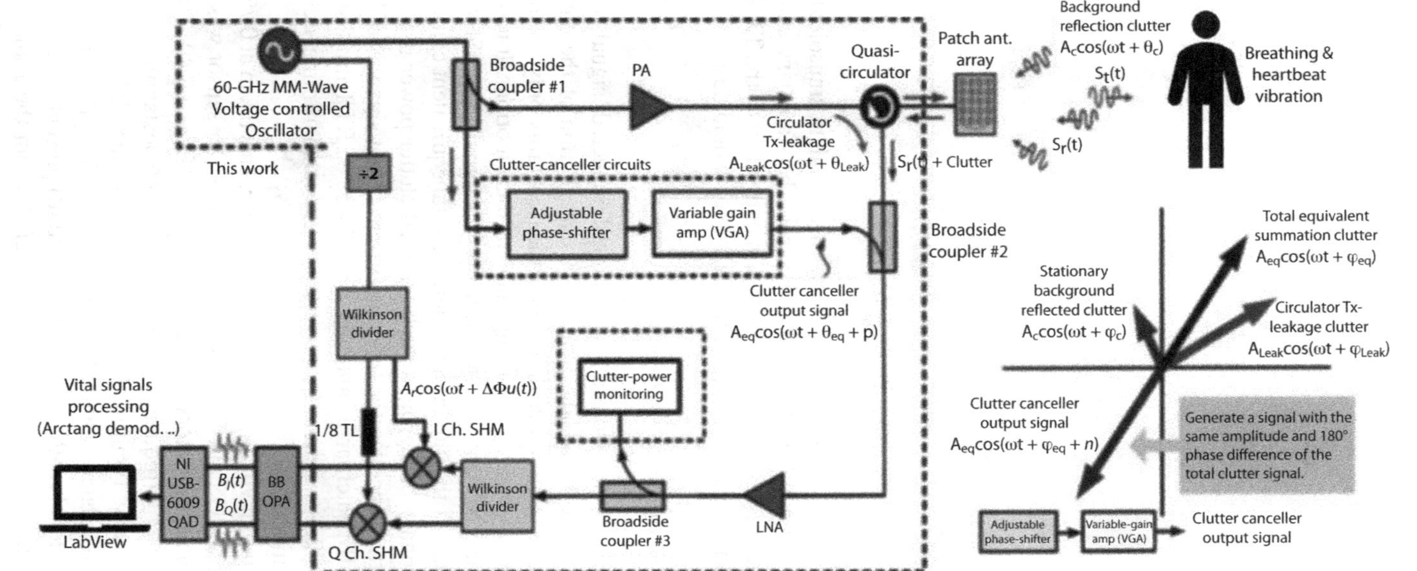


**FIGURE 7.79** Schematic diagram of 60 GHz CMOS direct-conversion Doppler radar RF sensor with clutter canceller circuits for single-antenna noncontact human vital-signs detection. The Doppler radar chip sensor has a high isolation QC and a clutter canceller circuit. It consists of a VCO, FD, PA, and QC, clutter canceller with a low phase-variation VGA and a full 360 continuously adjustable PS, LNA, I/Q subharmonic mixer (SHM), and three directional couplers. The inset figure to the right illustrates the principle of clutter cancellation. (Courtesy of Tzuen-Hsi Huang, National Cheng Kung University.)

which may be expressed as

$$V_{eq}(t) = C\cos(\omega t) + D\sin(\omega t) = A_{eq}\cos(\omega t + \theta_{eq}) \tag{7.17}$$

where $A_{eq}$ and $\theta_{eq}$ are the amplitude and phase of the equivalent summation signal, respectively and are given by

$$A_{eq} = \sqrt{|C|^2 + |D|^2} \tag{7.18}$$

and

$$\theta_{eq} = -tan^{-1}\frac{D}{C} \tag{7.19}$$

with

$$C = A_{Leak}\cos(\theta_{Leak}) + A_c\cos(\theta_c) \tag{7.20}$$

$$D = A_{Leak}\sin(\theta_{Leak}) - A_c\sin(\theta_c) \tag{7.21}$$

Note that if there are several stationary clutters, an equivalent sinusoidal clutter signal with the same frequency can still be formed from the stationary clutter signals. Hence, according to Eq. (7.17), to cancel the sum equivalent of the TX leakage and clutter signals, the output signal of the clutter canceller should be

$$V_{cancel}(t) = A_{eq}\cos(\omega t + \theta_{eq} + \pi) \tag{7.22}$$

$V_{cancel}(t)$ is combined with the received backscattered (reflected) signal, TX leakage and clutter signals in the broadside coupler for cancellation of the equivalent $V_{eq}(t)$ clutter. The output of the broadside coupler then contains only the received phase-modulating signal reflected by breathing and heartbeat motions. It is followed with amplification by the LNA and mixing with the LO signal in the SHM. Tests showed that when turning off the clutter canceller, the total equivalent clutter signal of TX leakage and stationary background backscattered clutter power is 5–7 dBm. After turning on the clutter canceller, the total equivalent clutter signal is reduced to –35 dBm. A 60 GHz 17 dBi patch-array antenna ($4 \times 2.2$ cm) on RT/Duroid substrate (0.127 mm thick and $\varepsilon_r = 2.2$) was used for testing. The expected minimal detectable displacement is 15–20 $\mu$m at 30 cm.

In the experimental human vital-sign detection measurements taken at 0.75 m, the fully integrated 60 GHz CMOS direct-conversion Doppler radar sensor was able to provide clear heartbeat and respiratory signals, as shown in Figure 7.80. The measured heartbeat and respiration frequency are about 1.1 Hz (66 beats/min) and 0.4 Hz (24 breaths/min), respectively. Figure 7.80(a) and (b) depict the CMOS radar sensor measured time and frequency domain heartbeat signals from the I and Q channels while the subject held its breath. Figure 7.80(c) and (d) present the radar sensor measured time and frequency domain respiration signals from the I and Q channels while the subject breathed normally. It can be seen from the I- and Q-channel

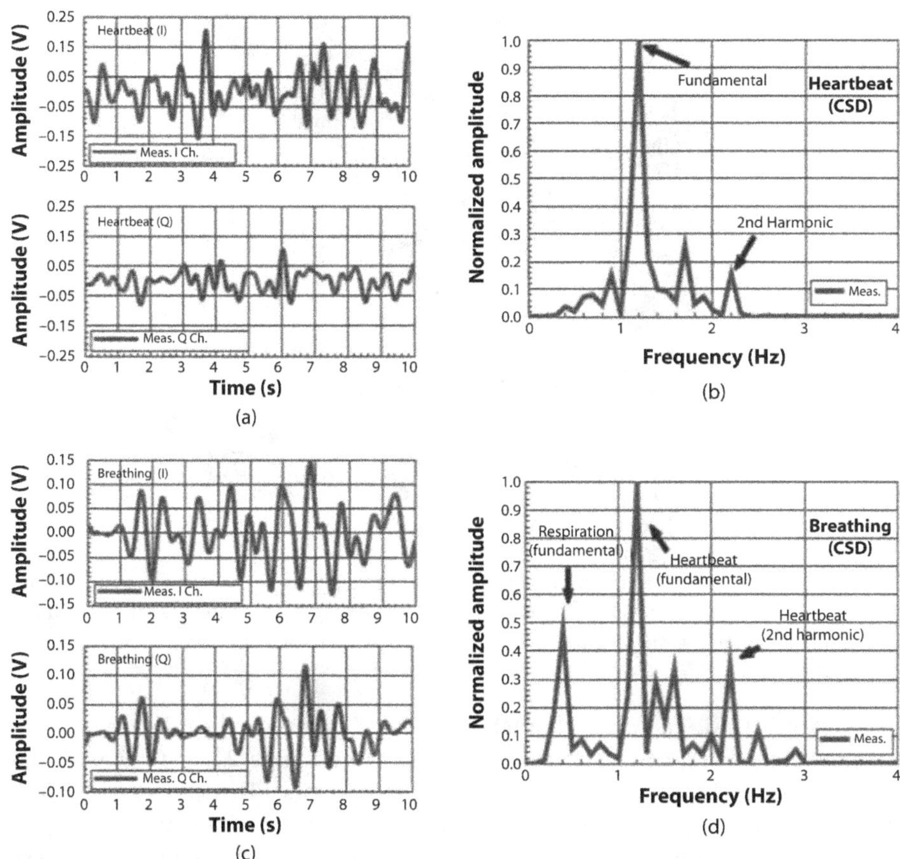


**FIGURE 7.80** Measured respiration and heartbeat signals of the human subject at 0.75 m: (a) Time-domain I/Q signal of the heartbeat signal, (b) Frequency spectrum of the heartbeat signal, (c) Time-domain I/Q signal of the breathing signal, and (d) Frequency spectrum of the respiration signal.

time-domain waveforms of Figure 7.80(a) and (c) that the two channels are somewhat different as expected. The frequency spectrum showed obviously visible vital signs with plainly distinguishable heart signals. Apparently, the detectability has benefited from arctangent demodulation of I/Q signals [Park et al., 2007] in the related series of experiments. In addition, there are several minor but lower peaks, suggesting that the clutter canceller is less than perfect. It is estimated that the CMOS radar sensor chip with a transmitted power of 3 dBm the detection distance is 1.5 m if the effective radiated power (ERP) is increased by 10 dB, the detection distance can be increased to 3 m. The ERP is higher than the power that is radiated because it takes the directional characteristics of the antenna into account.

More recently, the design of a mmW logarithmic power detector (PD) integrated in a 60 GHz CMOS vital-sign Doppler radar sensor incorporated with a microprocessor control unit (MCU) for fast automatic clutter cancellation was presented

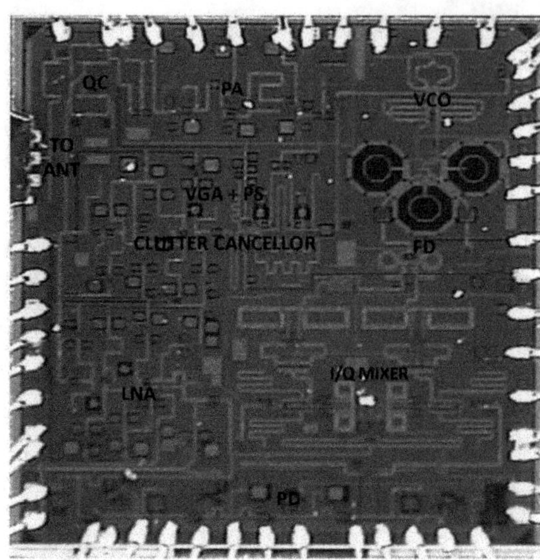


**FIGURE 7.81** Photomicrograph of 60 GHz CMOS Doppler radar sensor integrated with a V-band PD. The chip size is 2 × 2.34 mm. (Courtesy of Huey-Ru Chuang, Tzuen-Hsi Huang, National Cheng Kung University.)

[Chou et al., 2018]. The radar chip fabricated in 90 nm CMOS consumes 243 mW of DC power with a chip size of 2 × 2.34 mm (see Figure 7.81). To achieve low minimum detectable power and high dynamic range for the PD, the successive detection logarithmic amplifier (SDLA) topology was used, and the limited amplifiers are replaced by mmW linear amplifiers. The PD (integrated in the radar chip) exhibited a dynamic range and logarithmic errors about 35 dB and within ±2 dB at 60 GHz. The minimum detectable power level is −45 dBm. Unlike the slower manual tuning process for clutter cancellation [Kuo et al., 2016], by feeding the PD output voltage, which indicates the clutter power strength, to the A/D pin of the MCU, the automatic clutter cancellation function for the vital sign radar can be performed rapidly.

Figure 7.82 shows the I and Q channel outputs from the integrated CMOS Doppler radar package and frequency spectrum. The measured heartbeat and respiration frequency of a seated human subject are 1.1 Hz (66 beats/min) and 0.4 Hz (24 breaths/min), respectively. Aside from the respiration and heart-rate peaks, there are fewer and lower minor peaks compared to Figure 7.80. The measured heartbeat signal and frequency spectrum of a human subject holding its breath are given in Figure 7.83. It shows a singular heartbeat component without any breathing artifact. Note that in the experimental test, the radar chip and a 60 GHz 17 dBi patch-array antenna was integrated by bond-wire interconnection on a compact carrier board. The total loss of the bond-wire interconnection was reduced to 3.1 dB, less than half of the cable connection loss (7 dB) [Kuo et al., 2016]. Hence, the detection range can be extended from 0.75 to 1.2 m of the same power. Overall, the fast automatic clutter cancellation incorporated with MCU for the CMOS radar chip (integrated with a PD) bond-wired with the planar mmW antenna is achieved for practical human vital sign detection application.

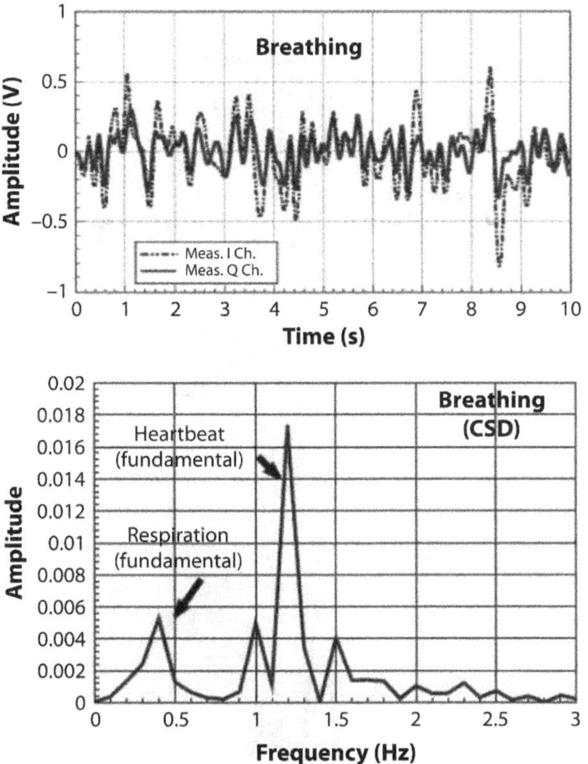


**FIGURE 7.82** V-band Doppler radar-measured respiration and heartbeat signals of the human subject with normal breathing at 1.2 m: (a) Time-domain I/Q channel signals and (b) Frequency spectrum.

In summary, the fully integrated 60 GHz CMOS direct-conversion Doppler radar sensor and the flip-chip integrated CMOS radar discussed in the previous section clearly indicate the importance of quadrature scheme in ensuring robust detection of vital signs in humans. The quadrature configurations allowed arctangent demodulation of the output signal and have contributed to enhanced detectability. When displacement of the chest wall is comparable to or greater than the wavelength $\lambda$, both random body movement and clutter due to presence of multiple targets can severely complicate phase modulation and seriously degrade vital-sign detectability and accuracy. The two different approaches invoked have found success either through software algorithm or hardware cancellation. The results suggest hardware mitigation in circuitry at the front end is straightforward and effective in cleaning up the signal, albeit at a greater system complexity.

#### 7.7.4.4 CW Doppler CMOS Radar-On-Chip at 100 GHz

The first fully chip-integrated 100 GHz Doppler radar transceiver using double-sideband low-IF architecture for vital-sign detection was implemented in 65 nm CMOS process [Ma et al., 2020]. Figure 7.84 shows the fully integrated 100 GHz CW

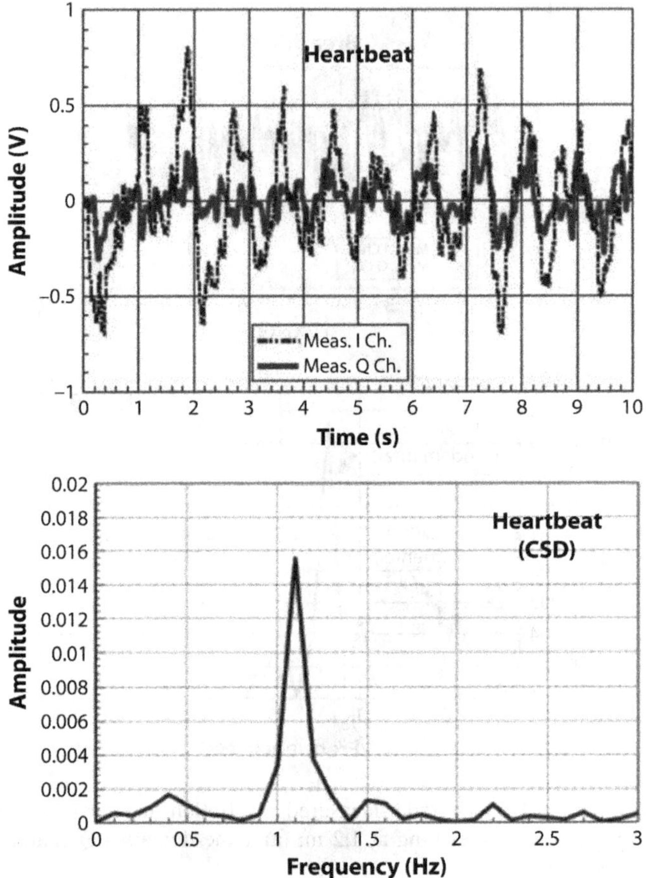


**FIGURE 7.83** V-band radar sensor measured heartbeat signals of a human subject holding its breath at 1.2 m: (a) Time-domain I/Q channel signals and (b) Frequency spectrum.

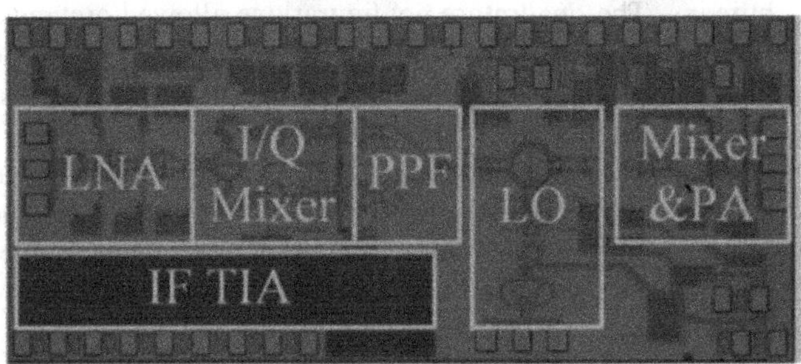


**FIGURE 7.84** Photomicrograph of 65 nm CMOS 100 GHz radar system on chip with dimensions of 0.9 × 2.0 mm including circuit blocks: LNA, I/Q down-conversion mixer, polyphase filter (PPF), IF transimpedance amplifier (TIA), LO generation, up-conversion mixer, and power amplifier (PA) and surrounding test pads. (Courtesy of Lianming Li, Southeast University.)

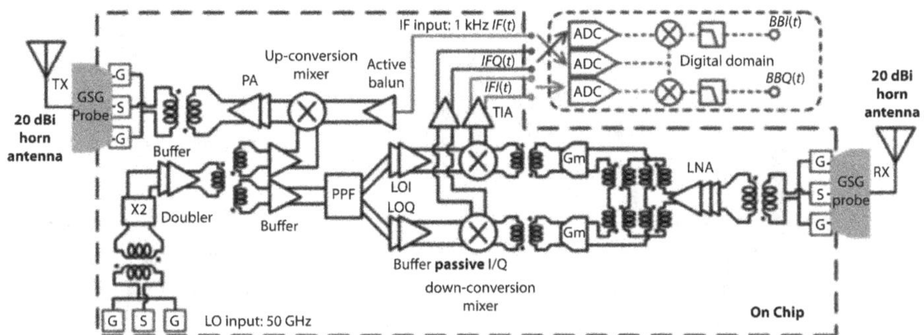


**FIGURE 7.85** Schematic diagram of the 100 GHz double-sideband low-IF continuous wave Doppler radar system-on-chip with transceiver chip, two horn antennas, and the off-chip digital signal processing. (Courtesy of Jenshan Lin, University of Florida.)

Doppler radar transceiver with the double-sideband low-IF architecture. The chip radar transceiver consumed 262 mW and measured 0.9 × 2.0 mm. Instead of a fundamental 100 GHz VCO, a push–push frequency doubler with a 50 GHz external source was used to drive the transceiver. The radar chip can transmit 4 dBm saturated power over 93–105 GHz with a 40 mV 1 kHz IF carrier and achieve good I/Q performance of phase mismatch < 1° and amplitude mismatch <1 dB over 95–104 GHz. With a 36 dBm microwave input from 99–104 GHz, the IF differential output amplitude varied from 470–680 mV.

A schematic diagram of the double-sideband low-IF CW radar system is given in Figure 7.85. It shows three major modules: the 100 GHz radar transceiver chip, two horn antennas with GSG probes for interconnection, and an off-chip digital signal processor [Ma et al., 2020]. To exploit the range correlation feature for oscillator phase noise cancellation, the same LO was shared in the TX and RX operations, and the IF signal from the TX is digitally sampled to demodulate the quadrature IF outputs from the RX. In this low-IF radar system, 1 kHz IF and 10 kHz sample frequencies were chosen. Both 1 kHz IF carrier IF(t) and quadrature IF outputs IFI(t) and IFQ(t) were sampled simultaneously for the synchronous demodulation operation. Calibration studies have shown that the detection accuracy of the CW radar could reach submicrometer level, based on the attributes of high operation frequency, and I/Q demodulation and SNR performances.

In general, the ADC's sampling frequency should be at least 10 times the IF frequency to fully sample the IF signal. With a 10–20 second time window (TW), the 1-Hz vital sign frequency can be recovered by implementing an FFT in the digital domain. A lower IF helps to reduce the amount of data required for processing. In contrast, to mitigate the flicker noise and to improve the system SNR, a higher IF is preferrable. Thus, there is a trade-off for IF selection between the amount of data processing and flicker noise immunity.

Vital sign detection experiments were conducted with the radar sensor at 2 m away from the chest of a human subject. A finger oximeter served as reference for heartbeat measurement. Results are shown in Figure 7.86. The subject was breathing normally for 25 seconds and then was asked to hold the breath for 20 seconds.

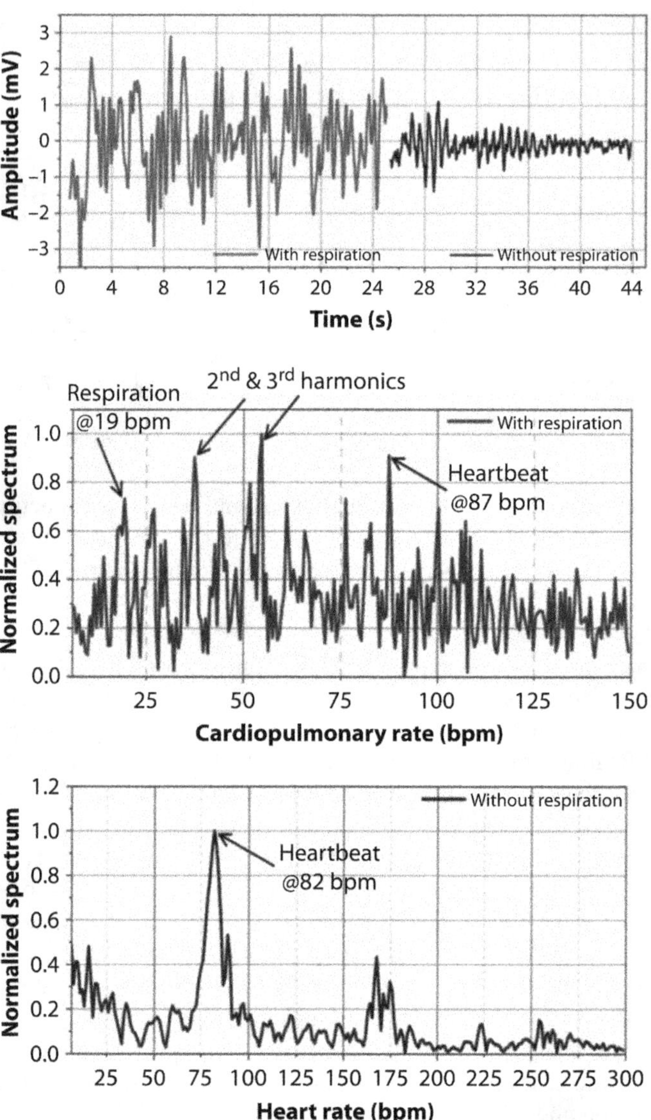


**FIGURE 7.86** Human vital-sign detection results from 2 m: (a) Two segments of time domain signals detected with and without respiration, (b) Normalized spectrum distribution showing breathing and heartbeat rates with respiration, and (c) spectrum distribution showing heart rate without respiration.

A digital Butterworth bandpass filter with cutoff frequencies of 0.1 and 5 Hz was used to remove DC offsets. Figure 7.86(a) shows two segments of time domain signals detected with and without respiration. Normalized spectrum distributions after FFT are given in Figures 7.86(b) and (c) showing breathing and heartbeat rates with and without respiration. A respiration rate at 19 breath/min, and second and third harmonics are visible in Figure 7.86(b). The heartbeat at 87 beats/min is consistent with the oximeter reading. A much cleaner heartbeat at 82 beats/min is obtained from the breath-holding waveform as shown in Figure 7.86(c), with possibly a second harmonic at 168 beats/min. The low-frequency components are associated with interference from random body motions.

It is interesting to note use of the 100 GHz chip radar in demonstrating detection of vital sign signal from small animals [Ma et al., 2020]. In this case, the signal SNR was reduced as were the target's size and related RCS. The 100 GHz radar was able to detect an adult bullfrog's hybrid respiration (buccal ventilation and lung burst) motion from 40-second records. It shows that the chip radar system is capable of detecting tiny vital signs from biological subjects.

#### 7.7.4.5 FMCW Radar with Antenna Lens at 120 GHz

The march toward using higher frequency bands for better receiver sensitivity has ushered in a problem with heart-rate detection, which, at 100 GHz, can be easily interfered with by the respiratory harmonics. Moreover, software and hardware approaches developed to alleviate the difficulties were explored on fully integrated CMOS chip systems with varying success at 60 GHz. To help resolve the issue of accuracy and robustness, especially for contactless human vital-sign monitoring, the use of a 120 GHz narrow beam mmW radar and an adaptive notch filter was proposed [Lv et al., 2021]. The use of the higher 120 GHz frequency potentially could afford better receiver sensitivity. The system was based on FMCW radar architecture connected to a pair of low sidelobe and small-size lens attached to the receiving and transmitting antennas. The narrow beam radar reduces the interference caused by backscattering from other objects in the measurement scene and improves the signal-to-clutter ratio of the intermediate frequency signal.

Furthermore, an adaptive notch filter was used to filter respiratory harmonics before applying FFT to extract the respiration and heart rates. The system revealed some serious limitations. The modest experimental results were obtained from measurement with restricted body and chest motions. It was difficult to obtain reliable results using the proposed system even with mode decomposition and fast independent component analysis algorithm. Thus, it is not apparent that further improvements in signal processing are the remedy.

It should be noted that software and hardware approaches to alleviate some of the difficulties have been explored on fully integrated CMOS chip systems with noticeable success at 60 GHz. The design and performance of higher frequency mmWe radar sensors remain as challenges with respect to robustness and accuracy of signal detection. The potential higher sensitivity also elicits more pronounced noise sources to interfere with vital-sign detection, including the presence of higher harmonics of vital-sign signals and other bodily motions. Techniques such as those applied for cancellation of interfering respiration harmonics and backscattered clutters (see Sections 7.7.4.1 and 7.7.4.3) could be useful for vital-sign radar sensors operating at frequencies in the mmW region. Furthermore, quadrature configurations would allow arctangent demodulation of the output signals, which could contribute to enhanced detectability, if they have not done so already. The higher mmW frequencies (including 100 and 120 GHz) may not be appropriate or optimal for human vital-sign sensing because the short wavelength may be too sensitive for the relatively large displacement. Displacement of the human chest wall is comparable to or greater than a wavelength $\lambda$. However, 100 GHz and mmW chip radars could facilitate remote detection of vital signs from small and tiny animal subjects.

## 7.8 SUMMARY AND PERSPECTIVE

Irrespective of the challenges encountered by the higher mmW vital-sign detection architectures, the emphasis on hardware research toward smaller integrated radar sensors with low power consumption and higher vital-sign detection sensitivity would likely continue. In this regard, it is noteworthy that the recent achievement of integrated 60 GHz CMOS vital-sign Doppler radar sensors may boost the technology to be incorporated into smartphones and other handheld devices — with the interest in and pace of 5G deployment and the impinging 6G wireless technology developments that may happen sooner than later. When that happens, it will enable the research on noninvasive microwave physiological measurement and sensing that began decades ago to bring useful wireless healthcare applications and remote physiological monitoring technology to the life and benefit of multitudes of ordinary people, if implemented judiciously.

## REFERENCES

Al-Naji, A., Gibson, K., Lee, S. H., Chahl, J., 2017. Monitoring of cardiorespiratory signal: Principles of remote measurements and review of methods. IEEE Access, 5:15776–15790

Baldi, M., Cerri, G., Chiaraluce, F., Eusebi, L., Russo, P., 2014. Non-invasive UWB sensing of astronauts' breathing activity. Sensors (Basel). 15(1):565–591

Beltrão, G., Stutz, R., Hornberger, F., Martins, W. A., Tatarinov, D., Alaee-Kerahroodi, M., Lindner, U., Stock, L., Kaiser, E., Goedicke-Fritz. S., Schroeder, U., Bhavani Shankar, M. R., Zemlin, M., 2022. Contactless radar-based breathing monitoring of premature infants in the neonatal intensive care unit. Sci. Rep., 25;12(1):5150. doi: 10.1038/s41598-022-08836-3. PMID: 35338172; PMCID: PMC8956695

Benchimol, A., Dimond, E. G., 1963. The normal and abnormal apexcardiogram. Am. J. Cardiol., 8:368–382

Bernardi, P., Cicchetti, R., Pisa, S., Pittella, E., Piuzzi, E., Testa, O., 2014. Design, realization, and test of a UWB radar sensor for breath activity monitoring. IEEE Sens. J., 14(2):584–596

Boryssenko, A. O., Sostanovsky, D. L., Boryssenko, E. S., 2007. Portable imaging UWB radar system with two-element receiving array, Ultra-Wideband Short-Pulse Electromagnetics (Vol. 8, pp. 153–160), Springer

Bozhenko, B. S., 1961. Seismocardiography–a new method in the study of functional conditions of the heart. Ter. Arkh., 33:55

Brower, R. W., Meester, G. T., 1979. Quantification of left ventricular function in patients with coronary artery disease. In: Hwang, N. H. C., Gross, D. R., Patel, D. J., Eds., Quantitative Cardiovascular Studies (pp. 639–688), Baltimore: University Park Press

Byrne, W., Flynn, R., Zapp, R., Siegel, M., 1986. Adaptive filter processing in microwave remote heart monitors, IEEE Trans. on Biomed. Engg., 33: 717–722

Chan, K. H., Lin, J. C., 1985. An algorithm for extracting cardiopulmonary rates from chest movements. Proc. IEEE Eng. Med. Biol. Conf., 466–469

Chan, K. H., Lin, J. C., 1987. Microprocessor based cardiopulmonary rate monitor. Med. Biol. Eng. Comput., 25:41–44

Chen, K. M., Huang, Y., Zhang, J., Norman, A., 2000. Microwave life detection systems for searching human subjects under earthquake rubble and behind barrier. IEEE Trans. Biomed. Eng., 47(1):105–114

Chen, K. M., Misra, D., Wang, H., Chuang, H. R., Postow, E., 1986. An x-band microwave life-detection system. IEEE Trans. Biomed. Eng., 33:697–701

Chou, C. C., Lai, W. C., Hsiao, Y. K., Chuang, H. R., 2018. 60-GHz CMOS Doppler radar sensor with integrated V-Band power detector for clutter monitoring and automatic clutter-cancellation in noncontact vital-signs sensing. IEEE Trans. Microw. Theory Tech., 66(3):1635–1643

Chuang, H. R., Chen, Y. F., Chen, K. M., 1991. Automatic clutter-canceler for microwave life-detection systems. IEEE Trans. Instrum. Meas., 40(4):747–750

Chuang, H. R., Kuo, H. C., Lin, F. L., Huang, T. H., Kuo, C. S., Ou, Y. W., 2012. 60-GHz Millimeter-wave life detection system (MLDS) for noncontact human vital-signal monitoring. IEEE Sens. J., 12(3):602–609

Cotran, R. S., Kumar, V., Robbins, S. L., 1994. Pathological Basis of Disease, 5th ed, Philadelphia: Saunders

Denef, B., De Geest, H., Kesteloot, H., 1973. Influence of changes in myocardial contractility on the height and slope of the calibrated apex cardiogram. Am. J. Cardiol., 32(5):662–669

Droitcour, A. D., Boric-Lubecke, O., Lubecke, V., Lin, J., Kovacs, G. T. A., 2002. 0.25 m CMOS and BiCMOS single-chip direct-conversion Doppler radars for remote sensing of vital signs. In Int. Solid-State Circuits Conf. Dig., vol. 1, San Francisco, CA, 348

Droitcour, A. D., Boric-Lubecke, O., Lubecke, V., Lin, J., Kovacs, G. T. A., 2003. Range correlation effect on ISM band I/Q CMOS radar for noncontact sensing of vital signs. In IEEE MTT-S Int. Microwave Symp. Dig., vol. 3, Philadelphia, PA, pp. 1945–1948

Droitcour, A. D., Boric-Lubecke, O., Lubecke, V. M., Lin, J., Kovacs, G. T. A., 2004. Range correlation and I/Q performance benefits in single chip silicon Doppler radars for noncontact cardiopulmonary monitoring. IEEE Trans. Microw. Theory Tech., 52(3):838–848

Droitcour, A. D., Seto, T. B., Park, B. K., Yamada, S., Vergara, A., Hourani, C. F., Shing, T., Yuen, A., Lubecke, V. M., Boric-Lubecke, O., 2009. Non-contact respiratory rate measurement validation for hospitalized patients. Annu. Int. Conf. IEEE Eng. Med. Biol. Soc., 4812–4815

Edmonds, Z. V., Mower, W. R., Lovato, L. M., Lomeli, R., 2002. The reliability of vital sign measurements. Ann. Emerg. Med., 39:233–237

Gu, C., Li, J., Lin, J., Long, J., Huang, F., Ran, L., 2010. Instrument based noncontact Doppler radar vital sign detection system using heterodyne digital quadrature demodulation architecture. IEEE Trans. Instrum. Meas., 59(6):1580–1588

Gu, C., Li, R., Zhang, H., Fung, A. Y. C., Torres, C., Jiang, S. B., Li, C., 2012. Accurate respiration measurement using DC-coupled continuous-wave radar sensor for motion-adaptive cancer radiotherapy. IEEE Trans. Biomed. Eng., 59(12):3117–3123

Hong, H., Zhang, L., Gu, C., Li, Y., Zhou, G., Zhu, X., 2018. Noncontact sleep stage estimation using a CW Doppler radar. IEEE J. Emerg. Sel. Topics Circuits Syst., 8(2):260–270

Hong, H., Zhang, L., Zhao, H., Chu, H., Gu, C., Brown, M., Zhu, X., Li, C., 2019. Microwave sensing and sleep: Noncontact sleep monitoring technology with microwave biomedical radar. IEEE Microw. Mag., 20:1829

Horng, T., 2013. Self-injection-locked radar: An advance in continuous-wave technology for emerging radar systems, Asia-Pacific Microw. Conf. Proc., 566–569

Hui, X., Kan, E. C., 2018. Monitoring vital signs over multiplexed radio by near-field coherent sensing. Nat. Electron., 1:74–78

Hui, X., Kan, E. C., 2019. No-touch measurements of vital signs in small conscious animals. Sci. Adv., 5(2):1–7

Jiang, S. B., 2007. Technical aspects of image-guided respiration gated radiation therapy. Med. Dosim., 31(2):141–151

Kao, T. Y. J., Yan, Y., Shen, T. M., Chen, A. Y. K., Lin, J., 2013. Design and analysis of a 60-GHz CMOS Doppler micro-radar system-in-package for vital-sign and vibration detection. IEEE Trans. Microw. Theory Tech., 61(4):1649–1659

Khanam, F.-T.-Z., Perera, A. G., Al-Naji, A., Gibson, K., Chahl, J., 2021. Non-contact automatic vital signs monitoring of infants in a neonatal intensive care unit based on neural networks. J. Imaging, 7:122

Kim, H., Jeong, J., 2020. Non-contact measurement of human respiration and heartbeat using W-band Doppler radar sensor. Sensors, 20(18):5209

Kuo, H. C., Lin, C. C., Yu, C. H., Lo, P. H., et al., 2016. A fully integrated 60-GHz CMOS direct-conversion Doppler radar RF sensor with clutter canceller for single-antenna noncontact human vital-signs detection, IEEE Trans. Microw. Theory Tech., 64(4):1018–1028

Lee, Y. S., Pathirana, P. N., Steinfort, C. L., Caelli, T., 2014. Monitoring and analysis of respiratory patterns using microwave Doppler radar. IEEE J. Trans. Eng. Health Med., 2:1800912

Li, C., Lubecke, V. M., Boric-Lubecke, O., Lin, J., 2013. A review on recent advances in Doppler radar sensors for noncontact healthcare monitoring. IEEE Trans. Microw. Theory Tech., 61(5):2046–2060

Li, C. J., Wang, F. K., Horng, T. S., Peng, K. C., 2009. A novel RF sensing circuit using injection locking and frequency demodulation for cognitive radio applications. IEEE Trans. Microw. Theory Tech., 5(12):3143–3152

Li, C., Xiao, Y., Lin, J., 2008. A 5 GHz double-sideband radar sensor chip in 0.18 $\mu$m CMOS for non-contact vital sign detection. IEEE Microw. Wireless Compon. Lett., 18(7):494–496

Li, C., Yu, X., Lee, C. M., Li, D., Ran, L., Lin, J., 2010. High-sensitivity software-configurable 5.8-GHz radar sensor receiver chip in 0.13-$\mu$m CMOS for noncontact vital sign detection. IEEE Trans. Microw. Theory Tech., 58(5):1410–1419

Li, C., Lubecke, V. M., Boric-Lubecke, O., Lin, J., 2021. Sensing of life activities at the human-microwave frontier. IEEE J. Microw., 1(1):66–78. doi: 10.1109/JMW.2020.3030722

Lim, W. S., Carty, S. M., Macfarlane, J. T., Anthony, R. E., Christian, J., Dakin, K. S., Dennis, P. M., 2002. Respiratory rate measurement in adults—how reliable is it? Respir. Med., 96:31–33

Lin, J. C., 1975. Noninvasive microwave measurement of respiration. Proc. IEEE, 63:1530

Lin, J. C., 1985. Frequency optimization for microwave imaging of biological tissue. Proc. of IEEE, 72:374–375

Lin, J. C., 1986. Microwave propagation in biological dielectrics with application to cardiopulmonary interrogation. In: Larsen, L. E., Jacobi, J. H., Eds., Medical Applications of Microwave Imaging (pp. 47–58), New York: IEEE Press

Lin, J. C., 1989. Microwave noninvasive sensing of physiological signatures. In: Lin, J. C., Ed., Electromagnetic Interaction with Biological Systems (pp. 3–25), New York: Plenum

Lin, J. C., 1992. Microwave sensing of physiological movement and volume change - a review. Bioelectromagnetics, 13:557–565

Lin, J. C., 1993. Diagnostic applications of electromagnetic fields. In: Stone, R., Ed., Review of Radio Science 1992 (pp. 771–778), Oxford: Oxford University Press

Lin, J. C., 1999. Biomedical applications of electromagnetic fields and waves: Radio frequencies and microwaves. In: Stone, R., Ed., Review of Radio Science 1996–1999 (pp. 959–970), Oxford: Oxford University Press

Lin, J. C., 2004. Studies on microwaves in medicine and biology: from snails to humans. Bioelectromagnetics, 25:146–159

Lin, J. C., 2006. Biomedical applications of electromagnetic engineering. In: Bansal, R., Ed., Engineering Electromagnetics: Applications (pp. 211–233) Boca Raton, Taylor & Francis
Lin, J. C., Bassen, H. J., Wu, C. L., 1977. Perturbation effects of animal restraining materials on microwave exposure. IEEE Trans. Biomed. Eng., 24:80–83
Lin, J. C., Dawe, E., Majcherek, J., 1977, A noninvasive microwave apnea detector, Proc. San Diego Biomed. Symp., Academic Press, 441–443
Lin, J. C., Guy, A. W., Kraft, G. H., 1973. Microwave selective brain heating. J. Microw. Power, 8:275–287
Lin, J. C., Kantor, G., Ghods, A., 1982. A class of new microwave therapeutic applicators. Radio Sci., 17:119S–123S
Lin, J. C., Kiernicki, J., Kiernicki, M., Wollschlaeger, P. B., 1979. Microwave apexcardiography. IEEE Trans. Microw. Theory Tech., 27:618–620
Lin, J. C., Salinger, J., 1975. Microwave measurement of respiration. IEEE International Microwave Symposium, Palo Alto, California, 285–287
Lin, J. C., Wu, C. L., 1976. Scattering of microwaves by dielectric materials used in laboratory animal restrainers. IEEE Trans. Microw. Theory Tech., 24:219–233
Liu, H., Allen, J., Zheng, D., Chen, F., et al., 2019. Recent development of respiratory rate measurement technologies. Physiol. Meas. 40(7):07TR01
Lovett, P. B., Buchwald, J. M., Stürmann, K., Bijur, P., 2005. The vexatious vital: Neither clinical measurements by nurses nor an electronic monitor provides accurate measurements of respiratory rate in triage. Ann. Emerg. Med., 45:68–76
Lv, W., He, W., Lin, X., Miao, J., 2021. Non-contact monitoring of human vital signs using FMCW millimeter wave radar in the 120 GHz band. Sensors, 21(8):2732
Ma, X., Li, L., Ming, S., You, X., Lin, J., 2018. Envelope detection for an ADC-relaxed double-sideband low-IF CW Doppler radar. IEEE Trans. Microw. Theory Tech., 66(12):5833–5841
Ma, X., Wang, Y., Lu, L., Zhang, X., et al., 2020. Design of a 100-GHz double-sideband low-IF CW doppler radar transceiver for micrometer mechanical vibration and vital sign detection, IEEE Trans. Microw. Theory Tech., 68(7):2876–2890
McBride, J., Knight, D., Piper, J., Smith, G. B., 2005. Long-term effect of introducing an early warning score on respiratory rate charting on general wards. Resuscitation, 65(1):41–44
Moskalenko, L. Y., 1960. Application of EM radio waves for non-contact recording of changes in volume of biological specimen. Biofizika (English transl.), 5:225–228
Mostafanezhad, I., Boric-Lubecke, O., 2014. Benefits of coherent low-if for vital signs monitoring using doppler radar. IEEE Trans. Microw. Theory Tech., 62(10):2481–2487
Muñoz-Ferreras, J. M., Peng, Z., Gómez-García, R., Li, C., 2017. Review on advanced short-range multimode continuous-wave radar architectures for healthcare applications. IEEE J. Electromagn., RF Microw. Med. Biol., 1(1):14–25
Papp, M. A., Hughes, C., Lin, J. C., Pouget, J., 1987. Doppler microwave, a clinical assessment of its efficacy as an arterial pulse sensing technique. Invest Radiol., 22:569–573
Park, B. K., Boric-Lubecke, O., Lubecke, V. M., 2007. Arctangent demodulation with DC offset compensation in quadrature Doppler radar receiver systems. IEEE Trans. Microw. Theory Tech., 55(5):1073–1079
Peng, Z., Muñoz-Ferreras, J. M., Tang, Y., Liu, C., Gómez-García, R., Ran, L., Li, C., 2017. A portable FMCW-interferometric hybrid radar with programmable low-IF architecture for short-range localization and vital sign tracking. IEEE Trans. Microw. Theory Tech., 65(4):1334–1344
Popovic, M. A., Chan, K. H., Lin, J. C., 1984. Microprocessor-based noncontact heart rate/respiration monitor. IEEE Eng. Medicine Biol. Conf., Los Angeles, 754–757
Rabbani, M. S., Ghafouri-Shiraz, H., 2017. Ultra-wide patch antenna array design at 60 GHz band for remote vital sign monitoring with Doppler radar principle. J. Infrared Milli Terahz Waves, 38:548–566

Rozzell, T., Lin, J. C., 1987. Biomedical application of electromagnetic energy. IEEE Eng. Med. Biol. Mag., 6:52–57

Seals, J., Crowgey, S. R., Sharpe, S. M., 1987. Electromagnetic vital signs monitor, Georgia Tech. Res. Inst., Atlanta, GA, Final Rep. Project A-3529-060

Seals, J., Sharpe, S. M., Schaefer, D. J., Studwell, M. L., 1983. A 35 GHz FM-CW system for long-range detection of respiration in battlefield casualties. Abstract of the Bioelectromagnetic Society Meeting, 35

Seals, J., Crowgey, S. R., Sharpe, S. M., 1987. Electromagnetic vital signs monitor, Georgia Tech. Res. Inst., Atlanta, GA, Final Rep. Project A-3529-060

Sharpe, S. M., MacDonald, A., Seals, J., Crowgey, S. R., 1986. An electromagnetic-based non-contact vital signs monitor, Georgia Tech. Res. Inst., Biomed. Div., Atlanta

Silverthorn, D. U., Human Physiology: An Integrated Approach, 7th ed., Upper Saddle River, NJ: Pearson

Skolnik, M. E., 1980. Introduction to Radar Systems, 2nd ed., New York: McGraw-Hill

Sørensen, K., Schmidt, S. E., Jensen, A. S., Søgaard, P., Struijket, J. J., 2018. Definition of fiducial points in the normal seismocardiogram. Sci. Rep., 8, 15455. doi: 10.1038/s41598-018-33675-6

Stuchly, S. S., Smith, A., Goldberg, M., Thansandote, A., Menard, A., 1980. A microwave device for arterial wall motion analysis. Proc. 33rd Annual Conf. Eng. Med. Biol., 22:47

Subbe, C., Davies, R., Williams, E., Rutherford, P., Gemmell, L., 2003. Effect of introducing the modified early warning score on clinical outcomes, cardio-pulmonary arrests and intensive care utilisation in acute medical admissions. Anaesthesia, 58:797–802

Tang, M. C., Kuo, C. Y., Wun, D. C., Wang, F. K., Horng, T. S., 2017. A self and mutually injection-locked radar system for monitoring vital signs in real time with random body movement cancellation. IEEE Trans. Microw. Theory Tech., 64(12):4812–4822

Tavel, M. E., Campbell, R. W., Feigenbaum, H., and Steinmetz, E. F., 1965. The apex cardiogram and its relationship to haemodynamic events within the left heart. Brit. Heart J., 27:829–839

Tseng, C. H., Yu, L. T., Huang, J. K., Chang, C. L., 2018. A wearable self injection-locked sensor with active integrated antenna and differentiator based envelope detector for vital-sign detection from chest wall and wrist. IEEE Trans. Microw. Theory Tech., 66(5):2511–2521

Uenoyama, M., Matsui, T., Yamada, K. S. S., Takase, B., Suzuki, S., Ishihara, M., Kawakami, M., 2006. Non-contact respiratory monitoring system using a ceiling-attached microwave antenna. Med. Bio. Eng. Comput., 44:835–840

Vander, A. J., Sherman, J. H., Luciano, D. S., 1990. Human Physiology, 5th ed, New York: McGraw-Hill

van Loon, K., et al., 2016. Wireless non-invasive continuous respiratory monitoring with FMCW radar: A clinical validation study, J. Clin. Monit. Comput., 30(6):797–805

Villarroel, M., Guazzi, A., Jorge, J., Davis, S., Watkinson, P., Green, G., Shenvi, A., McCormick, K., Tarassenko, L., 2014. Continuous non-contact vital sign monitoring in neonatal intensive care unit. Healthc. Technol. Lett., 1:87

Voigt, G. C., Friesinger, G. C., 1970. The use of apexcardiography in the assessment of left ventricular diastolic pressure. Circulation, 41:1015–1024

Walsh, J. A., Eric, J. T., Steinhubl, S. R., 2014. Novel wireless devices for cardiac monitoring. Circulation, 130:573–581

Wang, F. K., Li, C. J., Hsiao, C. H., Horng, T. S., 2010. A novel vital sign sensor based on a self-injection locked oscillator. IEEE Trans. Microw. Theory Tech., 58(12): 4112–4120

Wang, F. K., Horng, T. S., Peng, K. C., Jau, J. K., Li, J. Y., Chen, C. C., 2011. Single-antenna Doppler radars using self and mutual injection locking for vital sign detection with random body movement cancellation. IEEE Trans. Microw. Theory Tech., 59(12):3577–3587

Wang, F. K., Horng, T. S., Peng, K. C., Jau, J. K., Li, J. Y., Chen, C. C., 2013. Detection of concealed individuals based on their vital signs by using a see-through-wall imaging system with a self-injection-locked radar. IEEE Trans. Microw. Theory Tech., 61(1):696–704

Wang, F. K., Wu, C. T. M., Horng, T. S., Tseng, C. H., Yu, S. H., Chang, C. C., Juan, P. H., Yuan, Y., 2020a. Review of Self-Injection-Locked Radar Systems for Noncontact Detection of Vital Signs, IEEE Journal of Electromagnetics, RF and Microwaves in Medicine and Biology, 4(4):294–307

Wang, F. K., Juan, P. H., Chian, D. M., Wen, C. K., 2020b. Multiple range and vital sign detection based on single-conversion self-injection-locked hybrid mode radar with a novel frequency estimation algorithm. IEEE Trans. Microw. Theory Tech., 68(5):1908–1920

Wang, G., Munoz-Ferreras, J. M., Gu, C., Li, C., Gomez-Garcıa, R., 2014. Linear-frequency-modulated continuous-wave radar for vital-sign monitoring. Proc. IEEE MTT-S Radio Wireless Week, Newport Beach, CA, 37–39

Wang, F. K., Wu, C. T. M., Horng, T. S., Tseng, C. H., Yu, S. H., Chang, C. C., Juan, P. H., Yuan, Y., 2020a. Review of self-injection-locked radar systems for noncontact detection of vital signs. IEEE J. Electromagn., RF Microw. Med. Biol., 4(4):294–307

Wang, J., Karp, T., Muñoz-Ferreras, J. M., Gómez-García, R., Li, C., 2019. A spectrum-efficient fsk radar technology for range tracking of both moving and stationary human subjects. IEEE Transactions on Microwave Theory and Techniques, 67(12):5406–5416

Willems, J. L., De Geest, H., Kesteloot, H., 1971. On the value of apex cardiography for timing intracardiac events. Am. J. Cardiol., 28(1):59–67

Willems, J. L., Denef, B., Kesteloot, H., De Geest, H., 1979. Comparability and reproducibility of apex cardiogram recorded with six different transducer systems. Br Heart J., 41(6):716–727

Wu, P. H., Jau, J. K., Li, C. J., Horng, T. S., Hsu, P., 2013. Phase- and self injection-locked radar for detecting vital signs with efficient elimination of DC offset and null points. IEEE Trans. Microw. Theory Tech., 61(1):685–695

Xiao, Y., Lin, J., Boric-Lubecke, O., Lubecke, V. M., 2007. Frequency tuning technique for remote detection of heartbeat and respiration using low power double-sideband transmission in Ka-band. IEEE Trans. Microw. Theory Tech., 54(5):2023–2032

Zakrzewski, M., Vehkaoja, A., Joutsen, A. S., Palovuori, K. Y., Vanhala, J. J., 2015. Noncontact respiration monitoring during sleep with microwave Doppler radar. IEEE Sens. J., 15(10):5683–5693

Zhou, J., Sharma, P., Hui, X., Kan, E. C., 2020. A wireless wearable RF sensor for brumation study of chelonians. IEEE J. Electromagn. RF Microw. Med. Biol., 5(1):17–24

Zito, D., Pepe, D., Mincica, M., Zito, F., Tognetti, A., Lanatà, A., De Rossi, D., 2011. SoC CMOS UWB pulse radar sensor for contactless respiratory rate monitoring. IEEE Trans. Biomed. Circuits Syst., 5(6):503–510

# 8 Arterial Pulse Wave and Pressure Sensing

A variety of techniques have been developed over the years to study and measure the dynamic properties of the arterial pulse wave, arterial wall motion, and pulse pressure. Noninvasive measurement of pulse waves and the beat-to-beat blood pressure is useful for early detection of cardiovascular diseases [Avolio et al., 2010]. The important obtainable information includes regularity and rigor of the pulse, state and patency of the artery, and characteristics of the arterial pressure pulse wave. Several researchers have used microwave radar as a noninvasive method of measuring cutaneous and subcutaneous arterial wall movements. Furthermore, experimental validation of noninvasive pulse wave measurement using Doppler microwaves to detect pulse wave, arterial wall motion and pulse pressure have been reported [Lee et al., 1983; Lee and Lin, 1985; Lin and Lin, 2009; Papp et al., 1987]. The microwave technique can overcome some of the common wave propagation barriers in biological systems. Microwaves can propagate very effectively through bone and air as well as clothing and do not require a material, such as a coupling (gel) agent, to be applied to the skin. Therefore, a microwave radar front end may be applied by direct contact with the skin for noninvasive measurement of the subcutaneous arterial pulse. It may also be used in the near field, where noncontact modes of sensing pulse pressure waves, with a short separation between the radar sensor and the skin, includes sensing through clothing as a wearable device. The idea is to use microwaves to detect the movement of the arterial wall associated with the pressure pulse wave without interfering with the pulsing event or distorting features of the pulse wave contour.

Arterial blood pulse pressure — one of the four vital signs — is governed by several factors: (1) the force exerted on the blood as it is ejected by contraction of the left ventricle of the heart into the major arteries, (2) total blood volume, (3) the resistivity of lung tissues to the blood flowing out from the arterial compartment into the capillaries of tissues controlled by the small arteries, the terminal arterioles, and (4) the tension generated by the walls of large blood vessels in withstanding the pulse of blood ejected into the arteries by the heart. These four factors — cardiac output, blood volume, blood viscosity, and peripheral resistance — cooperate to affect blood pressure levels. When these factors increase, blood pressure also increases. Nevertheless, arterial blood pressure is maintained within normal ranges mostly by the fundamental hemodynamic quantities of cardiac output and peripheral resistance, which is related to lumen size. It is also essential to note the effects of neural and hormonal influences on contraction and dilation of arteries, which are related to movement of the arterial walls. It is important not to assume that adequate blood pressure is synonymous with adequate cardiac output.

As far back as recorded history, physicians have used palpation of the arterial pulse as a diagnostic tool during patient examinations [Ghasemzadeh and Zafari,


DOI: 10.1201/9781003315223-8

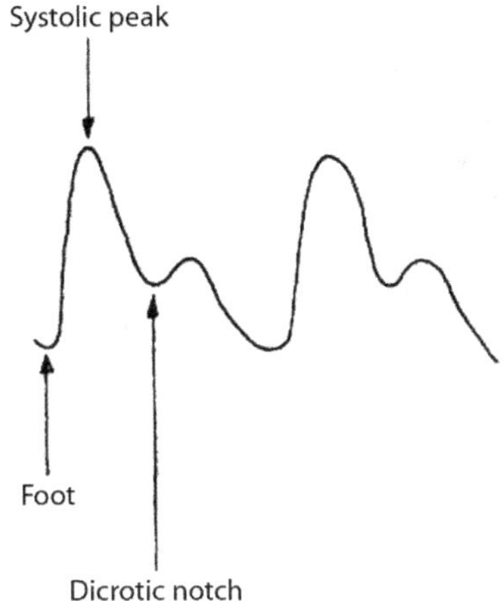


**FIGURE 8.1** Tracing of an arterial pulse wave illustrating the location of the foot, the systolic peak, and the dicrotic notch in the pulse waveform.

2011; Hajar, 2018]. The characteristic behavior of the pulse reflects the contraction and expansion of the artery and associated arterial-wall movement. Pulse diagnosis continues its important role in the practice of Chinese traditional medicine [Wang and Wu, 1973]. Great attention was and is paid to the character of the normal arterial pulse waveform (see Figure 8.1). Diagnosis of disease or assessment of the state of disease is based on the regularity, volume, and strength or weakness of the arterial pulse at the wrists. Contemporary physicians note the same; some palpate the pulse while others simply note the digital display of the pulse waveform on the screen, which often is considered more reliable than palpation. Techniques used to record and analyze the arterial pulse and its attributes have advanced, but the understanding of the various qualities of the arterial pulse continues to benefit from past experiences and observations on the specific changes that occur because of disease.

In recent years, extensive investigations have been made on the waveform and the propagation of the arterial pulse. Furthermore, studies have been carried out to examine the changes in the pulse wave contour because of such diseases as hypertension, arteriosclerosis, arterial stiffness, diabetes, and peripheral artery diseases [Alecu et al., 2008; Cruickshank et al., 2002; Eu, 2010; Gajdova et al. 2017; Garnier and Briet, 2016; Liao and Farmer, 2014; Stehouwer et al., 2008; Takemoto et al., 2021]. Indeed, pulse-wave analysis is recognized as a standard in cardiovascular risk evaluation for patients at risk, especially for diabetes [Gajdova et al., 2017]. Arterial stiffness assessment was found to be helpful in choosing more aggressive diagnostic and therapeutic strategies, particularly in younger patients, to reduce the incidence of cardiovascular disease in these patients. Moreover, it is noteworthy that pulse-wave amplitude has been observed to drop during sleep with clinical implications in the general population [Hirotsu et al., 2020]. The pulse-wave amplitude-drop feature during sleep seems to be an interesting biomarker that is independently associated with cardiometabolic outcomes in the general population.

Arterial stiffness has been described as an independent predictor for risk of mortality in patients with type 2 diabetes mellitus [Kim et al., 2020]. Also, an association between arterial stiffness, frailty, and fall-related injuries in older adults has been reported [Turusheva et al., 2020].

This chapter presents discussions of the research efforts to date on noninvasive microwave measurement and monitoring of arterial pulse waves. It summarizes earlier research and current advances and describes types of prototype devices and more sophisticated systems along with descriptions of various methodologies used for pulse wave analysis and experimental findings. It will be seen that arterial waves can be quickly acquired to assist noninvasive microwave examination of the pulse wave and pressure.

## 8.1 THE CIRCULATORY SYSTEM

A summary of the normal structure and function of the central and peripheral vascular circulation systems is presented in this section. Such information is important for a better understanding of the microwave sensing technique, process, and application.

The circulatory system or vascular system in the body is composed of large and small blood vessels: arteries, veins, and capillaries [Cotran et al., 1994; Grant, 1972; Silverthorn, 2016; Vander et al., 1990]. The arteries that transport blood from the heart to the capillaries are lined with endothelial cells and contain varying amounts of smooth muscle and elastic tissue in their walls. The veins that carry blood back to the heart have softer, thinner, less elastic walls, and are larger in diameter than the corresponding arteries. Arteries and veins are largest closer to the heart (Figure 8.2) and decrease in size and lumen away from the heart while they increase in number

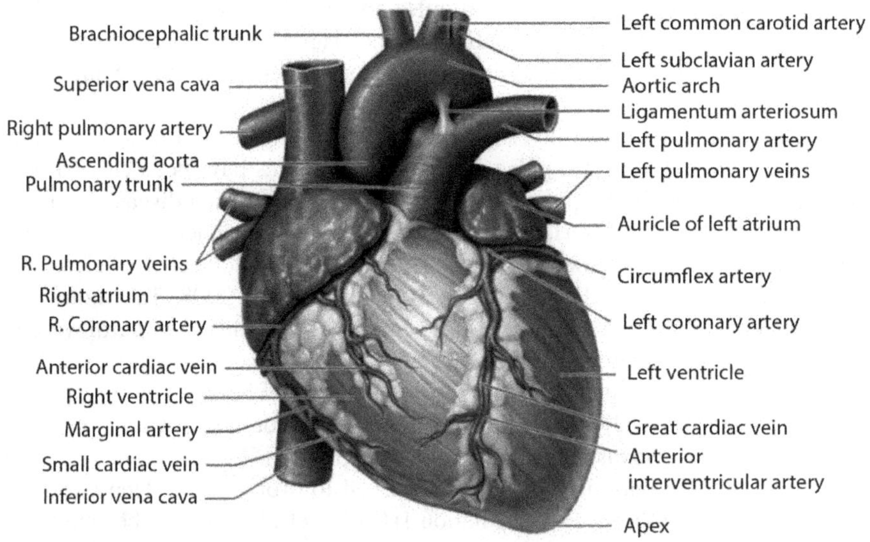


**FIGURE 8.2** Major blood vessels near the heart.

toward the capillaries. Some aspects of endocardial circulation and the blood vessels inside the heart are described in earlier chapters.

Normal functioning of cells, tissues, and organs is dependent on an intact blood supply. Blood transports nutrients and metabolic by-products to and from cells, tissues, and organs through large and small vessels. Local blood flow and blood pressure are regulated by changes in the lumen size and stiffness. Also, the widening or narrowing of blood vessels is subject to control by the autonomic nervous system and local tissue reactions. The resistance of vessels to blood flow is inversely proportional to the fourth power of its diameter. A decrease in diameter by a factor of two will increase the resistance by 16-fold. Thus, any change in the lumen size can have a significant impact on blood flow and pressure. Capillaries are the smallest blood vessels that have lumens approximately the size of a red blood cell (7–8 $\mu$m). They have different structures and functions at different sites. Changes in small vessels are typically subtle and are not easily or immediately detectable by externally applied microwaves in a typical situation.

Blood vessels including arteries and veins can be categorized according to their size, location, and functional features. The largest arteries comprise of the aorta and its major branches near the heart (Figure 8.2). The four main branches are the common carotid artery as the arteries of the head and neck, subclavian artery as the arteries of the upper extremity, descending aorta for the arteries of the trunk, and the abdominal aorta that continues as the femoral artery for the arteries of the lower extremity. The internal and external carotid arteries are branches of the common carotid artery in the head and neck region. The external carotid artery splits into two major arteries of the head: the superficial temporal artery and maxillary artery, among others (Figure 8.3). The two largest veins are

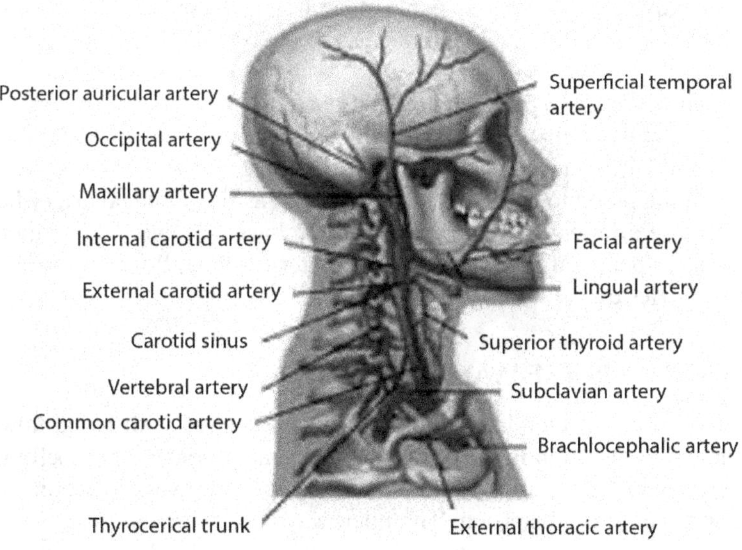


**FIGURE 8.3** Major arteries of the head and neck.

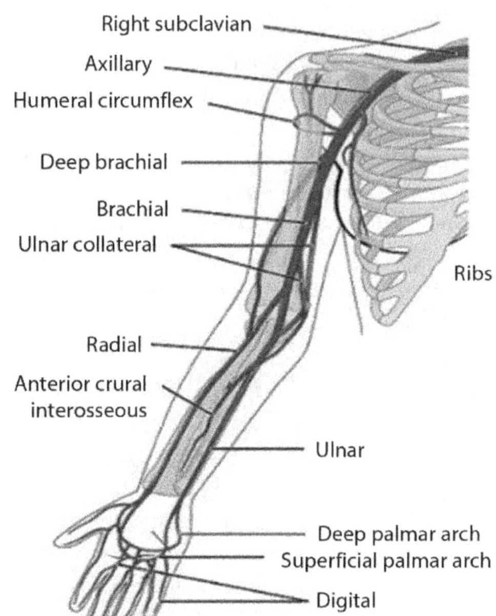


**FIGURE 8.4** Arteries in the arm and shoulder.

the superior vena cava and inferior vena cava that bring deoxygenated blood back to the heart.

Figure 8.4 depicts the arteries in the upper extremity or arm. The subclavian, axillary, and brachial arteries are the largest arteries bringing oxygenated blood to the shoulder and arm. The brachial artery runs down the upper arm and through the elbow before dividing into the radial and ulnar arteries below the elbow on their way to the wrist region. In the shoulder, branches of the brachial artery provide oxygenated blood to the muscles and bones.

As shown in Figure 8.5, the abdominal aorta branches into two common iliac arteries to travel down the legs before dividing into internal iliac and femoral arteries. The femoral artery is in the upper thigh, near the groin area. It is the major blood vessel supplying blood to each leg and it continues as the popliteal artery below the knee. The three arteries that supply blood to the lower leg and ankle region are all branches of the popliteal artery, namely, the anterior tibial, the posterior tibial, and the peroneal arteries.

## 8.2 ARTERIAL PULSE-WAVE MEASUREMENT

Microwave sensing of blood-vessel movements associated with blood-flow-related expansion and contraction in the circulatory systems provides a compelling noninvasive technique for measuring arterial pulse waves, blood-vessel motion, and pulse pressure with minimal distortion. The microwave hardware can vary from simple devices for pulse wave sensing to complex designs intended to minimize temporal drift, spatial clutter, and spurious noise for precision measurement. Because the

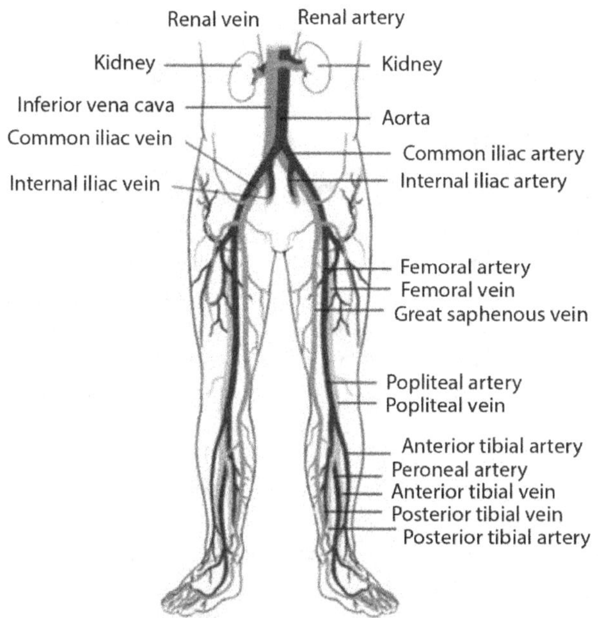


**FIGURE 8.5** Arterial and veinous circulation of the leg.

system employed in practice almost always operates with reflected energy, the transmission and reception functions usually share the same antenna.

Doppler microwave radars have been used to examine wall properties and pressure-pulse characteristics at a variety of arterial sites, including the head and neck, heart, and the upper and lower extremities (arms and legs) since the early 1980s [Lin, 1989, 1992]. The research showed that microwave Doppler radars have sufficient sensitivity to continuously measure pulse waves and blood pressure associated with small vascular movements. As mentioned earlier, the radiation pattern of an antenna determines the distribution of microwaves. This pattern is the same for transmitting and receiving operations. Antennas developed for biomedical applications usually have radiation patterns that give maximal intensity in the forward direction. The finite beamwidth permits microwaves to be directed to the biological target of interest and provides better spatial resolution. The output power is typically 5–10 mW in the frequency range of 2–60 GHz. The average power density of radiated microwaves from most systems ranges from 0.001–1.0 mW/cm$^2$. The low-power microwave transceivers not only transmit microwaves, but also receive the backscattered signal.

For application in pulse-wave measurements in which the extraction of fine features from the physiological signal is important, direct-contact methods that minimize scattered radiation are advantageous over remote, noncontact schemes. In contrast, backscattered radiation can be employed in many noninvasive remote sensing applications that use reflection measurement. The two methods and scenarios are described in the following sections.

### 8.2.1 Noninvasive Contact Pulse-Wave Measurement

The noninvasive microwave pulse wave sensing technique has been explored in several studies involving direct-contact application on the skin over the target artery using K-, X-, and S-band sources.

#### 8.2.1.1 Pulse Waves from K-Band Doppler Transceiver

A functional diagram of a contact Doppler radar arterial pulse-wave sensor and analyzer is shown in Figure 8.6. It consists of a K-band Doppler transceiver chosen as the microwave source operating at the frequency of 24.125 GHz. The wavelength in air is 1.25 cm. The depth of penetration in muscle-like tissue is 0.04 cm. The output power of the K-band transceiver is typically 5 mW. The radar sensor is intended to be placed directly in contact with the skin over the target pulse. The radiated microwaves are concentrated on an area of about 1 × 1 cm for a waveguide applicator (Figure 8.7). The direct contact mode of application reduces the clutter noise from reflections and can provide better spatial resolution of the biological target of interest. By positioning the radar sensor in light contact with the skin, it allows for examination of the pulse at close range without disturbing the arterial pulse itself.

Within the compact transceiver is a Gunn diode oscillator and Schottky mixer diode. The mixer diode combines the Doppler-shifted return signal with a portion of the microwave signal generated by the Gunn oscillator serving as reference signal (Figure 8.7). The output of the mixer is the Doppler shift frequency (see Chapter 5, Section 5.8), which is equal to the frequency difference between the reference signal and the signal reflected by the moving arterial wall. The output signal from the microwave

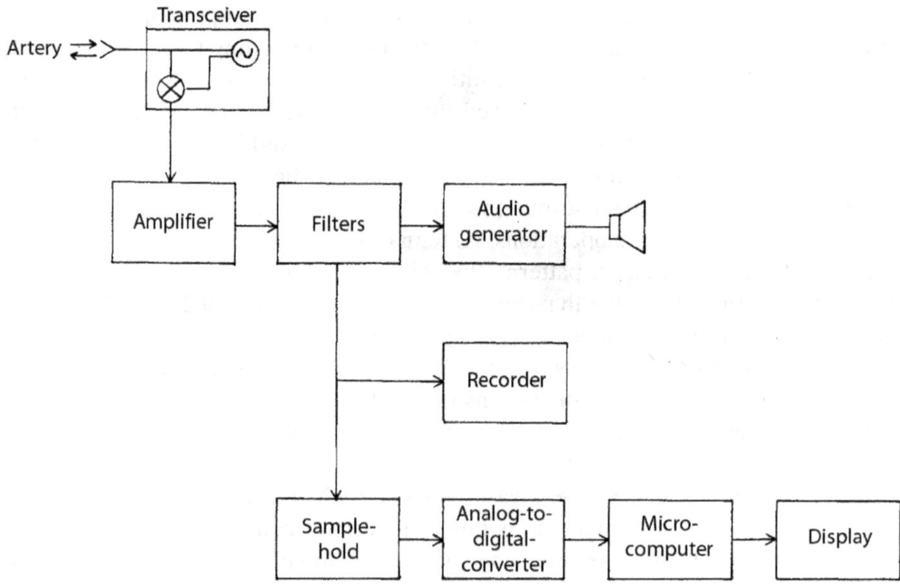


**FIGURE 8.6** Functional diagram of a contact Doppler K-band radar arterial pulse-wave sensor and analyzer.

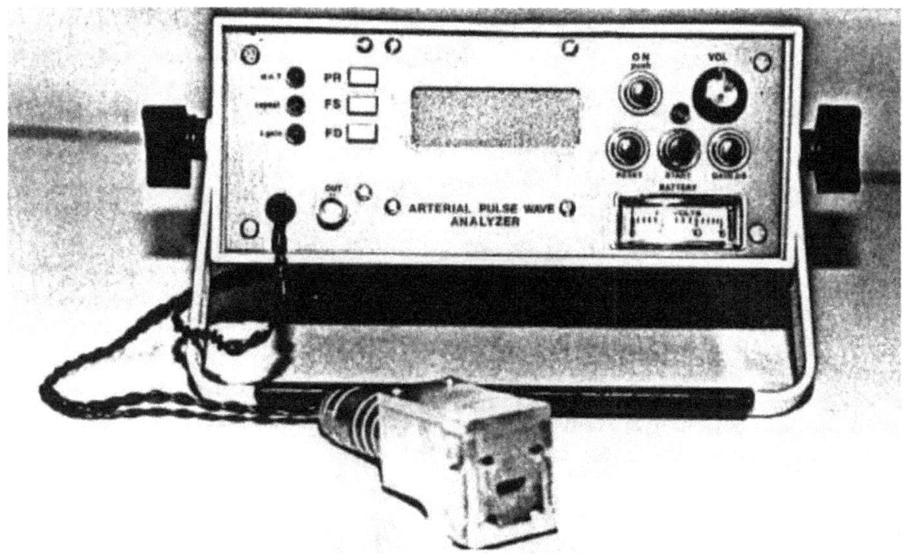


**FIGURE 8.7** A contact Doppler K-band radar arterial pulse-wave sensor and analyzer with $1 \times 1$ cm waveguide antenna applicator.

transceiver is amplified and filtered before being digitally coded for analysis by the microprocessor. The preprocessing stages include a fourth-order Butterworth bi-quad low-pass filter (100 Hz cutoff) and a 60 Hz notch filter. The high-pass filter (cutoff of 0.1 Hz) is used to remove the DC component of the transceiver output. The low-pass filter with a cutoff frequency of 100 Hz removes high-frequency noise but passes the high-frequency components, such as the dicrotic notch in arterial pulse waves. The output waveform from the notch filter is digitized and microprocessor analyzed using a feature extraction algorithm. One output from the notch filter generates an audio output to aid the operator in placing the transceiver waveguide applicator directly over the pulse site of interest. Another output channel from the notch filter is provided for analog recording or display. Note that the output $g(t)$ is proportional to the displacement of arterial wall movement, as shown in Chapter 5, Section (5.8), that is

$$g(t) = 4\pi G\left[\frac{x(t)}{\lambda}\right] \tag{8.1}$$

where $G$ is a constant gain factor, $x(t)$ is arterial-wall displacement, and $\lambda$ is microwave wavelength. Figure 8.8 gives the pulse waveforms detected by the sensor for carotid artery in the neck (see Figure 8.3) and brachial and radial arteries on the arm (see Figure 8.4). It is interesting to note that while there are characteristic differences, these arterial waveforms exhibit qualitative similarities in normal subjects. Figure 8.9 depicts the reproducibility of radial pulse recordings taken 4 months apart from the same subject. Note the similarity in the form of the pulse. These examples provide evidence of good reproducibility of the microwave pulse wave analyzer. The results presented indicate that the arterial pulse wave analyzer can accurately

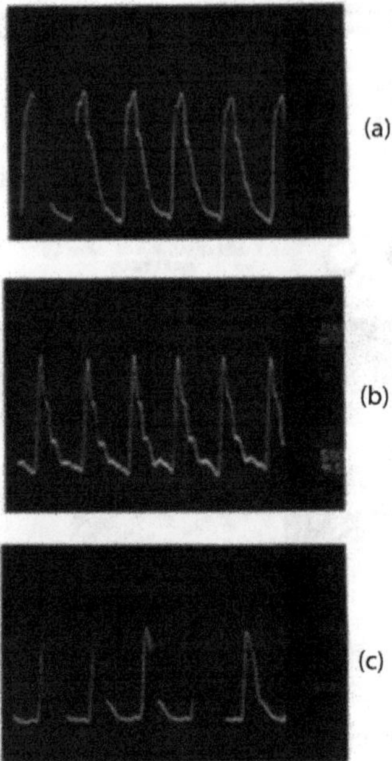


**FIGURE 8.8** Arterial pulse waveforms detected by the K-band Doppler pulse-wave sensor: (a) carotid pulse, (b) radial pulse, and (c) brachial pulse.

determine the movement of the arterial wall and can analyze and extract the pulse-wave contour for clinically important features.

The robustness and sensitivity of the 24 GHz Doppler sensor's transceiver and analog circuitry for arterial pulse measurement were investigated by extending the measurements and comparing them to records obtained from noncontact scenarios. In these measurements, the distances of separation between the pulse-wave sensor and moving skin surface over the artery were 0.6, 1.3, and 2.5 cm. The images in Figure 8.10 show the arterial pulse waveforms taken from the same subject for the

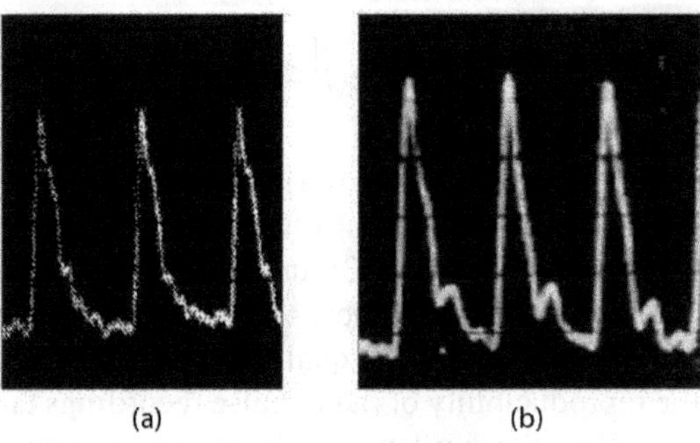


**FIGURE 8.9** Similarity of radial pulse waveform for the same subject: (a) Initial recording and (b) recording taken 4 months later.

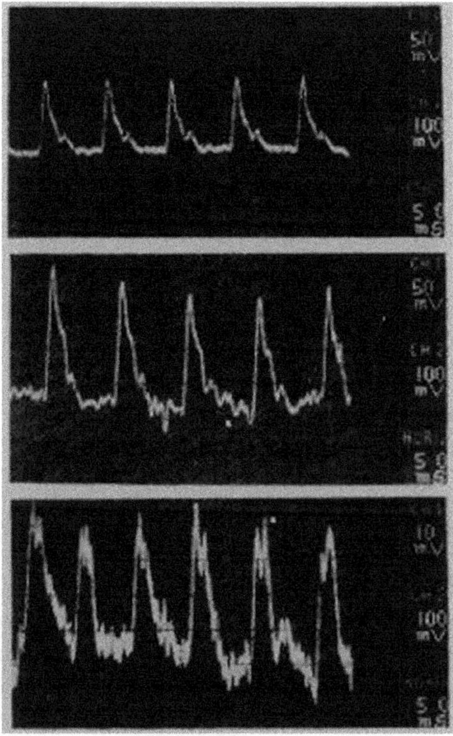

**FIGURE 8.10** Recordings of the radial pulse made at three test distances by the same microwave sensor: (top) 0.6 cm, (middle) 1.3 cm, and (bottom) 2.5 cm were used for the measurements.

three test distances. It can be seen from the photographs that the radial artery pulse wave can still be pulled out even when the Doppler sensor is 2.5 cm away. Clearly, the clutter noise increases with distance of separation when the sensor is operating in the near field under noncontact situations. One problem encountered is the difficulty in directing the microwaves on the target artery. A search maneuver is required to direct the microwave sensor to augment its ability to detect the arterial pulse from a short distance in the near field of the Doppler sensor. These findings suggest the importance of a direct-contact mode of application of a microwave pulse-wave sensor for diagnostic purposes. Nonetheless, the near-field-measured radial arterial pulse waveforms exhibit signal strengths that are well above the noise floor of the system and a morphology that is expected in an arterial pulse, thus suggesting that this radar sensor also can support operations in the near-field contactless measurement of the pulse at close range without disturbing the artery, avoiding potential distortions.

An important aspect of this investigation is the use of pattern-recognition and feature-extraction techniques. Through these signal processing approaches, key landmarks are located on the pulse contour. The pulse rate, foot-to-systolic peak time, and the foot-to-dicrotic notch time are calculated to analyze the pulse wave contour for clinically important features.

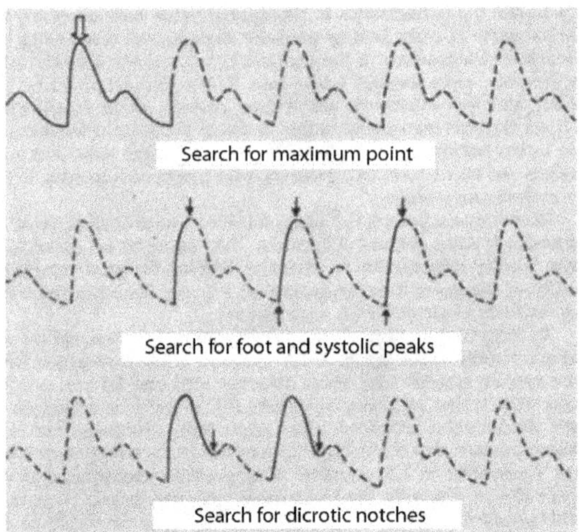


**FIGURE 8.11** Feature extraction algorithm for analysis of arterial pulse wave patterns.

Specifically, the feature extraction algorithm finds three peaks, two dicrotic notches, and two foots (Figure 8.11). From these data, the pulse rate, the foot-to-systolic peak time, and the foot-to-dicrotic notch time are calculated. The algorithm first locates three positive slopes. The beginning of each slope (i.e., potential foot) is designated as the point where the slope changes from a negative slope to a positive slope. Once the potential foot is located, the positive slope is tracked until a peak is found. The peak must be above a threshold to avoid recognizing an anacrotic notch as the systolic peak. If the peak found is greater than the threshold, then the foot and systolic peak are declared found and are stored for later use. If the systolic peak is less than the threshold, the search proceeds to seek another potential foot. If three systolic peaks are not located in the 6 seconds of data acquired, the analysis stops. In locating the systolic peak, the anacrotic shoulder is seen as a change in the ascending limb to a different upslope.

To find the dicrotic notch, two edge detectors (or operators) are used. The first operator performs a global search for the general area of the notch while the second operator performs a more localized search. For the global search, the algorithm begins by setting a search range to avoid erroneous fluctuations. The search range begins 21 samples (34 ms) after the systolic peak and ends either 70 samples (280 ms) after the systolic peak or one-half the distance between the systolic peak and the next foot, whichever comes first. To begin the global search, a pointer is placed at the beginning of the search range. Then, the 11 samples centered at the pointer are weighted using the following operator:

1, 0, 1, 0, 1,–6, 1, 0, 1, 0, 1.

A summation is made of the weighted samples and the sum is saved. The pointer is then advanced, and the weighting and summation is repeated until the end of the search range is reached. The sample point with the maximum sum is declared the potential dicrotic notch. The localized search for the dicrotic notch is performed over 10 sample points surrounding the potential dicrotic notch. The procedure used during the global search is repeated here, but the weighting only involves three sample points at a time. The three sample points are weighted with the following sequence of numbers:

1, −2, 1.

The summation performed in this instance produces the second difference. The sample point, which has the maximum second difference is the dicrotic notch. The performance of the arterial pulse-wave analysis algorithm was preliminarily tested on the radial pulse of eight healthy subjects. Comparison with visually identified pulse wave features (pulse rate, foot-to-systolic peak time, and foot-to-dicrotic notch time) on a screen display suggests that the algorithm can reliably and accurately detect the pulse waveform and to locate features in the waveform. However, efficacy of the feature extraction program needs further testing along with inclusion of subjects with abnormal pulse-wave characteristics to enhance its clinical utility for arterial pulse wave diagnosis.

#### 8.2.1.2 X-band Doppler Radar Sensors

Examples of 10.5 GHz microwave radar-sensed pulse waves from peripheral arteries in the human upper and lower extremities are shown in Figure 8.12. In each case, a 10.7 × 4.3 mm aperture antenna is placed directly in contact with the skin over the

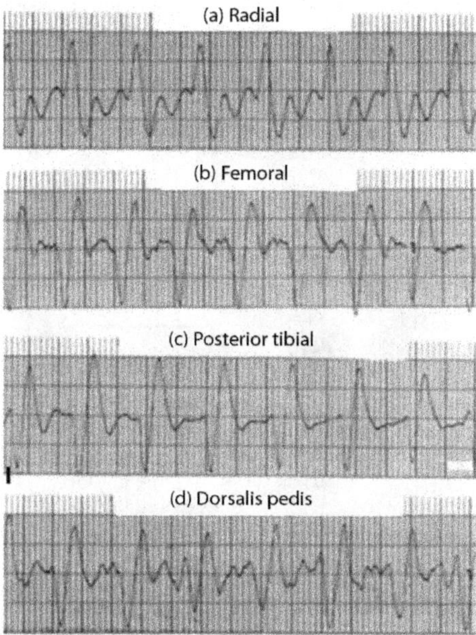


**FIGURE 8.12** Microwave-sensed pulse waves from peripheral arteries in the human upper and lower extremities: (a) Radial in the arm, and (b) femoral, (c) posterior tibial, and (d) dorsalis pedis arteries in the leg.

artery of interest [Stuchly et al., 1980; Thansandote et al., 1983]. This study used conventional X-band continuous wave (CW) Doppler microwave sensor architecture. Figure 8.12(a) shows the recorded radial artery on the arm and Figures 8.12(b)–(d) present the results from femoral, posterior tibial, and dorsalis pedis arteries in the leg of a human subject (see Figure 8.5 for anatomic sites of arteries). These results demonstrate microwave sensors can reliably detect and measure arterial pulse waves and wall motions in the arms and legs of humans. These measurements could provide valuable diagnostic information on the physical conditions of the peripheral arteries.

#### 8.2.1.3 Compact S-band Direct-Contact Sensors

An innovative compact pulse-wave sensor was developed by using a 2.45 GHz microwave oscillator integrated with a ribbon antenna. The S-band compact sensor consists of a bipolar transistor with a lightly coupled antenna serving as a load to the S-band microwave oscillator (Figure 8.13) [RCA Laboratories, 1987, Lin, 1989; 1993]. The front end (head) for the sensor is a modified transistor case, which measures 2.0 × 0.9 cm. In contact applications, the small time-varying artery wall will affect the oscillator's loading current due to changes in antenna coupling or impedance variation. The change in current is detected using an AC-coupled amplifier. In other words, the frequency of the free-running microwave oscillator is Doppler-shifted according to the displacement of the arterial wall. A frequency demodulator is then applied to the output of the oscillator to detect the motion. To minimize spurious signal and extraneous motion artifacts, the compact sensor is perfectly shielded with all microwave components residing within the sensing front end (head). This is accomplished by constructing the sensor as a two-piece assembly and housing the amplifier and power supply away from the sensing head in a separate package. This

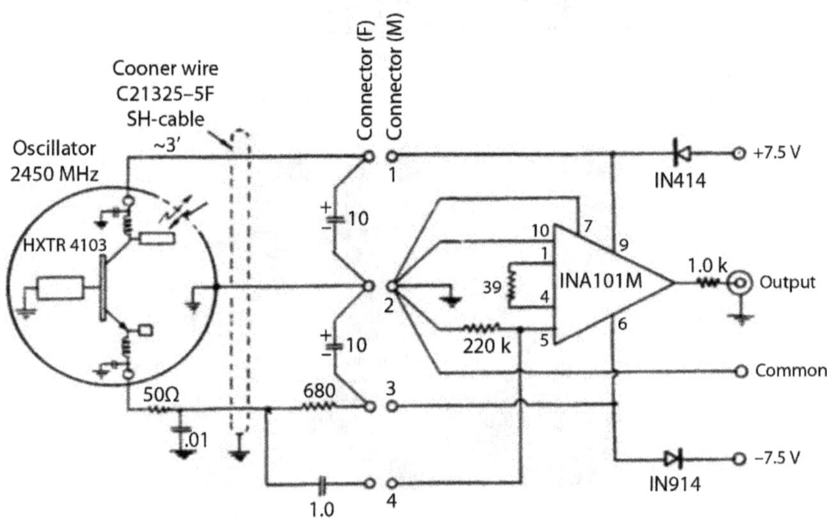


**FIGURE 8.13** Schematic diagram of a compact S-band microwave arterial pulse-wave sensor. The ribbon antenna is seen at the upper right corner within the transistor circle. (Lin, 1989.)

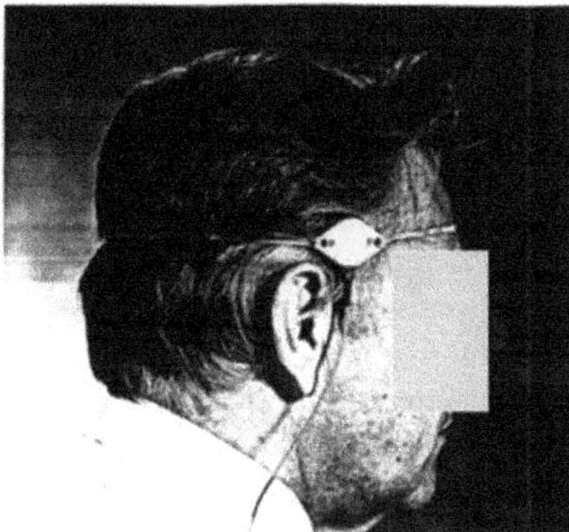

**FIGURE 8.14** A compact S-band microwave sensor held by an elastic headband for direct contact with the skin over the temporal region of the head.

design alleviates the frequently encountered microwave transmission and leakage through cabling and helps to minimize motion and other interference-generated artifacts. The device operates on a 9 V transistor battery to generate 0.5 mW of output power at 2.45 GHz for a power density of roughly 0.5 $W/m^2$ in air. The wearable sensing head ($2.0 \times 0.9$ cm) in a modified transistor case was held by an elastic headband to be in direct contact with skin over the temporal region of the head (Figure 8.14).

Figure 8.15 shows a compact S-band microwave sensor measure of a superficial temporal artery pulse wave. The clean, noise-free waveform, obtained by holding the head still, exhibits characteristics like the carotid pulse waves and that of other arteries in the upper extremities (see Figure 8.8) of normal subjects. This sensor is arguably the first wearable microwave arterial pulse monitor. The simple sensor design is unique in that it consumes low power, involves a miniature antenna, and uses a single microwave transistor as the microwave source. In essence, this compact S-band sensor is a predecessor to the self-injection locked (SIL) radars [Wang et al., 2010, 2011] described in earlier chapters under the topic of vital-sign sensing.

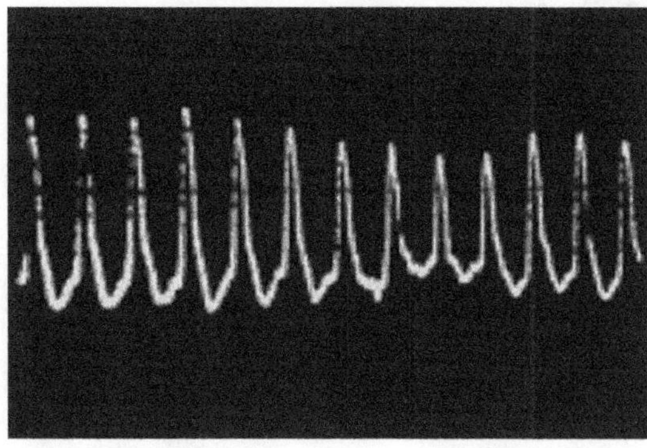

**FIGURE 8.15** A compact S-band microwave sensor measured superficial temporal artery pulse waves by direct contact with the scalp.

Indeed, recently, SIL radars have been proposed as a near-field contactless radial pulse monitor [Wang et al., 2016].

### 8.2.2 Near-Field Contactless Pulse-Wave Monitoring

As shown in Section 8.2.1.1 and Figure 8.10, the 25 GHz Doppler contact radar sensor can sense the pulse wave even when the Doppler sensor is 2.5 cm away from the radial artery. However, the clutter noise increased with distance of separation when the sensor is operating in the near field under noncontact scenarios. A challenging problem is the requirement of precisely aiming the microwave sensor on the target artery (line-of-sight operation) for quick and reliable pulse-wave measurements. Nonetheless, contactless extraction of the pulse wave from a returned microwave radar signal is feasible with simple signal processing, as demonstrated in Figure 8.10.

#### 8.2.2.1 Near-Field SIL Radar Pulse Sensors

In addition, some studies have reported using SIL radars for contactless sensing of the radial pulse from the wrist in a wearable mode [Kim et al., 2016; Tseng et al., 2018; Wang et al., 2016]. The application of SIL radar technologies for pulse-rate sensing in wearable devices uses an active antenna that consists of a SIL oscillator (SILO) and a patch antenna. The SIL sensing head is attached to an elastic band worn on the subject's wrist to monitor the radial pulse rate as a modulating Doppler signal. The SILO's output signal is received remotely for further processing. While the architectures are similar, the two prototype SIL radar systems described next differ. In one, the SILO output is demodulated by a remote frequency discriminator to provide pulse-rate information, and the other relies on amplitude demodulation of the SILO output with differentiator-based envelope detection.

A 5.2 GHz pulse-rate monitoring SIL radar system with two parts is shown in Figure 8.16 [Wang et al., 2016].The front end is an amplifier integrated antenna (AIA) on a wristband that consists of a patch antenna and a SILO. The SILO's output signal, $S_{out}(t)$, is transmitted by the patch antenna, and the reflected signal from the

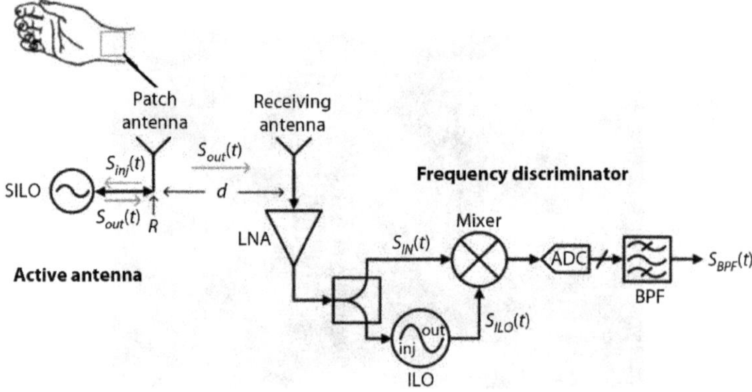


**FIGURE 8.16** Schematic diagram of the proposed self-injection locked radar architecture for a wrist pulse rate sensor.

wrist is received by the same antenna as $S_{inj}(t)$, which makes the SILO operate in an SIL state. Note the system does not include a buffer stage or any high-isolation components between the SILO and patch antenna to differentiate between $S_{out}(t)$ and $S_{inj}(t)$. The arterial motion-related Doppler effect appears as an FM signal. The second part is a wireless delay discriminator, which consists of the RX antenna, LNA, power splitter, mixer, and the ILO. The output signal from the SILO is received by the RX antenna, amplified, and divided into inputs for the mixer and ILO. The ILO serves as a variable delay element with frequency selectivity, and its output signal is used to feed the mixer. The output of the mixer is sampled by ADC and passed through the digital bandpass filter to define pulse rate.

Figure 8.17 gives a photograph of the noncontact radial pulse-rate monitor attached to the wrist with a wristband through light clothing. The 2.2 × 2.2 cm patch antenna is attached to the inner side of the wristband and the operating frequency is 5.2 GHz. The pulse-modulated Doppler microwave signal from the SIL antenna is transmitted remotely to a frequency discriminator at a distance up to 60 cm for demodulation. Figure 8.18(a) shows the bandpass-filtered results of time-varying pulse detected by the Doppler SIL radar. The noise level is considerably greater than that obtained using the conventional CW radar sensor shown in Figure 8.9 at longer distances (0.5–2.5 cm) from the wrist. While the SIL radar has difficulty in discerning the radial pulse in the time domain, Figure 8.18(b) indicates an accurate pulse rate of 93.6 beat/min, or 1.56 Hz, with a clear peak in the frequency spectrum. Clearly, considerable signal processing is required to isolate the pulse-wave signal using the SIL radar.

#### 8.2.2.2 Injection and Phase-Locked Loop Sensors

The technique of injection and a phase-locked loop (PLL) sensor for wrist pulse detection is a variant of the impedance variation and SIL structure mentioned in Sections 8.2.1.3 and 8.2.2.1. It consists of two main segments: a free-running oscillator and a PLL with a voltage-controlled oscillator (VCO, see Figure 8.19). The free-running oscillator is composed of a two-port interdigital-electrode microstrip line resonator, which acts as an antenna to transform the arterial motion into an impedance variation [Kim et al., 2016]. For the PLL portion, the frequency change is transformed to a variation in DC voltage (loop-control voltage) by injection of the modulated signal from the wrist pulse into a phase-locked oscillator. This sensor is placed close to the radial artery at the wrist. The output signal from the sensor is

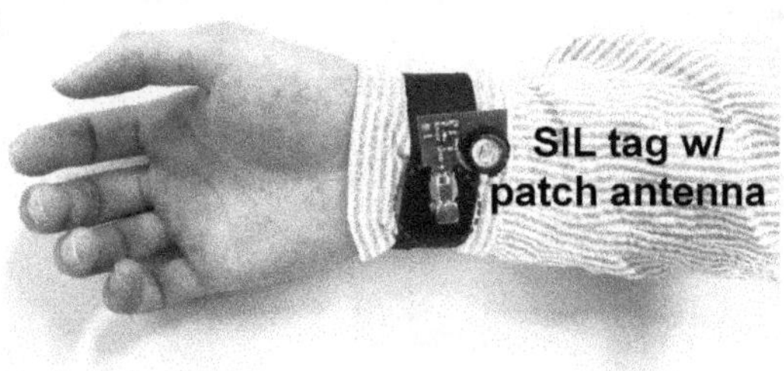


**FIGURE 8.17** Photograph of wrist pulse rate monitor attached through clothing with a wristband. (Courtesy of Fu-Kang Wang, National Sun Yat-Sen University.)

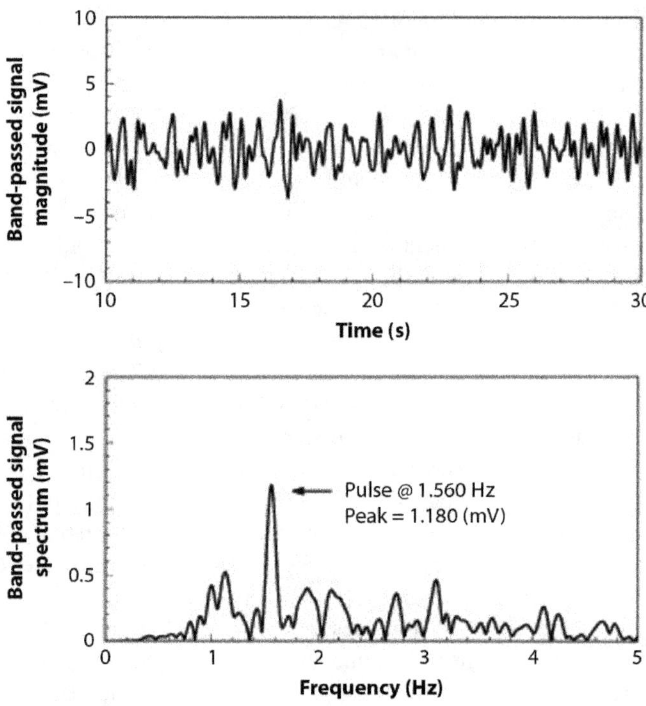


FIGURE 8.18 Radial pulse detected through a sleeved shirt from a subject: (a) Bandpass-filtered pulse signal and (b) frequency spectrum.

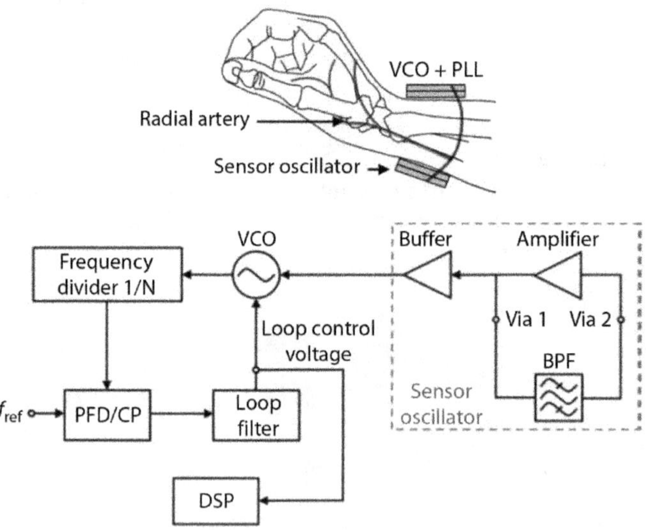


FIGURE 8.19 Schematic diagrams for a wrist pulse detection (a) and microwave sensor based on injection- and phase-locked loop (PLL) (b).

injected into the VCO through a microcoaxial cable. The PLL stabilizes the VCO frequency by applying a loop-control voltage, and the voltage variation from the loop filter is detected to yield the pulse-wave signal of interest.

For experimental tests, a 1 mm-thick layer of expanded polystyrene (Styrofoam) was inserted between the radar sensor and skin of the human subject wearing the sensor on the wrist. Figure 8.20 shows the time-domain data of the loop-control

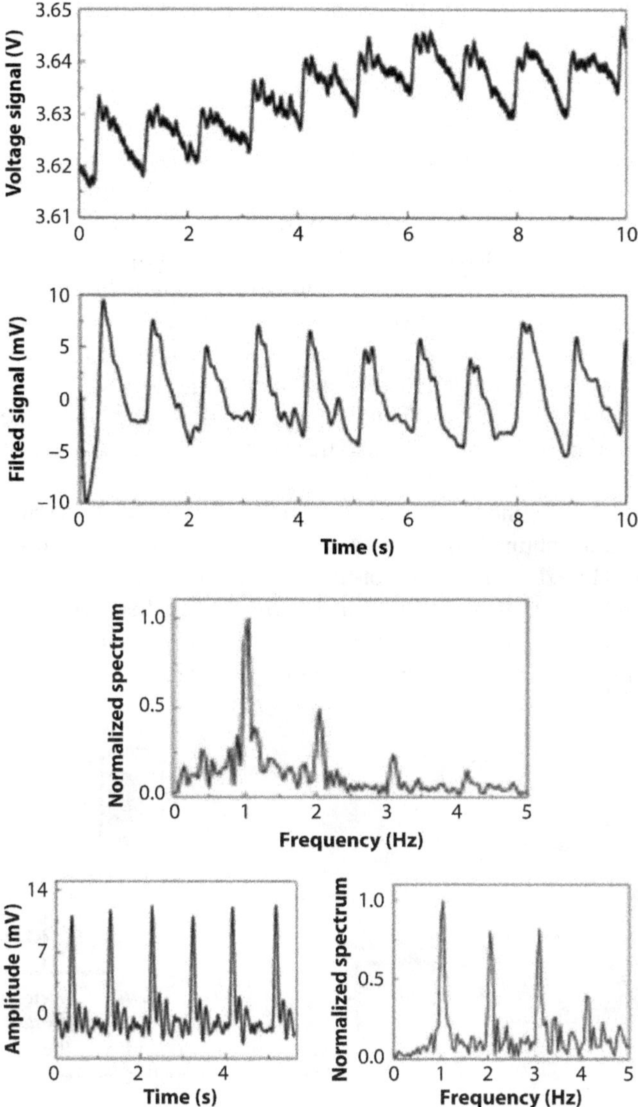


**FIGURE 8.20** Injection and phase-locked loop sensor-measured wrist pulse signal: (a) Time-domain bandpass-filtered signal from sensor, (b) frequency spectrum from radar sensor, and (c-bottom) bandpass-filtered data and frequency spectrum from piezoelectric transducer.

voltage of the sensor and bandpass (0.5–8 Hz) filtered data obtained after removal of DC-offset and 60 Hz noise. The output signal from a piezoelectric transducer is given for comparison. A pulse rate of 1 Hz is detected both by the radar sensor and piezoelectric transducer. In general, results obtained from the radar sensor show good agreement with the piezoelectric transducer data in the time and frequency domains. However, the results suggest that motion-related noise levels can be significant as a wearable device. The device operation is susceptible to distance between the sensor and skin. Also, the sensor oscillator's frequency may vary with temperature and moisture.

#### 8.2.2.3 SIL Pulse Sensor with Envelope Detection

Another variation of the SIL radar sensor incorporates a differentiator-based envelope detector for monitoring the radial artery at the wrist [Tseng et al., 2018]. The system block diagram of the wearable sensor is shown in Figure 8.21. The signal reflected from the target simultaneously introduces a variation in amplitude and a shift in the oscillation frequency. The output of AIA is a frequency-modulated carrier with an amplitude-varying envelope. Specifically, to acquire the pulse wave from the modulated signal an envelope detector is combined with a microwave differentiator to form a differentiator-based envelope detector to demodulate the pulse signal. The improvement in the demodulation scheme enabled the sensor to effectively detect radial pulse rates at 1.2–1.5 cm from the wrist. Information about the pulse wave can be converted into digital signals and transmitted via standard wireless interfaces such as Bluetooth or Wi-Fi.

Figure 8.22 depicts measured time-domain data along with the normalized frequency spectrum obtained via FFT. Note that the pulse waveforms clearly illustrate the 5.6 GHz SIL sensor's performance without additional digital-filtering for processing, in contrast to the results of Figure 8.17 in Section 8.2.2.1. The measured pulse rate of 87.5 beat/min agrees well with results from a finger pulse oximeter. Furthermore, the time-domain waveform is consistent with that obtained by

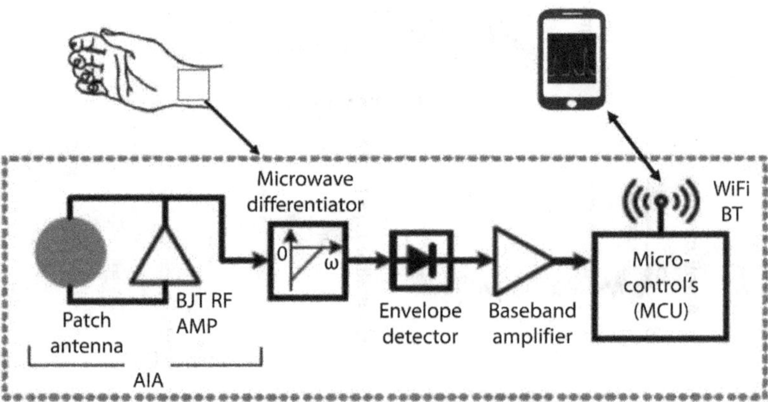


**FIGURE 8.21** Wearable self-injection locked radar pulse rate sensor with amplifier integrated antenna (AIA) and differentiator-based envelope detector.

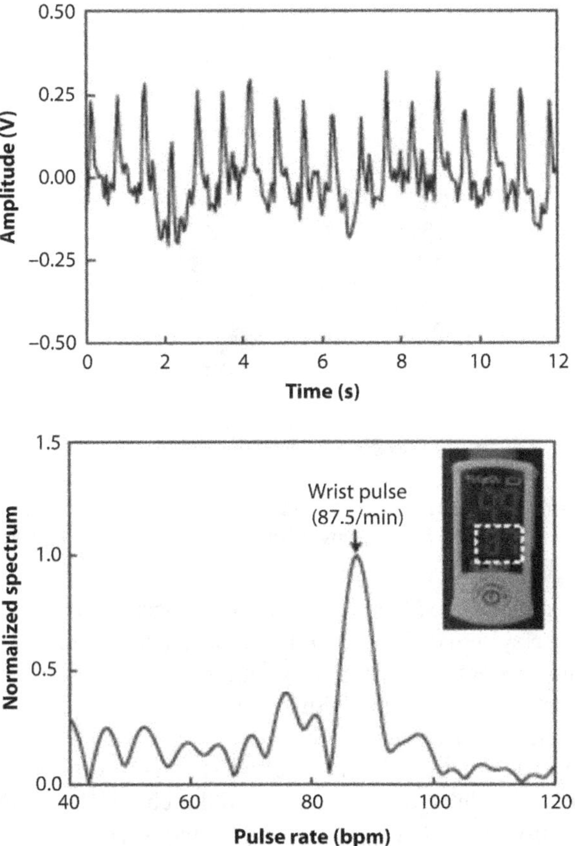


**FIGURE 8.22** Self-injection locked radar measured pulse-wave data: (top) Time-domain results of wrist pulse detection and (bottom) normalized spectrum.

the waveguide sensor described in Section 8.2.1.1 and shown in Figure 8.10. The sensitivity or SNR of the time-domain waveform is significantly increased for the differentiator-based wearable SIL AIA sensor with envelope detection. This sensor could become a fine contender for a near-field noncontact wrist pulse sensor for ambulatory or wearable application.

#### 8.2.2.4 Millimeter Wave Frequency-Modulated CW Radar Sensor

As described previously, a variety of noninvasive microwave radar techniques have been explored for monitoring arterial pulse waves to obtain a high-quality pulse signal noninvasively with minimal artifacts. The wavelength of 30–300 GHz electromagnetic waves in air ranges from 10 to 1 mm. It is, therefore, commonly referred to as mm-waves (mmW). At 60 GHz, the wavelengths are about 5 and 0.83 mm in air and muscle, respectively. Aside from reducing a device's physical size, a mmW radar sensor can potentially provide finer spatial resolution and greater sensitivity for accurate pulse wave measurement based on reflected signals from the small arterial

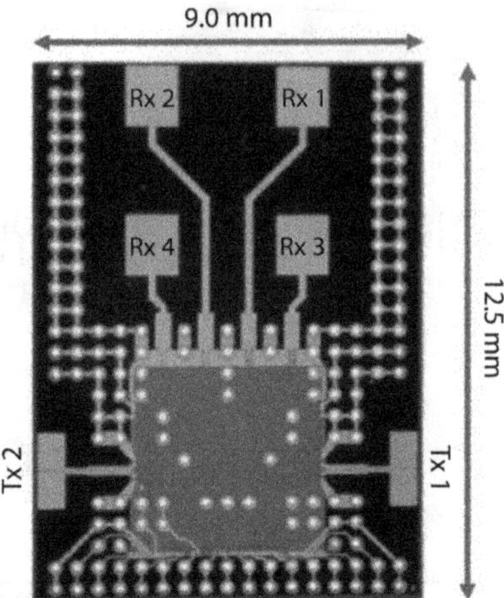


**FIGURE 8.23** Image of a frequency-modulated continuous wave mm-wave radar chip showing transmitter and receiver locations. (Courtesy of Jessi Johnson, Blumio, Inc.)

motions on the skin surface. (See Section 6.5.4 for discussions on contactless mmW vital-sign detection systems, chip implementations, and measurements.)

Recently, a noncontact, mmW radar system was developed to position the radar near the radial artery on the wrist without touching the skin, allowing for examination of the pulse at close range without disturbing the pulse itself. Figure 8.23 shows the integrated circuit's (ICs) architecture of a 57–63 GHz band, commercially available frequency-modulated CW (FMCW) radar chip [Johnson et al., 2019]. The device features fully integrated antennas with a maximum operating bandwidth of 6 GHz. As discussed in Section 6.2.3.4, the range resolution $\Delta R$ of Doppler radar systems is given by

$$\Delta R = \frac{v}{2B} \tag{8.2}$$

where $v$ is the speed of microwave propagation and $B$ is the system bandwidth. Therefore, at 6 GHz, the range resolution is 2.5 cm, which is a measure of the system's ability to spatially discriminate different targets in the same mmW beam.

For this study, TX1 was used as the transmitter and RX1 as the receiver, although multiple transmitter and receiver combinations are available from the radar chip. The small chip combined with the high sensitivity of mmW enabled the development of a wearable arterial-pulse sensing system. The PCB-mounted chip radar inside was held in place with a plastic cover. The enclosure was attached to a subject using a nylon strap and placed at 1 cm from the skin over the radial artery for near-field contactless measurement. A USB connection was employed for streaming the radar data.

Figure 8.24 gives the time domain radial artery waveforms and corresponding frequency domain plots for subjects with the strongest signal (Pat01) and the weakest signal (Pat02) in this study. The familiar dicrotic notch characteristic of a

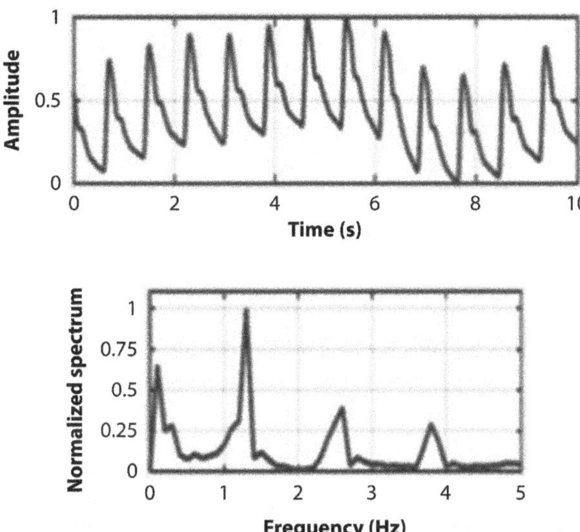


**FIGURE 8.24** Normalized time-domain waveform (top) and frequency spectrum (bottom) measured from the radial artery of a human subject.

radial arterial pressure pulse is clearly visible for both subjects. While the waveform shape and amplitude for the weaker signal exhibited greater influence of extraneous motion artifacts, it distinctly exhibits the pulse's spectral content. In general, these contactless recordings are consistent with those obtained using microwave radar sensing for radial arteries (see Section 8.2.1.1). Specifically, the distinct inflection points and dicrotic notch, features that are characteristic of a radial arterial pulse are comparable.

## 8.3 NONINVASIVE ARTERIAL-PRESSURE SENSING

An important parameter associated with the arterial-pulse wave that is of practical interest is blood pressure. In common sphygmomanometry, a pressure cuff is applied to the arm to measure blood pressure in the brachial artery with the aid of a stethoscope. However, sphygmomanometry is intermittent and is unable to extract beat-to-beat blood pressure or provide its variability as a function of time. From earlier discussions, it should be clear that arterial pulse detection using microwaves offers considerable promise for pulse-wave analysis. The extraction of essential arterial pulse features from both contact and contactless pulse-wave sensing may provide clinically important information to assist diagnosis of cardiovascular diseases. Furthermore, the significance of blood-pressure monitoring is well known, and blood-pressure monitoring has been essential for identifying hypertensive individuals and evaluating cardiovascular-related health risks such as impaired functioning of vital organs. Thus, knowledge of the quantitative relationship of pulse wave information to arterial blood pressure has immense clinical utility.

### 8.3.1 Arterial-Wall Movement and Pressure Pulse

The quantitative relationship of pulse waves measured from arterial-wall movement and arterial blood-pressure pulse may be shown through an examination of the blood-pressure-induced distension of cylindrical arterial walls. For a given pressure $P(z)$ in a cylindrical artery with radius $r(z)$ at point $z$,

$$P(z) = \mu A\left(\frac{v(z)}{r^2(z)}\right) \tag{8.3}$$

where $A$ is a constant, $\mu$ is the viscosity of blood, and the velocity of blood flow $v(z)$ can be expressed as [McDonald, 1974; Nichols and O'Rourke, 2005],

$$v(z) = B\left(\frac{\Delta r}{r(z)}\right) \tag{8.4}$$

where $B$ is a constant and $\Delta r$ is radial displacement. Combining Eq. (8.3) and Eq. (8.4) gives rise to an expression relating pressure to radial displacement such that

$$P(z) = \mu AB\left(\frac{\Delta r}{r^3(z)}\right) \tag{8.5}$$

Inverting (5) yields the radial displacement $\Delta r$ as directly proportional to blood pressure $P(z)$ such that

$$\Delta r \sim P(z) \tag{8.6}$$

Eq. (8.6) suggests that a microwave Doppler radar-measured arterial-pulse wave provides a direct measure of arterial-pulse pressure through measurement of the arterial-wall displacement. Thus, microwave Doppler radar can offer a viable method for beat-to-beat pulse-pressure monitoring. Indeed, the close correlation between noninvasive microwave-measured arterial-pulse wave and arterial blood-pressure pulse molds much of the discussion in several sections that follow. The application of propagation time of the pulse wave (i.e., pulse transit time, or PTT) for estimation of systolic and diastolic blood pressures will also be discussed.

### 8.3.2 Doppler Radar Measurement of Pulse Pressure

As seen in Section 8.2.1 and Figures 8.8 and 8.9, Doppler microwave radar has been employed to measure pulse-wave characteristics at a variety of arterial sites, including the carotid, temporal, brachial, radial, and femoral arteries. An example of a microwave-sensed carotid-pulse waveform in a patient by contact application of 25 GHz sensor to the carotid artery in the neck region is shown in Figure 8.25, along with simultaneously recorded intra-aortic pressure waves obtained from an invasive pressure transducer [Papp et al., 1987]. Note the resemblance of the characteristic features of microwave-measured carotid arterial pulse contour and the invasively recorded pressure pulse using the gold-standard catheter transducer for arterial blood pressure measurement. Indeed, a substantial portion of the two waveforms

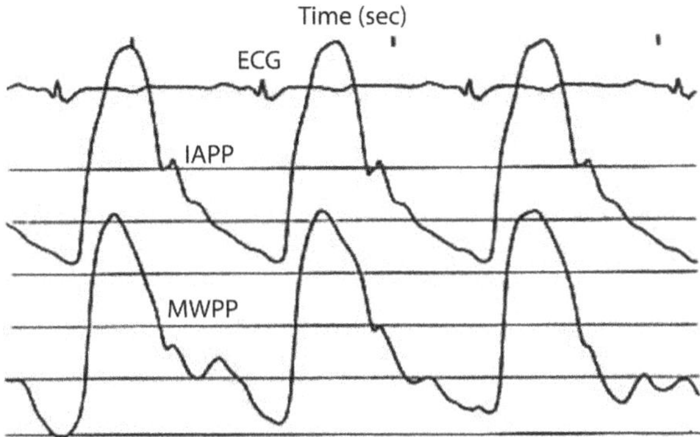


**FIGURE 8.25** Comparison of simultaneous intra-aortic pressure pulse (IAPP) and noninvasive microwave (MWPP) pulse pressure sensing.

have the same values, and the correlation coefficient is 0.98 [Lin, 1992]. The microwave tracings are faithful reproductions of the gold standard of invasive recordings of arterial pressure pulse contour.

It is noted that because of the CW Doppler method of arterial-wall motion detection, the microwave Doppler radar sensor can detect other localized displacements within its range of resolution. For example, the microwave tracings in Figure 8.25 have a characteristic positive ripple before each carotid upstroke, which results from a jugular venous artifact, which is not present in the corresponding intra-aortic catheter pressure pulse waves. The functional diagram of the microwave contact Doppler radar arterial pulse wave sensor is given in Figure 8.6. However, an independent calibration would be required for the Doppler radar sensor to provide an absoluate arterial pressure measurement.

The noninvasive Doppler microwave sensor designed for arterial pulse detection by assessment of arterial-wall motion was clinically evaluated [Papp et al., 1987]. Carotid pulse tracings obtained with the microwave sensor were compared with simultaneously obtained intra-aortic pressure pulse waves. The quality of the recording was also evaluated in 25 consecutive patients undergoing echocardiography. In 92% of the patients tested, good quality carotid pulse tracings could be obtained. Systolic time intervals and $T_{1/2}$ values (time required for a pressure pulse to reach one half of its maximum amplitude in milliseconds) calculated from these recordings correlated well with the known disease states of these patients, which ranged from aortic stenosis and aortic insufficiency to congestive heart failure (Table 8.1). A graphic illustration for the calculation of Pre-Ejection Period (PEP = QS2 – LVET) is given in Figure 8.26.

Table 8.2 lists the means and standard deviations of two derived quantities: $T_{1/2}$ and left ventricular ejection time (LVET). The $T_{1/2}$ values are significantly different for two subjects and the LVET value for one subject is significantly different ($P < .01$). In general, the results confirm that a noninvasive Doppler microwave sensor can successfully and reproducibly measure pressure pulse waveforms of diagnostic quality. With minimal training, a technician using the microwave sensor can usually obtain a good quality pulse waveform within 30–45 seconds. The pulse waves obtained

**TABLE 8.1**
**Diagnostic Indications from Patients with Various Disease States According to Pulse-Wave Features**

| Patient | Age | Diagnosis | LVEF | PEP/LVET=STI | $T_{1/2}$ |
|---|---|---|---|---|---|
| PGF | 53 | Aortic stenosis | 50% | 1.05/3.03 = 0.344 | 70 ms |
| PEC | 65 | Aortic insufficiency | 33% | 1.00/3.30 = 0.303 | 40 ms |
| PRA | 72 | Premature ventricular contraction | 60% | 0.85/2.65 = 0.320 | 50 ms |
| PJB | 53 | Congestive heart failure | 14% | 0.60/1.00 = 0.60 | 20 ms |

*Abbreviations:* LVEF = left ventricular ejection fraction, LVET = left ventricular ejection time, PEP = Pre-Ejection Period = QS2 – LVET, STI = systolic time interval, QS2 = Q wave to second heart sound time, $T_{1/2}$ = time for pulse to reach ½ of maximum amplitude in milliseconds (ms).

by the microwave sensor cannot be interpreted on an absolute scale since they are derived from the relative expansion of the target artery. Noninvasive Doppler microwave radar sensors can provide reliable reproductions of invasive recordings of arterial blood pressures when compared on the basis of LVET and pulse contour as well as pulse pressure waveforms. Used alone, microwave Doppler sensor can provide beat-to-beat pressure variations and relative numeric values for systolic and diastolic blood pressures. However, the microwave sensor could be used in conjunction with a blood pressure cuff, which could provide the necessary calibration for the pressure waves. Recently, measurement of the radial pulse wave noninvasively using piezoelectric tonometry combined with the central aortic pressure waveforms (see Figure 8.5 for anatomic site of the central aorta) has been shown to be applicable in estimating central aortic pressure [Qasem and Avolio, 2008]. The result suggests that microwave radar sensors of arterial pulse waves, especially the pulse waveform presented above and in Figure 8.25, are amenable to noninvasively estimate the central aortic pressure via arterial pulse-wave analysis.

In summary, noninvasive microwave arterial pulse detection has potential applications in pulse-wave analysis, continuous blood-pressure tracking, and arterial

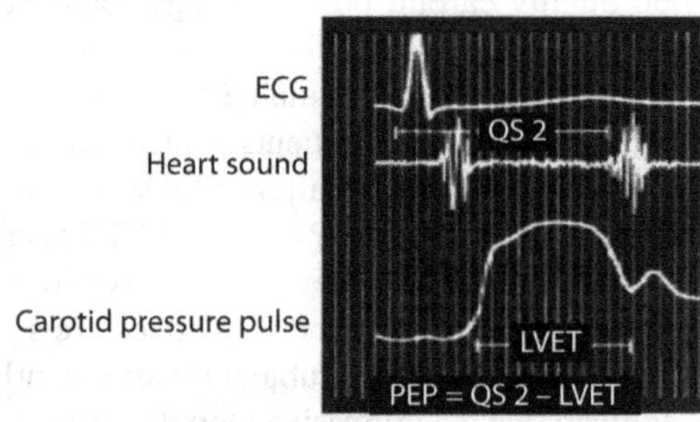


**FIGURE 8.26** Analysis of pulse wave diagnostic features: QS2 (Q wave to second heart sound time), LVET (Left Ventricular Ejection Time), PEP (Pre-Ejection Period) = QS2 – LVET.

**TABLE 8.2**
**Comparison of Intra-Aortic Catheter Pressure and Noninvasive Microwave Pulse-Wave Measurements for 5 Human Subjects**

| | | $^{a}T_{1/2}$ | | $^{b}$LVET | |
|---|---|---|---|---|---|
| **Patient** | **Measurement** | **Mean** | **S.D.** | **Mean** | **S.D.** |
| PEW | Intra-aortic | 48.4 | 2.87 | 336.0* | 5.96 |
| | Microwave | 45.8 | 5.38 | 359.6 | 9.20 |
| PMO | Intra-aortic | 49.6* | 0.80 | 265.0 | 5.47 |
| | Microwave | 42.0 | 1.89 | 261.0 | 2.74 |
| PMB | Intra-aortic | 46.8 | 2.92 | 286.0 | 5.83 |
| | Microwave | 39.6 | 1.49 | 275.6 | 3.38 |
| PAD | Intra-aortic | 38.2 | 3.06 | 322.0 | 6.78 |
| | Microwave | 36.0 | 2.00 | 330.0 | 7.07 |
| PJV | Intra-aortic | 49.4* | 3.38 | 406.0 | 6.63 |
| | Microwave | 41.2 | 1.47 | 402.0 | 5.10 |

[a] $T_{1/2}$ = Time required for a pressure pulse to reach one half of its maximum amplitude in milliseconds.
[b] LVET = Left ventricular ejection time in milliseconds.
* Significant at .01.

pressure measurement. Microwave sensors may be applied to patients and human subjects by direct contact, noncontact, near field, or remote methods with minimal intrusiveness, discomfort, or disturbance, including through clothing scenarios.

### 8.3.3 Blood Pressure from PTT

An estimation technique proposed recently uses PTT to indirectly derive arterial blood pressure [Buxi et al., 2017; Kuwahara et al., 2019; Rachim and Chung,, 2019; Zhao et al., 2018]. PTT is defined as the transit delay or the time for a pulse wave to travel from a proximal to a distal arterial site on the body [Mukkamala et al., 2015; Pitson and Stradling, 1998; Qasem and Avolio, 2008]. The method bases the estimation on calibrated systolic pressure (SBP) of each subject and derives the diastolic pressure (DSP) from a triangulated fitting-curve ratio of the arterial pulse wave such as those mentioned in the previous section.

An embodiment of the PTT method was demonstrated using contactless beat-to-beat blood-pressure measurement with a low-IF Doppler radar [Zhao et al., 2018]. The displacement on body surface induced by the central aortic artery near the sternum on the chest is acquired by a Doppler microwave radar sensor. The carotid PTT is extracted from the central aortic pulse. The procedure, as illustrated in Figure 8.27, enables measurement and estimation of both beat-to-beat SBP and DSP. Specifically,

$$PTT = \frac{ED - T1}{2} \tag{8.7}$$

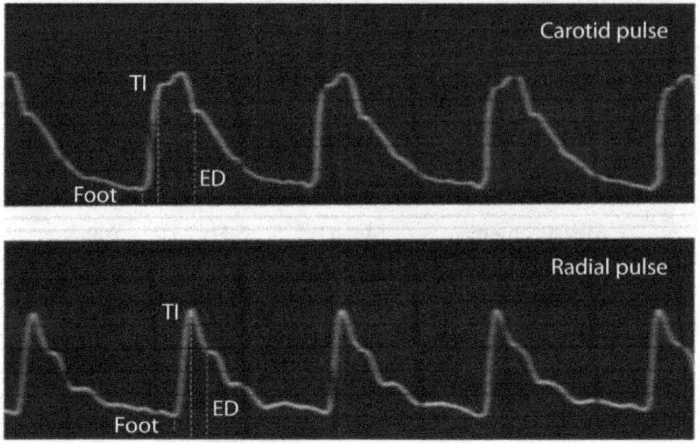


**FIGURE 8.27** Method of pulse transit time extraction from aortic and radial pulse waves measured by a microwave sensor.

where ejection duration (ED) and time to first systolic peak (T1) are measured from the systolic foot. The SBP and DSP are derived from PTT [Buxi et al., 2017; Zhao et al., 2018], such that

$$SBP = (a)PTT + b \tag{8.8}$$

and

$$DBP = \frac{SBP_0}{3} + \frac{2DBP_0}{3} + A\ ln\frac{PTT_0}{PTT} - \left(\frac{SBP_0\ -\ DBP_0}{3}\right)\left(\frac{PTT_0^{\ 2}}{PTT^2}\right) \tag{8.9}$$

where $a$ is the pressure rate and $b$ is a pressure parameter. A is a subject-dependent constant. $SBP_0$, $DBP_0$, and $PTT_0$ are quantities to be determined from the calibration procedure. Since these parameters are subject dependent, a calibration procedure is required to be performed before initiating the blood-pressure measurement.

A prototype system was tested with healthy human subjects lying in a supine position and the radar sensor mounted on a cantilever with its antenna directed toward the subjects' abdomens [Zhao et al., 2018]. For aortic pulse-wave acquisition, breathing was held for 5 seconds during measurement. Table 8.3 presents the calibration parameters of SBP-PTT and DBP-PTT for the subjects. The subjects' blood pressure was measured with a sphygmomanometer for comparison. As expected, values of the calibration parameters are subject-dependent and diverse. The final PTT value is the average of the PTTs extracted from the 5-second aortic pulse waves. The SBP and DBP values are derived using Eqs. (8.8) and (8.9) with the calibration parameters. Table 8.4 presents the result of SBP and DBP values using the Doppler radar sensor measurements, along with the sphygmomanometer reference. Three sets of data were collected on three different days, ending up with slightly different estimated blood pressure values or changes. Note that for SBP/DBP measurements, the errors are within 3 mm Hg.

**TABLE 8.3**
**Calibration Parameters of SBP-PTT and DBP-PTT for Human Subjects (S1, S2, and S3)**

| Parameters | S1 | S2 | S3 |
|---|---|---|---|
| $a$ (mm Hg/s) | –559.71 | –700.02 | –587.56 |
| $b$ (mm Hg) | 191.17 | 195.07 | 189.44 |
| $A$ | 70.85 | 203.02 | 49.32 |
| $DBP_0$ (mm Hg) | 65 | 66 | 75 |
| $SBP_0$ (mm Hg) | 102 | 104 | 118 |
| $PTT_0$ (s) | 0.1575 | 0.1309 | 0.1225 |

### 8.3.4 SIL Microwave Radar Arterial Pressure Sensor

The notion of PTT served as the basis for another scheme for measuring arterial blood pressure using a near-field microwave SIL radar (NFSILO) applied to arteries in the wrist [Tseng et al., 2020]. The wrist pulse sensor acquires an arterial pulse wave using a handheld SIL radar consisting of a split-ring resonator and amplitude demodulator (Figure 8.28). The arterial blood pressure is estimated through formulas based on derived relationships between the blood pressure and PTT. As previously mentioned, PTT is typically defined as the transit delay time for a pulse wave to travel from a proximal (aorta) to a distal arterial site. In the case of a brachial or radial artery, PTT is defined as the time interval between the peak of the arterial pulse wave and a characteristic point of the pulse wave, as shown in Figure 8.29, where S1 corresponds to the first systolic peak and S2 denotes the second systolic peak of the pulse pressure wave. R-PTT is the time interval between S1 and S2 and is used to estimate the SBP and DBP.

According to Bramwell and Hill, [1922a, b] and Tseng et al., [2020], the SBP from the artery can be represented as

$$SBP = \mathrm{DBP} + \frac{a}{R - PTT^2} \tag{8.10}$$

**TABLE 8.4**
**Result of SBP/DBP Measurements Using Microwave Doppler Radar for 3 Human Subjects**

| | Test 1 | | | Test 2 | | | Test 3 | | |
|---|---|---|---|---|---|---|---|---|---|
| **Subjects** | **Radar** | **Reference** | **Error** | **Radar** | **Reference** | **Error** | **Radar** | **Reference** | **Error** |
| S1 | 111/69 | 110/69 | 1/0 | 107/67 | 108/69 | 1/2 | 113/70 | 112/72 | 1/2 |
| S2 | 97/54 | 96/54 | 1/0 | 100/61 | 100/64 | 0/3 | 109/77 | 110/80 | 1/3 |
| S3 | 117/76 | 120/77 | 3/1 | 121/76 | 119/76 | 2/0 | 129/78 | 126/78 | 3/0 |

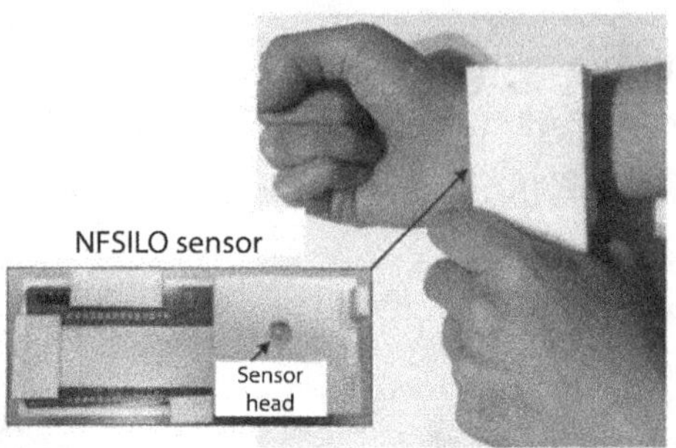


**FIGURE 8.28** Handheld self-injection locked radar arterial pulse pressure wave sensor. (Courtesy of Chao-Hsiung Tseng, National Taiwan University of Science and Technology.)

and

$$DBP = \frac{2}{0.031}\, ln \frac{b}{R - PTT} - \frac{1}{3} \frac{a}{R - PTT^2} \tag{8.11}$$

where $a$ and $b$ are calibration factors for the individual subject to be determined from the measured R-PTT and reference SBP and DBP from calibrations obtained independently.

A circuit view of the NFSILO sensor is shown in Figure 8.30 (see Figure 8.21 for a comparable system block diagram). The 5.7 GHz NFSILO sensor was implemented on a 20 mil-RO4003C substrate with a dielectric constant of 3.55 and a loss tangent of 0.0027. The handheld sensor is composed of a SILO, a differentiator, amplitude demodulator, a baseband amplifier, and a microcontroller unit (MCU) for analog-to-digital signal conversion. The output of the SILO is a frequency-modulated carrier of the wrist pulse, which is differentiated to enhance its amplitude-variation and facilitate acquisition by the envelope detector.

Performance of the contactless SIL radar arterial-pulse pressure sensor was tested by positioning the SILO sensor aperture with an air gap of 0.5 mm over the radial artery of a seated and resting normal subject. The separation is maintained by the SILO sensor casing lightly placed in contact with the wrist resting on a table. A 10-second record of radial artery pulse waveform obtained from the wrist is shown

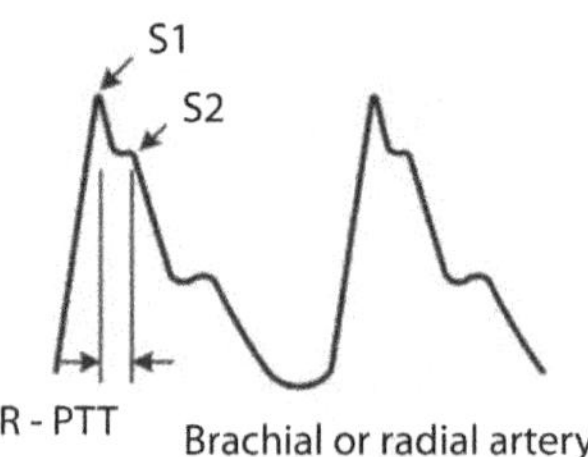


**FIGURE 8.29** Definition of S1, the first systolic peak and S2, second systolic peak of the arterial pulse wave and R-PTT, the time interval between S1 and S2.

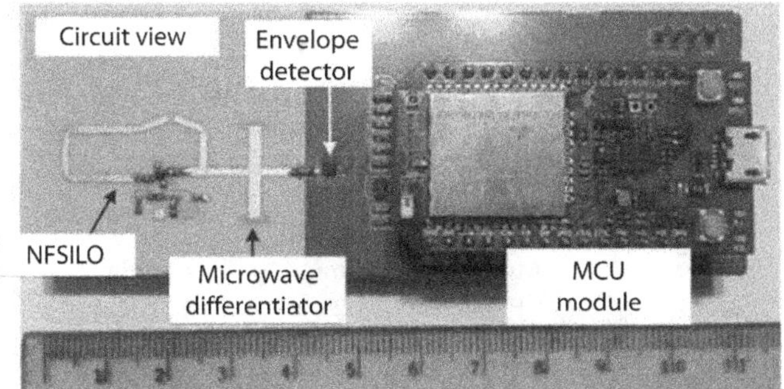


**FIGURE 8.30** Photographs of near-field microwave self-injection locked (NFSIL) radar sensor with a split-ring resonator, amplitude demodulator, and MCU module. (Courtesy of Chao-Hsiung Tseng, National Taiwan University of Science and Technology.)

in Figure 8.31. The spurious motion-related high-frequency noise visible in the raw waveform can be filtered to yield the figure displayed in the bottom of Figure 8.31. The first and second systolic peaks of each beat can be clearly identified for R-PTT calculation. Immediately following the wrist pulse measurement by the SILO BP sensor, reference SBP and DBP were acquired using a commercial sphygmomanometer for sensor calibration. The calibration and R-PTT are applied in the algorithm for the radial artery SBP and DBP determination in accordance with Eqs. (8.10) and (8.11). The calibration factors are $a = 1.2584$, $b = 0.6405$. Results indicated that compared to the reference blood pressure values, the maximum SBP deviation is 7.37 mm Hg, while the maximum DBP deviation is 8.35 mm Hg for the subject.

SILO sensor-measured blood pressure measurements of 10 subjects (4 male and 6 female) aged from 23 to 48 years are given in Table 8.5. It shows that

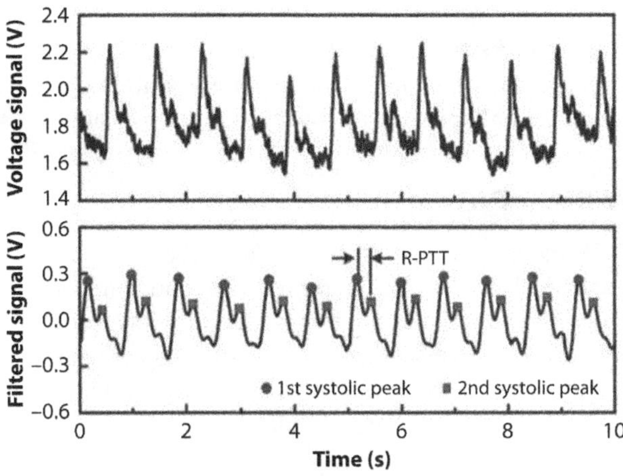


**FIGURE 8.31** Self-injection locked oscillator radar sensor measured raw (top) and filtered (bottom) arterial pulse waveforms from the wrist of normal subject.

**TABLE 8.5**
**SILO Sensor-Measured Arterial Blood Pressures of 10 Subjects Aged 23 to 48 Years: BMI (Body Mass Index)**

| Participants | Age | Gender | BMI | SBP (M+SD) | DBP (M+SD) |
|---|---|---|---|---|---|
| No. | Years | M/F | kg/m$^2$ | mm Hg | mm Hg |
| 1 | 23 | F | 22.2 | 1.82 ± 3.36 | 0.87 ± 1.68 |
| 2 | 23 | F | 20.3 | –4.39 ± 2.38 | –0.97 ± 7.54 |
| 3 | 23 | M | 19.3 | 0.44 ± 8.07 | –0.91 ± 7.54 |
| 4 | 32 | M | 22.6 | –6.82 ± 5.52 | –6.81 ± 5.32 |
| 5 | 35 | F | 18 | 2.02 ± 5.01 | –6.83 ± 4.5 |
| 6 | 39 | F | 19.5 | –10.04 ± 5.39 | –0.42 ± 6.66 |
| 7 | 44 | F | 28 | –4.48 ± 4.58 | 0.27 ± 7.05 |
| 8 | 44 | F | 18 | –10.58 ± 6.16 | –6.13 ± 7.52 |
| 9 | 46 | M | 28.5 | –5.93 ± 3.54 | –6.13 ± 7.52 |
| 10 | 48 | M | 24.3 | 0.07 ± 4.32 | –2.33 ± 6.01 |
| All | 35.7 | | 22.07 | | |

while there are some deviations in the multiple-subject experiment, most SBP and DBP values are within the 95% limit of agreement (LoA), except for two SBP and one DBP sets of measurements, presumably due to the wide age range and some sensing location uncertainty in applying the handheld wrist pulse sensor. It was suggested that if the SILO sensor is further miniaturized and can be worn on the wrist to detect the wrist pulses, the measurement accuracy could be effectively improved.

It is important to emphasize the need of independent or reference calibration in the previously mentioned blood pressure calculation algorithms that are predicated on PTT-related blood pressure sensors for noninvasive microwave arterial pressure estimation and measurement. Without the required calibration, PTT-based blood-pressure measurements only provide relative pressure estimates.

### 8.3.5 MMW Radar Pressure Sensor

The mmW FMCW radar pulse sensor discussed in Section 8.2.2.4 was shown to be well correlated with the waveforms of a commercial tonometer [Johnson et al., 2019]. In a test to measure blood pressure in humans, the mmW sensor was mounted inside a plastic cover and the package was attached to the subject using a nylon strap and placed over the radial artery as shown in Figure 8.32. Simultaneously, recordings of radial arterial pressure waves were obtained with a handheld tonometer on the contralateral wrist.

Measurements were conducted on 12 normal subjects (33 to 68 years) in a seated resting position to better maintain a stable heart rate and blood pressure. The computed root-mean-square (RMS) values of radar and electrocardiography (ECG)

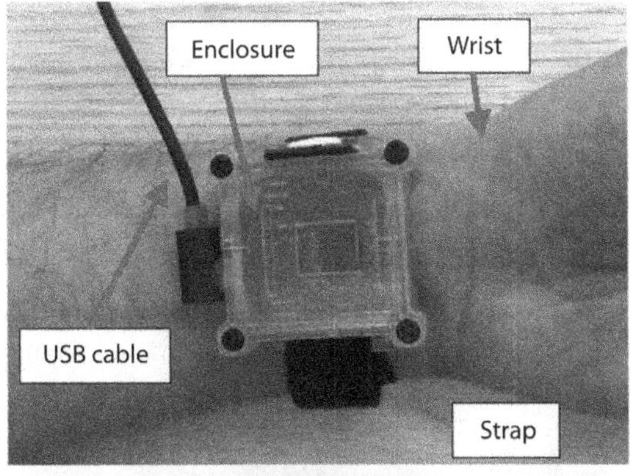


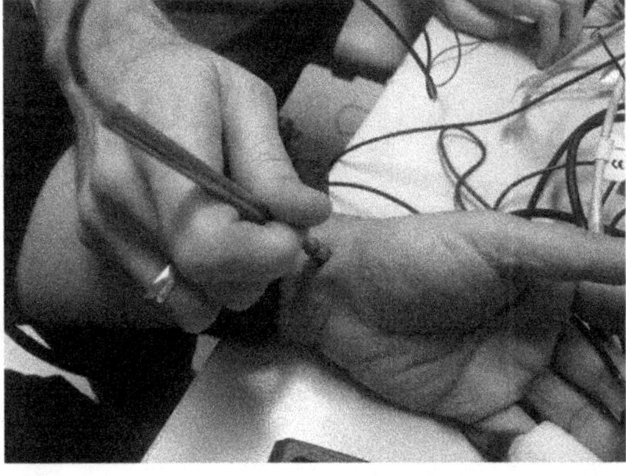

**FIGURE 8.32** Frequency-modulated continuous wave mm-wave radar sensor in a plastic cover attached to the subject using a nylon strap and placed over the radial artery (a). Simultaneous recordings of radial arterial pressure waves using a handheld tonometer on the opposite wrist (b). (Courtesy of Jessi Johnson, Blumio, Inc.)

measured HR for the 12 subjects are given in Table 8.6. A correlation coefficient ($R^2$) was computed by conducting a beat-by-beat comparison of the two waveforms over a 10-second window. The correlation coefficient for waveforms with $R^2$ values >0.90 are considered as "high," $R^2$ values <0.84 are considered as "low," and those values between them are considered as "typical."

Figure 8.33 provides three sets of comparisons of the mmW radar and tonometer measured signals over 10-second windows, which exhibit varying degrees of parallelism. For the subject with the lowest correlation of $R^2 = 0.72$ (#9), there are clear differences between the mmW radar and tonometer waveforms. The middle curves with $R^2 = 0.86$ (#3) are representative of typical signals. Both the wave shape and spectral content show similarly reproduced features. The bottom figure with $R^2 = 0.99$ (#12) demonstrates a set of well correlated signals in which the mmW radar and tonometer measurements are practically identical. However, the heart rates displayed a high degree of commonality (within 0.3 beat/min) among radar, ECG, and tonometer measurements.

**TABLE 8.6**
**Summary of Computed RMS Values of Radar and ECG-Measured HR for 12 Subjects**

| Subject # | Radar HR beat/min | ECG HR beat/min | Radar and Tonometer Waveform Correlation $R^2$ |
|---|---|---|---|
| 1 | 76.3 | 76.1 | 0.90 |
| 2 | 92.4 | 92.1 | 0.80 |
| 3 | 74.9 | 75.0 | 0.86 |
| 4 | 78.4 | 78.3 | 0.90 |
| 5 | 70.6 | 70.4 | 0.93 |
| 6 | 68.8 | 68.8 | 0.94 |
| 7 | 68.3 | 68.4 | 0.77 |
| 8 | 74.3 | 74.3 | 0.94 |
| 9 | 67.1 | 67.1 | 0.72 |
| 10 | 57.0 | 57.0 | 0.91 |
| 11 | 67.3 | 67.4 | 0.82 |
| 12 | 85.1 | 85.1 | 0.99 |
| Average | 73.4 | 73.3 | 0.87 |

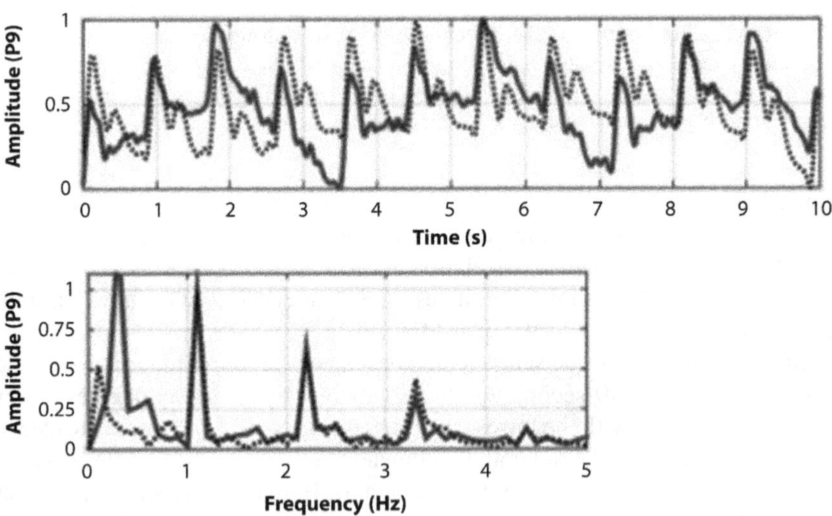


**FIGURE 8.33** Example waveforms and corresponding spectral distribution for subjects with varying $R_2$ values: (a) low, P9; (b) typical, P3; and (c) high, P12, obtained by mm-wave radar and tonometer (dotted line). *(Continued)*

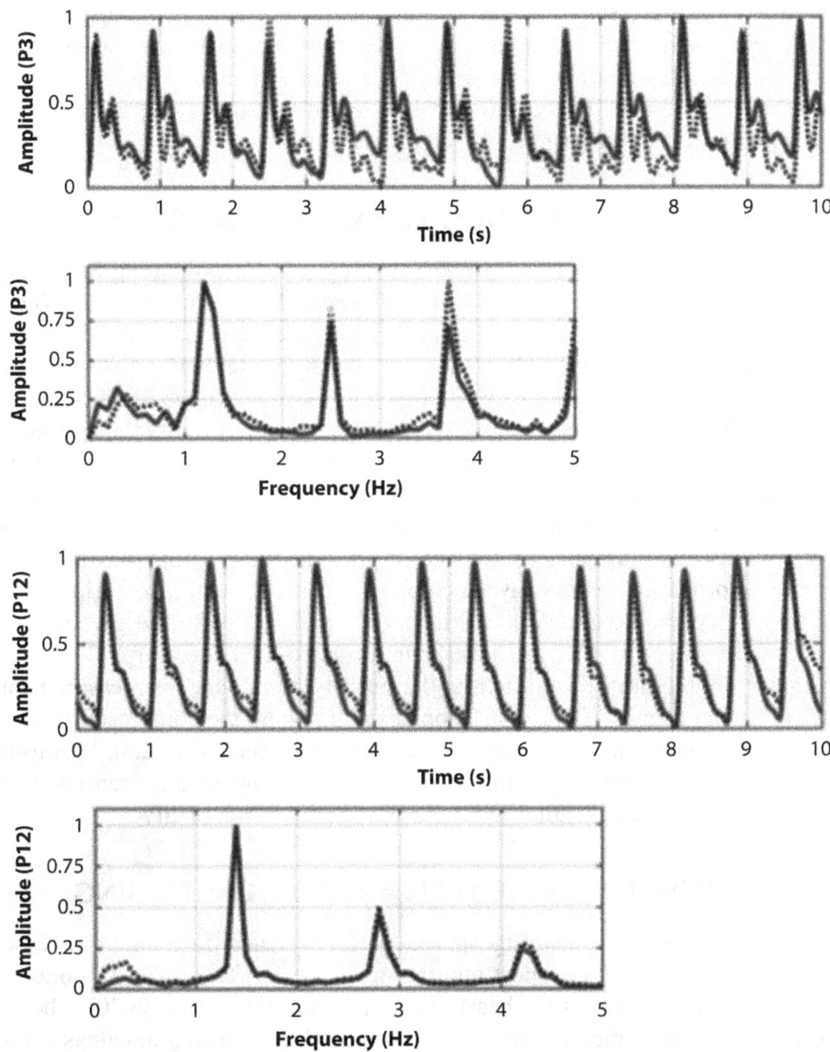


**FIGURE 8.33** *(Continued)*

For the subject with the lowest correlation coefficient and showing clear distinctions between the radar and tonometer measurements, the radar signal displays a prominent low-frequency element that can be accounted for by a respiratory component that is not present in the tonometer. However, significant differences in portions of the signal also can be observed from the radar signal, which is not present in the corresponding tonometer pressure pulse waves. The disparity or artifact potentially could be the result of radar reflections from veinous motions in the wrist region, as described in Section 8.3.2 and Figure 8.25, or some other spurious noise-related sources that would need further investigation.

In summary, the results and discussions in this section on the application of microwave radar in noninvasive arterial pressure sensing and monitoring strongly suggest the sustained interest and rigorous development of microwave radar technology in noninvasive arterial pressure sensing and monitoring alongside pulse wave analysis and PTT measurement for blood pressure tracking.

## 8.4 MULTIPARAMETER BLOOD PRESSURE SENSING

A different PTT-related contact method was proposed for estimating SBP using a combination of CW radar, ECG, and across-the-shoulder bioimpedance [Buxi et al., 2017]. The CW radar signal is used to acquire the arterial distension of the ventral side of the aorta by placing the CW radar antenna on the sternum. The three sensors are attached to the skin using sticky biopotential electrodes (6 cm in diameter). The PTT and pulse arrival times are measured and calibrated against the systolic and mean as well as DSP from a conventional oscillometer device. A signal processing technique like those described previously is used to estimate the PTT from the aorta to the common carotid arteries and used to estimate blood pressure from linear regression with the oscillometer reference. The results indicate that the multi-sensor architecture proposed in this investigation has some potential to estimate SBP. However, the Pearson correlation coefficients of pulse arrival time gave moderate values and the values for SBP are lower than those from the literature.

A major limitation of this system is the need for simultaneous measurement of electrical bioimpedance, ECG, and Doppler radar signal; the complexity renders it unsuitable for long-term monitoring. As described in Section (8.2.4), beat-to-beat blood pressure measurements using a single low-IF Doppler radar sensed PTT to overcome the drawback permit measurement of both SBP and DSP.

## 8.5 MULTIPOINT NEAR-FIELD BLOOD PRESSURE SENSING

An alternative microwave-sensing approach employs near-field microwave sensing, which can potentially support multipoint near-field assessment of motion and pressure at different parts of the heart inside the chest [Hui et al., 2020]. The technique enables cardiac measurement by placing multiple sensing antennas through clothing over the chest to allow near-field detection of heartbeat movement-induced modulations in the received microwave signal. The multipoint system is shown in Figure 8.34, which consisted of two software defined radios (SDR), denoted as SDR1 and SDR2. The two SDRs are synchronized by an external local oscillator (LO) with 10 MHz reference and 1 pulse per second (pps) baseband. The SDRs are connected to a host computer through USB cables.

Each port of the system consists of one radio frequency (RF) transmitter (TX) and one receiver (RX). For Port 1 (P1) in SDR1 (Figure 8.34), the sensing antenna pair is connected to TX1 and RX1. A field programmable gate array (FPGA) prepares the baseband signal to be fed to the TX1 chain, and the received RF signal modulated by the heartbeat is fed to RX1 and demodulated by the FPGA. The other three ports (P2, P3, and P4) are similarly configured with TX2 and RX2 to P2 in SDR1, TX3 and RX3 to P3 in SDR2, and TX4 and RX4 to P4 in SDR2. The RF

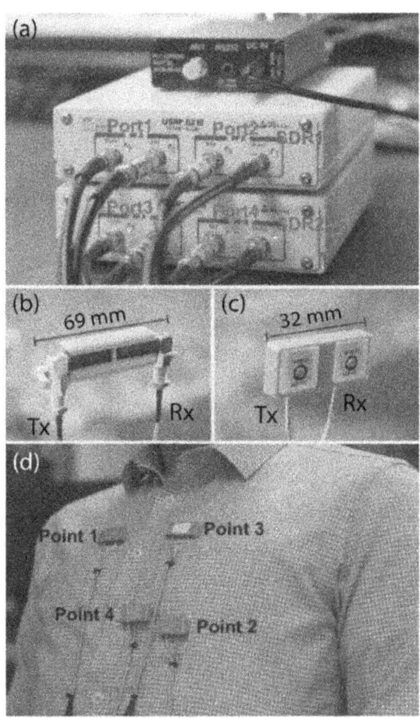


**FIGURE 8.34** Prototype multipoint near-field sensing system: (a) The transceiver by two software-defined radios (SDR1 and SDR2), (b) the sensing antenna pair at 1.8 GHz band, (c) the 900 MHz and 5 GHz bands, and (d) the sensing antenna placement when four antenna pairs are deployed to Points 1–4. The sensing antenna pairs are placed over the shirt. (Hui et al., 2020.)

signal at each TX can be multiplexed with time-division multiple access (TDMA), code division multiple access (CDMA) or, in the case of this work, frequency division multiple access (FDMA). The carrier frequency is 1.82 GHz with 0.71, 1.22, 1.71, and 2.33 MHz baseband offsets for TX1–TX4, respectively.

The four sensing antenna pairs are chosen to mimic the conventional auscultatory stethoscope for listening to the aortic, mitral, pulmonary, and tricuspid valves. Point 0 is chosen as Erb's point (Figure 8.35), a central area of the chest used as a reference position for timing comparison. The left and right leg ECG electrodes are pasted on the torso and connected to the host computer by USB. The ECG signal serves as a timing reference to highlight the feature points in the cardiac cycle. A digital stethoscope is placed at Point ST to record the S1 and S2 heart sounds. After channel demodulation, the signal is down-sampled to 50 kSps, which is slightly higher than 44.1 kSps of the digital stethoscope so that the system can contain all information from the audible signal. The SDR sampling rates of the data converter are set as 5 MSps, which is above the Nyquist rate of 2 times the highest baseband offset at 2.33 MHz. Furthermore, the cardiac signals are processed using frequency-time transforms to derive beat-to-beat blood pressure waves.

Figure 8.36 presents the results of blood pressure extraction from the channel of TX1-to-RX1 (C11) where the subjects are instructed to be still and control their breathing rhythm. During systole, C11 waveforms are dominated by the aortic

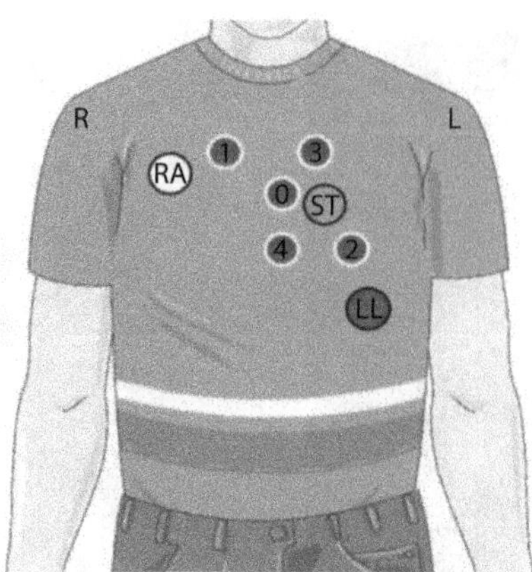


**FIGURE 8.35** The multipoint microwave system for near-field sensing. Placement of the sensing points (1–4): 0 (Erb's point), ST (stethoscope), LL and RA (ECG electrodes). (Hui et al., 2020.)

movement and are used for blood pressure derivation. Furthermore, C11 is more closely related to the central blood pressure of the aortic artery than the branchial blood pressure from arm cuffs, although their values are closely correlated when the cuff is at the same level of the heart. The high-frequency components in C11 during systole would contain features of aortic movement, which may be used to estimate the central SBP and DSP. Therefore, blood pressure derivation requires high resolution in both frequency and time domains with a broad bandwidth.

In this study, the Hilbert-Huang transform (HHT) was used to obtain the frequency time spectrum [Huang, 2014], where the instantaneous frequency is calculated at each sampling time point for the nonstationary oscillation analysis. The time resolution depends on the sampling rate in the time domain, which can be above 106 samples per second (Sps) by the analog-to-digital converter (ADC) in the chosen SDR. The high ADC sampling rate can also spread noise over a larger spectrum to reduce the noise floor and increase SNR. This frequency resolution was chosen to conserve computation time.

The HHT frequency time analysis of a single heartbeat obtained from C11 with the subject seated on the floor is depicted in Figure 8.36. The blue curve is the synchronized ECG signal for timing, and the ventricular ejection period is between the dashed lines. The sampling rate for the waveform is 103 Sps, producing a 1 ms time resolution. The highest frequency response is half of the sampling rate at 500 Hz. The frequency resolution is set to 0.125 Hz, 1/8000 of the sampling rate. All signals were filtered using a zero-phase finite impulse response (FIR) filters to cancel the phase shift and maintain the linear phase response. The down-sampled signal was further bandpass filtered (1.5–16 Hz) to attenuate the fundamental heartbeat tone and extraneous noise. The resulting waveform was processed as a part of the HHT algorithm.

Each point in Figure 8.36 represents the instantaneous frequency at the corresponding time, and its color shows the instantaneous amplitude in the dB scale normalized

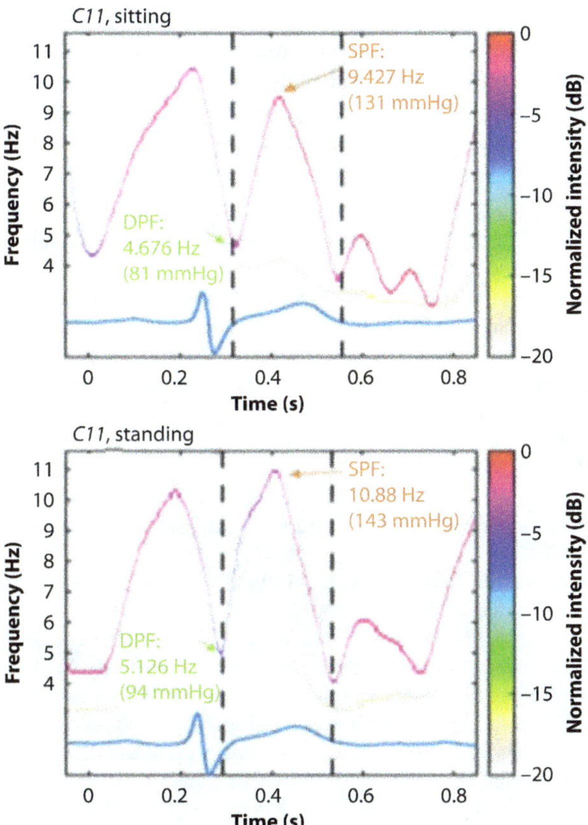


**FIGURE 8.36** Central blood pressure analysis based on Hilbert-Huang transform frequency-time analysis of near-field backscattering channel C11 during systole: (Top) Subject sat on the floor; (bottom) subject was in a standing posture. The synchronized ECG signal (blue) indicates timing. (Hui et al., 2020.)

by the respective maximum value. The horizontal and vertical axes are time and frequency, respectively. The maximum frequency point at 9.427 Hz, denoted as the systolic pressure frequency (SPF), is aligned with the SBP point. The minimum at 4.676 Hz, denoted as the diastolic pressure frequency (DPF), is aligned with the DSP point at the beginning of systole. The concurrent brachial blood pressures measured by an arm-cuff monitor are 131 mm Hg and 81 mm Hg. The experiment was repeated with the subject standing. The SPF and DPF in this case are 10.88 Hz and 5.126 Hz, and the corresponding arm-cuff blood pressures are 143 mm Hg and 94 mm Hg. The frequency resolution is 0.125 Hz, corresponding to 1.0 mm Hg resolution for the SBP and 3.6 mm Hg for the DSP. Two-point linear interpolation can transform the two SPFs to SBP, and similarly, for the two DPFs to DSP, as shown in Figure 8.36. The linear interpolation scheme allows the near-field sensing system to estimate central blood pressure from arterial pulse waves of individual subjects. Thus, the multipoint sensing method can potentially provide position-specific sensing, in which multiple antennas offer different sets of information to analyze the heartbeat motion and circulatory phenomena, albeit with considerably more instrumentational and analytical complexity as well as practical limitations when compared to Sections 8.2 and 8.3.

## REFERENCES

Alecu, C., Labat, C., Kearney-Schwartz, A., Fay, R., Salvi, P., Joly, L., Lacolley, P., Vespignani, H., Benetos, A., 2008. Reference values of aortic pulse wave velocity in the elderly. J Hypertens, 26:2207–2212

Avolio, A. P., Butlin, M., Walsh, A., 2010. Arterial blood pressure measurement and pulse wave analysis—Their role in enhancing cardiovascular assessment. Physiol. Meas., 31(1):Art. no. R1–47

Bramwell, J. C., Hill, A. V., 1922a. The velocity of the pulse wave in man. Proc. Roy. Soc. London B, 93(652):298–306

Bramwell, J. C., Hill, A. V., 1922b. Velocity of transmission of the pulse-wave. Lancet, 199(5149):891–892

Buxi, D., Redout, J. M., Yuce, M. R., 2017. Blood pressure estimation using pulse transit time from bioimpedance and continuous wave radar. IEEE Trans. Biomed. Eng., 64(4):917–927

Cotran, R. S., Kumar, V., Robbins, S. L., 1994. Pathological Basis of Disease, 5th ed, Philadelphia: Saunders

Cruickshank, K., Riste, L., Anderson, S. G., Wright, J. S., Dunn, G., Gosling, R. G., 2002. Aortic pulse-wave velocity and its relationship to mortality in diabetes and glucose intolerance: An integrated index of vascular function? Circulation, 106:2085–2090

Eu, H. J., 2010. The reference values for arterial stiffness' collaboration, determinants of pulse wave velocity in healthy people and in the presence of cardiovascular risk factors: 'establishing normal and reference values. Eur. Heart J., 31(19):2338–2350

Gajdova, J., Karasek, D., Goldmannova, D., Krystynik, O., Schovanek, J., Vaverkova, H., Zadrazil, J., 2017. Pulse wave analysis and diabetes mellitus. A systematic review. Biomed. Pap. Med. Fac. Univ. Palacky Olomouc. Czech. Repub., 161(3):223–233

Garnier, A., Briet, M., 2016. Arterial stiffness and chronic kidney disease. Pulse, 3(3–4): 229–241

Ghasemzadeh, N., Zafari, A. M., 2011. A brief journey into the history of the arterial pulse. Cardiol. Res. Pract., 2011:164832

Grant, I. L. B., 1972. Grant's Atlas of Anatomy, 6th ed, Baltimore, MD: Williams & Wilkins

Hajar, R., 2018. The pulse from ancient to modern medicine: Part 3. Heart Views, 19(3):117–120

Hirotsu, C., Betta, M., Bernardi, G., Marques-Vidal, P., Vollenweider, P., Waeber, G., Pichot, V., Roche, F., Siclari, F., Haba-Rubio, J., Heinzer, R., 2020. Pulse wave amplitude drops during sleep: Clinical significance and characteristics in a general population sample. Sleep, 43(7):322

Huang, N. E., 2014. Hilbert-Huang Transform and Its Applications, Singapore: World Scientific

Hui, X., Sharma, P., Kan, E. C., 2019. Microwave stethoscope for heart sound by near-field coherent sensing, in IEEE MTT-S Int. Microw. Symp. Dig., pp. 365–368

Hui, X., Conroy, T. B., Kan, E. C., 2020. Multi-point near-field RF sensing of blood pressures and heartbeat dynamics. IEEE Access, 8:89935–89945

Johnson, J. E., Shay, O., Kim, C., Liao, C., 2019. Wearable millimeter-wave device for contactless measurement of arterial pulses. IEEE Trans. Biomed. Circuits Syst., 13(6):1525–1534

Kim, B., Hong, Y., An, Y., et al., 2016. A proximity coupling RF sensor for wrist pulse detection based on injection-locked PLL. Trans. Microw. Theory Tech., 64(5):1667–1676

Kim, J. M., Kim, S. S., Kim, I. J., Kim, J. H., Kim, B. H., Kim, M. K., Lee, S. H., Lee, C. W., Kim, M. C., Ahn, J. H., Kim, J., Relationship between Cardiovascular disease and brachial-ankle pulse wave velocity (bapwv) in, 2020. Patients with type 2 diabetes (REBOUND) study group. Arterial stiffness is an independent predictor for risk of mortality in Patients with type 2 diabetes mellitus: The REBOUND study. Cardiovasc. Diabetol., 19(1):143

Kuwahara, M., Yavari, E., Boric-Lubecke, O., 2019. Non-invasive, continuous, pulse pressure monitoring method, in Proc. Annu. Int. Conf. IEEE Eng. Med. Biol. Soc., pp. 6574–6577

Lee, J. Y., Lin, J. C., 1985. A microprocessor based non-invasive pulse wave analyzer. IEEE Trans. Biomed. Eng., 32(6):451–455

Lee, J. Y., Lin, J. C., Popovic, M. A., 1983. Microprocessor-Based Arterial Pulse Wave Analyzer. IEEE Conference of Engg. in Medicine and Biology Society, Columbus, OH, p. 79

Liao, J., Farmer, J., 2014. Arterial stiffness as a risk factor for coronary artery disease. Current Atherosclerosis Reports, 16(2):387

Lin, J. C., 1989. Microwave noninvasive sensing of physiological signatures. In: Lin, J. C., Ed., Electromagnetic Interaction With Biological Systems (pp. 3–5), Plenum

Lin, J. C., 1992. Microwave sensing of physiological movement and volume change. Bioelectromagnetics, 13:557–565

Lin, J. C., 1993. Diagnostic applications of electromagnetic fields. In: Stone, W. R., Ed., Review of Radio Science (pp. 771–778), Oxford: Oxford University Press

Lin, J. Y., Lin, J. C., 2009. Contact microwave noninvasive continuous monitoring of blood pressure, DARPA Workshop on Continuous, Non-Invasive Monitoring of Blood Pressure, Coronado, California

McDonald, D. A., 1974. Blood Flow in Arteries, 2nd ed, London: Arnold

Mukkamala, R., Hahn, J. O., Inan, O. T., Mestha, L. K., Kim, C. S., Toreyin, H., Kyal, S., 2015. Toward ubiquitous blood pressure monitoring via pulse transit time: Theory and practice. IEEE Trans. Biomed. Eng., 62(8):18791901

Nichols, W., O'Rourke, M., 2005. McDonald's Blood Flow in Arteries: Theoretical, Experimental and Clinical Principles, 5th ed, London: Hodder Arnold

Papp, M. A., Hughes, C., Lin, J. C., Pouget, J., 1987. Doppler microwave, a clinical assessment of its efficacy as an arterial pulse sensing technique. Invest Radiol., 22:569–573

Pitson, D. J., Stradling, J. R., 1998. Value of beat-to-beat blood pressure changes, detected by pulse transit time, in the management of the obstructive sleep apnoea/hypopnoea syndrome. Eur. Respir. J., 12(3):685–692

Qasem, A., Avolio, A., 2008. Determination of aortic pulse wave velocity from waveform decomposition of the central aortic pressure pulse. Hypertension, 51(2):1188–1195

Rachim, V., Chung, W., 2019. Multimodal wrist biosensor for wearable cuff-less blood pressure monitoring system. Sci. Rep., 9(1):7947

RCA Laboratories, 1987. Miniature superficial temporal artery monitor, Report, Princeton, New Jersey

Silverthorn, D. U., 2016. Human Physiology: An Integrated Approach, 7th ed, Upper Saddle River: Pearson

Stehouwer, C. D. A., Henry, R. M. A., Ferreira, I., 2008. Arterial stiffness in diabetes and the metabolic syndrome: A pathway to cardiovascular disease. Diabetologia, 51(4):527–539

Stuchly, S. S., Smith, A., Goldberg, M., Thansandote, A., Menard, A., 1980. A microwave device for arterial wall motion analysis. Proc. 33rd Ann. Conf. Eng. Med. Biol., 22:47

Takemoto, R., Uchida, H. A., Toda, H., Okada, K., Otsuka, F., Ito, H., Wada, J., 2021. Total vascular resistance, augmentation index, and augmentation pressure increase in patients with peripheral artery disease. Medicine (Baltimore), 100(32):e26931

Thansandote, A., Stuchly, S. S., Smith, A. M., 1983. Monitoring variations of biological impedances using microwave Doppler radar. Phys. Med. Biol., 28:983–990

Tseng, C. H., Yu, L. T., Huang, J. K., Chang, C. L., 2018. A wearable self-injection-locked sensor with active integrated antenna and differentiator-based envelope detector for vital-sign detection from chest wall and wrist. IEEE Trans. Microw. Theory Techn., 66(5):2511–2521

Tseng, C. H., Tseng, T. J., Wu, C. Z., 2020. Cuffless blood pressure measurement using a microwave near-field self-injection-locked wrist pulse sensor. IEEE Trans. Microw. Theory Techn, 68(11):4865–4874

Turusheva, A., Frolova, E., Kotovskaya, Y., Petrosyan, Y., Dumbadze, R., 2020. Association between arterial stiffness, frailty and fall-related injuries in older adults. Vasc. Health Risk Manag., 6:307–316

Vander, A. J., Sherman, J. H., Luciano, D. S., 1990. Human Physiology, 5th ed, New York: McGraw-Hill

Wang, J., Wu, L., 1973. The Doctorine of the Pulse. History of Chinese Medicine; Being a Chronicle of Medical Happenings in China from Ancient Times to the Present Period, 2nd ed, New York: AMS Press

Wang, F. K., Li, C. J., Hsiao, C. H., Horng, T. S., Lin, J., Peng, K. C., Jau, J. K., Li, J. Y., Chen, C. C., 2010. A novel vital-sign sensor based on a self-injection-locked oscillator. IEEE Trans. Microw. Theory Tech., 58(12):4112–4120

Wang, F. K., Horng, T. S., Peng, K. C., Jau, J. K., Li, J. Y., Chen, C. C., 2011. Single-antenna doppler radars using self and mutual injection locking for vital sign detection with random body movement cancellation. IEEE Trans. Microw. Theory Tech., 59(12):3577–3587

Wang, F. K., Tang, M. C., Su, S. C., Horng, T. S., 2016. Wrist pulse rate monitor using self-injection-locked radar technology. Biosensors (Basel), 6(4):54

Zhao, H., Gu, X., Hong, H., Li, Y., Zhu, X., Li, C., 2018. Non-contact beat-to-beat blood pressure measurement using continuous wave Doppler radar, in IEEE/MTT-S International Microwave Symposium, pp. 1413–1415

# 9 Sensing of Tissue Volume Change and Redistribution

It was decades ago when the use of changes in microwave reflectance and transmittance as measures of physiologically significant parameters, such as circulatory and respiratory volume changes, was first suggested [Moskalenko, 1960; Susskind, 1973]. For example, excessive fluid retention would increase the dielectric permittivity of lung tissue, which may allow detection using noninvasive microwave techniques. Furthermore, as shown in previous chapters, a comparison between the results of noninvasive microwave-sensed respiration and anemometer measurement revealed the possibility of using microwaves to assess pulmonary air volume changes alongside respiration rates [Lin, 1975]. Specifically, microwave measurement may be correlated with the output voltage of the hot-wire anemometer flow meter, which is typically calibrated in volt/liter/min (see Chapter 7, Figures 7.4 and 7.5). It is noted that common airflow-based instruments for respiration or lung volume measurement such as spirometry are cumbersome, and their usefulness and accuracy are limited.

Recently, the issue of whether the amplitude of microwave radar signals can be used to estimate respiratory depth has become a subject of discussion. The ability to distinguish between respiration progression such as respiratory depth or tidal volume quickly and reliably, and to ascertain rapid shallow breathing versus rapid deep breathing are clinically important for assessing a patient's pulmonary reserve capacity. Radar amplitude patterns observed in some patients suggested that this might be the case [van Loon et al., 2016]. It can be seen from Chapter 7, Figure 7.24, that spontaneous respiration with different breathing patterns is measurable using microwave radar. Each inspiratory cycle is characterized by a first peak (chest-wall expansion during inhalation) and followed by a curved peak (during exhalation). Since a patient in the supine position would produce different radar amplitudes compared to the lateral position measuring actual tidal volumes may require use of more than one radar or a radar with scanning capability.

The volume of air inhaled or exhaled in a single breath during quiet breathing is referred to as tidal volume. It is the amount of air that moves in or out of the lungs with each respiratory cycle. Changes in tidal volume and chest-wall dimension are relatively consistent among human subjects. The normal total lung air volume at functional residual capacity is about 1.8–2.2 L with a tidal volume of 500 mL per inspiration, or approximately 7 mL/kg of body mass. Furthermore, in normal subjects breathing at rest in the seated posture, displacements of the rib cage during inspiration are in the cranial, lateral outward, and ventral directions, but expansion of the abdomen is confined to the ventral direction [de Groote et al., 1997].

DOI: 10.1201/9781003315223-9

Changes in tidal volume are obtained on a breath-by-breath basis and can serve as indicators of respiratory disorders during sleep and help to diagnose other medical conditions such as pulmonary reserve capacity and chronic obstructive pulmonary disease (COPD). Airflow can be extracted from tracheal sounds and movements, which are used for assessing the severity of sleep apnea.

Respiratory tidal volumes are known to change on a breath-by-breath basis. The use of Doppler continuous wave (CW) microwave radars for quantitative contactless and unobtrusive measurement of tidal volume in human subjects has shown that Doppler radar output is related linearly to tidal volume [Dei et al., 2009; Lee et al., 2014; Massagram et al., 2013]. Figure 9.1 presents a comparison of the 30-second records of AC-coupled Doppler radar, reconstructed waveform, and spirometer output from a human subject [Massagram et al., 2013]. A close relationship is seen between microwave sensor measurements and spirometer-measured tidal volume. Numerical results of the radar-measured and reference tidal volumes from eight subjects showed average mean difference of –39.9 mL in seated subjects and 23.5 mL in supine subjects. In comparison, other types of chest-wall displacement measurements, namely piezoelectric sensors at the upper and lower torso positions reported considerably higher differences: 40.6 mL and –54.8 mL in seated subjects and 246.6 mL and 69.5 mL in supine subjects. However, tidal volume is not often monitored in practice as the previously mentioned results demonstrate common

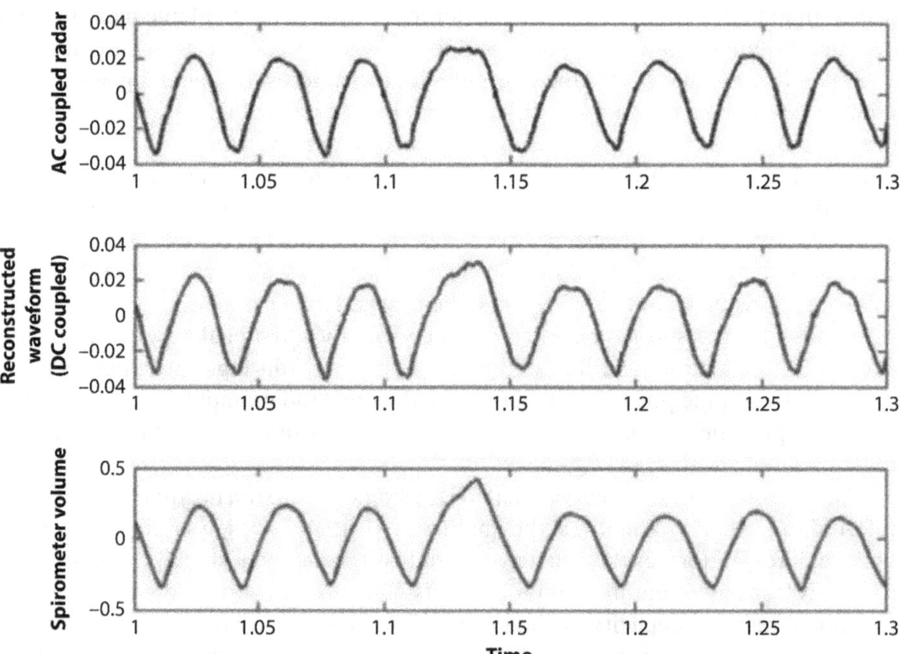


**FIGURE 9.1** Comparison of 30-second records of AC coupled Doppler microwave radar sensed respiratory volume signal (top), reconstructed waveform (middle), and spirometer transducer output (bottom).

techniques are not as reliable and difficult to apply. It requires a sealed mask or intubation for accurate measurement. Thus, Doppler microwave radar sensing could provide a valuable tool for contactless measurement of tidal volume in human subjects, noninvasively and unobtrusively.

Currently, X-ray chest radiography remains the most readily available tool in routine clinical practice or screening test for detection of pulmonary edema, the accumulation of abnormal amounts of fluid in the lungs [Lange and Schuster, 1999]. While X-ray computed tomography (CT) is the most accurate and reproducible, it is also the most expensive and difficult to implement outside the hospital. Concerns on risk of excessive X-ray exposure also limit X-ray CT's ability to be used as a monitoring option. Noninvasive systems that can effectively sense and record physiological parameters such as pulmonary edema in outpatient settings are especially desirable.

Similarly, cerebral edema occurs when an abnormal amount of fluid builds up in and around the brain, causing an increase in intracranial pressure (ICP). Cerebral edema is often accompanied by clinical complications such as herniation of the brain with potential lethal consequences. Cerebral tissue redistribution arises when brain matter, blood, and cerebrospinal fluid (CSF) shift from their normal position inside the skull. The current diagnostic procedures of choice for assessing cerebral edema involve either CT or magnetic resonance imaging (MRI) [Shah and Kimberly, 2016]. An MRI scan is most reliable for visualizing and identifying the extent and location of cerebral edema. However, these types of imaging modalities are associated with a high cost for routine examinations, and in the case of X-ray CT, it is often excluded for short-term follow-up procedures because of the ionizing-radiation burden. Therefore, it is important to investigate new noninvasive modes of imaging or sensing, based on nonionizing energy and low cost. A microwave transmission technique for detection and monitoring of cerebral edema was reported [Lin and Clarke, 1982]. It was shown by the use of a phantom head model that the microwave signal correlates with various quantities of excess water. The noninvasive microwave technique can detect fluid-volume changes as small as 1%.

The discussions that follow will begin with a brief description of the pertinent physiology and pathophysiology of the pulmonary and cerebral organs and related systems. For more comprehensive discussions the reader is referred to available textbooks [Cotran et al., 1994; Grant, 1972; Silverthorn, 2016; Vander et al., 1990].

## 9.1 PATHOPHYSIOLOGIC RESPIRATORY AND FLUID VOLUME CHANGES

As mentioned, the lungs fill up most of the chest cavity. They can be expanded and contracted by elevation and depression of the ribs to increase and decrease the anteroposterior diameter of the chest cavity by as much as 5 mm. Healthy human lungs in most people contain 450–500 mL of blood. The extravascular compartment normally contains another 250–650 mL of fluid. It is estimated that the normal intrathoracic fluid content ranges between 20% and 35% of the total volume. When lung water content is greater than 75–100% above these levels, physiological impairment such as pulmonary edema can occur, and it is often associated with congestive heart failure. Sensors that can effectively capture a patient's congestion status have the potential to reduce hospitalizations due to heart failure if they are sufficiently sensitive and specific. Continuous monitoring could allow earlier detection that may help to improve hospital care of presymptomatic patients and identify vulnerability in the outpatient population.

### 9.1.1 Pulmonary Edema and Pleural Effusion

Pulmonary edema and pleural effusion result when fluid builds up in and around the lungs. The pleura are the thin membranes that line the lungs. Pleural effusion occurs when fluid builds up in the layers of tissue that line the outside of the lungs. Edema refers to swelling due to trapped fluid anywhere in the body. Pulmonary edema can develop following blockages in the upper airway that cause negative pressure in the lungs from intense efforts to breathe despite the blockage. However, with prompt treatment, this type of pulmonary edema resolves in about a day. Pleural effusion is detectable on a chest X-ray and CT scan.

The more serious cardiogenic pulmonary edema is the result of fluid accumulation in the lungs caused by the left ventricle's failure to pump out enough of the blood it gets from the lungs, causing pressure in the heart go up. Thus, in this case, the pulmonary edema is caused by increased pressure in the heart, which is often associated with congestive heart failure. Typically, symptoms of heart failure are present in patients when there is greater than 50% change in lung fluid on thoracic CT. Figure 9.2 shows two X-ray CT images of the coronal section through the human chest. The CT in Figure 9.2(a) shows dry lungs in a nonheart-failure ambulatory subject, while Figure 9.2(b) depicts pulmonary edema in a patient with congestive heart failure.

### 9.1.2 Cerebral Edema

Cerebral edema, brain edema, or brain swelling refers to pathological accumulation of fluids or water in brain tissues. While the terms are often used interchangeably, they do have different pathological implications. Cerebral edema results from abnormal accumulation of water within the brain tissue. Brain swelling is caused by an increase in brain volume, and can result from hemorrhage or tumorous growth.

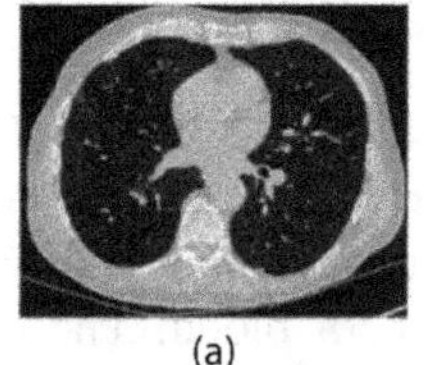
(a)

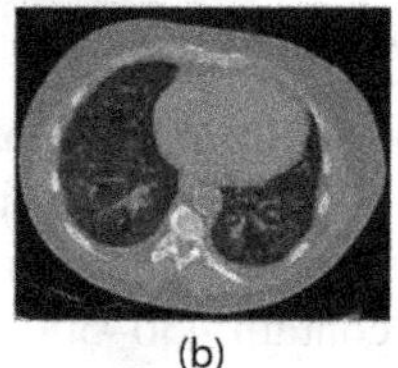
(b)

**FIGURE 9.2** Computer X-ray tomographic (CT) images of the coronal section of the human chest: (a) CT of ambulatory subject with dry lungs (non-heart failure), and (b) CT of a patient showing pulmonary edema in congestive heart failure.

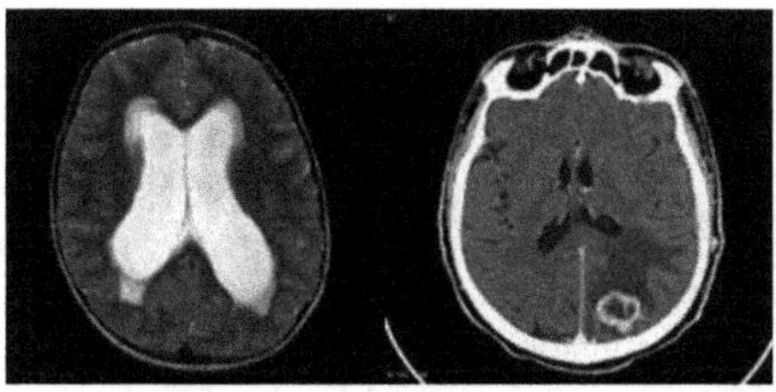

**FIGURE 9.3** Magnetic resonance image of cerebral edema: (Left) Ventricular edema and (right) tumorigenic brain edema.

Cerebral edema occurs when fluid builds up in and around the brain and is a major contributor to the increase in intracranial volume. It produces elevation in ICP and is often accompanied by clinical complications such as herniation of the brain with serious medical manifestations, including death. The main causes of cerebral edema include vasogenic stroke, traumatic brain injury, metabolic disease, infections like encephalitis and meningitis, ingestion of neurotoxic chemicals, or brain tumors (see Figure 9.3). Indeed, cerebral edema accounts for significant morbidity and mortality in many related neurologic conditions. Thus, its proper clinical management is significant and consequential.

Since the focus of this section is sensing and monitoring for the presence of cerebral edema, it is noteworthy that cerebral edemas may be classified into three major types: (1) hydrocephalus resulting from increased fluid around the brain, (2) hypertensive brain hemorrhage because of bleeding in the brain from high blood pressure, and (3) intraventricular hemorrhage due to blood bleeding into the fluid-filled ventricles inside the brain. Global cerebral edema primarily results in a global rise in ICP, while focal cerebral edema can result in cerebral herniation with or without ICP elevation. Integrity of the blood-brain barrier (BBB) is valuable for normal functioning of the brain, since increased permeability of the BBB permits extravasation of water and plasma proteins and causes extracellular edema associated with vasogenic edema. The water channel aquaporin-4 (AQP4) has been observed to be an important determinant of cerebral water accumulation and interestingly, it is associated with the clearance of excess brain water as well [Amiry-Moghaddam et al., 2003].

ICP monitoring has been used for early detection of brain edema with intraventricular and subdural cup catheters in various neurosurgical conditions, especially in the head-injury setting. However, the procedure is often linked to risks of infection. Furthermore, the use of ICP monitoring is not as effective, since ICP increase frequently causes irreversible problems in brain tissues. CT imaging is most widely used for the detection of cerebral edema because of its wide availability. MRI can be helpful in assessing the development of edema. The need to use a contrast agent in these modalities often limits their use under clinical settings [Shah and Kimberly, 2016]. Therefore, a noninvasive sensor capable of early detection of cerebral edema is of great importance in clinical medicine, but it remains a major challenge.

In general, the product of pressure and volume is a constant, when the temperature remains stable. Pressure and volume have an inverse relationship — pressure increases, then volume decreases and vice versa. However, the relationship breaks if a space or volume is closed or nearly closed, such as the mammalian cranium.

### 9.1.3 Arterial-Wall Movement and Blood Pressure

Arterial blood pressure refers to the pressure exerted by flowing blood upon the walls of blood vessels. It is considered one of the four vital signs and is governed by several factors: (1) the force exerted on the blood as it is being ejected by contraction of the left ventricle of the heart into the major arteries, (2) total blood volume, (3) the resistivity of lung tissues to the of flow of blood out from the arterial compartment into the capillaries of tissues that is controlled by the small arteries (terminal arterioles), and (4) tension generated by the walls of large blood vessels in withstanding the pulse of blood ejected into the arteries by the heart. These four factors: cardiac output, blood volume, blood viscosity, and peripheral resistance cooperate to affect blood pressure levels. When these factors increase, blood pressure also increases. Most significantly, arterial blood pressure is maintained within normal range by changes in cardiac output and peripheral resistance. It is important not to assume that adequate blood pressure is synonymous with adequate cardiac output.

## 9.2 MICROWAVE SENSING OF FLUID BUILDUP IN THE LUNGS

Many respiratory abnormalities are associated with alterations in lung water content and/or water distribution. CT and chest X-ray are the most widely used diagnostic tools for lung fluid detection. However, X-ray radiography is insensitive to soft tissues and fluids inside the body. Its lack of contrast coupled with the risk of ionizing radiation burden prevent the use of CT and chest X-ray as a serial or long-term monitoring tool. Since dielectric properties of biological tissues at microwave frequencies are directly related to their water content, measurement of microwave transmission and reflection coefficients should provide explicit information on the quantity of water present in the lungs.

### 9.2.1 Earlier Pulmonary Edema Investigations

Microwave techniques applied to assess pulmonary edema use experimental measurement systems that are the same as shown in Chapter 1, Figure 1.3, except for the use of a network analyzer and a two-channel strip chart recorder in an early investigation [Pedersen et al., 1978]. A 13 × 13 cm square direct-contact microwave applicator was strapped to the right side of the chest just below the right forelimb. The frequency used was 915 MHz and the power density from the applicator was limited to less than 100 mW/m$^2$. Figure 9.4 depicts the change in the baseline of the amplitude of the microwave reflection coefficient and of the left atrial pressure during development of pulmonary edema in a 25 kg dog that was anesthetized and placed on a respirator.

Pulmonary edema was induced by inserting a balloon catheter into the left atrium. A fluid (2000 mL of isotonic saline solution) was infused over a 22-minute period with no significant changes in either left atrial pressure or microwave reflection.

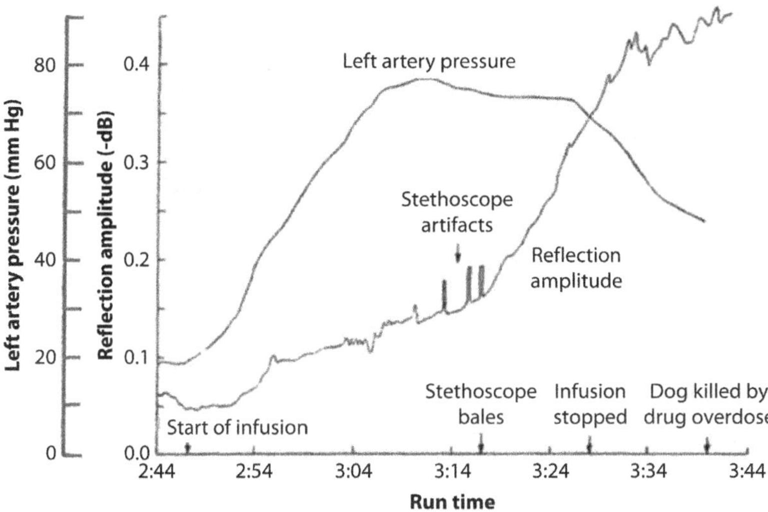


**FIGURE 9.4** Changes in the baseline of the amplitude of the microwave reflection coefficient and left atrial pressure during development of pulmonary edema in an anesthetized 25 kg dog on a respirator.

At 2:47 pm (see Figure 9.4), an infusion of Dextran 40 was initiated, which immediately produced a steadily increasing left atrial pressure and, 5 minutes later, a steadily changing baseline of the amplitude of the reflection coefficient. At 3:17 pm, crackles were heard with a stethoscope and, subsequently, the amplitude of reflected microwaves was rapidly increasing. At 3:28 pm, the infusion of Dextran 40 was stopped at which time a total of 2600 mL had been administered. The experiment was terminated at 3:40 pm. Autopsy revealed a grossly enlarged heart and severe edema of the lower lobes of the lungs. The amplitude change accompanying the progress of edema is clear and gives supportive evidence to the monitoring potential of the microwave reflection technique. Thus, the experimental results demonstrate the feasibility for the real-time microwave measurement of water buildup in and around the lungs inside of the chest.

In another experiment, a pair of 915 MHz stripline antennas was placed against the skin across the thoracic cavity and measured the amplitude and phase of the transmitted signal with respect to the source as a function of time [Durney et al., 1978]. The result obtained from artificially induced pulmonary edema in a dog is illustrated in Figure 9.5 where the phase of the transmitted microwave and the pulmonary arterial pressure are plotted against time. Clearly, phase changes in the microwave signal paralleled the physiological indicator of pulmonary edema. It is therefore feasible to use microwave transmission methods for noninvasive measures of changes in lung water.

A few years later, the group proposed a microwave radiometer approach to noninvasive monitoring of changes in lung-water content, in addition to the previously mentioned active microwave sensing [Iskander et al., 1984; Iskander and Durney, 1983]. The proposal was based on a planar theoretical model of the lungs.

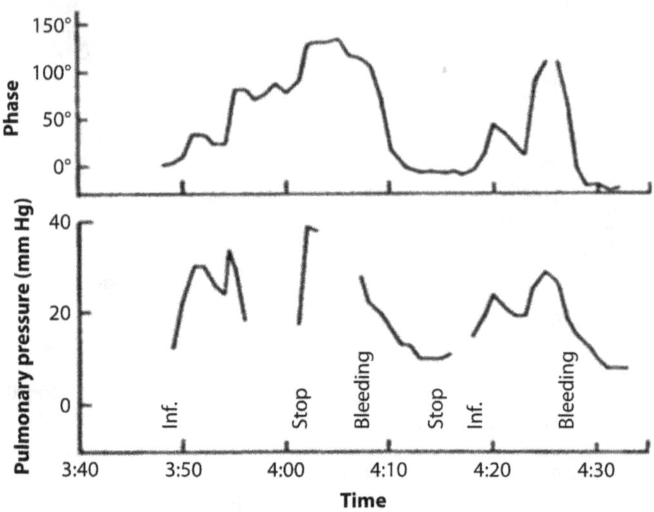


**FIGURE 9.5** Experimental results showing correlation between the phase of transmitted 915 MHz signal and the pulmonary arterial pressure in a dog during induction of pulmonary edema. (INF = infusion).

It suggested that a 1% change in lung-water content is within the radiometer's detection sensitivity limit. Preliminary experimental measurements at 1 GHz showed it was possible to detect 3–4% changes in water content in experiments by incorporating reflections at the tissue interfaces and attenuation in the chest wall (Figure 9.5). The planar phantom tissue model consisted of a flat 0.25 cm thick dielectric muscle layer and two 2 cm thick rectangular sponges. A punctured plastic tube for injecting room-temperature water was sandwiched between the two sponges. A $3 \times 3$ cm$^2$ open-ended waveguide was used to detect the emitted microwave radiation. The experimental results shown in Figure 9.6 illustrate that the injection of small amounts of water in the lung region beneath the chest-wall layer resulted in an immediate and definite change in the radiometric signature. It is important to note that the output signal tends to reach a new steady-state level after each injection. The peak that occurs after each injection is due to the initial squirt of water, which slowly diffuses into the sponge model.

Thus, both active microwave sensing and passive radiometry techniques are found to provide sufficient sensitivity for continuous monitoring of pulmonary edema in preliminary investigations. The feasibility of using the active microwave measurements has been demonstrated on phantoms, isolated dog lungs, and anesthetized dogs with induced pulmonary edema. The results clearly illustrated that the method is sensitive enough to measure small changes in lung water content. The model calculations and preliminary investigations in phantoms showed a passive radiometer measurement of changes in microwave emission with lung water content as little as 3–4%. The encouraging initial results from both active and passive sensing stimulated further development, especially, of the less complex active approach for clinical applications.

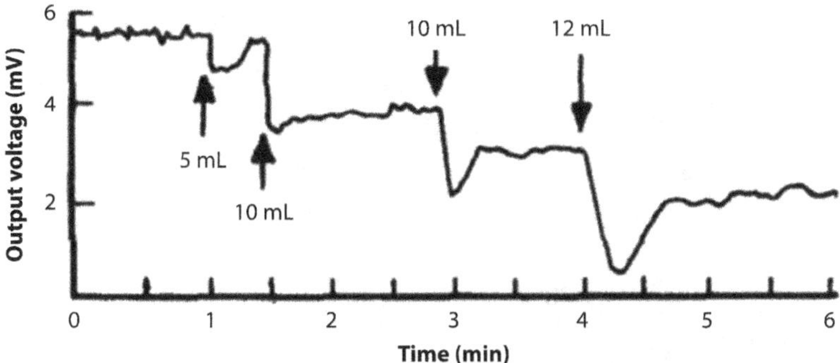


**FIGURE 9.6** Radiometric response to injections of water in a model of the human thorax. The phantom model's emissivity decreases as the volume of water increases.

### 9.2.2 Wideband Microwave Scanning

Recently, the basic concept of microwave sensing of pulmonary edema described previously and the results of feasibility studies using prototype systems have been extended through antenna design, instrumentation updates, and system upgrades, including the use of wideband microwave operation and automated scanning [Rezaeieh et al., 2014]. The wide-band system operates in the frequency range of 0.77–1 GHz from a microwave transceiver. The system's hardware comprises a custom-designed directional antenna, a controllable scanning stand, and a laptop with installed software algorithms for control, signal processing, and visualization. A functional component block diagram of the system is shown in Figure 9.7. A coax-coplanar-waveguide-fed slot antenna design with the configuration shown in Figure 9.8 provided the desired

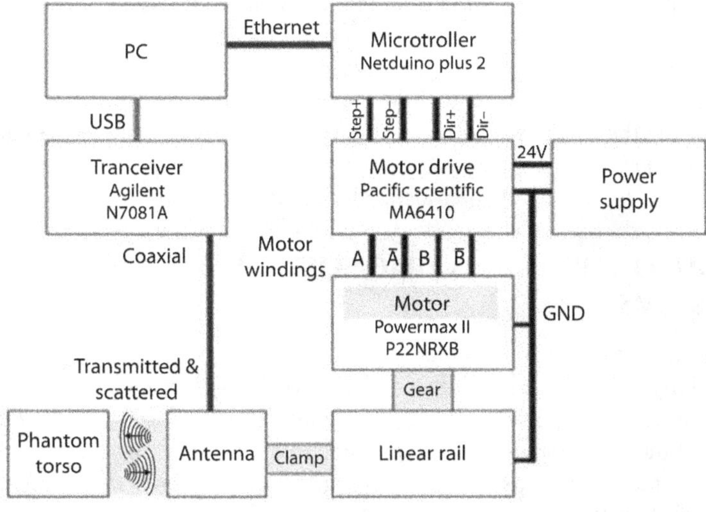


**FIGURE 9.7** A functional block diagram of the wideband microwave automated scanning system.

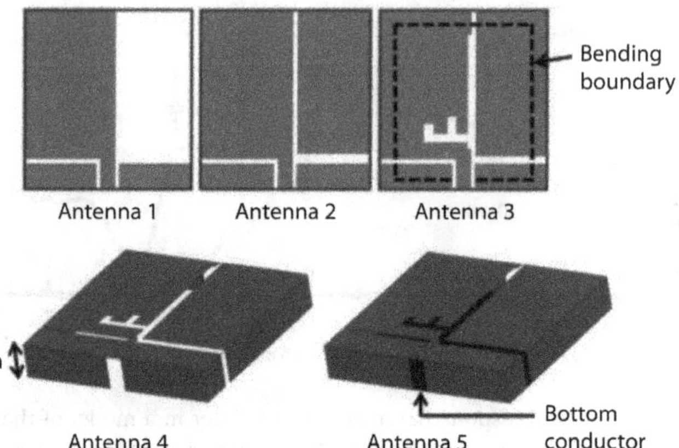


**FIGURE 9.8** Configuration of a coax-coplanar-waveguide-fed prototype slot antenna design: The evolution process of antenna 1 to antenna 5.

unidirectional radiation pattern. The system is controlled by a laptop computer, which is connected to a microwave transceiver on one side and to a stepper motor on the other side. The microwave transceiver is connected to the antenna that is attached to the automated vertical scanning platform in the form of a linear rail that is moved by the stepper motor. The antenna scans vertically along the back side of a human torso phantom and receives the backscattered signals in typical monostatic-radar mode.

The received signals are processed and then transformed into images showing the scattering profile inside the torso. Specifically, the frequency-dependent backscattered signals are converted to time-domain signals and then visualized as radar echo images. These images show the intensity of scattering within different regions in the torso and can be used to assess the fluid content of lungs inside the torso. In this case, for simplicity and to facilitate visualization, the differences between the scattering signal profiles received from the left and right lungs are obtained by subtracting them from each other. Figure 9.9 shows that the system can detect as low as 4 mL of water inside the lungs, which is close to the lowest level required for early detection of pulmonary edema. The result reinforces the noninvasive microwave system's potential to be an efficacious diagnostic and monitoring tool.

## 9.3 PULMONARY EDEMA DIAGNOSTIC AND MONITORING SYSTEMS

The previous discussions in this chapter indicate that low-power microwave systems are potentially valuable as a noninvasive diagnostic instrument and monitoring tool in the management of pulmonary diseases connected to lung function. The reports also suggest the need for further development in optimal frequency of operation and appropriate antenna designs for better coupling of the microwave signal into chest tissues, including the use of lower frequencies in the radio frequency (RF) range below 300 MHz, with less positional sensitivity. Smaller applicator profiles would offer patient comfort during sleep or under other long-term monitoring scenarios.

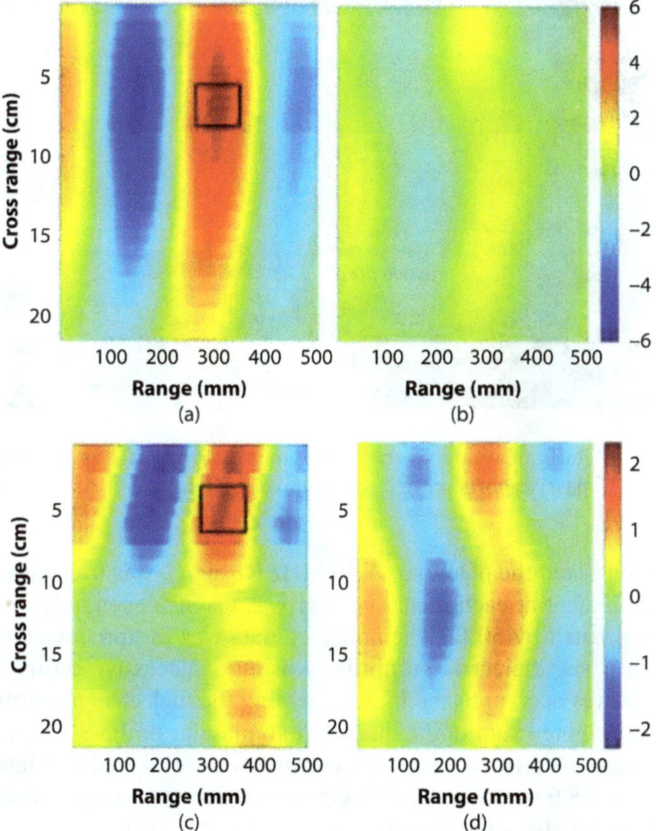


**FIGURE 9.9** Differential scattering profile of lowest detectable fluid compared to normal cases with identical scaling: (a) 10 mL water, (b) normal; and (c) 4 mL water, (d) normal. (Rezaeieh et al., 2014.)

### 9.3.1 Body-Area Network-Integrated RF Sensor

A prototype of a wearable noninvasive RF sensor front end for the diagnosis of pulmonary edema is shown in Figure 9.10. The sensor is intended to be placed on the human chest to detect water-content changes in the lungs by measuring the lung's average dielectric permittivity [Salman et al., 2014]. It is based on measurements of the fringe 40 MHz RF field scattered through chest tissues from an active port. The amplitude of the scattering parameters (S-parameters) received at each of the 15 ports are subsequently postprocessed to determine the tissue's permittivity changes.

The performance of the sensor was evaluated experimentally on a human torso phantom combined with porcine lungs to demonstrate its practicability and reliability in detecting abnormalities of the lungs. Fresh porcine lung tissues were secured in place using foam blocks and the sensor was placed on top of the cutaneous tissue mimicking gels (see Figure 9.11). The phantom was then laid in the prone position and remained as such throughout the measurement to ensure no air gaps existed

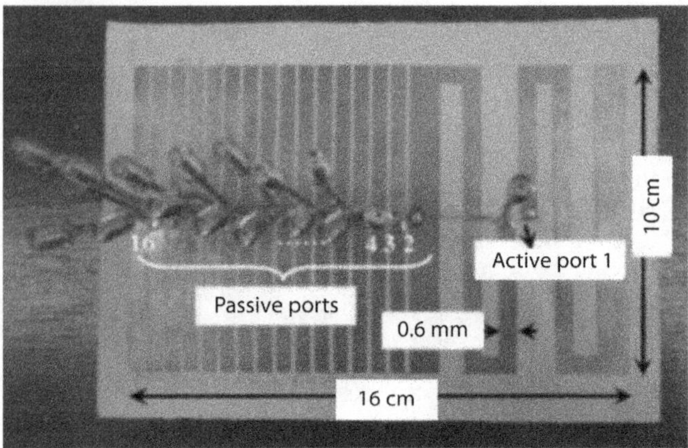


**FIGURE 9.10** Details of wearable sensor antenna: active port 1 is the radio frequency transmitter and 15 passive ports serve as the receivers. (Courtesy of Asimina Kiourti, Ohio State University.)

between the lungs and the phantom. A 40 MHz RF signal was transmitted from port #1, and measurement at each receiving port was taken sequentially, with the inactive ports terminated by 50 Ω. The collected data was postprocessed to determine the change in tissue dielectric permittivity using a successive estimation scheme. The extraction was accomplished by representing the dielectric permittivity at each depth using a weighted sum of the measured amplitudes of the S-parameters (transmission coefficients). Also, a body-area network was developed and integrated with the direct-contact RF sensors to enable continuous remote access of measured data.

Hollow plastic balls (diameter = 2 cm) filled with distilled water were inserted inside the porcine lungs to simulate pulmonary edema. RF transmission coefficients measured using the prototype sensor system are given in Figure 9.12 for porcine

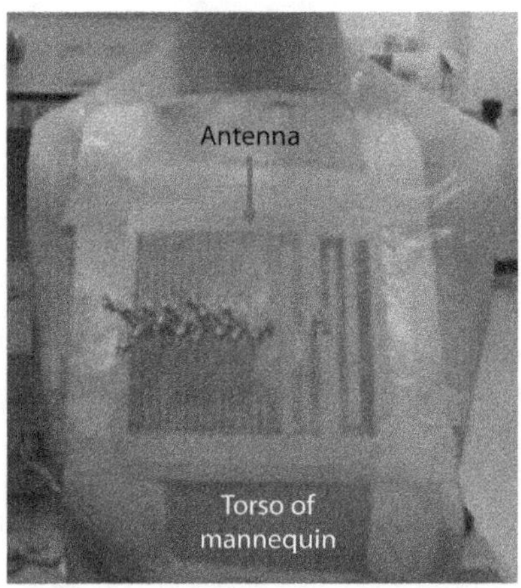


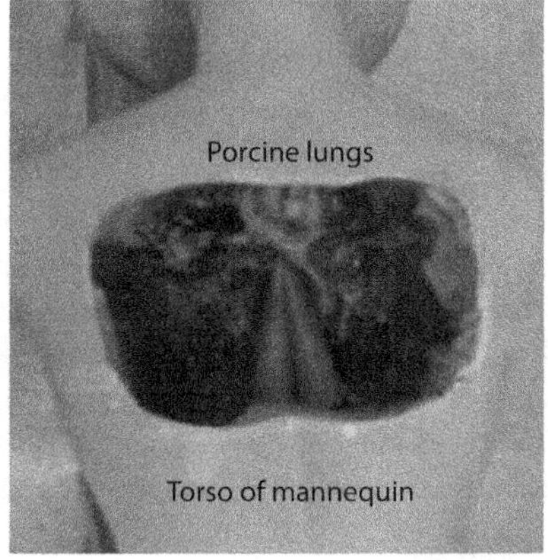


**FIGURE 9.11** Antenna placement on torso of mannequin and placement of porcine lungs inside the torso. (Courtesy of Asimina Kiourti, Ohio State University.)

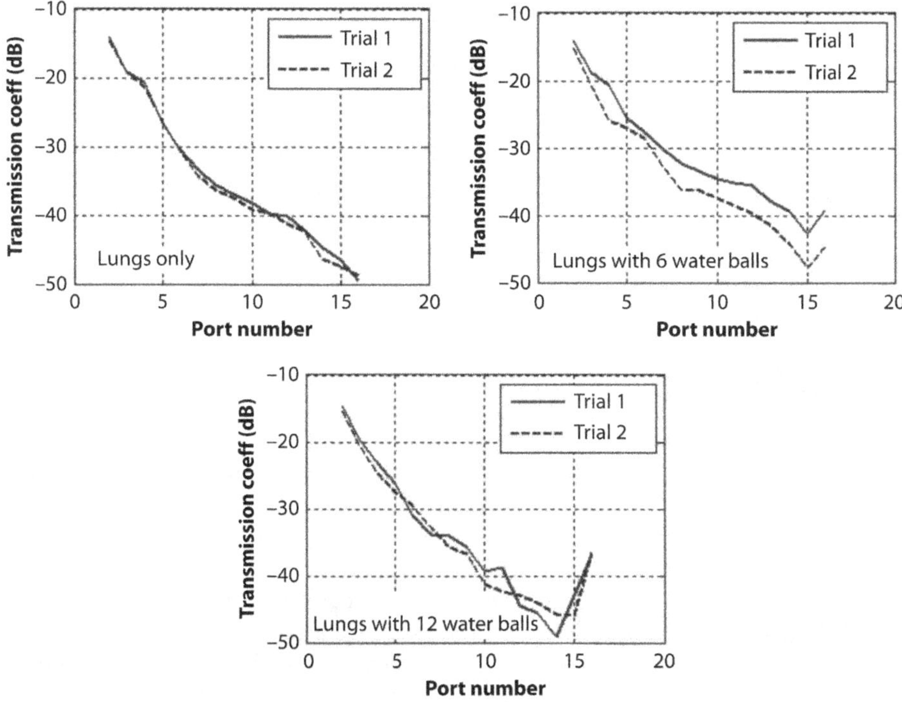


**FIGURE 9.12** Transmission coefficients of radio frequency signals measured using a prototype sensor system for diagnosis of pulmonary edema: (a) with porcine lung alone, (b) with six water balls inserted into the porcine lungs, and (c) with 12 water balls inserted into the porcine lungs.

lungs alone, with six plastic balls of water, and with 12 plastic balls of water inserted into the porcine lungs. As expected, the transmission coefficients varied from port to port. However, comparable results are obtained between the two sets of measurements in each case. Dielectric probe measurements of normal lung tissue permittivity, estimates of abnormal lung tissue permittivity using volumetric proportions between lung tissue and water, and sensor-detected results are compared in Table 9.1. It is seen that the differences are within 11%. These results demonstrate the feasibility of RF sensors in detecting lung-water content changes based on the dielectric permittivity variations. Distilled water was used in this study. It would have been a better or more appropriate model if physiological saline was used instead, although it may not have any effect concerning the outcome of feasibility assessment.

### 9.3.2 Wideband Near-Field Microwave Detection

A noninvasive microwave system for near-field detection of pulmonary edema using a foam-based bed platform that contains two linear arrays of wideband antennas operating over the band 0.7–1 GHz has been reported in a preclinical investigation [Rezaeieh et al., 2015]. The directional antennas consist of a meandered loop, a

**TABLE 9.1**
**Comparison of Dielectric Probe Measured, Estimated, and Sensor-Detected Values of Dielectric Permittivity from 2 Different Trials**

| Experimental Trials | Probe Measured or Estimated Permittivity | Sensor Detected Permittivity | % Error |
|---|---|---|---|
| Lung tissue only #1 | 106.80 | 96.40 | 9.74 |
| Lung tissue only #2 | 106.80 | 99.92 | 6.44 |
| 6 lungs/water balls #1 | 99.67 | 89.47 | 10.44 |
| 6 lungs/water balls #2 | 99.67 | 94.06 | 3.70 |
| 12 lungs/water balls #1 | 95.30 | 89.37 | 6.22 |
| 12 lungs/water balls #2 | 95.30 | 89.39 | 9.82 |

L-shaped monopole, and a parasitic patch. The computed front-to-back ratio of the microwave fields gave a value of 4:1, which bolsters the directivity of the antenna across its operating band. The platform is designed for the subject to lie on the bed with the back of the torso in front of the antenna arrays during tests (Figure 9.13). The system consists of a hardware unit for data acquisition and software unit for signal processing and image formation. Two antenna arrays separated by 11 cm are located between the left and right lungs. They are connected to a vector network analyzer, which generates the microwave signal and serves as the transceiver for the system. It transmits the microwave signal to the antenna arrays and receives the backscattered signals from the torso through the antenna arrays. The scanning of the torso area takes place along the central lines of the two lungs and results are sent as

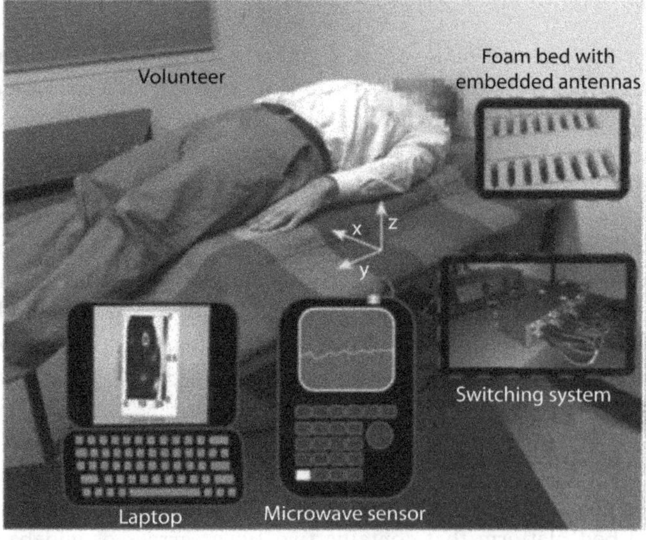


**FIGURE 9.13** Experimental arrangement of a near-field microwave pulmonary edema sensing system with an antenna array embedded inside a foam bed. (Rezaeieh et al., 2015.)

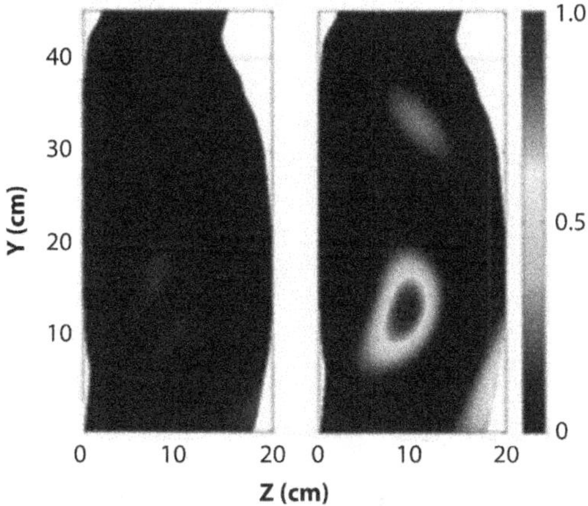


**FIGURE 9.14** Images obtained using an 8 × 2 array configuration for a torso phantom: (Left) Normal artificial lungs without water and (right) abnormal artificial lungs with 1 mL inserted water.

digital data to a laptop. A frequency-based imaging algorithm is used to process the received signals and generate an image of the scattered field inside the torso to reveal accumulated fluids in the lungs. Essentially, the received signal intensity as a function of the distance and angle of each point within the imaged domain (torso) relative to the antenna's position is summarized over all the antennas from each array and displayed as variations of dielectric permittivity inside the torso.

The system and algorithm were tested using a phantom torso with artificial and animal lungs. Figure 9.14 presents the difference values obtained after subtracting the scattering profiles of right and left sides of phantom torso from each other. Data are from two arrays of eight antennas each. The subtraction images for normal and abnormal (artificial lungs with 1 mL water content) cases are shown. Note the high contrast region at the lower portion of the phantom showing presence of water in the artificial lungs.

The system's ability to monitor different volumes of accumulated fluid was assessed by inserting varying amounts of water into the artificial lungs. The scattered signal intensity is shown in Figure 9.15. The intensity of the reconstructed scattered field is seen to increase linearly with the amount of water inside the artificial lungs. Thus, the data shown in Figure 9.15 suggest that the near-field microwave approach may be used to evaluate changes of fluid accumulation at different stages of edema development. Note that zero volume is for the typical lungs, and the intensity values are normalized to the value at 100 mL fluid volume.

In further experimentation with the system, the artificial lungs in the phantom torso were replaced with lamb lungs for a more realistic model scenario. To simulate pulmonary edema, 1 mL of water was injected into the lower side of the left lung. A display of the variations of "dielectric permittivity" inside the torso is depicted in Figure 9.16. While the images showed some differences from the artificial lungs, the enhanced signal intensity showing water presence is obvious and is considerably

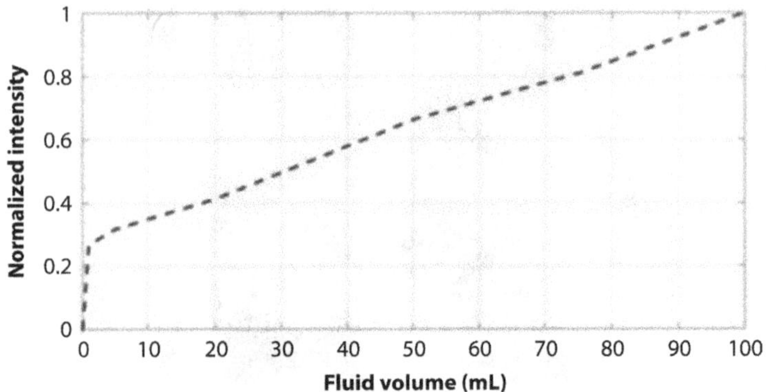


**FIGURE 9.15** Variation of the intensity of differential scattered field with the increase of water volume in the lungs using arrays of eight antennas (normalized with respect to the field value at 100 mL fluid volume).

stronger at the location of lung tissues with increased water content by as much as a ratio of 2.5:1.

As a feasibility study, a series of preclinical tests were conducted on normal (volunteer) particpants to help determinate the type or nature of the reconstructed images. A further goal was to investigate the range of acquired intensity levels for the scattering profile of the torso. Examples of the images obtained are depicted in Figure 9.17 for participants with different body dimensions. The images are normalized to the maximum field intensity obtained over all volunteers. In each image, a high scattering location is seen in the upper region of the torso. The location of this scatterer and the high dielectric permittivity of organs in the upper torso indicate that the high intensity is due to the blood inside the heart. This suggests the system's capacity to detect strong scatterers within the chest. As a corollary, when presented

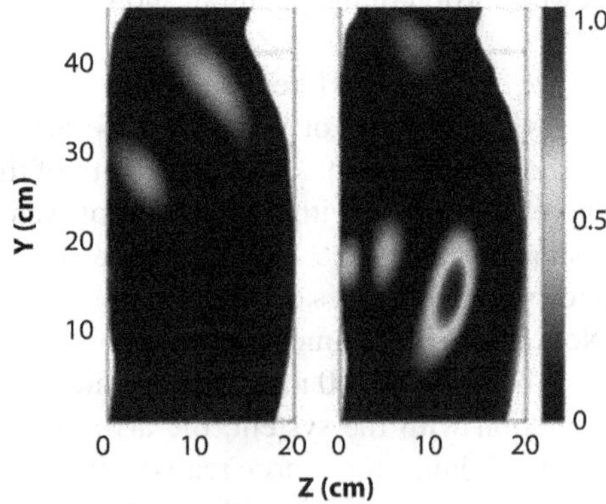


**FIGURE 9.16** Images from using 8 × 2 antenna array configuration for a phantom torso with animal lungs: (Left) normal lamb lungs and (right) abnormal lamb lungs with 1 mL injected water.

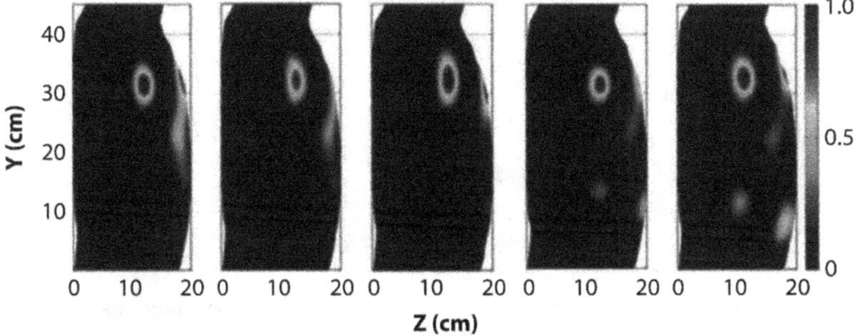


**FIGURE 9.17** A set of scattered field intensity images obtained from healthy volunteers. The high-intensity area corresponds to the location of the heart in the human volunteers.

with lungs with accumulated fluid, it is expected that the field images would show the water inside the lungs as the high-intensity scatterer. Moreover, a 10% variation in field intensities was observed from the limited set of images inside the upper body.

In summary, although preliminary, these results from phantom modeling and preclinical studies are encouraging and present the possibility of a noninvasive microwave system and platform for early detection and monitoring of pulmonary edema, regardless of its cardiogenic causes such as congestive heart failure, or others, like respiratory infection and distresses, that can lead to fatal consequences.

## 9.4 COMMERCIAL WEARABLE SENSING SYSTEMS

In recent years, some innovative wearable noninvasive systems have been introduced commercially for early detection of pulmonary edema using microwaves in the lower RF band. Interestingly, the microwave technique applied in the commercial devices for sensing pulmonary edema use the simple functional designs that are fundamentally the same as those shown in Chapter 1, Figure 1.3 and as discussed in the previous chapter on vital-sign sensing. From the perspective of sensor front ends, they are akin to the prototype two-antenna transmission and reflection microwave sensing system described previously, instead of the more sophisticated systems presented in Section 9.3. In one case, it applies the transmission mode of operation and in another, it uses the backscattered signal or reflection scheme. Aside from the low power demand and remote access through wireless data links, salient features of the devices include integrated component designs and streamlined and compact forms, as well as the convenience and simplicity in operation for body attachment or placement of sensors.

### 9.4.1 Wearable Near-Field RF Sensing System

A noninvasive RF sensor for the measurement of lung fluid using specially designed radar sensors in a wearable vest was tested to validate its efficacy in providing absolute percentage readings of fluid in a patient's lungs [Amir et al., 2016]. The sensor with two antennas embedded in a wearable vest is fitted to the body: one anteriorly

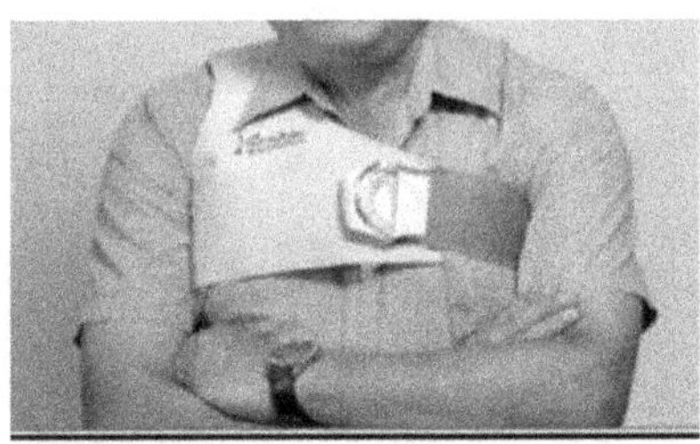

**FIGURE 9.18** A commercial noncontact near-field sensor with antennas embedded in a wearable vest over clothing. (Amir et al., 2016.)

on the chest and the other posteriorly on the patient's back (see Figure 9.18). Each antenna is a small round sensor capable of transmitting and receiving the RF signal through the lungs. Dielectric permittivity of the segment of lungs between the antennas is obtained from the signals that propagate between the two antennas.

The wearable RF sensor [ReDS, 2016] was tested to assess its accuracy in measuring lung fluid content by comparing it with that measured by chest CT, currently the most accurate method for quantitating lung fluid content in humans. Patients with and without acute heart failure (AHF) were recruited to represent lung fluid contents spanning the range expected in clinical use. Each participant underwent RF sensor and CT measurements by a trained technologist to quantify lung fluid content according to a standardized protocol. During the measurements, a spirometer was used for the registration of a breathing pattern to enable comparison between the two modalities at the same stage of respiration. CT images were converted to percentage units for comparison with the ReDS readings on 16 AHF and 15 non-AHF participants. The analyses were performed by an independent observer blinded to RF sensor outcomes.

A comparison of CT and RF sensor-detected pulmonary fluid content is given in Figure 9.19. The average and standard deviation (SD) for the non-AHF group were $29.7 \pm 5.9\%$ and $29.3 \pm 6.6\%$ and for the AHF patients $40.7 \pm 9.8\%$ and $39.8 \pm 6.8\%$ (CT and RF, respectively). Intraclass correlation was found to be 0.90 (95% CI:0.8–0.95). Regression analysis yielded a slope of 0.94 (95%, CI: 0.77–1.12) and intercept 3.10 (95%, CI: −3.02–9.21). The absolute mean difference between the quantification of the two methods was 3.75% with SD of 2.22%. An interesting observation is that the percentage reading of fluid in the lungs from RF sensing may not depend on its baseline reading. The findings of a high correlation between the CT and noninvasive RF in both AHF and non-AHF participants suggest RF sensing using the ReDS system could be helpful in managing pulmonary edema of patients with AHF.

### 9.4.2 Noncontact Near-Field Patch Sensor

The ability of a noninvasive RF near-field device ($\mu$Cor, Zoll, USA) to sense pulmonary edema was recently evaluated in hospitalized patients both with and without AHF [Wheatley-Guy et al., 2020]. In this validation study, the wearable RF patch sensor measured lung-fluid content was compared to thoracic CT-determined fluid

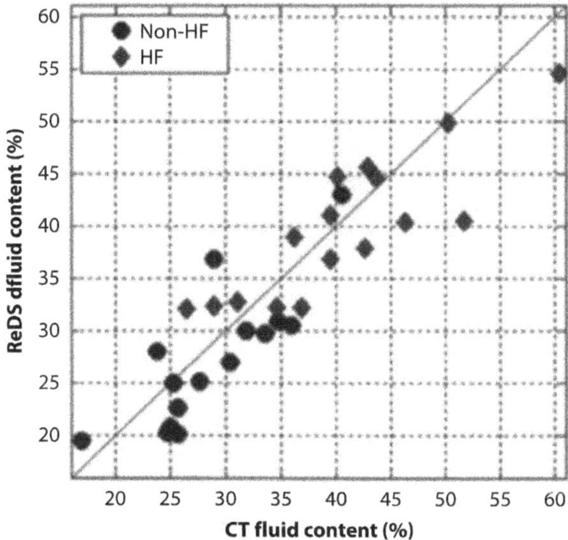


**FIGURE 9.19** Comparison of lung fluid level in participants (N = 31) quantitated using computerized tomography and noninvasive radio frequency sensing.

volume. The average time between the CT scan and RF measurements was 2 hours or less. The CT values were converted to a percentage rating to calculate fluid content by expressing lung fluid as a percentage of the lungs. This allows for comparison of CT lung fluid and RF lung fluid in the same units of measure.

The noninvasive RF system consists of an adhesive patch and a removable antenna sensor. The sensor is placed in the patch via snap-in clip and positioning tabs (Figure 9.20). The patch along with antenna sensor is placed on the body in the left anterior axillary position (Figure 9.21). A pulsed RF signal is transmitted from the antenna, which propagates primarily through the left lung in the thoracic cavity, as it is limited by tissue attenuation characteristics of the RF propagation channel. The backscattered signal is received by the same antenna as a reflected signal from tissues. The amplitude, phase, and time of arrival of the reflected RF pulse are used to measure lung fluid content. The RF-measured fluid contents in the sitting and supine body positions are shown in Figure 9.22. A strong correlation (0.96, $p < 0.01$) was found between the two positions, suggesting the short duration in the supine position did not cause sufficient shifts in fluid distribution. Accordingly, only the supine position RF fluid content was used to compare to the fluid content from CT. So, the body positions are identical for both methods of measurement.

Both CT and RF measured fluid content had a sensitivity of 70% and specificity of 80%. A comparison of the fluid contents measured by CT and RF is given in Figure 9.23. The correlation between fluid content measured by two modalities is $r = 0.7$ ($p < 0.001$). RF measured fluid content in the AHF group was 20.7 ± 5.6% compared to 15.6 ± 3.3% in the non-AHF group ($p < 0.05$). Fluid content in the left lung was not different between stable AHF and healthy participants (19.0 ± 1.8% vs. 16.3 ± 1.5%, $p = 0.16$). Thus, the lung-fluid contents measured noninvasively

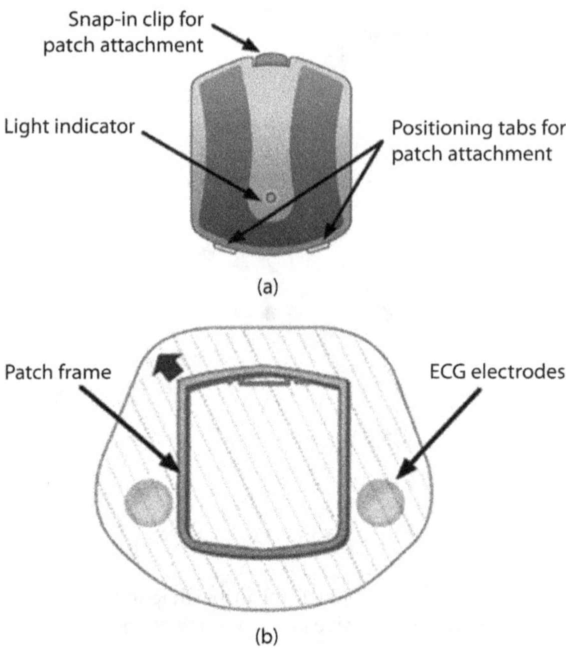


**FIGURE 9.20** A noninvasive radio frequency pulmonary edema sensing system with an adhesive patch and a removable antenna sensor: (a) Sensor's front view and (b) adhesive patch. (Wheatley-Guy et al., 2020.)

showed similar sensitivity and specificity as thoracic CT in discriminating AHF patients from normal subjects. These results validate the capability of the noninvasive RF sensor in assessing lung fluid content associated with pulmonary edema. The noninvasive RF sensor provides a potential alternative to other modalities for diagnosing and monitoring pulmonary edema and for managing AHF patients with fluid problems.

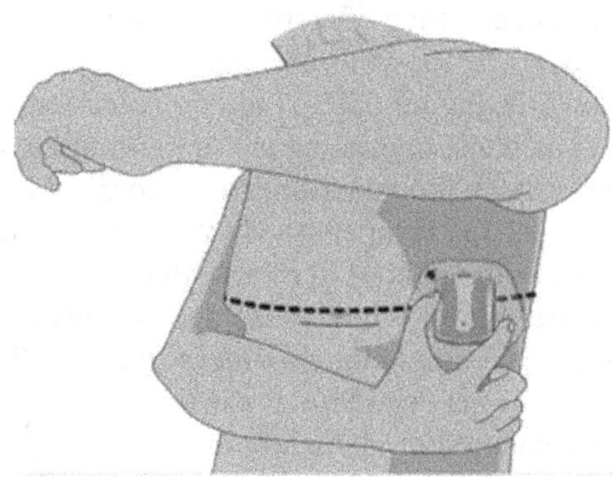

**FIGURE 9.21** Placement of the sensor and patch in the left anterior axillary. (Wheatley-Guy et al., 2020.)

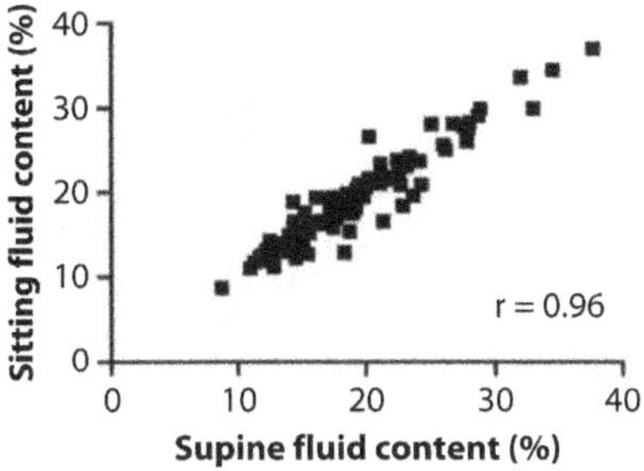


**FIGURE 9.22** Comparison of radio frequency-measured pulmonary fluid content based on subject's sitting versus supine body position.

## 9.5 NEAR-FIELD RESPIRATORY VOLUME SENSING

Despite the efforts discussed previously, respiratory volume changes remain difficult to measure with accuracy as it is influenced by body posture and sensor design, position, and orientation. Recently, a different measurement technique — placing multiple sensing antennas through clothing over the upper torso — was proposed that enable near-field detection of respiratory movements induced by modulations on the microwave signal [Sharma et al., 2020]. The noninvasive approach works by transmitting a low-power CW microwave signal into the body using software-defined radio (SDR) transceivers. The prototype system involves the belting of two lightweight, near-field microwave sensors (NCS) on a subject through clothing. One wearable antenna sensor is strapped close to the heart on the chest and the other below the xiphoid process of the sternum to monitor heart, lungs, and diaphragm movements to measure respiratory rate (RR) and volume (RV). Figure 9.24 shows the experimental arrangement of the prototype system and test instruments. It exhibits the attachment, data collection, and signal flow of all sensors including commercial BIOPAC ECG, chest belts, and a pneumotachometer (PTM) connected to a facemask. It also shows the participant in a sitting posture instrumented with all sensors including the two wearable NCS sensors.

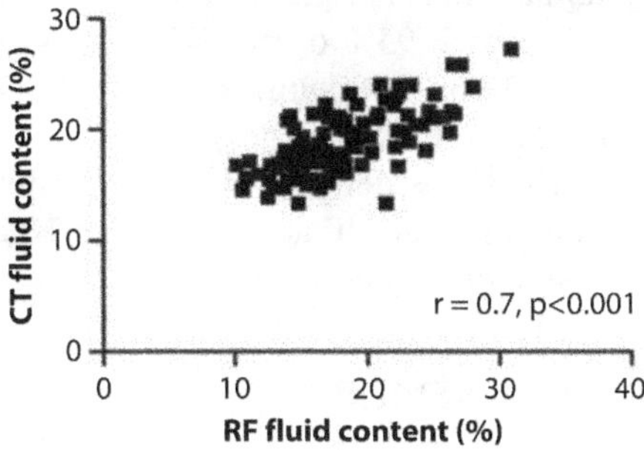


**FIGURE 9.23** Correlation between computerized tomography and radio frequency-measured fluid contents in the lungs.

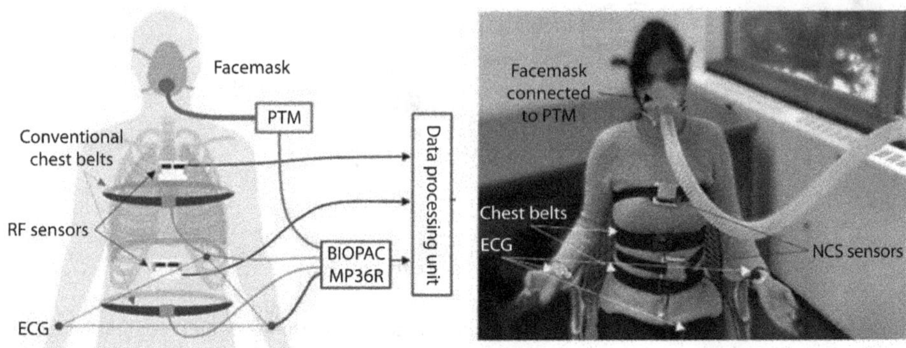


**FIGURE 9.24** Experimental arrangement of the prototype system and test components, attachments, data collection, and signal flow of all sensors including commercial BIOPAC devices, chest belts, and a pneumotachometer (PTM) connected to a facemask. (Sharma et al., 2020.)

Experimental data were obtained from 20 healthy participants (14 females and 6 males) with varying body mass index (BMI). Since RV is sensitive to body posture and breathing modes, the data were analyzed for various postures, and according to conscious and spontaneous breathing exercises with a wide breathing range (0–45 breath/m) and a resting hear rate in the range of 50–90 beat/m. A brief calibration was performed using a standard PTM for each subject and posture, and the corresponding values were used for both NCS and chest belt sensors. Figure 9.25 shows the results for NCS and PTM measured RV across three postures with different breathing modes including conscious normal, deep, fast and breath-hold (BH), as well as spontaneous breathing in relaxation and attention states. The scatter plot (top) displays the RV data with a Pearson's correlation coefficient $r = 0.84$ indicating a high-level of correlation between the two sensors.

The Bland-Altman (B&A) plot related to the mean m and standard deviation $\sigma$ of the measurement differences was employed to assess the agreement between NCS and PTM. B&A plots can also identify possible outliers in an XY scatter plot with the Y axis as the pairwise difference and the X axis as the mean of the two measurements. Any systematic bias is evaluated as the mean difference m. Limits of agreement (LoA) within which 95% of the differences are expected to lie are approximated as $\text{LoA} = m \pm 1.96\ (\sigma)$, assuming a normal distribution. Figure 9.25 (bottom) shows good agreement between the sensors with a low mean deviation mRV = 9.6 mL and narrow LoA, as denoted by the dashed lines around the mean value. Thus, the results demonstrated that noninvasive NCS microwave sensors can estimate RV with satisfactory accuracy.

## 9.6 CEREBRAL EDEMA AND ICP

Cerebral edema signifies excess fluid within the brain. It occurs when fluid builds up in and around the brain through, for example, extravasation of blood from the cerebral vasculature, causing increases in ICP and volume. Cerebral edema, elevated

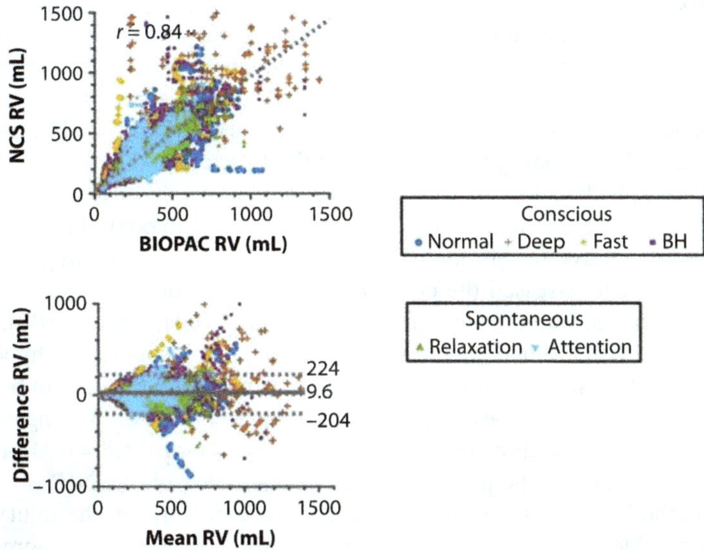


**FIGURE 9.25** Correlation and agreement between near-field microwave sensors (NCS) and pneumotachometer (PTM) measured respiratory volume (RV) for all participants. The label shows a marker for each breathing mode, including conscious normal, deep, fast and breath-hold (BH), as well as spontaneous breathing in relaxation and attention states. Also shown are the scatter plot (top) with Pearson's correlation coefficient r, and Bland-Altman plot (bottom) showing bias m at the center (solid line), and the corresponding limits of agreement (dash lines) given by m ± 2.24 ($\sigma$). (Sharma et al., 2020.)

ICP, and cerebral volume change are interrelated. Thus, cerebral herniation or tissue redistribution as a resulting medical condition can happen, where brain tissues are forced to move from one part of the brain to another adjacent part of the brain. It is usually caused by swelling or pressure elevation inside the brain. In general, cerebral edema contributes to an increase in intracranial volume. Global cerebral edema primarily results in a global rise in ICP, while focal cerebral edema can result in cerebral herniation with or without ICP elevation. The three major types of cerebral edema are classified as: 1) hydrocephalus from increased fluid around the brain, 2) hypertensive brain hemorrhage from bleeding in the brain from high blood pressure, and 3) intraventricular hemorrhage from bleeding into the fluid-filled ventricles inside the brain.

CT and MRI are commonly used for detection and assessment of cerebral edema because of their wide availability. However, a noninvasive and dependable sensor capable of early detection of cerebral edema is clinically important and remains a technological challenge.

A noninvasive near-infrared (NIR) light-scattering method was investigated for the early detection of brain swelling in mice [Thiagarajah et al., 2005]. Brain tissue was illuminated through the intact skull with NIR light at 850 nm, and the scattered light intensity was monitored at an angle of 90 degrees at a position on the skull approximately 10 mm from the illuminated site. It was reported that NIR light scattering reversibly increased with brain swelling, but was insensitive to changes in cerebral blood flow, blood oxygenation, or blood flow-related changes in ICP. However, the early kinetics of brain swelling in normal and aquaporin-4 protein (AQP4)-deficient mice showed that NIR signal increase was preceded by measurable increases in ICP, suggesting the potential of the NIR method to detect early brain edema before ICP elevation.

Recently, a newborn piglet (large animal) model of hypoxic brain injury was investigated to study the ability of NIR technology to detect hypoxia-induced cerebral edema and assessed the correlation of the NIR-derived water signal with increases in cerebral water content in the piglet brain [Malaeb et al., 2018]. Changes in NIR-derived water signal was detectable as early as 2 hours after hypoxia, and provided a five-fold signal amplification, representing a 10% increase in brain water content and a six-fold increase in AQP4, 4 hours after hypoxia. Changes in water signal correlated well with changes in cerebral water content ($R = 0.74$) and AQP4 expression ($R = 0.97$) in the piglet brain. The data indicated that NIR offers a non-invasive method to detect and monitor cerebral edema early in the injury process and could provide an opportunity to initiate therapy at an earlier and more effective time-point after an injury to the brain.

### 9.6.1 Microwave Transmission for Cerebral Edema in a Phantom Model

A novel microwave-transmission technique for noninvasive detection and monitoring cerebral edema was first reported by Lin and Clarke [1982]. The technique demonstrated that microwave signals are correlated with various quantities of excess water in a phantom head model. The noninvasive microwave technique can detect fluid volume changes as little as 1%. Specifically, it involves microwave energy at 1000–3000 MHz, which has an effective penetration depth of 2–10 cm for soft tissues and 5–18 cm for bone (see Chapter 3). Since the human skull ranges in radius from 7–10 cm, a significant amount of the impinging microwaves can be transmitted through the skull. The signature of the transmitted microwave is characterized both by the geometry and the composition of intervening tissue structures. Therefore, it provides a noninvasive method that could be useful in early detection and monitoring of cerebral edema, which may lead to a more optimal therapy that achieves maximal benefit with minimal side effects.

The use of microwaves has advantages over conventional skull X-ray radiography in that it is continuous and, at the power levels required (less than 10 $\mu W/cm^2$), has minimal health hazards. (Indeed, these power levels are about 1000 times less than the exposure to cellular mobile telephones.) Microwaves are also superior to ultrasound in imaging and sensing of the internal structures of the head. Unlike ultrasonic energy, microwaves are capable of penetrating both bone and air, allowing a significant fraction of microwaves to be transmitted through tissues of the head. Nevertheless, a nondestructive technique for diagnosis of brain edema has been reported, which is based on the characteristics of mechanical vibrations of the head system [Kostopoulos et al., 2006].

The rest of this section discusses a series of microwave transmission experiments using a phantom head model to determine the feasibility of contactless noninvasive sensing of cerebral edema. It will be followed in the next section by a detailed description of related animal investigations, indicating the ability of the microwave method to noninvasively detect cerebral edema in rats.

A three-component spherical phantom model was used to simulate a human head. It involved a 9.4 cm radius glass sphere. Inside the skull-equivalent glass sphere, a rubber balloon was filled with water to an initial volume of 550 mL to simulate CSF. The balloon was surrounded by 1150 mL of ethanol to simulate brain tissue. The ethanol and water compartments are connected to two separate 30 mL syringes through plastic tubes to allow manipulation of the relative quantity of ethanol and water. The head model was positioned on a polyform or wooden support (see Figure 9.26).

The instrumentation consisted of a microwave source, a directional coupler, two microwave applicators or antennas, an amplitude/phase detector (vector voltmeter), and a recording device, like that depicted in Chapter 1, Figure 1.3. The complete system was surrounded by microwave absorbers to reducc potential interference in the laboratory (see Figure 9.26). The technique involved transmitting a beam of 2.4 GHz CW microwave signal from one side, through the phantom head model, and receiving it on the opposite side of the microwave propagation channel. The received microwave signal was compared with the reference signal from the directional coupler, processed by the vector voltmeter, and displayed or recorded as a function of time. The transmittance variation in amplitude and phase of the received signal (transmission coefficient) is related to the variable amounts of excess water. Because of the superior sensitivity of the phase of microwave transmittance to changes of fluid contents, most experiments were conducted with phase detection.

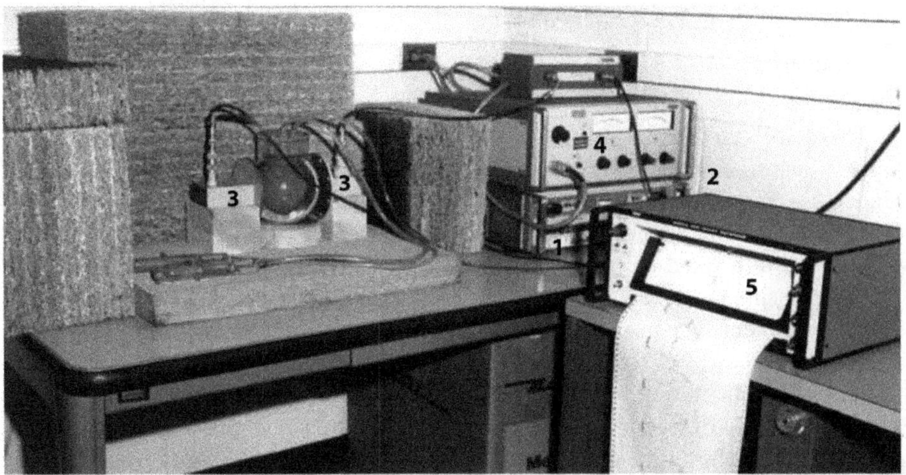


**FIGURE 9.26** Microwave instrumentation for detection and monitoring of cerebral edema: 1) Microwave signal generator, 2) directional coupler, 3) antennas, 4) vector voltmeter, and 5) chart recorder.

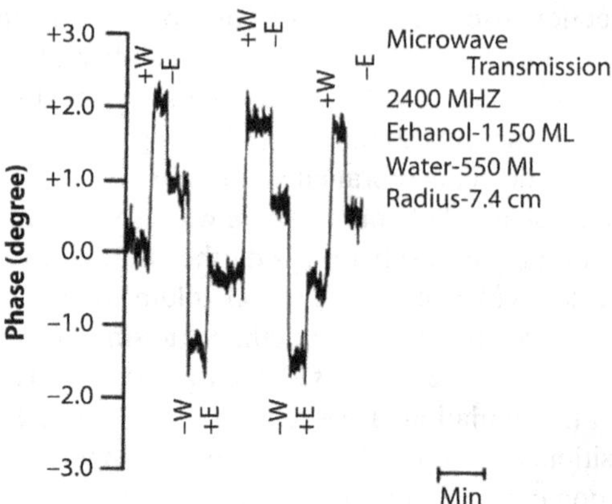


**FIGURE 9.27** Changes in the phase of microwave signal transmitted through the phantom head model. The ± signs associated with W and E correspond to addition or subtraction of 10 mL of water and ethanol.

Experimental results obtained using 2.4 GHz microwaves are shown in Figure 9.27. It is seen that phase changes in the microwave signal correlated with the addition and subtraction of water and ethanol. A change of ± 2.0° in the phase is paralleled by the addition or subtraction of 10 mL of water. Similarly, a change of 1.0° corresponded to a 10 mL change in the volume of ethanol. Clearly, this microwave technique is capable of monitoring changes as low as 1% or less in the phantom model. It is emphasized that the results are highly reliable and have been repeated over many experimental sessions. Note that the phantom head experiments are highly repeatable. The head model may be removed and then put back to achieve the same phase indications. A record of phase changes in microwave signal transmitted through a phantom head model in response to successive additions of measured amount (in mL) of saline, which mimics CSF, is given in Figure 9.28. The minute-to-minute changes in the saline addition–derived microwave phase signal was detectable instantaneously.

There are at least two possible scenarios for clinical application of this microwave transmission technique for detection and monitoring of cerebral edema. Under one scenario, the antennas may be attached to two sides of the subject's head, and the other where the subject's head is positioned between two antennas spaced at a fixed distance. The first approach is more amenable to continuous monitoring, whereas the second is more applicable for periodic assessment. With the advent of conformal, wearable antennas, the distinctions of these two scenarios become blurred or non sequitur. While definitive answers must await further experimentation, these results indicate that both approaches are feasible. For example, small lightweight microstrip antennas have been designed and fabricated in many laboratories for direct-contact uses. Noninvasive microwave sensing is envisioned to be most suited for direct contact continuous monitoring situations. In this case, motion artifacts could become a potential difficulty. However, motion-related artifacts usually are transient in nature, so they may not seriously disrupt the measurement or could be mitigated through realistic signal-processing

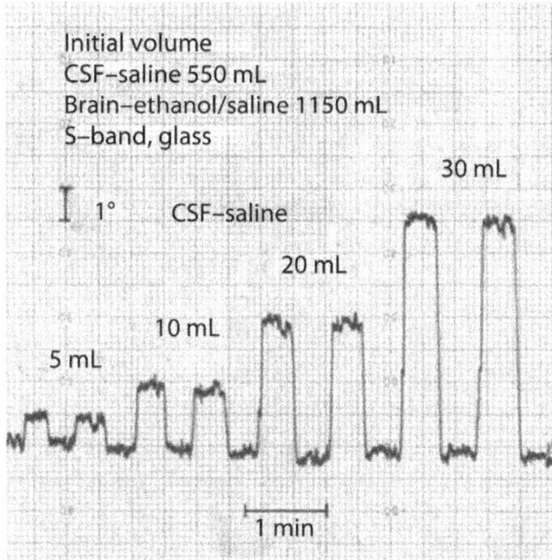


**FIGURE 9.28** Phase changes in microwave signal transmitted through a phantom head model in response to successive additions of a measured amount (in mL) of saline (mimicking cerebrospinal fluid [CSF]).

schemes. As with any new procedure, considerable data and experience must be accumulated before introduction into the medical clinic.

### 9.6.2 Microwave Sensing of Cerebral Edema in Animal Model

Although results from the phantom modeling study are encouraging and the microwave properties of the phantom model closely resemble those of mammalian cranial tissues, applicability of the noninvasive microwave technique in humans and laboratory animals needs confirmation. Note that this technique involves low levels of nonionizing microwaves and can cost effectively support continuous monitoring on a long-term basis with minimal health hazard. The initial animal experiments [Clarke and Lin, 1983] showed that microwave sensing can detect small volume and pressure changes, indicating that pathologic pressures inside the brain may be sensed *in vivo* noninvasively.

Adult Wistar Rats (550 g) were anesthetized with Nembutal (40/mg/kg, IP). A tracheotomy was performed and the animal intubated with a cannula 3 mm in diameter. A midline insertion on the dorsal surface of the skull was made and extended laterally on both sides, forming two flaps of skin. The tissue on the skull was dissected away. The exposed bone on the dorsal and lateral sides was thoroughly cleaned for bonding purposes. A small burr hole was made through one of the lateral sides of the skull. A 1 mm outer diameter catheter was inserted through the burr hole, 2 mm beneath the skull in the epidural space for aliquot injections and infusion of 2% saline. A second burr hole was made through the dorsal surface of the skull on the contralateral side. Another catheter (1.1 mm OD) filled with saline was inserted 2 mm beneath the skull in the epidural space and connected to a Statham pressure transducer for recording ICP. A dental compound was applied to the surface of the skull to seal the catheter in place. A paralytic dose of Curare (3 mg/kg) was administered to stabilize the baseline recording.

Microwave absorbers were placed on all sides of the experimental setup to eliminate potential interference in the laboratory, as shown in Figure 9.26. Two coaxial or waveguide antennas are positioned firmly against the skull on either side served as the transmitting or receiving antennas. A beam of 2.4 GHz CW microwave was propagated through the rat's head. The phase of transmittance was compared with the reference input signal, following appropriate conditioning and processing, the phase signal was displayed as the output, along with ICP and ECG. A schematic diagram of the experimental system is shown in Figure 9.29.

A previously published procedure [Wilkinson et al., 1981] was employed in performing the step volume tests. Specifically, rapid injections of an aliquot of 2% saline equaling 0.4%, 0.8%, 2%, 2.8%, and 4% of the rat's brain volume (approximately, 2.5 mL) were used. In another 4 animals, 2% saline was infused at the rates of 0.09, 0.16, 0.33, and 0.4 mL/min. Suction tests, performed in 5 experiments, consisted of a rapid withdrawal of the syringe plunger to volumes of 0.02 and 0.05 mL, respectively. All steps of injection and infusion were performed in the lower region of the pressure volume curve, so that viability of the animal preparation was maintained throughout the experiment.

Representative recordings of relative phase and ICP for an injection of an aliquot of saline (0.07 mL) followed by another injection (0.05 mL) are given in Figure 9.30. A sharp increase in ICP is paralleled by a negative increase in phase. While ICP returns exponentially to a low level, a smaller and slower secondary negative increase occurred in the phase. Both relative phase and ICP approach levels that are elevated relative to normal. Following the second injection, the phase and ICP responses are similar to those of the first injection.

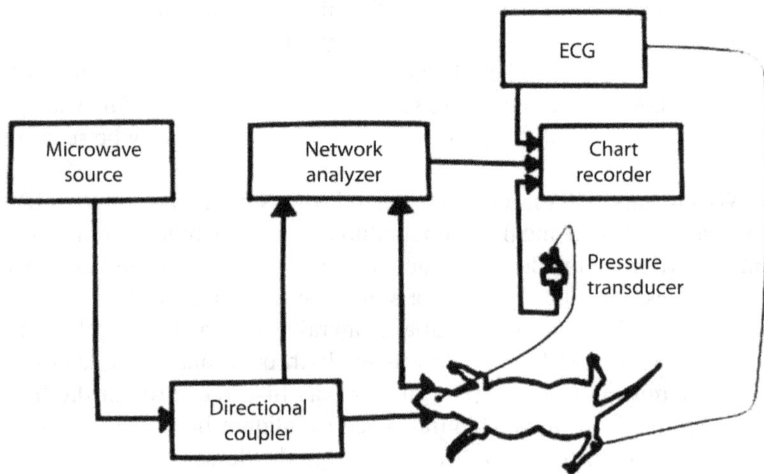


**FIGURE 9.29** Schematic diagram of experimental setup for recording microwave phase change, electrocardiogram, and intracranial pressure.

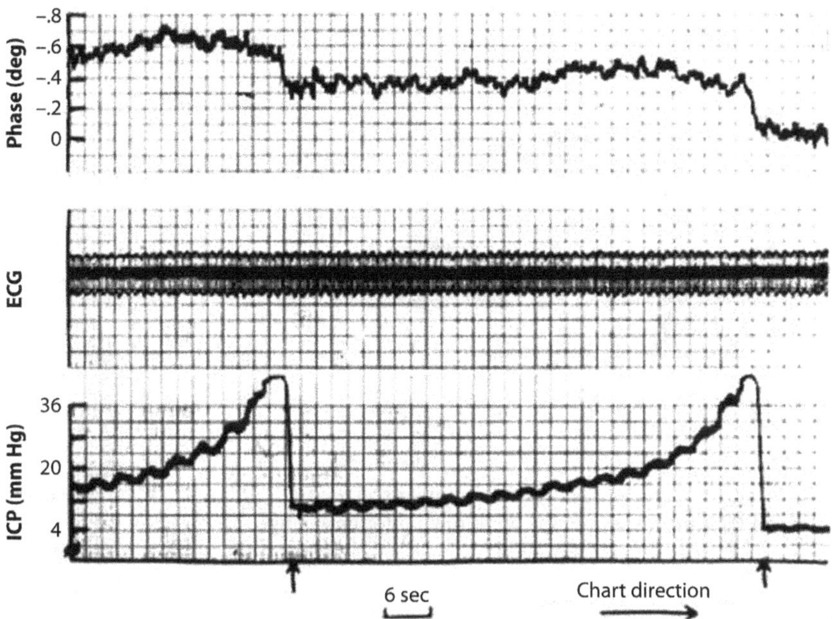


**FIGURE 9.30** Changes in relative phase, electrocardiogram (ECG), and intracranial pressure (ICP) following saline injections (see arrows) of 0.07 mL and 0.05 mL, respectively.

Typical phase and ICP changes after suction are shown in Figure 9.31. Relative phase reaches a maximum value in the positive direction as ICP decreases by approximately by 1 mm Hg relative to normal. Figure 9.32 presents a graph of the maximum phase change versus maximum ICP change for a series of aliquot injections in one experiment.

Figure 9.33 depicts representative recordings of phase and ICP during the continuous infusion. Before the start of infusion (upward arrow), the phase and ICP are stable for several minutes. During the infusion of saline (0.16 mL/min), the phase and ICP slowly approach values of –3 and 10 mm Hg, respectively. The large value of phase change, –3, when compared with maximum phase changes in the step volume experiments is consistent with the relative amount of saline infused (0.44 mL after 3 minutes vs. 0.07 mL and a maximum phase change of 0.7 for the step volume injection) (Figure 9.32). However, the maximum level of pressure reached in the infusion test, 10 mm Hg, is comparable to the lower level of maximum ICP reached in the step volume experiments. After a volume of 0.5 mL had been infused, the infusion pump was turned off (see downward arrow in Figure 9.34). The phase and ICP slowly returned to normal levels, at a slightly different rate, over a period of several minutes. Figure 9.35 is a representative recording taken 1 minute after the respirator had been turned off, showing a period of hypoxia. It is seen that associated with each heartbeat, there is a transient change in the phase and ICP recordings alongside bradycardia.

Aliquot injection and continuous infusion of saline at constant rates produces increased intracranial water content that was detectable in the microwave phase

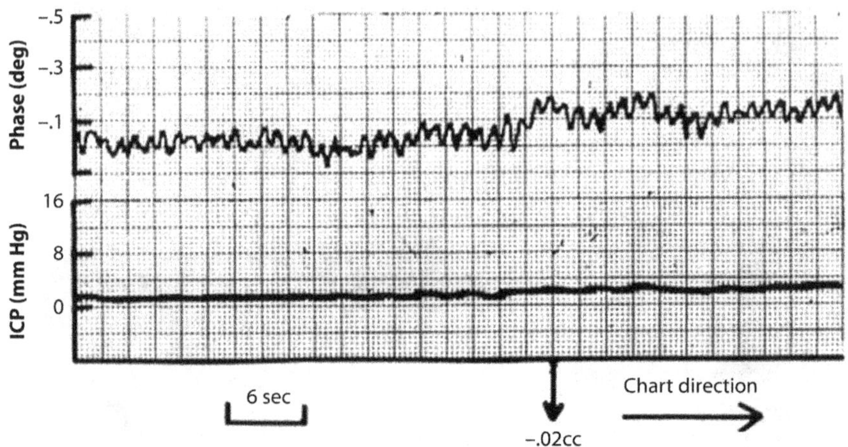


**FIGURE 9.31** Relative phase and intracranial pressure (ICP) following suction (see arrow). A volume of 0.02 mL of saline was withdrawn into the syringe.

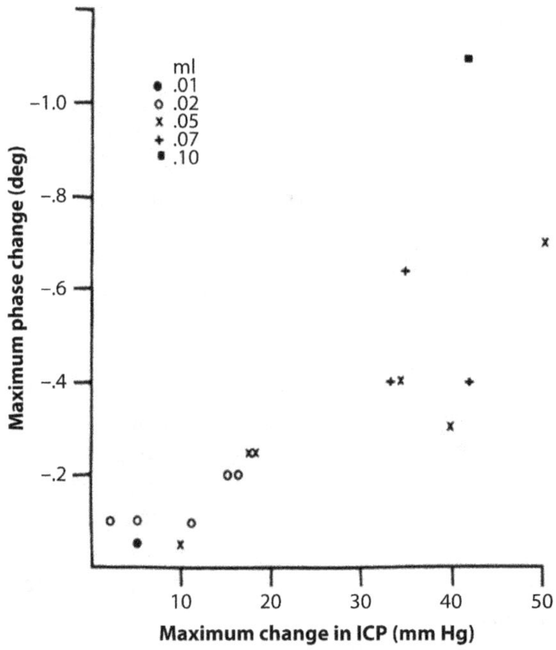


**FIGURE 9.32** Maximum phase change versus maximum intracranial pressure (ICP) change for injection of aliquots. Volumes of aliquot are shown by symbols.

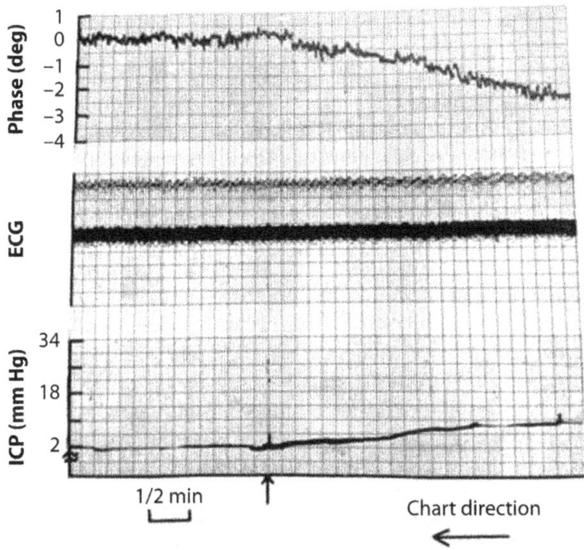


**FIGURE 9.33** Change in phase, electrocardiogram (ECG), and intracranial pressure (ICP) following a saline infusion (see upward arrow) of 0.16 mL/min.

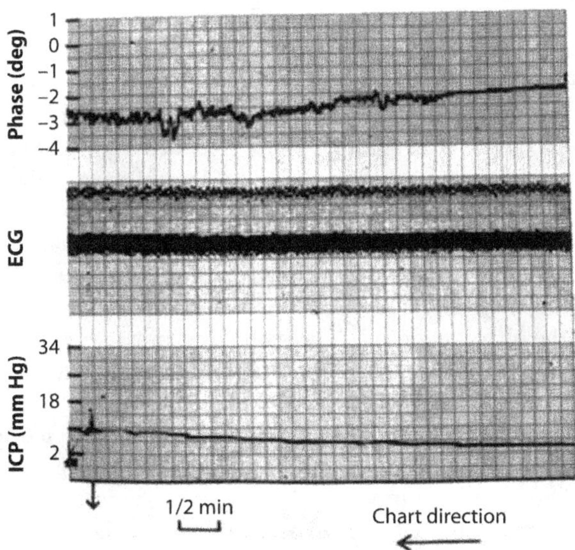


**FIGURE 9.34** Return of relative phase toward the baseline after cessation of a saline infusion (see downward arrow).

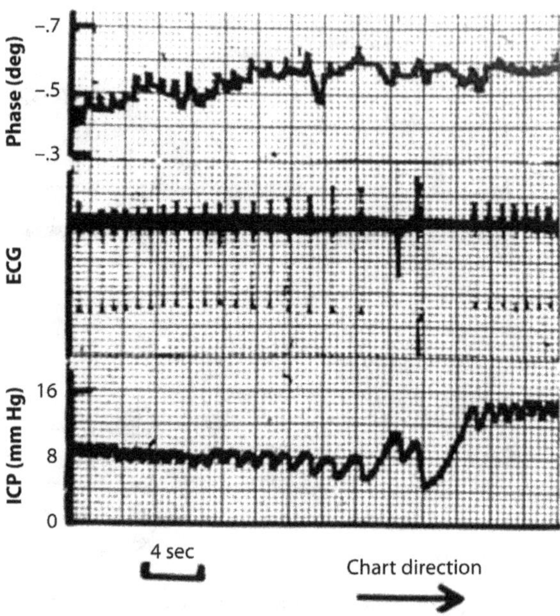


**FIGURE 9.35** Transient changes in phase and intracranial pressure (ICP) associated with each heartbeat during a period of hypoxia.

recording. Increase in intracranial water content on the order of 1% was detectable via this sensing technique. Some researchers [Cervos-Navarro and Ferszt,1980; Penn, 1980] have reported typically increased water content in brain matter on the order of 9%. This level of increased water content is well within the range of detectability of microwave sensing. The water contents of white and gray matter in a normal human brain are 0.71 and 0.01 and 0.83 and 0.03 g/mL, respectively [Whittall et al., 1997].

Note that the low frequency oscillations, about 18/min, seen in the ICP and phase recordings of Figure 9.35 could correspond to pathologic pressure variations in the rat. After the respirator was turned off, phase variation is clearly correlated with the ICP variations and heartbeat during bradycardia. The results of these experiments indicate that small pressure variations having a magnitude of few mm Hg, are detectable in the phase recording. The pathologic pressure waves in humans are significantly larger in amplitude than the pressure variations discussed previously.

The maximum phase change in a series of aliquot injections in the experiment is roughly proportional to the amount of saline injected. As depicted in Figure 9.32, for injections of 0.05 mL of saline, the maximum phase change is also related to the maximum pressure change produced by a given volume of saline. The significant lower ICP reached in the infusion experiment and the large phase values when compared with the maximum attained in the step volume injection series suggest the phase change is primarily due to increased water. A possible explanation for the proportionally large phase change, relative to the pressure change, after maximum levels were attained in the aliquot and infusion tests, is the phase may be more sensitive to increased intracranial water content than ICP recording. Since phase change relative to control level is associated temporarily with change in ICP, relative phase is also associated with ICP. The levelling off of relative phase and ICP after several minutes, while the infusion proceeded at a constant rate, may be related to some reported experimental findings [Lundberg et al., 1975]. Specifically, during experimental infusion of CSF in cats, a constant brain ICP was reached after 1 hour. The rate of infusion in that experiment was considerably less than the rates used in the microwave experiments.

Microwave sensing provides a noninvasive technique to monitor brain edema and detect increased intracranial water content. Measurement of the phase variations of transmitted microwave signals indicates that increases in intracranial water content on the order of 1% are detected *in vivo* with potential clinical applications. The findings suggest that the progression of brain edema on a long-term basis can be assessed using microwave sensing. Furthermore, phase changes related to small ICP variations are observed, indicating that the detection of pathologic pressure variations such as Traube-Hering-Mayer waves and plateau waves [Best et al., 1990; Barnett et al., 2020] is possible by the noninvasive microwave technique.

Further development of this technique would involve calibration studies to be performed on animal subjects and human participants. The baseline values of phase variations are functions of several factors such as head size, structure, geometry, the optimal position of the transmitting and receiving antennas on the head, ventricular dimensions, and the category of cerebral edema or brain swelling. Dynamic calibration requires measurements of the change in phase as a function of brain tissue water content. The antenna to be employed could be of the flexible contact type. The antennas could be placed on a patient suffering from brain edema and long-term monitoring of phase performed without interfering with conventional forms of treatment. In this case, microwave sensing may have immediate medical benefits. For example, before surgical implantation of a ventricular catheter to monitor ICP, pathologic pressure variations such as the Traube-Hering-Mayer waves and plateau waves [Lemaire et al., 2002; Lundberg et al., 1968] could be detected by using contact antennas.

## 9.7 MICROWAVE TOMOGRAPHIC IMAGING OF HEMORRHAGIC HEAD PHANTOM

Recently, a tomographic imaging system using microwaves was described for detection of hemorrhagic bleeding associated with traumatic brain injuries [Mobashsher et al., 2014; 2016a, b]. The system includes a small ultrawideband (UWB) antenna, a compact microwave transceiver, a 360° scanning system, signal processing, and a back-projection image reconstruction algorithm. The low-profile folded-structure antenna covers the band of 1.1–3.4 GHz with a directional radiation pattern. The system was tested on a 3-D head phantom with realistic dielectric permittivity for head tissues. The performance of the system was demonstrated using datasets recorded at 32 antenna positions around the head, and the back projection algorithm reconstructed images of the scanned phantom head. Note that 2-D microwave tomographic imaging of biological bodies has been a long-standing research topic. The interested reader is referred to extensive publications on the subject available in the open literature.

The complexity of the instrumentation and process of image formation for microwave tomographic imaging of cerebral edema or hemorrhagic bleeding in the brain would likely be less than those especially of X-ray CT and perhaps, MRI scanning. Moreover, it is not obvious that the efficiency of microwave tomographic imaging in detecting cerebral edema would surpass that of X-ray radiography, CT, or MRI. A microwave imaging would be less bulky and not as expensive, since it would require less power to operate, but it would be a challenge to make it easily portable and practical. Thus, continued development of the straightforward real-time microwave sensing, as discussed previously may turn out to be more advantageous and efficacious. Nonetheless, a computer simulation study of microwave scattering from a 3-D anthropomorphic human head model for hemorrhagic and ischemic brain stroke detection has been initiated [Munawar Qureshi et al., 2018]. The two common types of brain stroke at various locations inside the head model could be analyzed for possible detection and classification by developing an image reconstruction algorithm.

## 9.8 MICROWAVE THERMOACOUSTIC TOMOGRAPHY AND IMAGING

Several other tomographic techniques for tissue imaging are currently under investigation that exploit the cost differential and at the same time, utilize the nonionizing and noninvasive advantages of microwave radiation. It is noted that the emerging microwave thermoacoustic tomography (MTT) imaging technique uses microwave-pulse-induced thermoelastic pressure waves to form body tissue images [Lin 2021a,b; Lin and Chan, 1984; Manohar and Razansky, 2016; Olsen and Lin, 1983; Zhang et al., 2023].

The generation and detection of thermoacoustic pressure waves in biological materials depend on the dielectric permittivity and acoustic properties of tissue materials. Thus, MTT imaging possesses the characteristic features of a duel-modality imaging system. The attributes of high contrasts afforded by differential dielectric absorption of microwaves and the fine spatial resolution furnished by ultrasonic wave propagation in biological tissues are being explored to provide a unique duel imaging modality for noninvasive characterization of tissues, especially for the early detection of soft-tissue tumors such as breast cancer [Kruger et al., 2000], among others. Indeed, the same rationale applies to measurement of changes in fluid contents inside the brain and lungs. Therefore, MTT could provide an imaging modality capable of early detection of cerebral and pulmonary edemas and volume changes with a potential to offer it on a more widely available basis and without any ionizing radiation risk to the patient. The research being conducted in developing MTT for medical diagnosis are described in the following references [Lin 2021a,b]. The discussions also provide further details on the science of thermoelastic wave generation and propagation in biological tissues; the design of prototype MTT imaging systems; and the reconstruction of tomographic images using filtered-back projection algorithms; as well as the performance of prototype systems in phantom models and human subjects.

## 9.9 HEMORRHAGIC BLOOD VOLUME CHANGE

As discussed in earlier chapters, a noninvasive, contactless, remote Doppler microwave sensing technique was developed to measure precordial displacements of the chest wall and vibrations in response to ventricular contraction — microwave apexcardiography (MACG) [Lin et al., 1979]. The microwave remote sensing approach eliminates any change in sensitivity and discomfort caused by attaching acoustic sensors to the chest in conventional apexcardiography (ACG). It was suggested that the complex ACG tracings can reveal not only intracardiac pressures, but changes in left ventricular compliance, position, and volume as well [Voigt and Friesinger, 1970]. Furthermore, MACG recordings closely resemble the characteristics of seismocardiography (SCG) signals recorded by attaching an accelerometer to the skin over the apex, near the sternum [Bozhenko, 1961; Elliott et al., 1954; Mounsey, 1957; Sørensen et al., 2018]. Interestingly, a recent study demonstrated that SCG-derived characteristic timing events in the cardiac cycle such as pre-ejection period (PEP) and left ventricular ejection time (LVET) are more sensitive in detection of early-stage hemorrhage compared to pulse pressure and heartbeat [Tavakolian et al., 2014]. Indeed, the LVET and PEP features extracted from SCG are well correlated with different stages of graded lower-body negative pressure, which was used to create a hemodynamic response similar to hemorrhage. As previously mentioned, the noninvasive Doppler microwave sensor can successfully and reproducibly measure cardiovascular signal waveforms and timing intervals (such as LVET, PEP, and STI) of diagnostic quality [Lin, 1992; Papp et al., 1987]. Thus, the sensitivity and unique contactless character of MACG or remote Doppler microwave sensing suggest further investigations to explore its viability as a noninvasive measurement technique, not only for cardiac health and performance, but also as a nonintrusive monitor for early-stage or moderate hemorrhage detection, especially in emergency and trauma settings where contactless sensing may be more advantageous. It is interesting to note that microwave radar signals were investigated as a potential method, using hemorrhagic rabbits, to extract time-frequency characteristics associated with survival periods of hemorrhagic victims during disaster rescue missions [Matsui et al., 2004; Yu et al., 2021].

## REFERENCES

Amir, O., Azzam, Z. S., Gaspar, T., Faranesh-Abboud, S., Andria, N., Burkhoff, D., Abbo, A., Abraham, W. T., 2016. Validation of remote dielectric sensing (ReDS™) technology for quantification of lung fluid status: Comparison to high resolution chest computed tomography in patients with and without acute heart failure. Int. J. Cardiol., 221:841–846

Amiry-Moghaddam, M., Otsuka, T., Hurn, P. D., Traystman, R. J., Haug, F. M., Froehner, S. C., Adams, M. E., Neely, J. D., Agre, P., Ottersen, O. P., Bhardwaj, A., 2003. An alpha-syntrophin-dependent pool of AQP4 in astroglial end-feet confers bidirectional water flow between blood and brain. Proc. Natl. Acad. Sci. USA, 100:2106–2111

Barnett, W. H., Latash, E. M., Capps, R. A., et al., 2020. Traube–Hering waves are formed by interaction of respiratory sinus arrhythmia and pulse pressure modulation in healthy men. J. Appl. Physiol., 129(5):1193–1202

Best, C. H., Taylor, N. B., West, J. B., 1990. Best and Taylor's Physiologic Basis of Medical Practice, 12th ed, Baltimore, Md: Williams & Wilkins

Bozhenko, B. S., 1961. Seismocardiography–a new method in the study of functional conditions of the heart. Ter. Arkh., 33:55

Cervos-Navarro, J., Ferszt, R., 1980. Brain Edema, New York: Raven

Clarke, M. J., Lin, J. C., 1983. Microwave sensing of increased intracranial water content. Invest. Radiol., 18:245–248

Cotran, R. S., Kumar, V., Robbins, S. L., 1994. Pathological Basis of Disease, 5th ed, Philadelphia: Saunders

de Groote, M., Wantier, M., Cheron, G., Estenne, M., Paiva, M., 1997. Chest wall motion during tidal breathing. J. Appl. Physiol., 83(5):1531

Dei, D., Grazzini, G., Luzi, G., Pieraccini, M., Atzeni, C., Boncinelli, S., Camiciottoli, G., Castellani, W., Marsili, M., Dico, J. L., 2009. Noncontact detection of breathing using a microwave sensor. Sensors, 9:2574–2585

Durney, C. H., Iskander, M. F., Bragg, D. G., 1978. Noninvasive microwave methods for measuring changes in lung water content, in Proc IEEE Electro/78 30/6, Boston, pp. 1–7

Elliott, R. V., Packard, R. G. A. Y., Kyrazis, D. T., 1954. Acceleration ballistocardiography: Design, construction, and application of a new instrument. Circulation, 9:281–291

Grant, I. L. B., 1972. Grant's Atlas of Anatomy, 6th ed, Baltimore, MD: Williams & Wilkins

Iskander, M. F., Durney, C. H., 1983. Microwave methods of measuring changes in lung water. J. Microw. Power, 18(3):265–275

Iskander, M. F., Durney, C. H., Grange, T., Smith, C. S., 1984. Radiometric technique for measuring changes in lung water. IEEE Trans. Microw. Theory Tech., 32(5):554–556

Kagawa, M., Tojima, H., Matsui, T., 2016. Non-contact diagnostic system for sleep apnea-hypopnea syndrome based on amplitude and phase analysis of thoracic and abdominal Doppler radars. Med. Biol. Eng. Comput., 54(5):789–799

Kim, J. Y., et al., 2021. New unobtrusive tidal volume monitoring system using channel state information in wi-fi signal: Preliminary result. IEEE Sens. J., 21(3):3810–3821

Kostopoulos, V., Douzinas, E. E., Kypriades, E. M., Pappas, Y. Z., 2006. A new method for the early diagnosis of brain edema/brain swelling. An experimental study in rabbits. J. Biomech., 39(16):2958–2965

Kruger, R. A., Miller, K. D., Reynolds, H. E., Kiser, W. L. Jr, Reinecke, D. R., Kruger, G. A., 2000. Breast cancer in vivo: Contrast enhancement with thermoacoustic CT at 434 MHz-feasibility study. Radiology. 216:279–283

Lange, N. R., Schuster, D. P., 1999. The measurement of lung water. Crit. Care, 3(2):R19–R24

Lee, Y. S., Pathirana, P. N., Steinfort, C. L., Caelli, T., 2014. Monitoring and analysis of respiratory patterns using microwave doppler radar. IEEE J. Transl. Eng. Health Med., 2:1–12

Lemaire, J. J., Khalil, T., Cervenansky, F., et al., 2002. Slow pressure waves in the cranial enclosure. Acta Neurochir. (Wien), 144:243–254

Lin, J. C., 1975. Noninvasive microwave measurement of respiration. Proc. IEEE. 63:1530

Lin, J. C., 1992. Microwave Sensing of Physiological Movement and Volume Change. Bioelectromagnetics, 13:557–565

Lin, J. C., 2021a. Microwave thermoacoustic tomographic (MTT) imaging, Phys. Med. Biol., 66(10):10–30

Lin, J. C., 2021b. Auditory Effect of Microwave Radiation, Switzerland, Springer

Lin, J. C., Chan, K. M., 1984. Microwave thermoelastic tissue imaging–system design. IEEE Trans. Microwave Theory Tech. 32:854–860

Lin, J. C., Clarke, M. J., 1982. Microwave imaging of cerebral edema. Proc. IEEE, 70: 523–554

Lin, J. C., Kiernicki, J., Kiernicki, M., Wollschlaeger, P. B., 1979. Microwave apexcardiography. IEEE Trans. Microwave Theory and Tech., 27:618–620

Lundberg, N., Cronquist, S., Kjallquist, A., 1968. Clinical investigations on the inter- relationships between intracranial pressure and intracranial hemodynamics. Prog. Brain Res., 30:69–75

Lundberg, N., Pontén, U., Brock, M., 1975. Intracranial Pressure II, Germany: Heidelberg

Malaeb, S., Izzetoglu, M., McGowan, J., et al., 2018. Noninvasive monitoring of brain edema after hypoxia in newborn piglets. Pediatr. Res., 83:484–490

Manohar, S., Razansky, D., 2016. Photoacoustics: A historical Review. Adv. Opt. Photon., 8(4):586–617

Massagram, W., Hafner, N., Lubecke, V., Boric-Lubecke, O., 2013. Tidal volume measurement through non-contact Doppler radar with DC reconstruction. IEEE Sens. J., 13:3397–3404

Matsui, T., Ishizuka, T., Takase, B., Ishihara, M., Kikuchi, M., 2004. Non-contact determination of vital sign alterations in hypovolaemic states induced by massive haemorrhage: An experimental attempt to monitor the condition of injured persons behind barriers or under disaster rubble. Med. Biol. Eng. Comput., 42(6):807–811

Mobashsher, A. T., Abbosh, A. M., Wang, Y., 2014. Microwave system to detect traumatic brain injuries using compact unidirectional antenna and wideband transceiver with verification on realistic head phantom. IEEE Trans. Microw. Theory Tech., 62(9):1826–1836

Mobashsher, A. T., Bialkowski, K. S., Abbosh, A. M., Crozier, S., 2016a. Design and experimental evaluation of a non-invasive microwave head imaging system for intracranial haemorrhage detection. PLoS ONE, 11(4):e0152351

Mobashsher, A. T., Mahmoud, A., Abbosh, A., 2016b. Portable wideband microwave imaging system for intracranial hemorrhage detection using improved back-projection algorithm with model of effective head permittivity. Sci. Rep., 6(1):20459

Moskalenko, Y. E., 1960. Application of centimeter radio waves for electrodeless recording of volume changes of biological materials, Biophysics (USSR):259–264

Mounsey, P., 1957. Praecordial ballistocardiography. Br. Heart J., 19:259

Munawar Qureshi, A., Mustansar, Z., Mustafa, S., 2018. Finite-element analysis of microwave scattering from a three-dimensional human head model for brain stroke detection. R. Soc. Open Sci., 5(7), 180319. doi: 10.1098/rsos.180319

Olsen, R. G., Lin, J. C., 1983. Acoustical imaging of a model of a human hand using pulsed microwave irradiation. Bioelectromagnetics 4:397–400

Papp, M. A., Hughes, C., Lin, J. C., Pouget, J. M., 1987. Doppler microwave: A clinical assessment of its efficacy as an arterial pulse sensing technique, Invest. Radiol, 22:569–573

Pedersen, P. C., Johnson, C. C., Durney, C. H., Bragg, D. C., 1978. Microwave reflection and transmission measurements for pulmonary diagnosis and monitoring. IEEE. Trans. Biomed. Eng., 25:40–48

Penn, R. D., 1980. Cerebral edema and neurological function in human beings. Neurosurgery. 6(3):249–254

Rezaeieh, S. A., Bialkowski, K. S., Abbosh, A. M., 2014. Microwave system for the early stage detection of congestive heart failure. IEEE Access, 2:921–929

Rezaeieh, S., Zamani, A., Bialkowski, K., et al., 2015. Feasibility of using wideband microwave system for non-invasive detection and monitoring of pulmonary oedema. Sci. Rep., 5:14047

ReDS, 2016. Remote Dielectric Sensing, Sensible Medical Innovations. Israel: Kfar Netter

Salman, S., Wang, Z., Colebeck, E., Kiourti, A., Topsakal, E., Volakis, J. L., 2014. Pulmonary edema monitoring sensor with integrated body-area network for remote medical sensing. IEEE Trans. Antennas Propag., 62(5):2787–2794

Shah, S., Kimberly, W. T., 2016. The modern approach to treating brain swelling in the neuro ICU. Semin Neurol., 36(6):502–507

Sharma, P., Hui, X., Zhou, J., et al., 2020. Wearable radio-frequency sensing of respiratory rate, respiratory volume, and heart rate. NPJ Digit. Med., 3:98. doi: 10.1038/s41746-020-0307-6

Silverthorn, D. U., 2016. Human Physiology: An Integrated Approach, 7th ed., Upper Saddle River: Pearson

Sørensen, K., Schmidt, S. E., Jensen, A. S., Søgaard, P., Struijket, J. J., 2018. Definition of fiducial points in the normal seismocardiogram. Sci. Rep., 8:15455. doi: 10.1038/s41598-018-33675-6

Susskind, C., 1973. Possible uses of microwaves in the management of lung diseases. Proc. IEEE, 61:673–674

Tavakolian, K., Dumont, G. A., Houlton, G., Blaber, A. P., 2014. Precordial vibrations provide noninvasive detection of early-state hemorrhage. Shock, 41(2):91–96

Thiagarajah, J. R., Papadopoulos, M. C., Verkman, A. S., 2005. Noninvasive early detection of brain edema in mice by near-infrared light scattering. J. Neurosci. Res., 80(2):293–299

Vander, A. J., Sherman, J. H., Luciano, D. S., 1990. Human Physiology, 5th ed, New York, McGraw-Hill

van Loon, K., et al., 2016. Wireless non-invasive continuous respiratory monitoring with FMCW radar: A clinical validation study. J. Clin. Monit. Comput., 30(6):797–805

Voigt, G. C., Friesinger, G. C., 1970. The use of apexcardiography in the assessment of left ventricular diastolic pressure. Circulation, 41:1015–1024

Wheatley-Guy, C. M., Sajgalik, P., Cierzan, B. S., Wentz, R. J., Johnson, B. D., 2020. Validation of radiofrequency determined lung fluid using thoracic CT: Findings in acute decompensated heart failure patients. Int. J. Cardiol. Heart. Vasc., 30:100645

Whittall, K. P., MacKay, A. L., Graeb, D. A., Nugent, R. A., Li, D. K., Paty, D. W., 1997. In vivo measurement of T2 distributions and water contents in normal human brain. Magn. Reson. Med., 37(1):34–43

Wilkinson, H. A., Rosenfeld, S., Denherder, D., Bronson, R., 1981. The linearity of the volume/pressure response during intracranial pressure "reserve" testing. J. Neurol. Neurosurg. Psychiatry, 44:23–28

Xia, Z., Shandhi, M. M. H., Inan, O. T., Zhang, Y., 2018. Non-contact sensing of seismocardiogram signals using microwave doppler radar. IEEE Sens. J., 18(14):5956–5964

Xia, Z., Shandhi, M. M. H., Li, Y., Inan, O. T., Zhang, Y., 2021. The delineation of fiducial points for non-contact radar seismocardiogram signals without concurrent ECG. IEEE J. Biomed. Health Inform., 25(4):1031–1040

Yamaura, I., 1977. Measurement of 1.8-2.7 GHz microwave attenuation in the human torso. IEEE Trans. Microw. Theory Tech., 25:707–710

Yu, X., Yin, Y., Lv, H., Zhang, Y., Liang, F., Wang, P., Wang, J., 2021. Non-contact determination of vital sign alterations in hypovolemic states induced by massive hemorrhage: An experimental attempt to monitor the condition of injured persons behind barriers or under disaster rubble. Prog. Electromagn. Res., 100:23–34

Zanetti, J. M., Salerno, D. M., 1991. Seismocardiography: A technique for recording precordial acceleration. Computer-Based Medical Systems, in Proceedings of the Fourth Annual IEEE Symposium, pp. 4–9

Zhang, H., Ren, M., Zhang, S., Liu, J., Qin, H., 2023. Microwave-induced thermoacoustic imaging for biomedical application. Phys. Scr., 98:032001

# 10 Wearable Devices and Sensors

Wearable sensors and devices are attracting considerable research and development interest and are becoming increasingly popular because they promise to offer seamless and continuous monitoring at a low cost. They are becoming available in various forms, shapes, and configurations and can be worn on different parts of the body. Wearable devices can be classified as wearable bands (such as rings, watches, bracelets, and chest, head, and arm bands), wearable textiles (clothing, t-shirts, and socks), wearables gear (glasses, hats, and helmets), and other sensory devices for health monitoring. A few of them have been popularized and are widely available as consumer electronic products. Many of them are lightweight and convenient to wear on the wrist or carry on the body. They have achieved considerable popularity owing to recent advancements in miniaturization in electronic technology and materials processing. Technological innovations in microelectronics and wireless communications along with microelectromechnical systems (mems) design and fabrication expertise are providing smaller, smarter, and cheaper sensors appropriate for integration into compact wearable devices. Many consumer-electronics enterprises and information technology companies worldwide have launched their own products and are capitalizing on the sustained consumer pivot toward health and wellness. The number of such applications is expected to increase, and the market size of wearable devices associated with physical wellness and fitness is likely to further expand. Many wearable devices also allow real-time connectivity to the Internet through mobile phone via Bluetooth and the Internet of Things (IoT).

Wearable noninvasive microwave and wireless sensors for measuring arterial pulse waves and vital signs have attracted considerable interest for biomedical applications in recent years [Chow and Yang, 2020; Costanzo et al., 2023; He et al., 2015; Seneviratne et al., 2017; Yilmaz et al., 2010] and are beginning to have significant impact on the practice of medicine and healthcare delivery. Indeed, direct contact and contactless Doppler microwave radar technology for sensing vital signs and physiological motions noninvasively has expanded to sports medicine, fitness sensing, and security monitoring and, in some cases, the technology has reached the commercialization stage [Li et al., 2021].

Most wearable wireless sensors are small devices designed for on-body applications (for carrying on or attachment to a body strap) and can be categorized according to where they are worn, such as the wrist, head, limb, or body. Furthermore, the noninvasive technology may be broadly classified into contact and contactless types. In contact applications, the sensor is in contact with the skin through a thin dielectric or air gap, and microwaves are transmitted into the tissue without intervening air space or material substance. Under contactless scenarios, the sensor may be attached to clothing or other wearable materials on the body. Microwaves are transmitted

DOI: 10.1201/9781003315223-10

through clothing and similar material to the body in the near field of a microwave radar device or through layers of clothing from a distant far field location.

At times, the term wearable sensors are used to refer to prototype multipoint wireless sensors for cardiovascular and respiratory parameters (see Chapter 8, Sections 8.3, 8.4, and 8.5). These devices can be worn over clothing for sensing cardiopulmonary parameters noninvasively in laboratory or test environments. Also, some early "wearable" devices typically used large backpacks or waist bags, or were otherwise difficult or ergonomically inconvenient to carry because of limitations of electronics and component packaging technologies. Even so, more recent approaches in related situations have made it simpler to explore wearable sensing using customized devices and systems. Nevertheless, ergonomics, unobtrusiveness, and portability remain issues to be overcome.

Indeed, the interest in research and development of wearable physiological measurement systems has witnessed extensive growth during the past two decades [Cheng et al., 2021; Daskalaki et al., 2022; Guk et al., 2019; Seneviratne et al., 2017]. Aside from applications in medicine and healthcare, there has been increasing recognition of the efficacy in monitoring the health status of individuals in their daily routine, including the elderly, ambulatory, and in-hospital patient populations. Implementation of wireless mobile healthcare technology promises to enhance the quality of life for patients with chronic diseases and promote the fitness and well-being of healthy individuals. Moreover, there is also a gradual shift toward technology that prioritizes ergonomics and user comfort.

It should be noted that the fundamental objective of active sensing is to couple sufficient energy into the target of interest and make reliable and accurate observations using principles provided by the most appropriate information transmission and detection channel. The emergence of wireless technologies and on-body sensor design are enabling wearable healthcare devices and systems to center on the individual. It may also bring about transformational changes to the conventional healthcare delivery system. Wearable noninvasive monitoring systems can potentially provide continuous physiological data such as vital-sign monitoring and improved information regarding the general health of individuals by advancing disease prevention, enabling better disease management, and enhancing quality of life with better ergonomics and patient well-being.

## 10.1 FITNESS AND SLEEP TRACKERS

At present, the best-known wearable devices are fitness trackers and wristwatches. Wearable fitness trackers can monitor activity such as workout routines, step- and distance-tracking, as in pedometers, and can help to support and motivate behaviors toward improved health. Monitoring could take place during walking, running, cycling, swimming, or other healthcare application scenarios, such as during sleep [Cao et al., 2022; Dixon et al., 2021]. Typically, accelerometers are used for sensing body movement and activity assessment. Tracked information is displayed in real-time on the tracker's screen or wristwatch's digital crown. Recently, some of the wearable fitness trackers have moved beyond their original purpose of fitness tracking and wellness monitoring to that of sleep tracking and vital-sign monitoring, and are becoming trendy for health maintenance and a chosen tool in athletic training practices.

Sleep trackers most often use electrodes and accelerometers to sense heart rate (HR) and body movement as wearable devices. They may also offer data on body temperature and oxygen consumption. For continuous monitoring, the device must remain on the person throughout the night to evaluate sleep patterns. For others, such as activity tracking or health monitoring, the device needs to stay on the person throughout the day and night to monitor daily physical activity. Typically, the collected information or data are uploaded to a device (mobile phone or laptop computer) that assesses the data and displays the estimated results on-board or offline on a screen. Examples of sleep-tracking results for an adult male are given in Figures 10.1 and 10.2. The screen display in Figure 10.1 shows the various stages and associated durations of sleep a person cycled through during the night. Also, the tracker's algorithm provides a summary assessment of 7-day sleep patterns and compares them to the prior 14-day average (Figure 10.2).

In addition to sleep tracking, some models of wearable trackers can act as a health monitor by sensing and displaying vital signs such as respiration rate (RR), HR, heart rate variability (HRV), and skin temperature (see Figure 10.3). Also, some wearables can provide information on daily activity such as a comparison of "recovery" or routine weekly levels as shown in Figure 10.4.

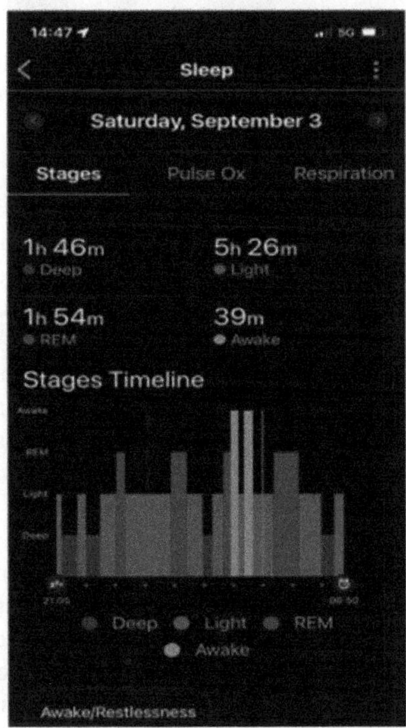


**FIGURE 10.1** Sleep stage, duration, and timeline cycled through during the night on a screen display.

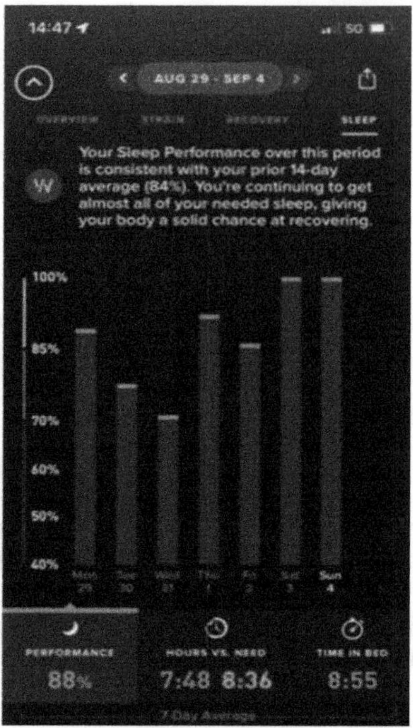


**FIGURE 10.2** A screen display showing 7-day sleep patterns compared to the prior 14-day average.

## 10.2 SMARTWATCH HEART-RATE SENSORS

Many smartwatch sensors offer capabilities as wearable devices to provide continuous health-related biometric monitoring. They can potentially be integrated into medical practices to facilitate diagnosis and management of disease, complement routine medical assessments, and monitor and prevent disease in primary care. For example, most currently marketed smartwatches come with electrocardiogram (ECG) monitoring for HR and HRV, including arrhythmias (abnormal heartbeats or irregular rhythms such as atrial fibrillation). The sensor typically uses electrical measurement through conductive electrodes in contact with skin surface to generate a single-lead ECG associated with lead-I in the conventional three-lead ECG recording configuration [Klabunde, 2021]. Recently, there has been some movement toward technology leading to the development of systems based on capacitive coupling for indirect or noncontact ECG sensing to monitor HR. Furthermore, the accelerometer and HR data may be integrated on-board to provide information for activity classification such as exercise intensity and fall detection [Prawiro et al., 2016].

The three-lead configuration is the most common of all cardiac monitoring lead systems [Klabunde, 2021]. ECG recordings use the standard limb lead configurations shown in Figure 10.5. By convention, the lead-I configuration measures the voltage difference between electrodes on the left arm (LA) and right arm (RA). In the lead-II configuration, the voltage difference is measured between electrodes on

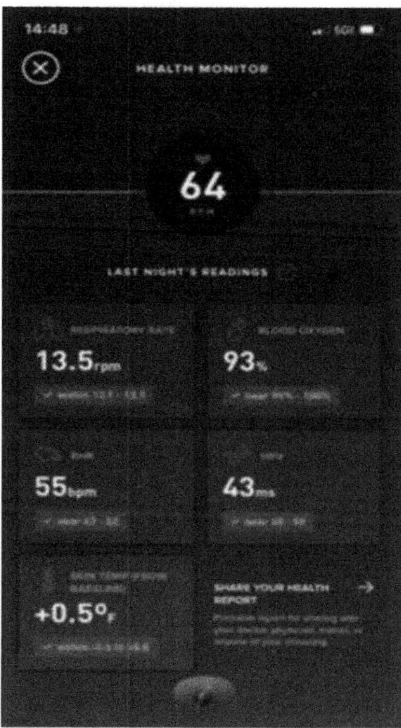


**FIGURE 10.3** A wearable tracker as health monitor for vital signs such as respiration rate, heart rate, heart rate variability, and skin temperature.

the left leg (LL) and on the RA. Lead-III measures the voltages between LL and LA electrodes. In single-lead ECG, only recordings from one lead is displayed. Whether the conductive electrodes are attached to the end of the limb (wrists and ankles) or at the attachment point of the limb (shoulder or lower abdomen) makes little difference in the recording because biological tissues serve as volume conductors of the electrical signal originating from the heart in the upper torso of the body. The three leads roughly form an equilateral triangle (with the heart at the center) that is referred to as Einthoven's triangle in honor of Willem Einthoven who developed the scheme for ECG recordings in the early 1900s.

Current models of the smartwatch can provide ECG monitoring such as HR and HRV by applying electrodes in contact with skin on the wrist to acquire a single-lead ECG (Figure 10.6). In this case, it is typically the "lead-I" in the conventional three-lead ECG recording configuration, although, on rare occasions, the lead-II recording from the leg may yield a stronger signal or higher voltage reading when appropriate or desirable. Single-lead ECGs are often prescribed for ambulatory patients (people at home) or in-hospital patients to obtain a clearer understanding of the nature and consistency of the underlying rate and rhythm of the heart.

Under most scenarios, the watchband needs to fit snuggly to ensure the conductive electrodes are in good electrical contact with the wrist's skin to ensure uninterrupted low-frequency voltage measurement by the electrodes. Body movement

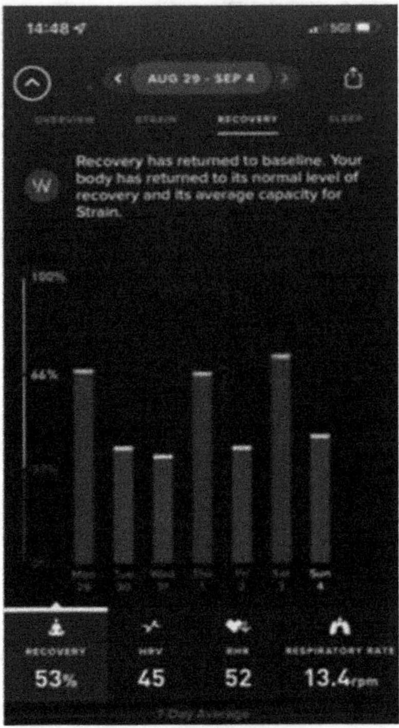


**FIGURE 10.4** Daily activity and comparison to "recovery" to normal weekly levels.

should be minimized, and arms should rest on a table or in the lap while making a measurement, which normally takes about 30 seconds. Most wearable smartwatch devices come with an ECG software application (app). The wearable sensor's recording is combined with on-board data processing methods and artificial intelligence (AI) algorithms in a smart decision support system with simple diagnostic outcomes [Bae et al., 2022]. At the end of the measurement and decision process, the ECG

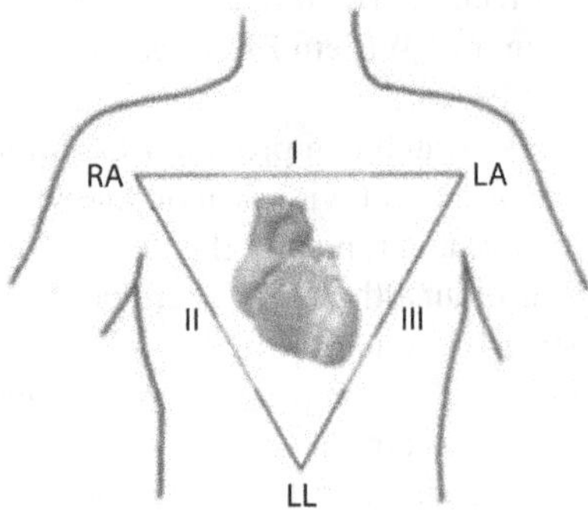


**FIGURE 10.5** The standard three-lead configuration (I, II, and III) for electrocardiogram recording.

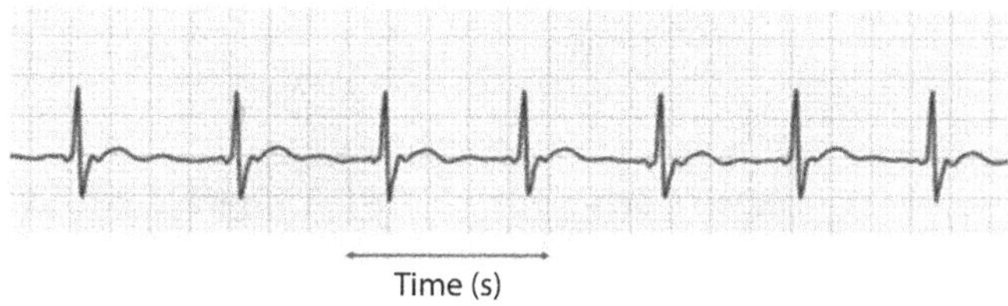


**FIGURE 10.6** Normal single lead (lead I) electrocardiogram from a wrist-worn smartwatch sensor.

app provides a notification on the classification of the measured cardiac rhythm, including inconclusive or unclassified readings due to poor ECG recordings. While the ECG app can record heart rhythms and pulse rates using the resistive electrode sensors and can check the recording for irregular rhythms, the ECG app cannot provide medical or clinical quality diagnosis for heart failures or reliably detect a heart attack.

It is noteworthy that while many people may use various wearable health-related wellness products such as smartwatches and fitness trackers, and they may also provide this data to their physicians to include in evaluations to help improve their healthcare, these products are not regulated by the Food and Drug Administration (FDA) in the U.S. The FDA has authority to regulate devices intended for use in the diagnosis of disease or other conditions, or in the cure, mitigation, treatment, or prevention of diseases. At present, these wearable devices are regarded by the FDA as health-related consumer products. This means that these products generally fall outside medical-device regulation unless the manufacturer plainly intends the product to be used as a medical device and markets it as such. Otherwise, manufacturers can advertise without FDA regulation. It is important to recognize there are legal uncertainty and unresolved liability questions for wearable health-related products that may arise as the technology and application proliferate [Simon et al., 2022].

Several commercial wearable and compact body-worn ECG monitors are registered with the FDA prior to marketing the devices for longer wear through FDA's notification process, at present, they may not be functioning the same way as an approved medical device, such as a modern Holter monitoring system, for diagnosis of a potential cardiac rhythm issue. Holter monitors are known for accurate and reliable analysis of complex ventricular arrhythmias by providing a choice of three to seven leads, enabling multiple simultaneous views of cardiac electrical activity. The modern battery-operated Holter monitors are roughly the size of a cellphone (see Figure 10.7). The patient usually wears it via a strap around the neck or an elastic band around the waist. Typically, there are multiple ECG leads that attach to the chest. The data recorded from a Holter monitor are analyzed offline after the completion of monitoring. A cardiologist would analyze the data before meeting with the patient to discuss the results.

It is noted that an exploratory analysis to perform ambulatory atrial fibrillation (AF) detection in a cohort of participants using smartwatch data from standard, commercially available wristwatches was reported [Tison et al., 2018]. HR data from the photoplethysmography (PPG) sensor were accessed by the available mobile

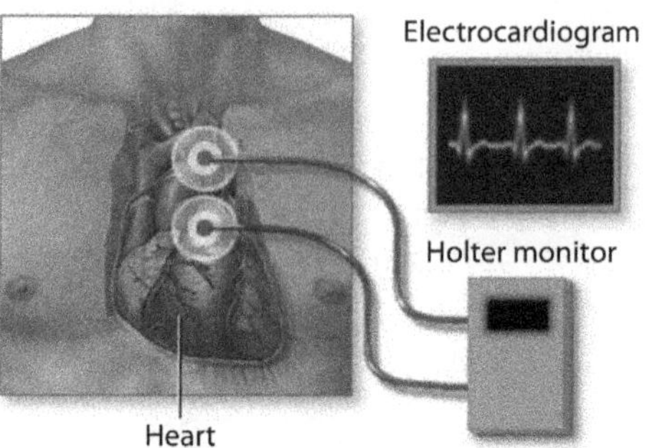


**FIGURE 10.7** A modern Holter monitoring device for cardiac rhythm diagnosis. (From Medical Encyclopedia, Holter heart monitor, MedlinePlus [Internet]. Bethesda (MD): National Library of Medicine (US); [updated Jun 24; cited 2020 Jul 1]. Available from: https://medlineplus.gov/.)

application program and fed into an AI neural network in which the AI network approximated representations of the R–R interval between heartbeats. This proof-of-concept study found that smartwatch PPG paired with an AI neural network can passively detect AF but with some loss of sensitivity and specificity against a reference standard ECG–diagnosed AF.

Several versions of capacitive coupling ECG for noncontact HR monitoring using electric voltage sensing arrays have been reported. In this case, measurements are made without any direct electrical contact with the skin, but multichannel ECG monitoring can be accomplished using conventional ECG recording cables [Harland et al., 2005; Oehler et al., 2008]. Capacitive sensors represent an appealing choice for noninvasively monitoring ECG by embedding sensor arrays in a support system or even a garment worn by neonates in the intensive care unit (ICU). Their use could help to prioritize a subject's comfort, reduce pain, facilitate better recovery, and lessen potential scars caused by adhesive electrodes. Sensor arrays have been successfully applied for unobtrusive ECG monitoring in the neonatal ICU when embedded in a neonatal support mattress [Atallah et al., 2014] and to provide reliable ECG signals when embedded in a smart chair for indirect contactless measurement [Baek et al., 2012]. However, in most cases, the bulky capacitive sensors were applied in an array. While they are promising with noninvasive and unobtrusive attributes, they may not be directly translatable to the wrist-worn scenario unless the challenge of miniaturization is properly met.

Note that measurements of ECG activity using insulated electrodes (see Figure 10.8) for capacitive coupling, including through-clothing recordings, have been reported [Matthews et al., 2005]. They have been used for the measurement of ECG signals without conductive electrical contact with skin, but not as a wearable from the wrist. Furthermore, a small (15 mm diameter) electrode that represents a significant decrease over other capacitive electrodes for recording bio-potential signals including ECG was reported [Portelli and Nasuto, 2017]. However, details on its performance as a capacitive electrode on a printed circuit board (PCB) that can potentially rival conventional recording methods for ECG are not available.

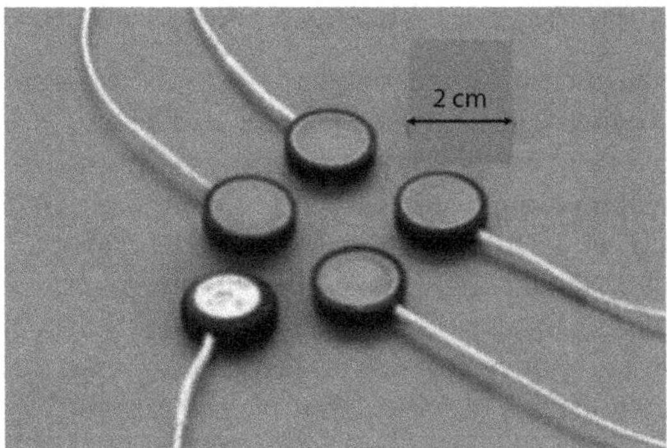


**FIGURE 10.8** Insulated electrodes for capacitive coupling sensors.

## 10.3 WEARABLE MICROWAVE VITAL-SIGN SENSING

The monitoring of vital signs by smartwatches and fitness trackers requires use of electrodes in contact with the skin. Recent advances in wireless communication and microelectronics technologies have ushered in new opportunities to leverage developments in wireless microwave technologies that may provide a convenient channel to transmit information about vital signs, but also enable small wireless sensors to detect and measure physiological parameters of interest.

Research in wireless microwave sensing and monitoring of heartbeat, arterial pulse rate, and respiratory activity in humans and animals has been discussed in previous chapters. With some exceptions, many of the results were obtained using low-power prototype microwave systems that were assembled from larger laboratory equipment and test instruments and components. The prototypes have demonstrated the capability for continuous monitoring of the time-dependent changes in vital signs through direct contact or noncontact modes from distances of a few millimeters, through layers of clothing, and with varying skin or surface coverings including animal pelts and shells. It is significant to note that many of the noninvasive measurement systems discussed are useful for wearable applications when miniaturized.

The goal of wearable microwave sensing is to leverage current research and advances in wireless technology, and ultimately enable wireless vital-sign sensing and monitoring applications to benefit a broad range of the population in an ergonomically appealing and functionally more efficient manner. However, while the use of common technological platforms is envisioned, the particular configuration and hardware implementation may vary depending on specific application or functional realms. It is interesting to note, in this regard, the development of a lightweight, low-power, minimally invasive wearable wireless sensor for the continuous vital-sign monitoring of turtles in various stages of brumation or hibernation for cold-blooded animals [Zhou et al., 2020]. The vital signs were recorded unobtrusively with minimal animal handling. It was found that the turtle's heartbeat was correlated with the ambient temperature, while the breath rate did not significantly reduce during brumation.

### 10.3.1 A Miniature Wearable Microwave Arterial Pulse Sensor

As shown previously, microwave-measured arterial pulse rates are related directly to the heartbeat. Accordingly, some papers may refer to devices that can extract pulse rates off data logged from arteries on the arm as wrist-worn HR sensors. The earliest reported wearable microwave arterial pulse monitor was an S-band microwave oscillator integrated with a ribbon antenna [RCA Laboratories, 1987]. The small sensor consisted of a bipolar transistor with a lightly coupled antenna serving as a load to the S-band microwave oscillator [Lin, 1989]. The simple sensor design is exceptional in that it consumes low power, involves a miniature antenna, and uses a single microwave transistor as the microwave source. The device operated on a 9 V transistor battery to generate 0.5 mW of output power at 2.45 GHz for a nominal current drain of less than 15 mA (Figure 10.9). The front end or sensing head is less than 3 cm in diameter. In contact applications, the small time-varying arterial wall movements will influence the oscillator's loading current due to changes in antenna coupling or impedance variation. The change in current is detected using an AC-coupled amplifier.

Consequently, the frequency of the free-running microwave oscillator is Doppler-shifted according to displacements of the arterial wall. A frequency demodulator is applied to the output of the oscillator to detect the motion. To minimize spurious signal and extraneous motion artifacts, the miniature sensor was completely shielded with all microwave components residing within the sensing front end (head). This is accomplished by constructing the sensor as a two-piece assembly and housing the amplifier and power supply away from the sensing head in a separate package. This design alleviates the commonly encountered microwave transmission

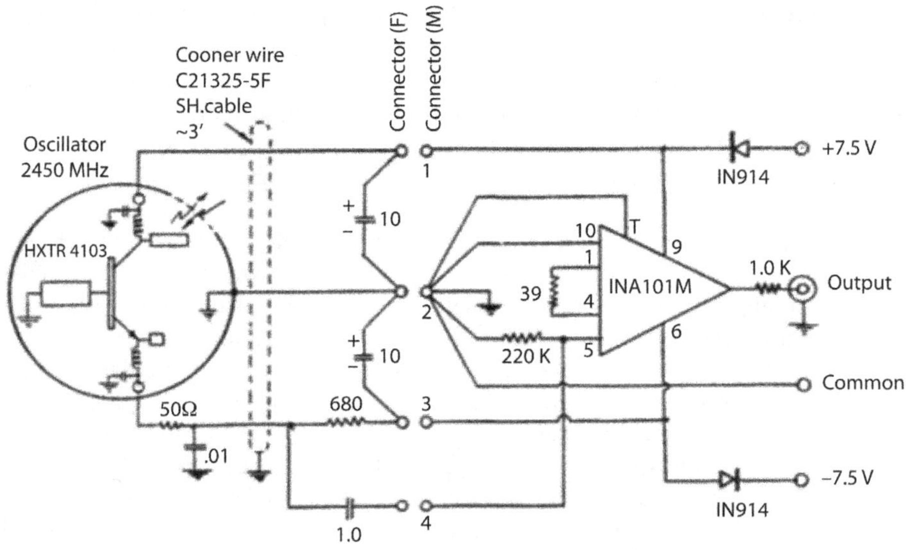


**FIGURE 10.9** Schematic diagram of a miniature S-band microwave arterial pulse-wave sensor. The ribbon antenna is seen at the upper right corner within the transistor circle.

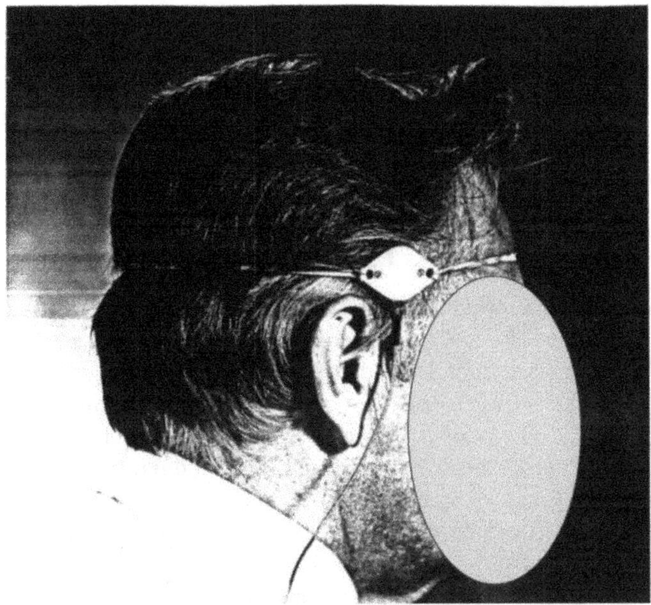

**FIGURE 10.10** A wearable microwave sensor held in direct contact with the skin over the right temporal artery of the head using an elastic headband.

and leakage through cabling and helps to minimize motion and other interference generated noise or artifacts.

Figure 10.10 shows the wearable microwave sensor held in contact through a thin dielectric gap with skin over the right temporal artery by an elastic headband. An example of the compact S-band microwave sensor-measured superficial temporal arterial pulse wave is given in Figure 10.11. The clean, noise-free waveform exhibits

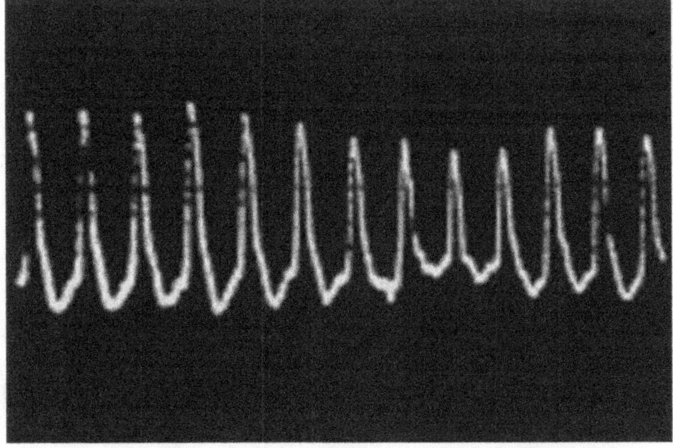

**FIGURE 10.11** A wearable miniature S-band microwave sensor measuring superficial temporal artery pulse waves by direct contact through a thin dielectric with the scalp.

characteristics like the carotid pulse waves and that of other arteries in the human upper extremities. This sensor is arguably the first wearable microwave arterial pulse monitor. Moreover, in essence, the tiny S-band sensor is a predecessor of the self-injection locked (SIL) radars [Wang et al., 2010, 2011] described in earlier chapters. Indeed subsequently, SIL radar devices have been proposed as a near-field contactless radial pulse monitor [Wang et al., 2016].

### 10.3.2 Wearable SILO Radar Pulse Sensors

Numerous studies have reported using SIL radars for contactless sensing of radial pulse from the wrist in a wearable manner [Kim et al., 2016; Tseng et al., 2018; Wang et al., 2016]. The application of SIL radars for pulse rate sensing in wearable devices involves the use of an active antenna that integrates a patch antenna with a SIL oscillator (SILO). The SILO sensor is typically strapped to the subject's wrist using an elastic band and monitors the radial pulse rate as a modulating Doppler signal. The SILO's output signal may be received remotely for further signal processing. While the hardware and architecture are similar, the technology applied in the two prototype SIL radar systems vary. In one, the SILO output is demodulated by a remote frequency discriminator to provide pulse-rate information [Wang et al., 2016] and the other relies on amplitude demodulation of the SILO output with differentiator envelope detection [Tseng et al., 2018]. A follow-up development on the handheld near-field SILO radar arterial pulse sensor suggested that the small near-field SILO sensor can be further miniaturized to be worn on the wrist to detect arterial pulse waves, with possible gains in measurement accuracy along with less noise [Tseng et al., 2020; Tseng and Wu, 2020]. More detailed discussions on using SIL radars for noninvasive sensing of the radial pulse from the wrist in wearable scenarios are described in Chapter 8 on pulse wave sensing.

### 10.3.3 Another Prototype Wearable Pulse Monitor

A protype sensor for wrist-worn microwave pulse waves using a voltage-controlled oscillator (VCO) circuit was recently proposed [McFerran et al., 2019]. By injection-locking the sensor oscillator to a phase-lock loop (PLL) circuit, the VCO frequency would change with variations of the PLL control voltage caused by movements associated with arterial pulses. The operating principles are akin to the SILO sensor discussed in Chapter 8. It relies on the established association of a change in the load impedance of an oscillator triggering a corresponding change to its free running frequency and, consequently, a change to its DC bias current [Kim et al., 2016]. The pulse rate can be extracted from the voltage variation across a resistor placed in series with the DC power supply. (See also Section 10.3.1 for related discussion.)

Figure 10.12 illustrates positioning of the prototype microwave sensor and a subject's wrist. The sensor is in contact with the skin directly over the radial artery. The VCO was tuned to 2.42 GHz, with a DC bias-voltage fluctuation of up to 10 mV, representing the heart or pulse rate. The arrangement allowed the subject to remain in the test position for prolonged measurement periods with reduced sensor movement-related noise. The prototype sensor is required to be consistently placed, such as with

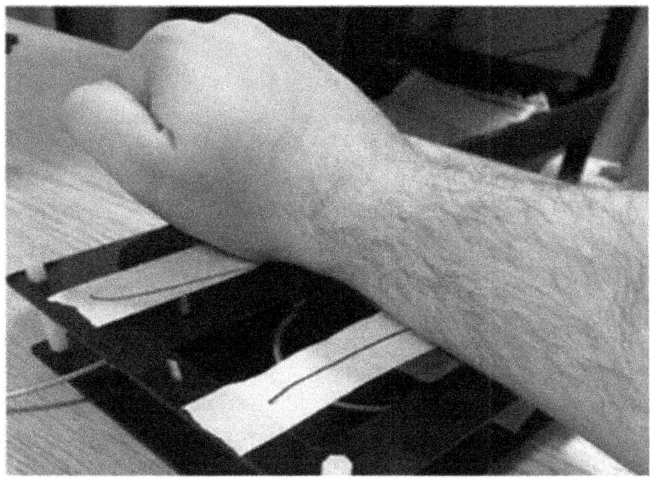

**FIGURE 10.12** Positioning of the prototype microwave sensor and a subject's wrist. (McFerran et al., 2019.)

the subject's wrist placed over the sensor, to reliably measure the subject's heart or pulse rate. It is obvious that the prototype is not ready or suitable to be wrist-worn or wearable on the wrist for pulse sensing.

Examples of measured results for a human subject are shown in Figure 10.13. The results are consistent with those obtained from using a commercial photo plethysmograph optical sensor-based pulse rate monitor. The data gave an average HR of 60 beats/min(bpm) in this case. The results show that the simple VCO/resonator detector can produce comparable results as PPG. However, the level of clutter noise

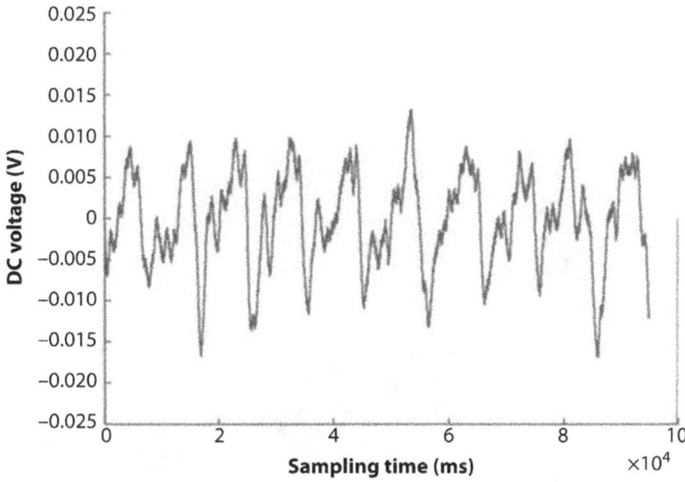


**FIGURE 10.13** Measured radial artery results from a human subject's wrist using a voltage-controlled oscillator.

is greater compared to some of the related results described earlier and in previous chapters. The signal quality can be substantially degraded by the insufficient directivity of the antenna and echo signals from the skin of monitored subject, although the clutter phenomenon could potentially be mitigated with further filtration and postprocessing of the signal. Indeed, other investigations using designs closely related to the VCO/resonator approach, such as the near-field contactless SIL sensors described earlier, have made further advances, and can offer superior performances in comparison as wearable pulse monitors.

## 10.4 WEARABLE MICROWAVE HR SENSORS

Displacements of the precordium overlying the apex of the heart and chest are related to mechanical movements in the left ventricle and echoes the hemodynamic events within the left ventricle. A prototype microwave sensor discussed in Chapter 7, Section 7.5, based on the well-known concept of Doppler radar, involved the detection of phase variation in the low-power microwave signal reflected using an antenna located in the near field (at 3 cm) over the apex of the heart [Lin et al., 1979]. However, the prototype system made use of a laboratory microwave antenna and test equipment that are not portable. In 2010, a small wearable microwave sensor for ambulatory cardiac monitoring was developed using low-cost Doppler radars [Fletcher and Kulkarni, 2010a, 2010b]. While the detection electrical system matches the earlier prototype, the principal advantage of the wearable device includes it being light weight and low cost. The clip-on microwave sensor can be placed on the subject's chest over clothing (Figure 10.14). A 2.45 GHz microwave oscillator was implemented using a single transistor oscillator circuit with a microstrip resonator. A low-power 8-bit microcontroller with 12-bit ADC was used to digitize the signal for minimal processing. A photograph of the microwave Doppler radar sensor is given in Figure 10.15 showing the integrated microwave circuit, patch antenna, filter, and microcontroller in a transparent plastic clip-on badge holder. The sensor includes a wireless data link for sending data to a remote

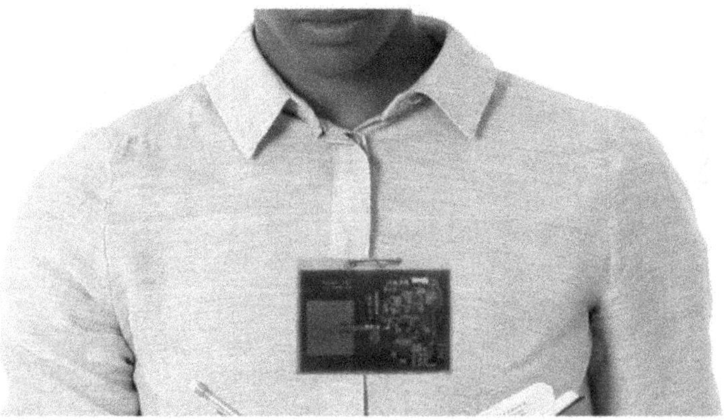

**FIGURE 10.14** A wearable clip-on microwave sensor inside a plastic sleeve over clothing.

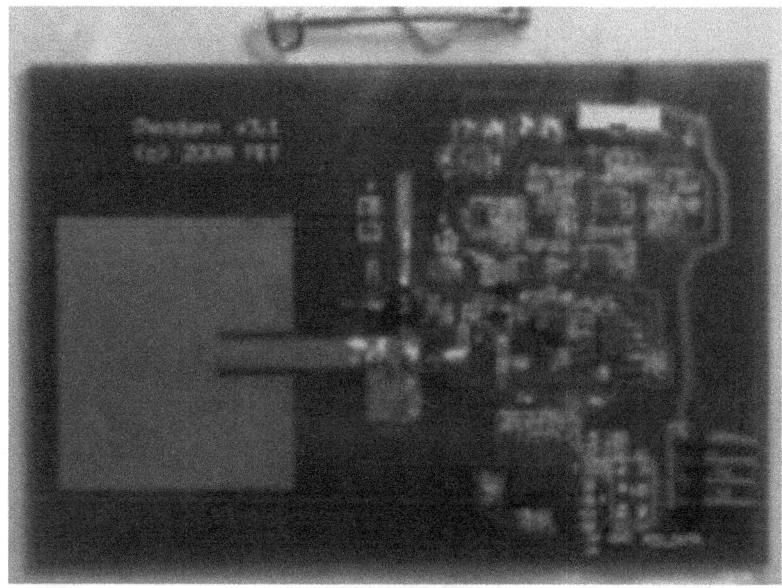

**FIGURE 10.15** Microwave sensor board including integrated microwave circuit, patch antenna, filter, and microcontroller in transparent plastic clip-on badge holder.

computer or mobile phone. The power consumption of the microwave sensor is roughly 30 mA when operating.

Some test results are given in Figures 10.16 and 10.17 for several subjects. Results are compared to data obtained from a commercial ECG monitor. Figure 10.16 shows several significant features that are much the same as those shown in Chapter 7, Section 7.5 for heart-movement signals measured by near-field microwave Doppler sensors in earlier investigations. Results exhibited in Figure 10.17 indicate that measurements from the wearable microwave sensor are generally

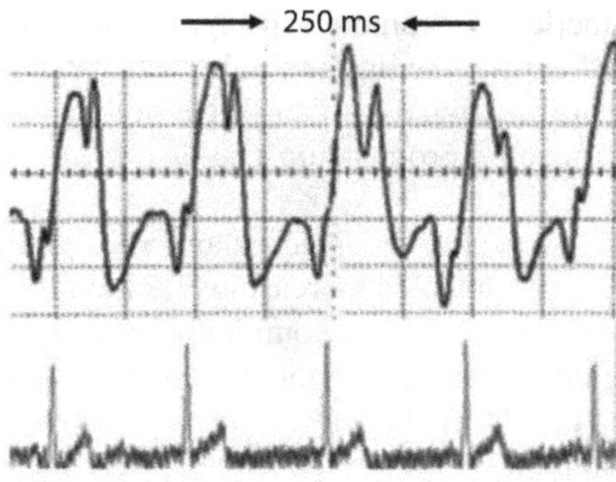


**FIGURE 10.16** Comparison between clip-on wearable microwave Doppler sensor (top) and commercial electrocardiogram monitor (bottom)-measured heart signals.

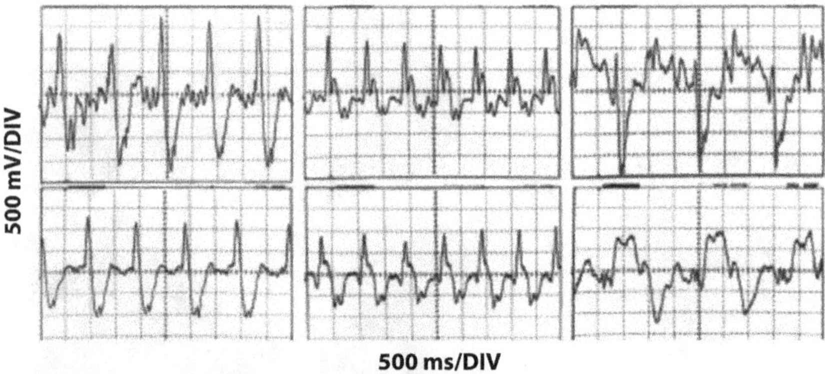


**FIGURE 10.17** Clip-on wearable microwave sensor measurements taken from three different subjects. The top row of tracings was taken with horizontal polarization and the bottom row corresponds to vertical polarization. The right-most data are for a subject with medically diagnosed Wolff-Parkinson-White syndrome.

reproducible, showing a significant number of unique features identifiable with various phases of cardiac contraction. However, a comparison between the wearable microwave sensor and results published decades ago for microwave apexcardiography (MACG) using laboratory-grade instrumentations [Lin et al., 1979] suggests that the data obtained from the wearable microwave sensor may have additional signal components that are linked to relative motions of the clip-on sensor, chest wall, other body movements caused by strong clutter from antenna coupling, and the reception of the echo signals.

## 10.5 CHEST-WORN SILO TAG SENSOR FOR HR MONITORING

Doppler microwave radars are vigorously investigated for use in the noninvasive monitoring of vital signs, circulatory phenomena, and respiratory activities through contact, contactless, or remote sensing. Except for contact applications, the quality of acquired cardiovascular and pulmonary signals are often degraded by the antenna's lack of directivity or other target body movements. The spurious scattered signals can become problematic clutter even for near-field contactless situations.

Recent advances in wearable Doppler radars based on SIL technology that avoid stationary clutter have enabled increasing attention for noncontact vital-sign monitoring applications. However, the commonly used broad-beam antennas for sensing heartbeat signals often have poor directivity toward the target area. A design was introduced to replace the antenna in SIL Doppler radar with a complementary split-ring resonator (CSRR) to generate a more focused electric field pattern [Tseng and Wu, 2020]. The design succeeded in demonstrating high-quality wrist or finger (see the next section) pulse-wave detection with better accuracy and lower noise levels.

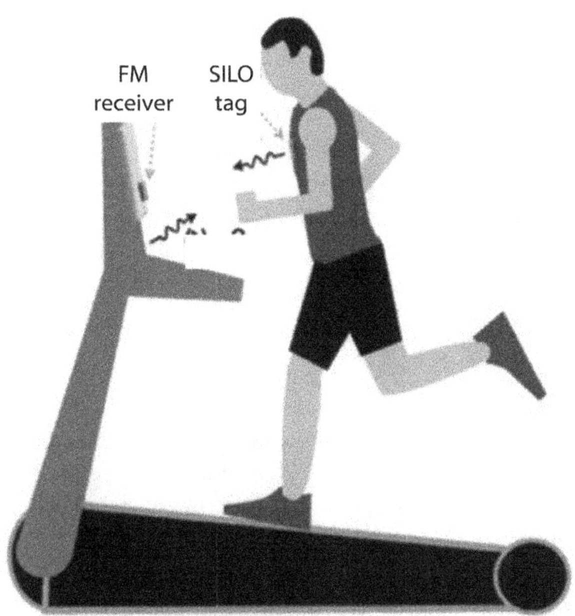


**FIGURE 10.18** Wearable microwave radar sensor with a self-injection locked oscillator (SILO) tag for monitoring the heartbeats of a person in motion.

Interestingly, a SILO tag worn on the chest of a subject to monitor heartbeat was recently reported [Arif et al., 2022]. The investigation builds on the novel concept of coupling an SIL radar with a split-ring resonator (SRR) for finger and wrist pulse detection [Tseng and Wu, 2020]. The 5.8 GHz sensor transmits the output signal (0.5 dBm) of a SILO that is frequency modulated (FM) by the Doppler effect of chest movement via the tag antenna to a remote FM receiver (Figure 10.18). The system architecture is shown in Figure 10.19. The chest-worn SILO tag senses the movement of the chest wall by injecting the Doppler-shifted signal into the SILO via its output port. A circularly polarized antenna in a stacked structure combined

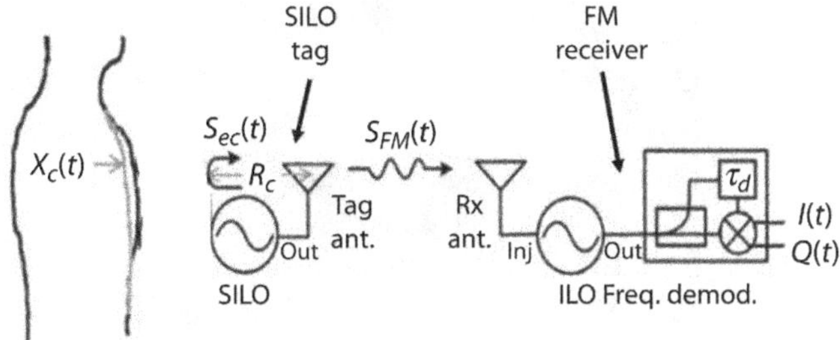


**FIGURE 10.19** The system architecture for a chest-worn self-injection locked oscillator (SILO) tag sensor for heart-rate monitoring.

with a CSRR enables simultaneous sensing and transmission. The tag is designed to use the SRR as a sensing interface to allow a greater transmitted field from the antenna with SRRs arranged in an array to enhance sensing directivity. The SILOs of the tag and the injection-locked oscillator (ILO) of the FM receiver are of the same circuit design. The antennas in both are circularly polarized to reduce interference due to noise clutter by rejecting the clutters associated with other moving objects through orthogonal polarization. The heartbeat signal is obtained using arctangent detection, i.e., by taking the arctangent of the in-phase and quadrature signals I(t) and Q(t) at the output of the demodulator.

The prototype HR sensor was laboratory tested using the experimental setup shown in Figure 10.20. A wearable SILO tag was attached to the subject's clothing. The FM receiver was located about 30 cm away on a tripod. Figure 10.21 compares the microwave signal at the output of the FM receiver with the reference ECG signal for a subject sitting quietly and holding breath for 15 seconds. As expected, the output microwave signal patently displays the cardiac motions with characteristics that correlate with those of the ECG signal. The microwave signal is clear and devoid of any body and respiratory motion artifacts.

Measurements recorded from a subject wearing the SILO tag while performing three successive activities — standing still for 50 seconds, walking in place for 40 seconds, and running in place for 30 seconds — are presented in Figure 10.22. There is little resemblance between the Doppler microwave signal and the reference

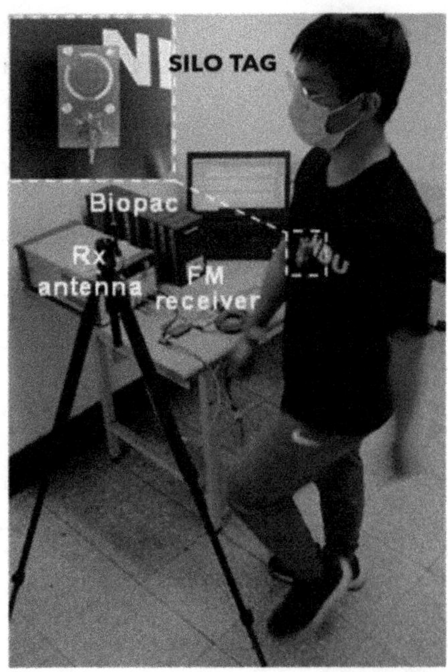


**FIGURE 10.20** A wearable self-injection locked oscillator (SILO) tag attached (see inset) to the subject's clothing. The FM receiver is located 30 cm away on a tripod along with a BIOPAC electrocardiogram monitor. (Courtesy of T.-S. Jason Horng, National Sun Yat-Sen University.)

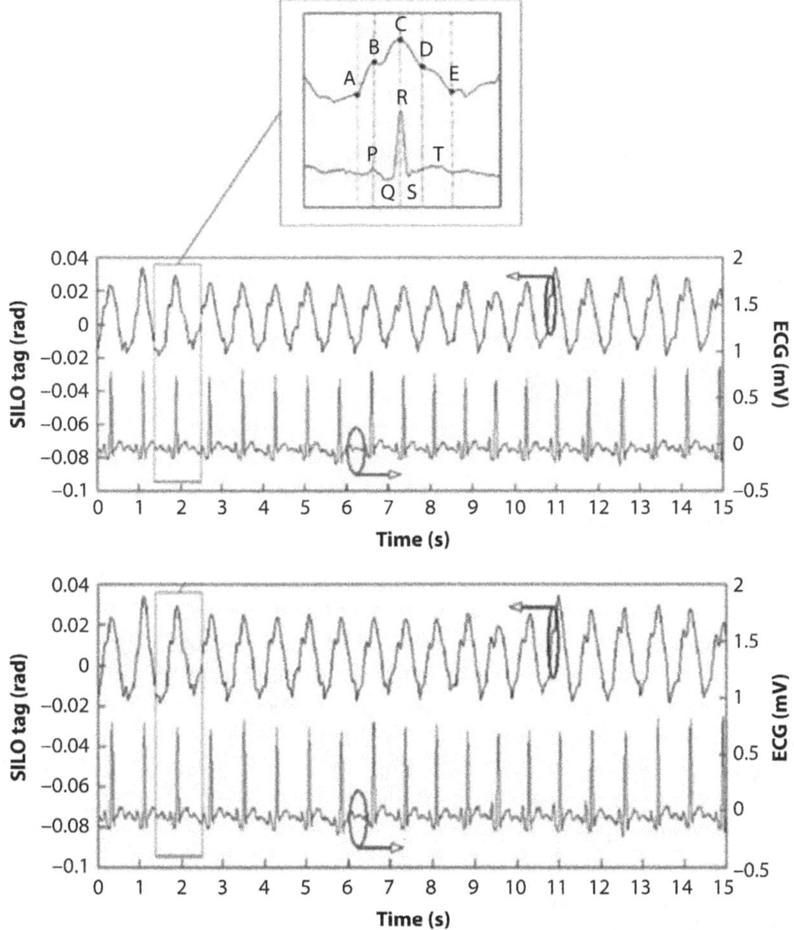


**FIGURE 10.21** Comparison of the Doppler microwave signal detected by the SILO tag (Upper trace in each panel) with the reference ECG signal (Lower trace) in a seated subject. The figure at top shows five characteristic points, A, B, C, D, and E, identifiable in a cycle of the Doppler waveform. Specifically, A - corresponds to the middle of the T-P interval, B - the peak of the P wave, C - the peak of the R wave, D - the beginning of the T wave, and E - the end of the T wave in the ECG.

ECG signal. A direct comparison between these two signals in Figure 10.22 is difficult. Apparently, the heartbeat is overwhelmed by respiratory and other body motions from the wearable microwave SILO tag sensor. Nonetheless, the report suggested that an empirical mode decomposition (EMD) method may be applied to remove the unwanted motion artifacts that involve nonlinear or nonstationary behavior [Mostafanezhad et al., 2013]. However, the use of the EMD method often suffers from a mode-mixing problem, which results in the spread of HR information around different intrinsic mode functions (IMFs). For further improvement, the well-known principal component analysis (PCA) algorithm may be combined with EMD method to extract HR from the Doppler microwave signal to yield fairly accurate estimates of HRs.

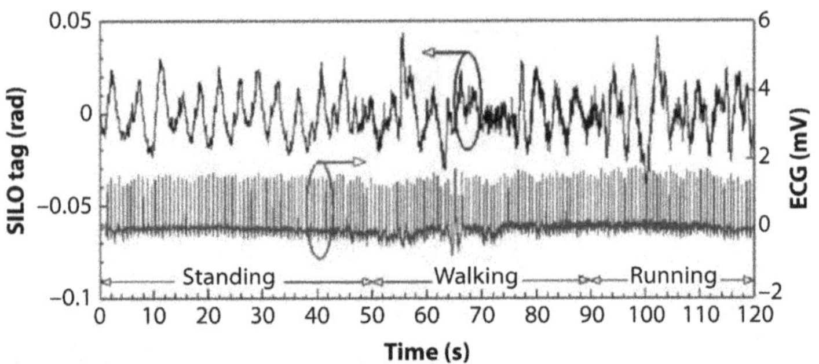


**FIGURE 10.22** Comparison of the Doppler signal detected by the self-injection locked oscillator (SILO tag) (upper) with the reference electrocardiogram ECG signal (lower) in phase 2 of the experiment.

## 10.6 CONTACT SENSING OF FINGERTIP AND WRIST PULSE WAVES

Many techniques using noninvasive sensing with microwaves have emphasized the efficacy and advantages of remote and contactless applications. The recent introduction of perturbation self-injection-locked oscillator (SO or ILO) with a complementary split-ring resonator (CSRR) for pulse sensing from the fingertip or wrist spotlights the attention on noninvasive contact applications such as vital-sign and arterial pulse-wave sensing [Tseng and Wu, 2020]. CSRRs can help produce a more focused electric-field pattern into a small area and work most effectively within the near field or in contact with the skin. Figure 10.23 presents a computational simulation of 5.6 GHz electric-field distributions on virtual observation planes as functions of distance in front of the CSRR. Note the electric field concentration in the near field region is well confined within the CSRR's 5 mm footprint (see related discussions in Chapter 8, Section 8.2 on Arterial Pulse-Wave Measurement and Figure 8.10).

The design succeeded in demonstrating detection of high-quality finger and wrist pulse waves with better accuracy and lower noise levels [Tseng and Wu, 2020]. A system block diagram of the ILO-CSRR/SO-CSRR sensor is given in Figure 10.24, showing the main circuit components. The output from the ILO-CSRR sensor is a frequency-modulated signal. Thus, the demodulation performance of the PLL in the ILO-CSRR sensor is superior compared to that of amplitude-based demodulation. Although the ILO-CSRR sensor does not include a voltage gain amplifier, it can provide better sensitivity and noise immunity than ILO or SIL sensors without CSRR.

The measured vital-sign (pulse) signals are sent to a laptop computer for signal processing and display. A photograph showing the top and bottom views of the ILO-CSRR sensor is given in Figure 10.25. In this configuration, the top view shows a microcontroller unit (MCU) used to control the PLL. The bottom view shows the location of the sensor opening for finger/wrist pulse sensing.

The performance of the CSRR sensor was tested with the measurement setups shown in Figure 10.26 for finger and wrist pulse sensing. The sensor with a 1 mm thick Styrofoam sheet cover to emulate the separation caused by sensor packaging

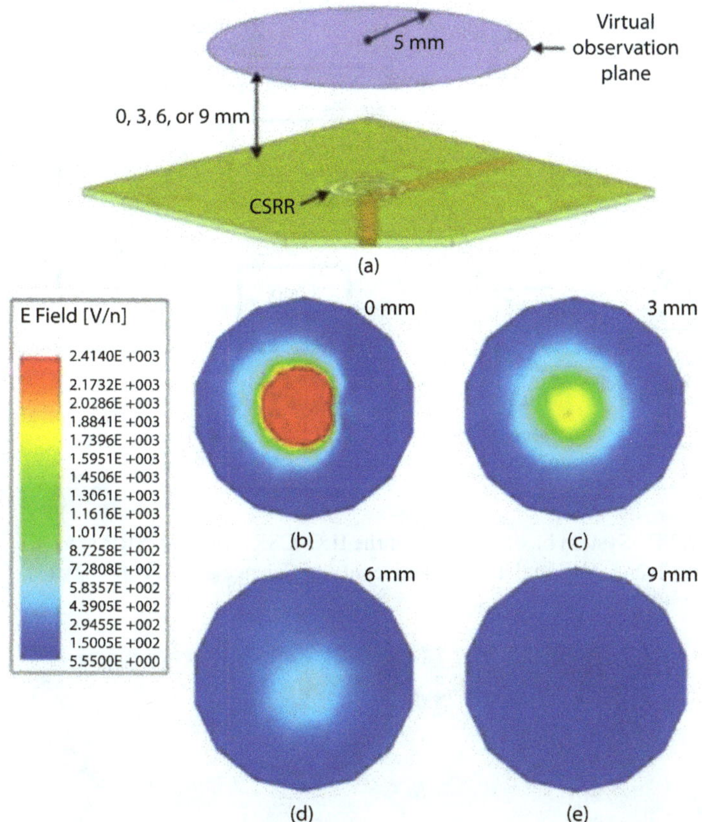


**FIGURE 10.23** Computational simulation of 5.6 GHz electric-field distributions on virtual observation planes in front of the CSRR: (a) Simulation configuration for observations at distances of (b) 0.0, (c) 3.0, (d) 6.0, and (e) 10.0 mm. (Courtesy of Chao-Hsiung Tseng, National Taiwan University of Science and Technology.)

was positioned on a table. The subject was instructed to press the index finger lightly on the CSRR (top figure). A record of the acquired time-domain waveform of the finger pulse is shown in Figure 10.27 along with the reference PPG finger pulse waves and respiration signal obtained using a respiration sensor belt strapped on the chest. The figures suggest that the finger pulse waveforms are similar, and the heartbeat rates are the same as measured by either the ILO-CSRR or PPG sensors. In addition, the respiration waveform appears as a slowly varying envelope over the CSRR finger pulses via amplitude modulation.

The measurement setup for wrist pulse sensing is shown in the bottom of Figure 10.26. As for finger pulse detect, the ILO-CSRR sensor was positioned on a table with a 1 mm thick Styrofoam sheet cover. The subject aligns the radial artery at the wrist with the CSRR sensor opening and then lightly presses the wrist over the sensor. Examples of the measured time-varying wrist pulse waves are shown in Figure 10.28. The reference PPG finger pulse and respiration waveforms are also

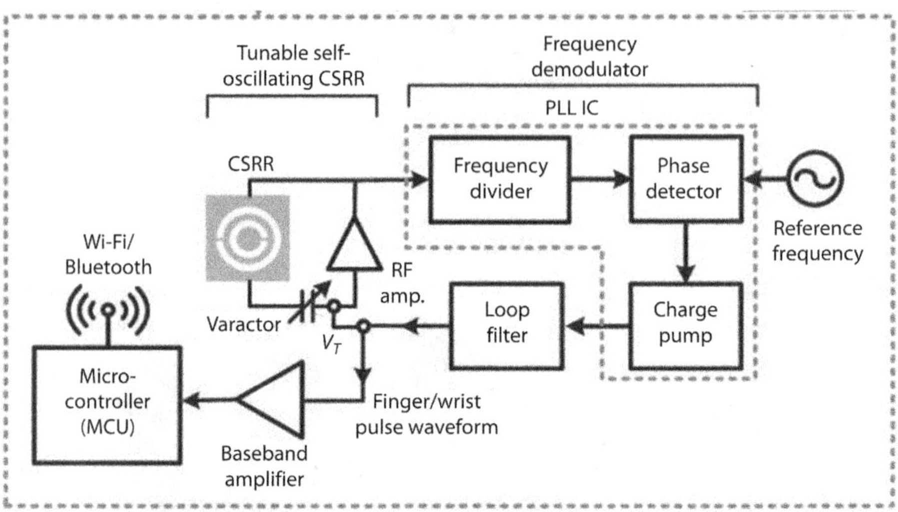


**FIGURE 10.24** System block diagram of the ILO-CSRR or SO-CSRR sensor. (Courtesy of Chao-Hsiung Tseng, National Taiwan University of Science and Technology.)

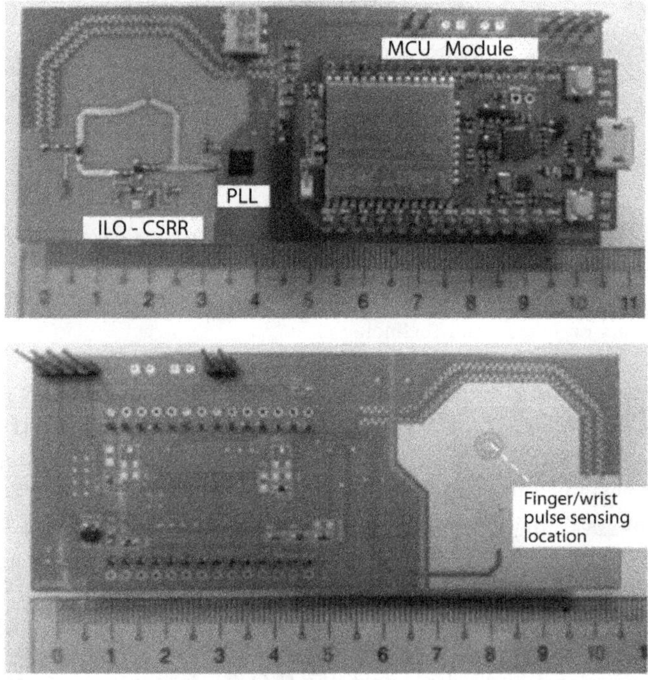


**FIGURE 10.25** Photograph of ILO-CSRR sensor: (a) Top view showing microcontroller unit (MCU) used to control the phase-lock-loop (PLL IC) and (b) the bottom view showing the finger/wrist pulse sensor location. (Courtesy of Chao-Hsiung Tseng, National Taiwan University of Science and Technology.)

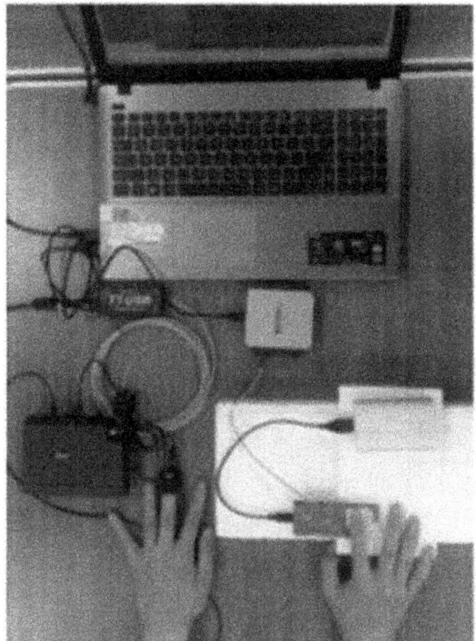
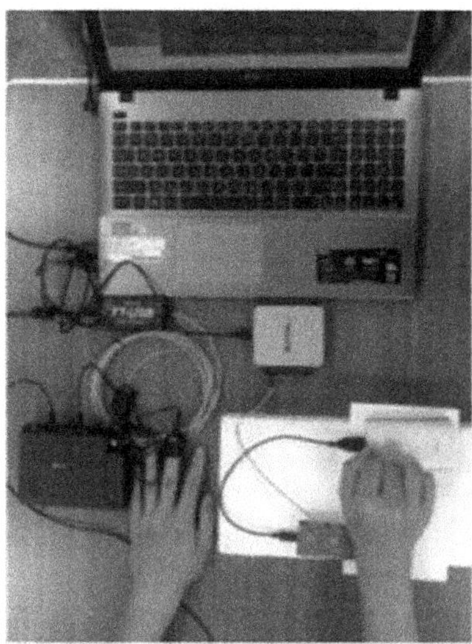

**FIGURE 10.26** Measurement setups for finger (a) and wrist (b) pulse sensing. (Courtesy of Chao-Hsiung Tseng, National Taiwan University of Science and Technology.)

shown in the same figure for comparison. Both the waveform and rate of the CSRR-measured wrist pulse waves are like those of the reference PPG recordings. In addition to the slowly varying envelope of the wrist pulse associated with the respiratory modulation, the wrist pulse waveform exhibits greater structural details that seem to correlate with vascular motion of the radial artery pulse.

In brief, the novel microwave ILO-CSRR or SO-CSRR sensor design has been experimentally demonstrated for successful noninvasive detection of finger and wrist pulse waves. The key resonator component in CSRR was employed to produce

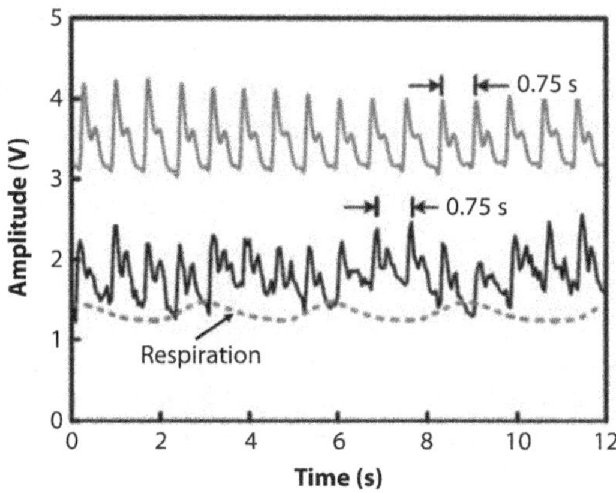


**FIGURE 10.27** Measured time-domain results of finger pulse detection using ILO-CSRR and photoplethysmography sensor (upper).

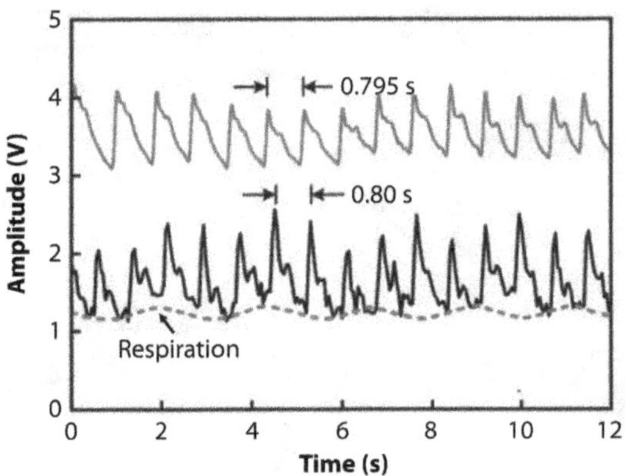


**FIGURE 10.28** Examples of the measured time-varying wrist pulse wave detection using an ILO-CSRR sensor (lower) compared to photoplethysmography sensor (upper).

a focused electric field in the near-field region. Since the electric field could be effectively targeted in the sensing area, it significantly improves the sensitivity for finger/wrist pulse detection as compared to antenna-based SIL sensors [Tseng et al., 2018; Wang et al., 2016]. Furthermore, the PLL frequency-demodulation scheme helped to improve detection sensitivity and noise immunity. The widely adopted PPG sensor for finger-pulse sensing requires the PPG sensor to be fastened tightly to the finger [Khan et al., 2016]. In contrast, the microwave CSRR sensor only needs a gentle press of the fingertip on the sensor. Thus, microwave CSRR sensors may prove to be a viable competitor with great potentials for wearable healthcare applications as a finger pulse sensor.

## 10.7 WEARABLE MILLIMETER-WAVE ARTERIAL PULSE SENSOR

As described in Section 8.2.2.4, a noncontact, a 60 Hz mm-wave (mmW) frequency-modulated continuous wave (FMCW) radar sensor was designed and fabricated using commercially available FMCW radar integrated-circuit (IC) chips for sensing arterial pulse waves at close range without disturbing the artery itself [Johnson et al., 2019]. For wearable applications, an antenna-to-skin standoff distance was maintained to keep the target artery in the near field for noncontact monitoring. The model shown in Figure 10.29 illustrates a patch antenna on PCB aligned inside a plastic enclosure for mounting over skin tissue. The plastic enclosure allows the patch radar antenna to be positioned above the skin surface for consistent measurements of arterial pulse waves without contacting or disturbing the pulsing artery.

In human studies conducted with a normal subject, the prototype sensor in plastic enclosure was attached to the wrist of a seated subject using a nylon strap and positioned over the radial artery as shown in Figure 10.30. This permits the radar antenna to be placed on the wrist without touching the skin. Simultaneous ECG recordings were made for reference. Preliminary testing indicated that arm motions during the measurements could significantly distort the results. Thus, the subjects were instructed to remain still while data was being collected.

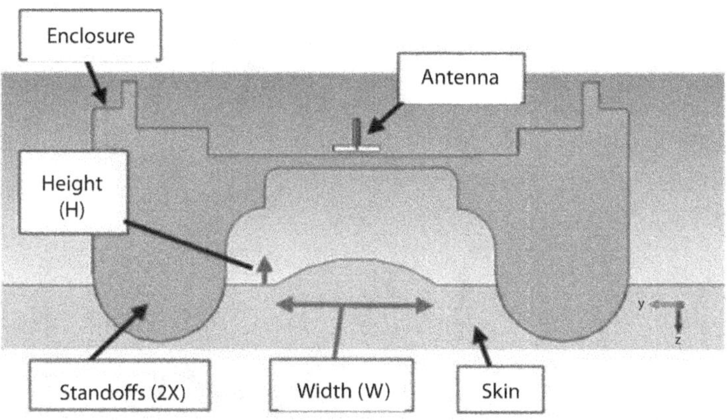


**FIGURE 10.29** Model of an antenna and enclosure positioned on the skin over an artery with H for artery height and W for width. Note that the extent of expansion (height and width) of the artery is exaggerated for illustration. (Courtesy of Jessi Johnson, Blumio Inc.)

Figure 10.31 presents normalized radial pulse waveforms and the corresponding frequency spectrum from two human studies, a subject with strong (Pat01) and one with weak (Pat02) signal. A low-frequency respiratory artifact is evident in both recordings. However, the pulse rates are consistent for both recordings, which suggests the mmW radar could provide viable monitoring of pulse rates for a variety of subjects noninvasively by wrist measurement without disturbing the arterial pulse itself. There are beat-to-beat variations in waveform shape and amplitude. The beat-to-beat and average pulse rate was computed using peak-to-peak timing over a 10-second sample window for the radar and ECG signals. Results showed a maximum difference of 0.05 Hz (0.3 bpm) was observed between the radar and ECG over a 10-second duration from an ensemble of 12 subjects. Thus, the

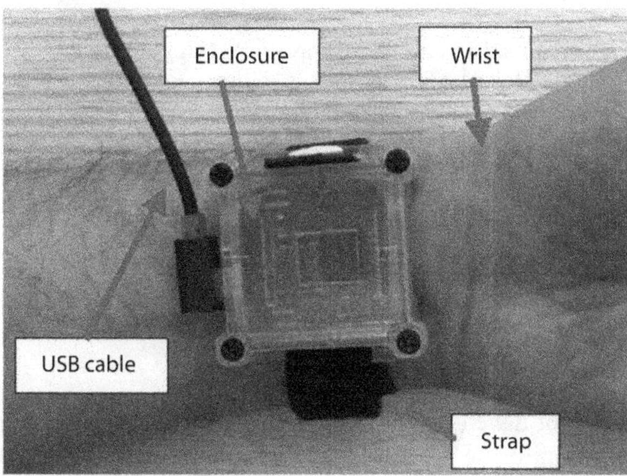


**FIGURE 10.30** Photograph of mm-wave arterial sensor strapped on wrist of a subject for radial artery pulse measurement. (Courtesy of Jessi Johnson, Blumio Inc.)

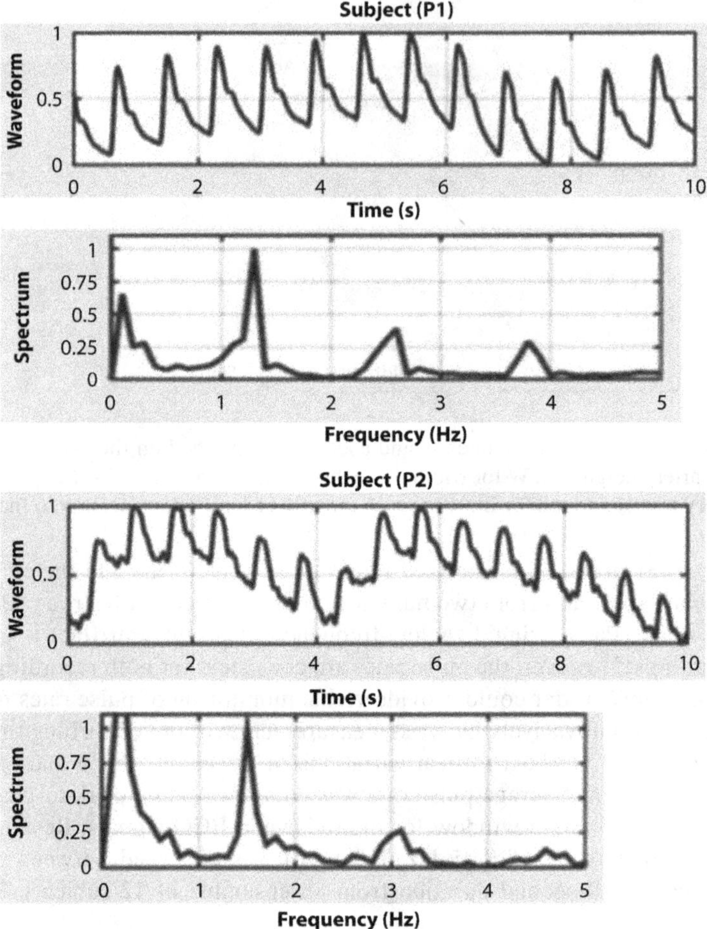


**FIGURE 10.31** Normalized radial artery waveform (Upper in each case) and frequency spectrum (Lower) obtained from a human subject with stronger signal (P1) and a subject with weaker signal (P2).

beat-to-beat tracking of the pulse rate was comparable between radar and ECG. This suggests that the mmW radar system is a feasible approach for characterizing both HR and HRV.

## 10.8 CHEST-WORN 5.8 GHz SILO FOR RESPIRATION MONITORING

Recently, the design of a wearable SILO respiration sensor was validated for operation at 5.8 GHz in monitoring breathing activities of human subjects [Costanzo et al., 2023; Paolini et al., 2022]. The chest-worn respiration sensor in a plastic holder is strapped on the torso using an elastic band over clothing. The spacing is roughly 2.5 cm between the SILO sensor antenna and torso (Figure 10.32).

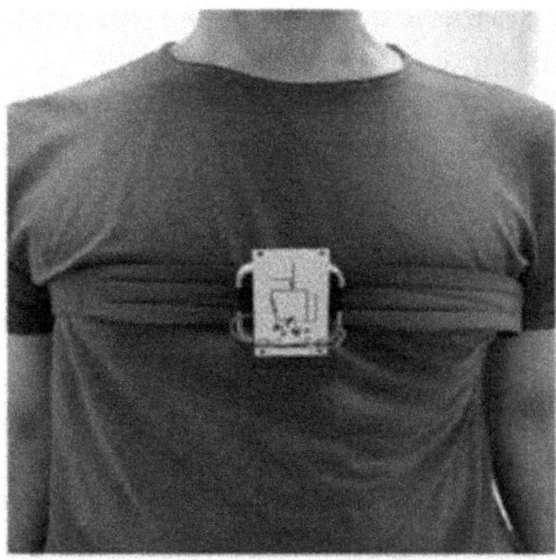

**FIGURE 10.32** Wearable self-injection locked oscillator radar sensor positioned on a subject's chest for measurement of breathing activity. (Costanzo et al., 2023.)

As a distinctive feature, the system's design includes an RF-to-DC rectifier to support energy harvesting to power an MCU and a transceiver to transmit respiration data to a laptop computer or a mobile phone. This device can harvest radio frequency (RF) energy from the modulated 5.8 GHz, while down-converting it to retrieve the respiratory signal of the subject from the SILO sensor. The overall estimated power consumption is 220 mW and the transmitted power is roughly 10 mW. With an antenna gain of 6.84 dBi, the corresponding effective isotropic radiated power (EIRP) is approximately 48 mW for the prototype.

Figure 10.33 presents a block diagram of the wearable respiration monitor for breathing-rate detection with RF energy harvesting via system-on-chip (SoC). The radiating component of the 5.8 GHz sensor is a dual-port, dual-polarized, aperture-coupled patch antenna connected to the input and output ports of the SILO circuit. A quarter-wavelength microstrip coupler connects the SILO output to a passive demodulator/rectifier to complete detection of the output voltage peaks for breathing rates for the prototype. The signal processing is performed on-board in real time. Compared to other existing designs or solutions, this wearable SILO sensor design offers a reduced dimensional profile for contactless respiratory rate measurements.

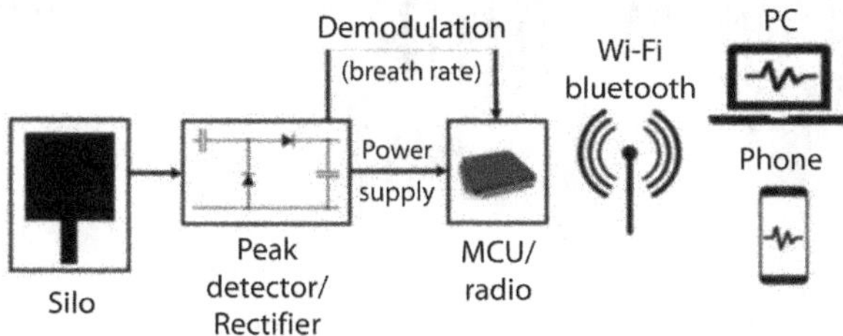


**FIGURE 10.33** Block diagram of wearable respiration monitor for breathing rate detection with radio frequency energy harvesting via system-on-a-chip.

The respiratory activity for a human subject breathing at two different rates recorded from the demodulator output is shown in Figure 10.34. Clearly, the wearable SILO sensor can detect a normal RR of 15 breath/min (bpm) or (0.25 Hz) and a faster tachypnea rate of 42 bpm (0.7 Hz). The waveforms contain significant levels of

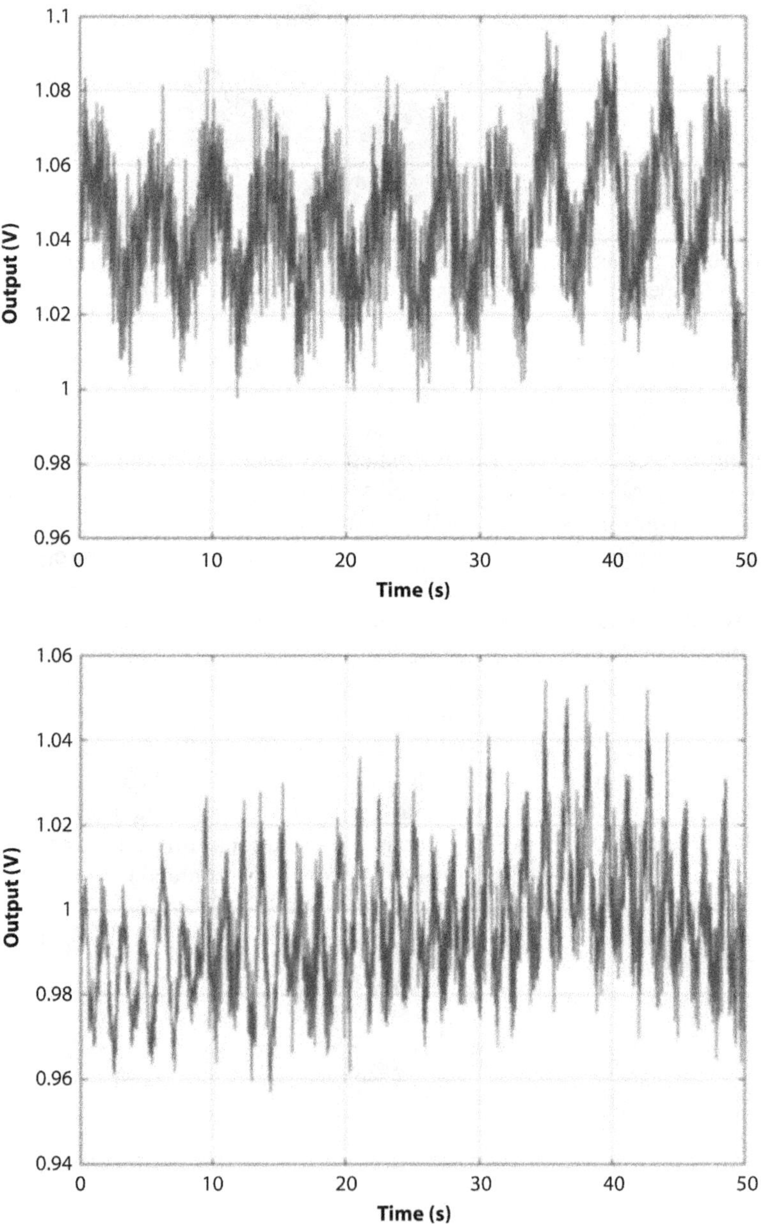


**FIGURE 10.34** Output voltage waveforms of the demodulator circuit: (a) normal breathing at 0.25 Hz (15 bpm) and (b) rapid breathing at 0.7 Hz (42 bpm).

high-frequency spurious noise from other bodily movements riding on the respiratory signal. While the high-frequency noise is apparent, the demodulated signal is still amenable to retrieval of respiratory signals, especially, extraction of minima and maxima corresponding to inspiration and expiration, without any filtration process. However, it was noted that the detected signal can vary significantly with the relative position of the sensor with respect to the chest.

Regarding the resulting monitor's energy harvesting performance, tests suggest that for an input power equal to 10 dBm, the power conversion efficiency (PCE) is roughly 36%, whereas the result for the same circuit is 20% with 0 dBm of input power. These values of PCEs are lower than tthose reported in the literature [Sabban, 2022 for energy harvesting]. Perhaps, the differences may stem from variances with the standard energy harvester design; note that a matching network is missing in this case.

## 10.9 WEARABLE CARDIOPULMONARY MOTION SENSORS

Recently, a multisensor technique for heartbeat and respiratory motion measurement was reported based on near-field microwave (1.82 and 1.9 GHz) sensing, named near-field coherent sensing (NCS) of chest movements through clothing [Sharma et al., 2020]. The small lightweight microwave sensors, which consist of microwave TX and RX antennas connected to the software-defined radio (SDR) transceiver in a 3D-printed package (Figure 10.35), can make measurements with a power consumption of roughly 10 dBm.

The laboratory setup to monitor heartbeat and respiration is illustrated in Figure 10.36. NCS sensors are placed on a participant, one close to the heart and the other below the xiphoid process of the sternum and close to the diaphragm, to detect the heart and lung motions that modulate the microwave signal. The figure shows the placement, data collection, and signal flow of all sensors including commercial BIOPAC ECG, chest belts, and a pneumotachometer (PTM) connected to a facemask. It also shows a subject in the sitting position instrumented with all sensors including the two wearable NCS sensors.

Experiments were performed with 20 healthy participants (14 females) in various postures and under different breathing conditions. Figure 10.37 shows the results for NCS and ECG measured HRs across three postures with different breathing modes including conscious normal, deep, fast, and breath-hold (BH), as well as spontaneous breathing in relaxation and attention states. The scatter plot (a-top) displays the HR data with a Pearson's correlation coefficient, r = 0.95, indicating an excellent correlation between the two sensors.

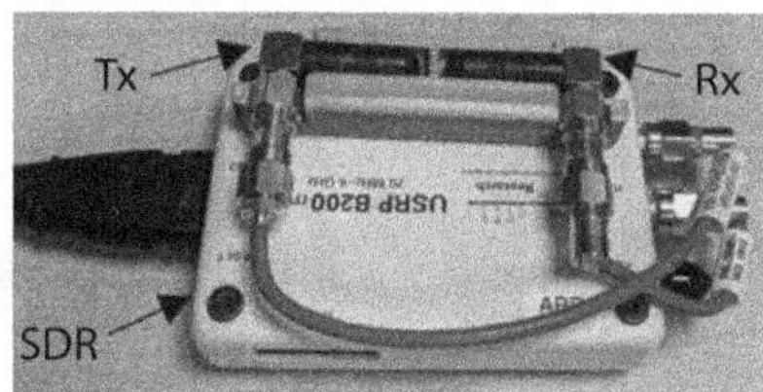


**FIGURE 10.35** Microwave TX and RX antennas connected to the software-defined radio (SDR) transceiver in a 3D-printed package. (Sharma et al., 2020.)

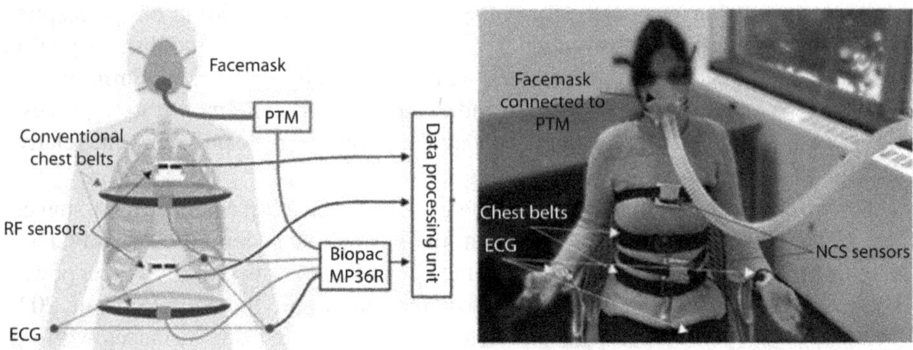


**FIGURE 10.36** The laboratory setup to monitor heartbeat and respiration. (Sharma et al., 2020.)

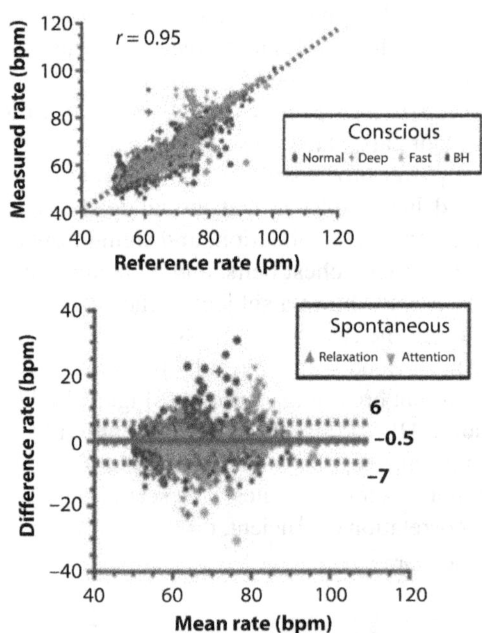


**FIGURE 10.37** Correlation and agreement between the near-field coherent sensing and electrocardiogram-measured heart rate for the entire dataset. The label shows a marker for each breathing mode, including conscious normal, deep, fast, and breath-hold (BH), as well as spontaneous breathing in relaxation and attention states. The scatter plot (top) with Pearson's correlation coefficient r and Bland-Altman plot (bottom) showing bias m at the center (solid line) and the corresponding limits of agreement (dashed line) given by $m \pm 1.96(\sigma)$.

The Bland-Altman (B&A) plot was employed to quantify the agreement between NCS and ECG, which can be used to estimate the mean m and standard deviation $\sigma$ of the measurement differences. B&A plots can also identify possible outliers in an XY scatter plot, with the Y axis as the pairwise difference, and the X axis as the mean of the two measurements. Any systematic bias is estimated as the mean difference m and limits of agreement (LoA) within which 95% of the differences are expected to lie, such as LoA = m ± 1.96 ($\sigma$), assuming a normal distribution. Figure 10.37 (b-bottom) shows good agreement (small differences) between the sensors with low mean deviation, mHR = −0.5 bpm and narrow LoA, as denoted by the dashed lines around the mean value.

As mentioned, the NCS sensors are designed also to measure respiratory changes from movements induced in the chest wall over clothing via SDRs. The results on RR shown in Figure 10.38 are from the same group of 20 healthy participants mentioned above and were obtained using the same instrumentation as those presented in Figure 10.36. The correlation coefficient and mean LoA for tests conducted on subjects performing voluntary breathing exercises in different postures are illustrated in Figure 10.38. A high correlation at r = 0.93 of the NCS sensor with the reference device for the respiratory rate was demonstrated. It also showed good agreement between the sensors with low mean deviations (mRR = 0.05 bpm) and narrow LoA around the mean value.

In short, suitable correlations of the over-clothing multiple NCS microwave sensor designs with the reference devices for heartbeat and RR can be achieved.

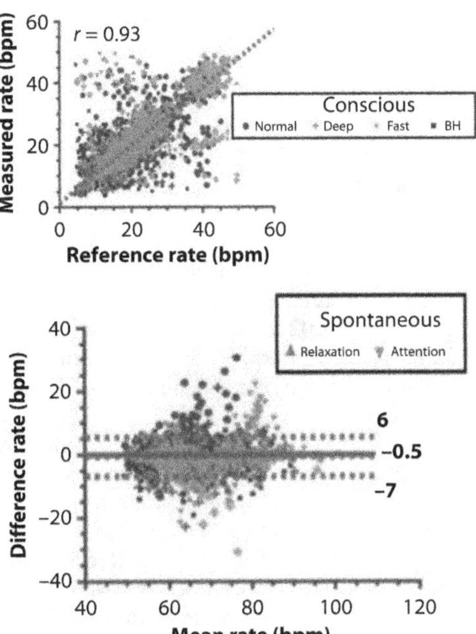


**FIGURE 10.38** Correlation (top) and limits of agreement (bottom) of the near-field coherent sensor compared to reference device for respiratory rate measurement (see also explanations in Figure 10.37).

By design necessity, the multiparameter technique demands more components and greater circuit complexity. It is a noninvasive approach that functions by transmitting a low-power continuous wave microwave signal into the body with over-clothing antennas. As with other near-field and contact modes of operation, especially when compared to far-field environments, the wearable NCS sensor design has high ambient motion tolerance, which makes NCS sensors less vulnerable to environmental clutter, where motion within the antenna radiation pattern can cause significant interference. Furthermore, multiple sensors can be placed on the body to couple to both respiratory and heartbeat motion with frequency multiplexing. It is conceivable that due to its transceiver architecture, the NCS sensor may be designed with compact form factors at lower costs.

An NCS technique for long-term wearable heart motion measurement by placing multiple sensing antennas over clothing on the chest was proposed that would enable near-field detection of heartbeat movement-induced modulations in the received microwave signal [Hui et al., 2020]. It is closely related to the multipoint system described previously, which uses SDRs. The NCS method enables position-specific sensing in which multiple antennas provide dynamic information to analyze complex heartbeat motions, including both systemic and pulmonary circulation with the participants in a still sitting position and a controlled breathing rhythm (see further details in Chapter 8, Section 8.5).

Note that additional discussions on near-field sensing and monitoring including patch antennas, wideband sensors, over-clothing, and wearable systems as well as applications for pulmonary edema and lung-fluid content detection can be found in Chapter 9, Sections 9.3, 9.4, and 9.5.

## REFERENCES

Arif, R. E., Su, W. C., Horng, T. S., 2022. Chest-worn heart rate variability monitor with a self-injection-locked oscillator tag. IEEE Trans. Microw. Theory Tech., 70(5):2851–2860

Atallah, L., Serteyn, A., Meftah, M., Schellekens, M., Vullings, R., Bergmans, J. W., Osagiator, A., Oetomo, S. B., 2014. Unobtrusive ECG monitoring in the NICU using a capacitive sensing array. Physiol. Meas., 35(5):895–913

Bae, S., Borac, S., Emre, Y., et al., 2022. Prospective validation of smartphone-based heart rate and respiratory rate measurement algorithms. Commun. Med., 40(2022). https://doi.org/10.1038/s43856-022-00102-x

Baek, H. J., Chung, G. S., Kim, K. K., Park, K. S., 2012. A smart health monitoring chair for nonintrusive measurement of biological signals. IEEE Trans. Inf. Tech. Biomed., 16(1):150–158

Cao, R., Azimi, I., Sarhaddi, F., Niela-Vilen, H., Axelin, A., Liljeberg, P., Rahmani, A. M., 2022. Accuracy assessment of oura ring nocturnal heart rate and heart rate variability in comparison with electrocardiography in time and frequency domains: Comprehensive analysis. J. Med. Internet Res., 24(1):e27487. https://doi.org/10.2196/27487

Cheng, Y., Wang, K., Xu, H., Li, T., Jin, Q., Cui, D., 2021. Recent developments in sensors for wearable device applications. Anal. Bioanal. Chem., 413(24):6037–6057

Chow, H., Yang, C., 2020. Accuracy of optical heart rate sensing technology in wearable fitness trackers for young and older adults: Validation and comparison study. JMIR. Mhealth. Uhealth., 8(4):e1470

Costanzo, A., Augello, E., Battistini, G., Benassi, F., Masotti, D., Paolini, G., 2023. Microwave devices for wearable sensors and IoT. Sensors, 23, 4356. https://doi.org/10.3390/s23094356

Daskalaki, E., Parkinson, A., Brew-Sam, N., Hossain, Z., O'Neal, D., Nolan, C. J., Suominen, H., 2022. The potential of current noninvasive wearable technology for the monitoring of physiological signals in the management of type 1 diabetes: Literature survey. J. Med. Internet. Res., 24(4):e28901

Dixon, M., Schneider, L. D., Yu, J., Hsu, J., Pathak, A., Shin, D., Lee, R. S., Malhotra, M., Mixter, K., McConnell, M. V., Taylor, J. A., Patel, S. N., 2021. Sleep-Wake Detection with a Contactless, Bedside Radar Sleep Sensing System Google Whitepaper

Fletcher, R. R., Kulkarni, S., 2010a. Clip-on wireless wearable microwave sensor for ambulatory cardiac monitoring. Annu Int Conf IEEE Eng Med Biol Soc. 2010:365

Fletcher, R. R., Kulkarni, S., 2010b. Wearable Doppler radar with integrated antenna for patient vital sign monitoring. 2010 IEEE Radio and Wireless Symposium (RWS), New Orleans, LA, USA, 2010, 276–279

Guk, K., Han, G., Lim, J., Jeong, K., Kang, T., Lim, E. K., et al., 2019. Evolution of wearable devices with real-time disease monitoring for personalized healthcare. Nanomaterials., 9(6):813. https://doi.org/10.3390/nano9060813

Harland, C. J., Clark, T. D., Peters, N. S., Everitt, M. J., Stiffell, P. B., 2005. A compact electric potential sensor array for the acquisition and reconstruction of the 7-lead electrocardiogram without electrical charge contact with the skin. Physiol. Meas., 26:939–950

He, D. D., Winokur, E. S., Sodini, C. G., 2015. An ear-worn vital signs monitor. IEEE Trans. Biomed. Eng., 62(11):2547–2552

Hui, X., Conroy, T. B., Kan, E. C., 2020. Multi-point near-field RF sensing of blood pressures and heartbeat dynamics. IEEE Access, 8:89935–89945

Johnson, J. E., Shay, O., Kim, C., Liao, C., 2019. Wearable millimeter-wave device for contactless measurement of arterial pulses. IEEE Trans. Biomed. Circuits Syst., 13(6):1525–1534

Khan, E., Al Hossain, F., Uddin, S. Z., Alam, S. K., Hasan, M. K., 2016. A robust heart rate monitoring scheme using photoplethysmographic signals corrupted by intense motion artifacts. IEEE Trans. Biomed. Eng., 63(3):550–562

Kim, B., Hong, Y., An, Y., et al., 2016. A proximity coupling RF sensor for wrist pulse detection based on injection-locked PLL. IEEE Trans. Microw. Theory Tech., 64(5):1667–1676

Klabunde, R. E., 2021. Cardiovascular Physiology Concepts, 3rd ed, Philadelphia: Wolters Kluwer

Li, C., Lubecke, V. M., Boric-Lubecke, O., Lin, J., 2021. Sensing of life activities at the human-microwave frontier. IEEE J. Microw., 1(1):66–78

Lin, J. C., 1989. Microwave noninvasive sensing of physiological signatures, In: Lin, J. C., Ed. Electromagnetic Interaction with Biological Systems (pp. 3–25), New York: Plenum

Lin, J. C., Kiernicki, J., Kiernicki, M., Wollschlaeger, P. B., 1979. Microwave Apexcardiography, IEEE Trans. Microwave Theory and Tech., 27:618–620

Matthews, R., McDonald, N. J., Fridman, I., Hervieux, P., Nielsen, T., 2005. The invisible electrode zero prep time, ultra low capacitive sensing. Proceedings of 11th International Conference on Human-Computer Interaction, Las Vegas, NV, pp. 22–27

McFerran, C., McKernan, A., Buchanan, N. B., 2019. Simplified wrist-worn heart rate sensor using microwave VCO. Electron. Lett., 55(7):370–372

Mostafanezhad, I., Yavari, E., Boric-Lubecke, O., Lubecke, V. M., Mandic, D. P., 2013. Cancellation of unwanted Doppler radar sensor motion using empirical mode decomposition. IEEE Sensors J., 13(5):1897–1904

Oehler, M., Ling, V., Melhorn, K., Schilling, M., 2008. A multichannel portable ECG system with capacitive sensors. Physiol. Meas., 29(7):783–793

Paolini, G., Shanawani, M., Masotti, D., Schreurs, M. M. P., Costanzo, A., 2022. Respiratory activity monitoring by a wearable 5.8 ghz silo with energy harvesting capabilities. IEEE J. Electromagn. RF Microw. Med. Biol., 6(2):246–252

Portelli, A. J., Nasuto, S. J., 2017. Design and development of non-contact bio-potential electrodes for pervasive health monitoring applications. Biosensors, 7(1):2. https://doi.org/10.3390/bios7010002

Prawiro, E., Yeh, C. I., Chou, N. K., Lee, M. W., Lin, Y. H., 2016. Integrated wearable system for monitoring heart rate and step during physical activity. Mob. Inf. Syst., Article ID 6850168, 10 pages. https://doi.org/10.1155/2016/6850168

RCA Laboratories, 1987. Miniature Superficial Temporal Artery Monitor. Final Laboratory Report, Princeton, New Jersey

Sabban, A., 2022. Wearable self-powered sensors for health care, 5G, energy harvesting, and IOT systems. Biomed. J. Sci. Tech. Res., 41(1):006550

Seneviratne, S., Hu, Y., Nguyen, T., Lan, G., Khalifa, S., Thilakarathna, K., et al., 2017. A survey of wearable devices and challenges. IEEE Commun. Surv. Tutor., 19(4):2573–2620

Sharma, P., Hui, X., Zhou, J., et al., 2020. Wearable radio-frequency sensing of respiratory rate, respiratory volume, and heart rate. NPJ Digit. Med., 3:98. https://doi.org/10.1038/s41746-020-0307-6

Simon, D. A., Shachar, C., Cohen, I. G., 2022. Unsettled liability issues for "prediagnostic" wearables and health-related products. JAMA. 328(14):1391–1392. https://doi.org/10.1001/jama.2022.16317

Tison, G. H., Sanchez, J. M., Ballinger, B., et al., 2018. Passive detection of atrial fibrillation using a commercially available smartwatch. JAMA Cardiol. 3(5):409–416. https://doi.org/10.1001/jamacardio.2018.0136

Tseng, C. H., Wu, C. Z., 2020. A novel microwave phased- and perturbation-injection-locked sensor with self-oscillating complementary split-ring resonator for finger and wrist pulse detection. IEEE Trans. Microw. Theory Tech., 68(5):1933–1942

Tseng, C. H., Tseng, T. J., Wu, C. Z., 2020. Cuffless blood pressure measurement using a microwave near-field self-injection-locked wrist pulse sensor. IEEE Trans. Microw. Theory Tech., 68(11):4865–4874

Tseng, C. H., Yu, L. T., Huang, J. K., Chang, C. L., 2018. A wearable self-injection-locked sensor with active integrated antenna and differentiator based envelope detector for vital-sign detection from chest wall and wrist. IEEE Trans. Microw. Theory Tech., 66(5):2511–2521

Wang, F. K., Li, C. J., Hsiao, C. H., Horng, T. S., Lin, J., Peng, K. C., Jau, J. K., Li, J. Y., Chen, C. C., 2010. A novel vital-sign sensor based on a self-injection-locked oscillator. IEEE Trans. Microw. Theory Tech., 58(12):4112–4120

Wang, F. K., Horng, T. S., Peng, K. C., Jau, J. K., Li, J. Y., Chen, C. C., 2011. Single-antenna Doppler radars using self and mutual injection locking for vital sign detection with random body movement cancellation. IEEE Trans. Microw. Theory Tech., 59(12)3577–3587

Wang, F. K., Tang, M. C., Su, S. C., Horng, T. S., 2016. Wrist pulse rate monitor using self-injection-locked radar technology. Biosensors (Basel). 6(4):54

Yilmaz, T., Foster, R., Hao, Y., 2010. Detecting vital signs with wearable wireless sensors. Sensors, 10(12):10837–10862. https://doi.org/10.3390/s101210837

Zhou, J., Sharma, P., Hui, X., Kan, E. C., 2020. A wireless wearable RF sensor for brumation study of chelonians. IEEE J. Electromagn. RF Microw. Med. Biol., 5(1):17–24

# 11 Advanced Topics and Contemporary Applications

The previous chapters of this book discussed developments in noninvasive microwave sensing for vital signs, pulse waves, arterial pressure, edema, and body fluid-volume changes. The emphasis has been on noninvasive physiological sensors for healthcare, wellness, and fitness sensing and monitoring. The discussions have concentrated on sensor design, device feasibility, prototyping, concept validation, laboratory evaluation, preclinical testing, efficacy study, and sensors that function as standalone systems. The sensing scenarios have included contact, noncontact, near-field, and remote stand-off protocols involving mostly a single subject or participant. In a few cases, the sensor development has reached the commercialization stage, and some are able to interface with wireless communication protocols to make use of the Internet system for additional analysis and decision-making. The important aims of these sensors and devices include flexibility, light weight, unobtrusiveness, and subject or patient acceptance and comfort that go beyond their functionality and noninvasiveness.

This chapter describes some advanced experiments and contemporary applications where the potential of wireless noninvasive sensing is explored for contactless remote sensing of vital signs from multiple subjects in a crowd, applications in medicine and health care, and monitoring driver alertness. The fundamental microwave radar designs are analogous to those discussed in previous chapters. The main antenna features of importance are comparable to those of single-target applications. However, advances and developments in radar hardware and architectures such as array antennas are especially beneficial for multiple-target application scenarios [Fang et al., 2020; Islam et al., 2022; Li et al., 2021; Xu et al., 2022]. In this regard, it is interesting to note the novel design of a four-element antenna array on a flexible 100 μm thick liquid crystal polymer (LCP) substrate ($\varepsilon_r = 3.35$). The compact 36.5 × 53 mm$^2$ antenna array was used in a 24 GHz radar system for contactless vital-sign monitoring of two human subjects from a distance of 60 cm at a radio frequency (RF) output power of –3 dBm [Kathuria and Seet, 2021].

Indeed, there are reported approaches for separating multiple vital signs from multiple subjects using separate transceivers for each subject as well as using ultra-wideband (UWB) impulse Doppler radars [Ren et al., 2015]. The use of array antennas offers the prospect for realizing compact advanced system with a well-established antenna technology base. Nonetheless, the major innovations that would be most essential include schemes for reliable individual target identification or resolution and effective signal processing, and decision-making algorithms for separation of vital signs coming from multiple subjects within the same radar

DOI: 10.1201/9781003315223-11 

beamwidth. Additionally, the discussions will involve a paradigm shift to put the spotlight on recent research into applications in sleep medicine, postoperation and anesthesia recovery, diabetes monitoring, and telehealth management through home healthcare delivery.

The chapter closes with a section on monitoring driver's vital signs inside a vehicle's cabin. Wireless noncontact sensing techniques for unobtrusive monitoring of vital signs, especially in electric vehicles, are gaining increasing attention in recent years. Indeed, for autonomous driving with higher levels of automation in vehicles, the need for robust driver monitoring systems increases. It is essential to ensure that the driver can intervene at any moment. While some of the studies have involved participants in simulated driving and others in road tests, most of the studies are proof-of-concept investigation. To date, a majority of the research is focused on sensor technology development for enhanced driving safety. The question of how the sensor-derived physiological data can be used to support the driver and driving functions remains as a research and development challenge.

## 11.1 REMOTE RADAR SENSING OF VITAL SIGNS OF MULTIPLE SUBJECTS

A major challenge in line-of-sight, vital-sign sensing, and health monitoring of a single subject is the suppression of noise and clutter associated with unwanted extraneous motions from other biological targets. In contrast, the sensing of vital signs of many subjects in a crowd, reflection, and scattering of microwave signals from multiple subjects in the target space are exploited. A typical Doppler radar sensor demodulates the received signal and extracts the vital-sign information associated with various body movements due to cardiorespiratory activities, arterial pulsations, and other bodily motions. However, as discussed in previous chapters, in most cases, noncontact microwave radar sensing of the heartbeat and respiration signals from chest movements is more robust and most efficacious.

In the related case of room-occupancy sensing, a straightforward approach for radar systems is to estimate occupant count based on the received signal strength, which varies significantly for different numbers of occupants and is directly related to radar echoes [Choi et al., 2017; Yavari et al., 2014, 2018]. However, the utility of the simple methodologies is limited since they do not provide information on subject location. Of course, it cannot yield vital signs or any motion-generated data, let alone the separation of individual physiological signatures from many subjects in a crowd. While the well-known Fourier Transform method or Fast Fourier Transform (FFT) approaches may be reliably applied to obtain the frequency spectrum of vital signs for any single isolated subject, they are ill-suited for the task of separating individual physiological signatures in complex overlapping mixtures of different vital signs from multiple subjects in a crowd. The partitioning of signals from multiple subjects may be accomplished through either hardware or software or a combination of both to achieve more effective subject separation and identification.

This section presents recent research on vital sign monitoring of multiple subjects using contactless microwave Doppler radar sensors. A common strategy is to locate or position subjects and extract physiological signals at each location [Chian et al., 2020].

The efforts characteristically incorporate various signal processing and decision-making algorithms for extracting and separating independent physiological signatures from the complex signals that arise from mutual interference or collision of phase components and create ambiguity in the various signal elements. Aside from frequency separation of individual physiological signals, other techniques include direction of arrival (DoA), range discrimination and spatial resolution, antenna beamwidth, and use of multiple antennas. The DoA techniques are beamforming algorithms that estimate the direction of the source relative to the location of the array. The technique separates multiple subjects by steering the antenna beam in the direction of each subject, assuming that there is only one subject within the steered antenna beamwidth. These methodologies may also be combined to provide more efficiency and better adoptability for signal extraction or subject separation dealing with different technologies or under specific circumstances. While the issue of separating independent physiological signatures entails the phenomenon of many-body interactions, the current research is primarily directed toward resolving the most imminent two-body problem. The discussion will begin with through-wall detection of the vital signs of two subjects involving the self-injection locked (SIL) radar system [Wang et al., 2013].

### 11.1.1 Detection of Subject Vital Signs Through Office Partitions

The SIL radar combined with the frequency-modulated continuous-wave (FMCW) and sum-difference pattern (SDP) detection methods was studied to establish the distance and azimuth from the radar to everyone in a scene behind a wooden partition wall (Figure 11.1). In this study, a subject is distinguished from a stationary object by using dynamic spectral subtraction to extract human motions or vital signs. Furthermore, two or more subjects can be distinguished from one another by decomposing the Doppler signal into contributions of individuals in a polar domain. A prototype through-wall detection system was tested to locate two participants behind an office panel wall [Wang et al., 2013].

A photograph of the experimental arrangement is given in Figure 11.2. The SIL radar in the FMCW mode sweeps the voltage-controlled oscillator (VCO) frequency from 2.4 to 2.7 GHz with a 30 MHz/ms scan rate. The line-of-sight beam direction

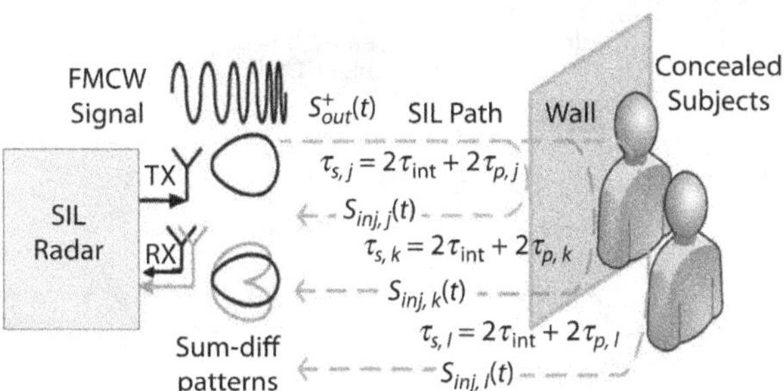


**FIGURE 11.1** A multisubject vital-sign sensing system combining self-injection-locked (SIL) radar with frequency-modulated continuous-wave (FMCW) and sum-difference pattern detection techniques.

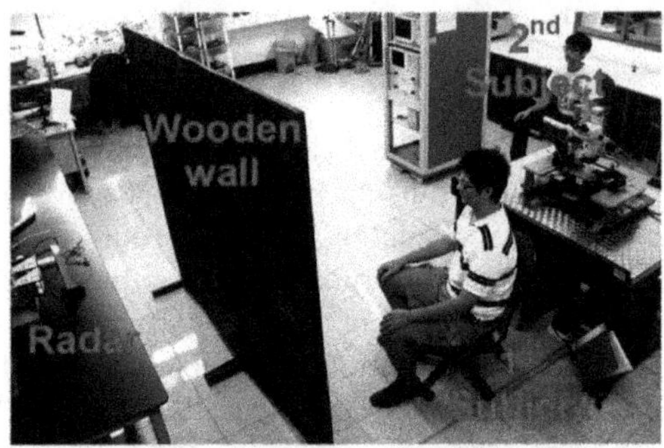


**FIGURE 11.2** Photograph of the experimental arrangement for detection of two test participants behind a wooden partition panel. (Courtesy of T.-S. Jason Horng, National Sun Yat-Sen University.)

is set at 90°.The two test participants were instructed to sit still and breathe normally behind a wooden partition panel. Various clutter-causing objects were placed within the radar's sensing range. Distances from the radar to the wooden partition wall, participant 1, stainless table, probe station, electronic cabinet, participant 2, and wood panel are 0.83, 1.86, 2.41, 3.4, 4.41, 5.28, and 6.5 m, respectively. The azimuth angle of participants 1 and 2 are 65° and 95°, respectively.

Figure 11.3 shows the 1-second cumulative FMCW spectra. The signatures located at 630, 836, 945, 1140, 1345, 1521, and 1760 Hz correspond to the TX/RX coupling signal and the echo reflections of the wooden partition wall, participant 1, stainless table, probe station, electronic cabinet, participant 2, and wood wall with windows for detected distances of 0.825, 1.855, 2.4, 3.375, 4.4, 5.28, and 6.475 m, respectively. The maximum range error is less than 3 cm. Furthermore, the range resolution could be improved by using a broader scanning bandwidth. The two large

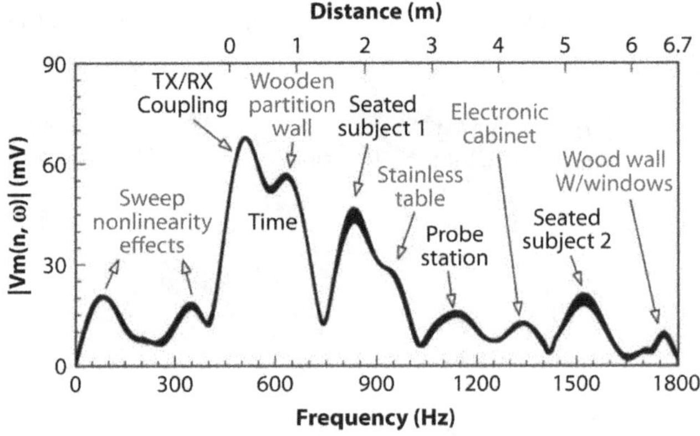


**FIGURE 11.3** Cumulative (1 s) frequency-modulated continuous-wave spectra for range (distance) detection.

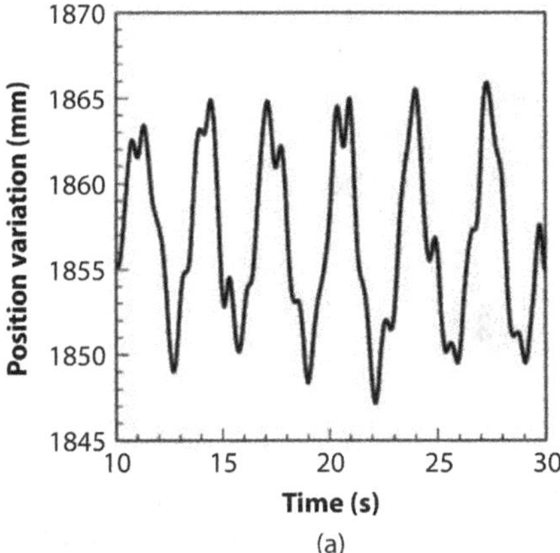


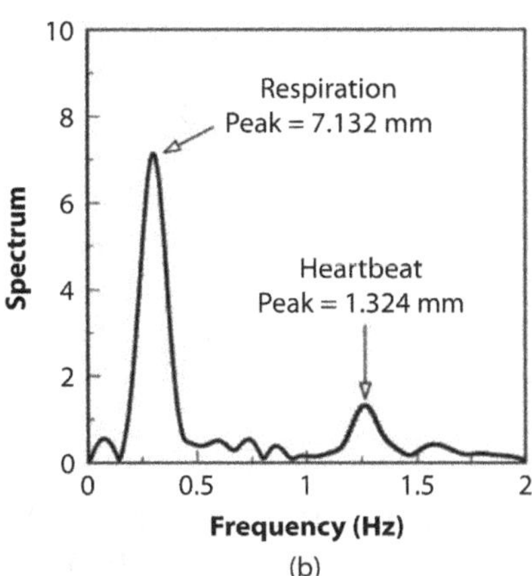


**FIGURE 11.4** Vital signs detected for participant 1: (a) Position fluctuations due to vital signs at participant position and (b) spectrum of position fluctuations corresponding to heartbeat and respiration.

spectral peaks occurring at the frequencies that represent the ranges of participants 1 and 2 from the radar and are associated with their respective vital signs during the 1-second measurement time. In addition, the amplitude of spectral peak for participant 1 is greater than for participant 2 because the former is at a closer range to the SIL radar. Figures 11.4 and 11.5 show the position fluctuations and the spectra of participants 1 and 2, respectively. The spectral peak values associated with respiration and heartbeat are 7.13 and 1.32 mm, respectively, for participant 1, and 8.47 and 1.76 mm, respectively, for participant 2. Moreover, Figures 11.4(b) and 11.5(b)

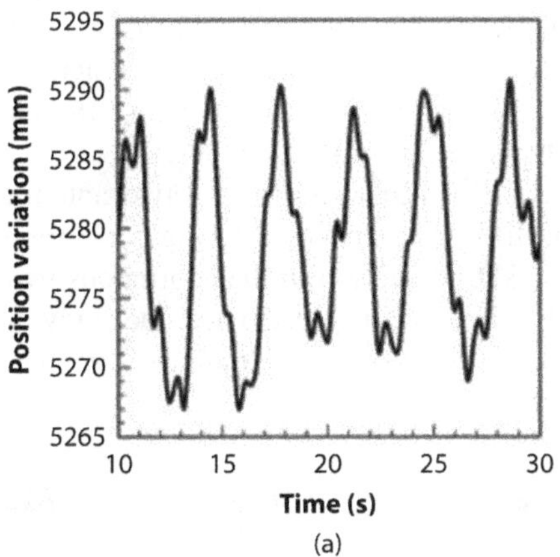


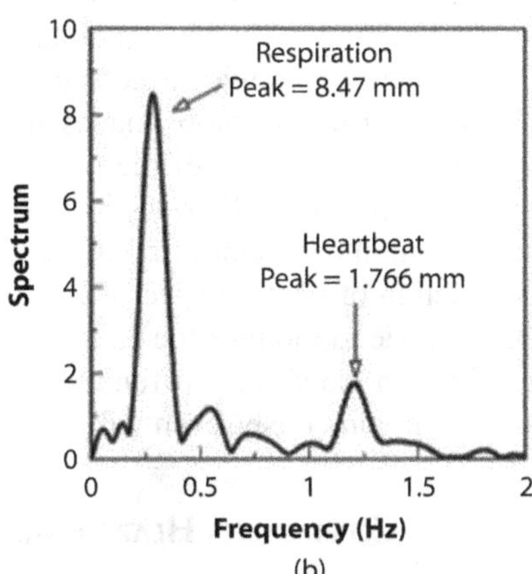


**FIGURE 11.5** Vital signs detected for participant 2: (a) Position fluctuations due to vital signs at participant position and (b) spectrum of position fluctuations corresponding to heartbeat and respiration.

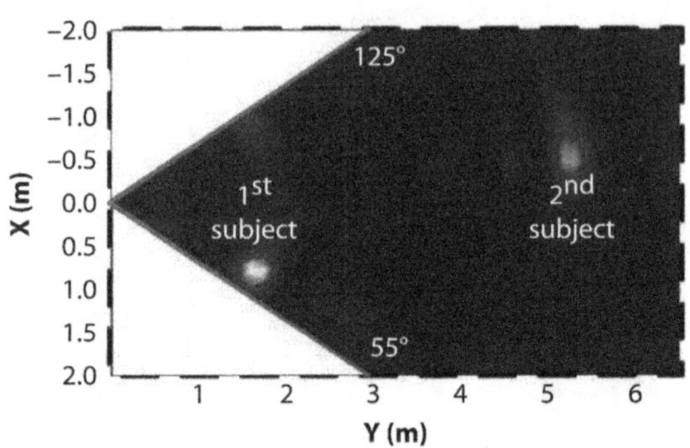


**FIGURE 11.6** Reconstructed image for positions of the two participants based on the range and azimuth information. (Courtesy of T.-S. Jason Horng, National Sun Yat-Sen University.)

clearly indicate a breathing rate of 18 breaths/min and a heart rate of 76 beats/min for participant 1, and a breathing rate of 17 breath/min and a heart rate of 72 beat/min for participant 2, respectively.

In this study, the azimuth tracking is scanned from 55° to 125°. The antenna beamwidth is sufficiently wide so that the received signal for various angles simultaneously contains the Doppler signal caused by the two participants located at different azimuth angles. An image showing the positions the participants may be reconstructed based on the range and azimuth information (see Figure 11.6). Since the tracking pattern is proportional to the measured voltage caused by the participants' cardiorespiratory signals within the sensing range, the strength by the closer participant 1 tends to dominate at an azimuth of 65°. Conversely, the blob image of participant 2 has a lower intensity due to its more distant position from the radar, hence a weaker returned signal. In principle, the blob images in Figure 11.6 may be improved by raising the spatial resolution with increased scanning bandwidth and antenna array elements. Notably, the brightness of the blob image varies with time according to the detected cardiorespiratory activity. Therefore, the two blob images would twinkle asynchronously because the cardiorespiratory signals of the two subjects have different frequencies.

In summary, a SIL radar with one antenna for transmission and two antennas for reception can achieve range detection of different subjects by using background subtraction of FMCW spectra and by way of SDP detection in the continuous wave (CW) mode to monitor the azimuth angle of individual subjects. Thus, the study has exhibited a capability to remotely sense multiple subjects and monitor their vital signs simultaneously, even with an intervening office partition.

### 11.1.2 Contactless Heart Rate Measurement Using X-Band Array Radar

A CW radar operating in the X-band (8.4 GHz) was used to demonstrate the feasibility of measuring a person's heart rate when two people are standing next to each other at roughly the same distance from the radar [Sakamoto et al., 2018]. The radar system consists of a four-channel network analyzer (Figure 11.7) and a planar

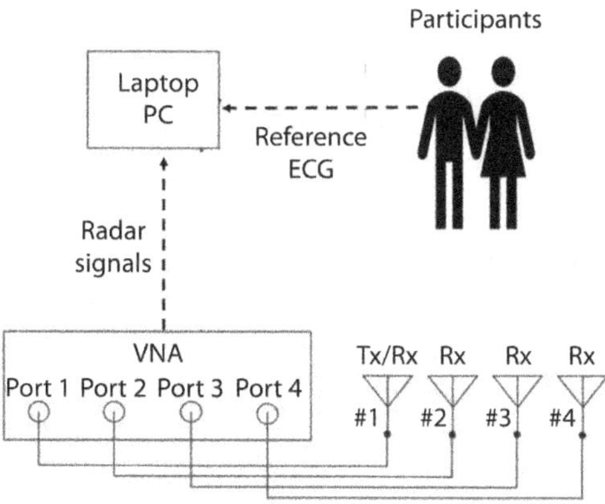


**FIGURE 11.7** Schematic diagram of a radar measurement system with four-channel network analyzer and a planar wide-beam array antenna and electrocardiogram (ECG) as a reference signal.

wide-beam 9 × 9 array antenna with a size of 14.5 × 14.5 mm for each antenna element. The antenna array has a beamwidth of 160° and 145° in the E- and H-planes, respectively.

The method involved the synthesis of a composite radar reflection signal from the two subjects by superposing the signals acquired separately from each subject. The synthesized signal was used to compare the measurements from different scenarios with a single subject or multiple subjects in a scene. Adaptive array processing algorithms are employed to locate and measure the heartbeat of a subject of interest by suppressing undesired reflections from the other subject. A directionally constrained minimization of power (DCMP) algorithm was applied to extract the subject's instantaneous heart rate. Figure 11.8 presents the normalized histograms of errors

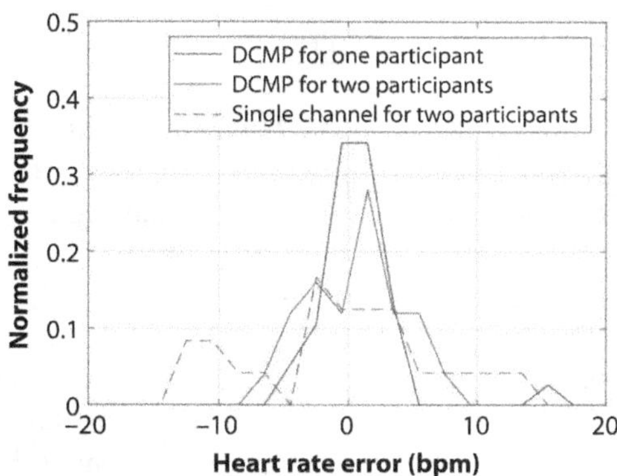


**FIGURE 11.8** Normalized histograms of errors in estimating the heart rate using the directionally constrained minimization of power (DCMP) for one participant (black), DCMP for two participants (light black), and a single channel for two participants (dashed) compared to electrocardiogram measurements.

in estimating the heart rate using DCMP for one participant and two participants and using a single channel for two participants. Electrocardiogram (ECG) measurements are used as references for heart rates. The error distributions when using the DCMP for two participants are narrower than that when using a single channel, which indicates the effectiveness of using multiple channels. The scheme did not require repeated measurements for the comparison because the sensing system can measure and store all signals received by the antenna elements and the adaptive array algorithms can be applied offline to multiple-channel data after the measurement.

Note that when there is a single participant, the root-mean-square (RMS) errors in estimating the inter-beat intervals using a single channel and the DCMP signals are 44.6 and 27.3 ms. When there are both participants, the RMS errors of a single channel and the DCMP signals are 64.4 and 20.9 ms. It was shown that in both cases, the use of the DCMP is effective in improving the accuracy of the estimation of the instantaneous heart rate. When applying the array beamforming technique to the signals from both participants in the scene, the RMS error in estimating the inter-beat intervals was found to be 53.4 ms, which is smaller than the error of the single channel, but larger than the error of the DCMP.

The performance of the prototype system demonstrated that it can selectively extract vital signs from a specific participant with the presence of another participant in the scene. The algorithm performed accurately in estimating the instantaneous heart rate and inter-beat interval. However, because the participants were separated by 0.6 m and were at about the same distance (0.5 m) from the radar antennas, in this case, their radar echoes could not be separated even when wideband signals were employed. Thus, the problem of mutual interference endures.

### 11.1.3 Hybrid Doppler Radars for Multisubject Vital-Sign Sensing

The challenge of efficiently and reliably identifying and isolating vital-sign features concurrently from multiple subjects persists as an important topic of investigation. This section examines the developments of hybridizing or combining two or more techniques to extract radar-measured vital signs.

#### 11.1.3.1 Dual-Beam Phased-Array CW Doppler Radars

A dual-beam phased-array Doppler radar was proposed and experimentally validated for concurrent short-range monitoring of human vital signs [Nosrati et al., 2019]. The dual-beam radar sensor exploits space diversity to mitigate the mutual interference problem in the presence of multiple subjects. The vital signs of more than one subject can be consistently detected, differentiated, and retrieved at the same time and with the same microwave source using a CW radar transceiver. A prototype phased-array radar designed and implemented using the hybrid beamforming architecture to generate two simultaneous beams with separate TX and RX antennas is shown in Figure 11.9. The system operates in CW mode at 2.4 GHz both for TX and RX. The transmitter uses a four-element array setup in a linear arrangement. The RF/microwave signal level at each antenna port is –11 dBm, and the equivalent isotropic radiated power is 0 dBm. The receiver architecture is direct conversion. The receiver antenna port sensitivity is –80 dBm.

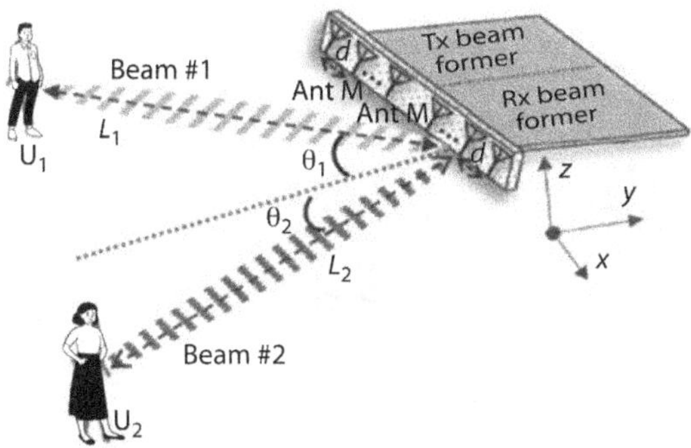


**FIGURE 11.9** Dual-beam phased array radar detection scenario for two subjects using multiple-input, multiple-output (MIMO) beamforming techniques. (Courtesy of Mehrdad Nosrati, Stevens Institute of Technology.)

A photograph of the fully assembled radar system including the TX and RX antenna arrays is shown in Figure 11.10. The microcontroller, transceiver, and the antenna arrays are marked. The rectangular patch antenna array elements are housed in a foam enclosure. The distance between adjacent elements is 8 cm, which is a little more than a half-wavelength, $\lambda/2$, at 2.4 GHz. Experimental measurements were performed in a typical classroom with 10 different two-person combinations of five healthy participants. The experimental setup is given in Figure 11.11 for the concurrent respiration monitoring via the dual-beam CW radar. The participants were separated by 2 m from each other and were 3 m away from the radar sensor. The positions

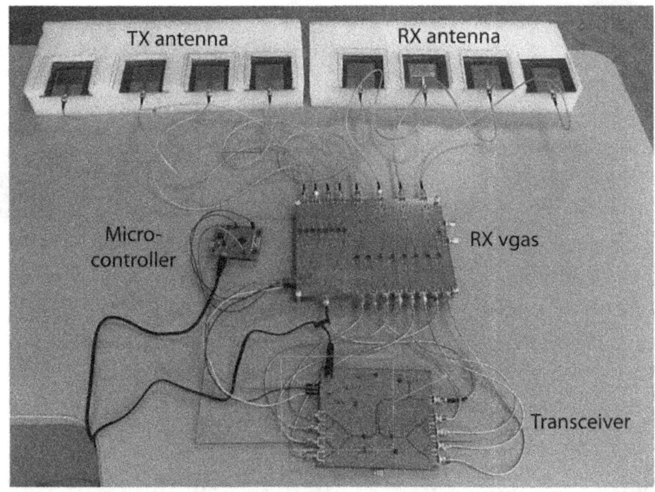


**FIGURE 11.10** Photograph of assembled dual-beam CW radar system including the transmitting and receiving patch antenna arrays. (Courtesy of Mehrdad Nosrati, Stevens Institute of Technology.)

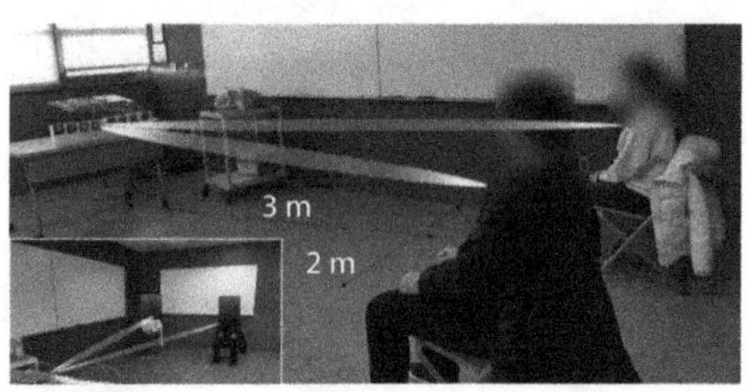


**FIGURE 11.11** Measurement setup for the concurrent respiration monitoring of two participants using the dual-beam phased array CW radar sensor. (Courtesy of Mehrdad Nosrati, Stevens Institute of Technology.)

were determined based on the direction of two distinct predefined beams. The respiratory rates of the participants were monitored for 1 minute.

Figure 11.12 illustrates the frequency spectrum of two sets of detected signals for radar operating in single-beam mode and in dual-beam mode. The true respiration rates for participants 1 and 2 were roughly 18 bpm (0.3 Hz) and 22 bpm (0.36 Hz), respectively. Clearly, when the radar operates in the single-beam mode, the output is a composite signal from two participants that collides and interferences with each other, so that no useful information can be recovered. A peak around 0.22 Hz is observed, which is associated with the harmonic mixing of signals from the two participants. The solid and dashed curves show the output of beam #1 and #2, respectively under the dual-beam operating mode. In contrast, it is seen that there are two persons present, and each participant's signal is easily recoverable because of the two independent receiving channels. Accordingly, each participant's respiratory rate can be identified and assigned. The interference of beam #2 (participant 2) on the peak of beam #1 (participant 1) is 15 dB lower than the peak of beam #1. This number is roughly 11 dB for the interference of beam #1 on the peak of beam #2, when the radar operates in the single-beam mode.

Thus, the study established that vital signs of two subjects can be detected, retrieved, and differentiated concurrently using a dual-beam phased array CW radar sensor and the multiple-input multiple-output (MIMO) beamforming technique for short-range vital sign (respiration) monitoring. Also, the study demonstrated that the sensor's signal-to-noise (SNR) performance versus distance to the subject (or range) is constrained by the antenna's radiation zone. However, the issue of signal interference within a beam (intra-beam interference or lateral spatial resolution) continues as an unsettled problem awaiting additional research. Aside from hardware approaches to support angular discriminations between equidistant subjects, the use of advanced signal processing techniques would be an option to isolate or separate the desired vital signs from other intra-beam signals.

#### 11.1.3.2 Phase Comparison Radar with ICA-JADE and DOA Algorithms

Recently, an effective combination of three signal processing techniques — the independent component analysis (ICA), joint approximation diagonalization of eigenmatrices (JADE), and DOA — was demonstrated to provide accurate and efficient

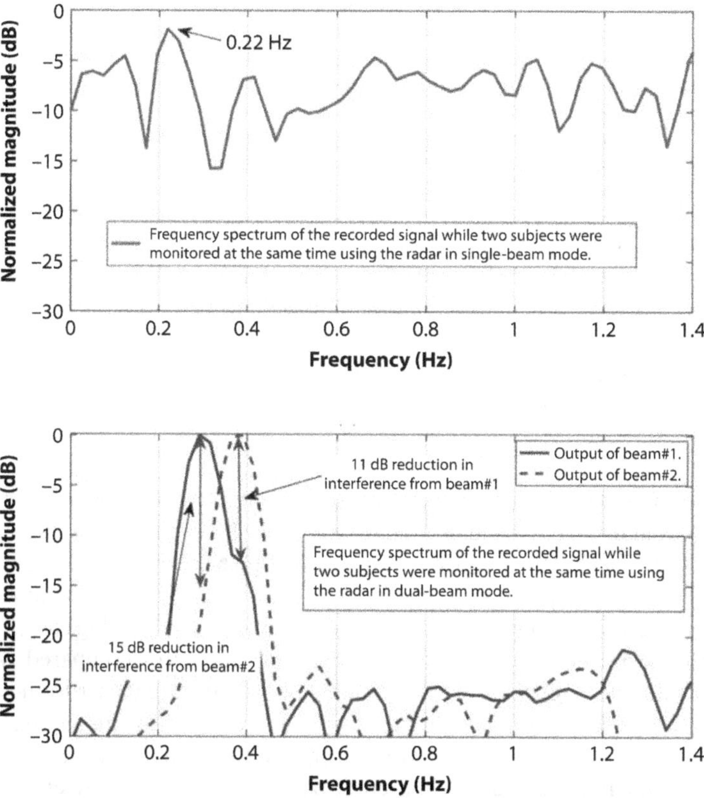


**FIGURE 11.12** Frequency spectrum of two sets of detected signals for radar operating in single-beam mode and in dual-beam mode: (a) Mixed colliding signal for radar operating in the single-beam mode and (b) solid and dashed curves showing the output of beam #1 and #2, respectively under dual-beam mode.

monitoring of multiple subjects across a broad range of subject separation scenarios [Islam et al., 2020]. The integrated decision algorithm was shown to be able to efficiently separate the physiological signatures of multiple subjects. A schematic diagram of the prototype monopulse CW Doppler radar system is given in Figure 11.13. The transmitter array has $4 \times 8$ patch elements, and the receiver is a $2 \times 8$ array. The 24 GHz phase monopulse Doppler radar applies ICA-JADE when the subjects are within the beamwidth (30°), and DOA when they are not. The radar module contains two coherent receivers with in-phase (I) and quadrature phase (Q) channels. The monopulse feature offers a technique through which information concerning the angular location can be obtained by comparing the phase properties between spatially separated receivers.

The experimental arrangement for human testing was set up in a microwave anechoic chamber. Figure 11.14 shows two participants in front of the radar. A commercial chest belt respiration monitor was strapped to the participants to serve as

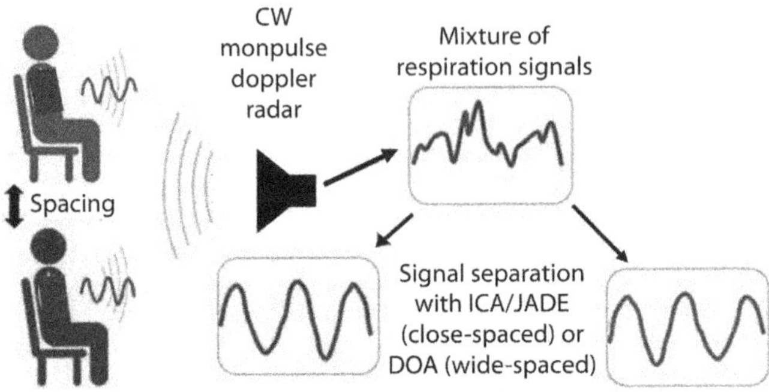


**FIGURE 11.13** Schematic diagram of a prototype monopulse CW Doppler radar system for concurrent respiratory monitoring of multiple subjects.

reference signals. The two participants were positioned at different angular discrimination ranges at different distances within the radar beamwidth.

Figure 11.15 depicts the extracted respiratory signatures from the combined mixture for two subjects at a range of 1 m with an angular discrimination of 0.4 m. The radar signatures closely match the chest-belt-captured breathing rates. Table 11.1 presents the performance of separated respiratory signatures compared with respiration-belt reference signals. It is seen that when subjects are closer to the radar and within the main beamwidth (30°) of the transceiver, thus having an angular discrimination limit within the beamwidth of the transceiver, the mean square error (MSE) between the separated signatures and chest-belt reference signals decreases and the cross-correlation coefficient increases. The reason is when the subjects are closer and the angular position is within the main beamwidth of the antenna pattern, the SNR level of the received signal is higher than that for subjects at the edge of the main radar beamwidth. The results confirm the effectiveness of the ICA-JADE algorithm for separating subjects that are closer to the radar sensor and within the main beamwidth of the antenna pattern of the transceiver as the probability of the received signal being degraded is less than it is for larger distances.

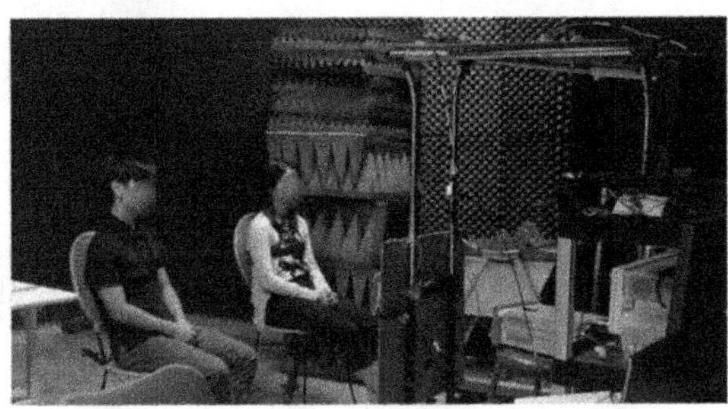

**FIGURE 11.14** Experimental setup showing two participants inside a microwave anechoic chamber. (Islam et al., 2020.)

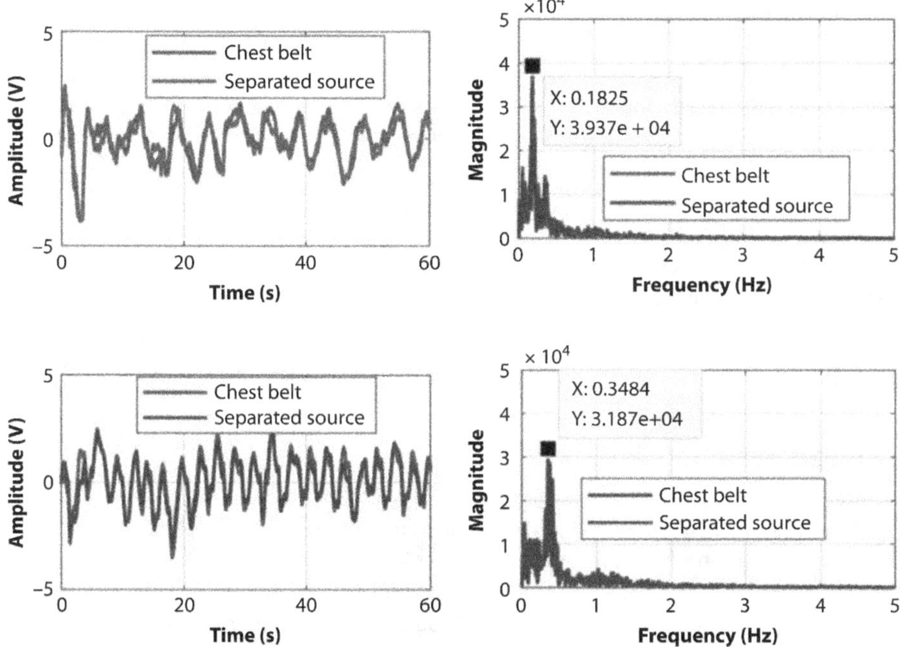


**FIGURE 11.15** Radar sensor separated respiratory signatures (gray) and chest belt signals (black) for: (a) subject-1 and (b) subject-2, along with corresponding frequency spectra used to extract respiration rates for: (c) subject-1 and (d) subject-2. Measured breathing rates are 0.18 Hz for subject-1 and 0.35 Hz for subject-2, both values closely match the chest belt reference.

**TABLE 11.1**

**Performance Evaluation of Separated Respiration Signatures with Reference Respiration-Belt Reference Signals at Range Distances (1–3 m) for Two Different Angular Discriminations**

| Slant Ranges (m) | Angular Discrimination Limit (m) | MSE (%) | Cross Correlation Coefficient |
|---|---|---|---|
| R = 1 | 0.4 (within beamwidth) | 0.055 | 0.99 |
| | 0.52 (edge of beamwidth) | 5.53 | 0.94 |
| R = 1.5 | 0.5 (within beamwidth) | 7.23 | 0.95 |
| | 0.78 (edge of beamwidth) | 12.86 | 0.93 |
| R = 2 | 0.7 (within beamwidth) | 15.86 | 0.94 |
| | 1.04 (edge of beamwidth) | 21.34 | 0.93 |
| R = 2.5 | 1.0 (within beamwidth) | 24.04 | 0.86 |
| | 1.29 (edge of beamwidth) | 30.52 | 0.82 |
| R = 3 | 1.25 (within beamwidth) | 32.22 | 0.81 |
| | 1.55 (edge of beamwidth) | 38.69 | 0.77 |

This hybrid method consisting of an SNR-based decision algorithm integrates two different approaches to isolate respiratory signatures of two subjects within the radar beamwidth separated by less than 1 m with a 93% accuracy. Thus, the hybrid method can separate independent respiratory patterns more accurately when subjects are more closely spaced than previously reported. The angular location of each subject is estimated by phase-comparison monopulse scheme, and the sensing system is endowed with an integrated beam switching facility. However, an intrinsic disadvantage of the technique is that it is computationally intensive as it needs to switch between the two different algorithms, which may counter the implicit advantage of contactless noninvasive sensing.

### 11.1.4 Sensors for Localization of Multiple Subjects in Cluttered Environments

A closely related issue of efficient separation of independent vital signs for multiple subjects is radar-based localization of subjects. Traditional solutions rely on a large bandwidth to achieve a desired range resolution, which is equally deployed to everything in the antenna field of view. For example, the extraction of vital signs of two subjects spaced 20 cm apart by using a 1 GHz bandwidth to achieve a range resolution 15 cm at greater costs to spectral, computational, and energy resources, instead of a more modest 250 MHz RF bandwidth.

This section discusses a dual-mode approach to efficiently track the vital-sign information of a human subject at a stationary location in an environment with limited clutter and the use of the high-resolution FMCW method to resolve the locations of different subjects when multiple objects are present in a cluttered environment. Also, a modulated waveform signal can be used in an environment with limited clutter for its operational simplicity and low bandwidth requirement. Lastly, it includes a description of 3-D MIMO radar with nonuniformly spaced array. It should be noted that UWB radars have high-range resolution because of the wide bandwidth available through its use of narrow impulses; thus, it can readily localize the target [Piotrowsky and Pohl, 2021]. However, it is inefficient in terms of complexity and cost for its use in vital-sign detection.

Nonetheless, it is noteworthy that sensing and tracking of both moving and stationary human subjects are of significant practical interest. In addition to medical monitoring and geriatric care, there are many potential areas of the application of radar sensors for short-range target localization and vital-sign tracking. They include, but are not limited to, driver assistance, security surveillance, occupancy sensing, hidden-intruder detection and tracking, emergency search and rescue operations, autonomous vehicles, factory automation, and navigation for the visually impaired, robots, and drones.

#### 11.1.4.1 Integrated FMCW and Interferometry Radar Sensor

The concept of combining two different radar operation modes by switching through an on-board microcontroller enables the attainment of a sensor capable of measuring both the absolute range and vital signs of human targets. The integrated system combines FMCW radar and Doppler interferometry [Peng et al., 2017a; Wang et al.,

2014]. FMCW radars can provide accurate target-range information and can extract radial velocity and displacement of targets. Interferometry radars can operate as unmodulated CW systems. They rely on a single-tone CW to find phase history of targets and like all CW Dopplers, they feature high precision in displacement and speed measurement. However, they do not yield absolute target range information.

A schematic diagram of the integrated 5.8 GHz FMCW interferometry radar system is given in Figure 11.16. The two radar modes are realized by sharing the same RF components and signal paths, both to simplify system complexity and minimize its cost. The FMCW radar uses operational-amplifier-based circuits to generate an analog sawtooth signal and a reference pulse sequence (RPS). The RPS is locked to the sawtooth signal to obtain coherence for the radar system. A low-intermediate-frequency (low-IF) modulation method is employed to avoid the slowly varying vital signs from being distorted by the high-pass filter for the interferometry mode. The low-IF design has the added advantage of mitigating flicker noise, which has a higher power level around the zero-frequency component of the baseband signal. Envelope detection is applied to retrieve the vital signs in interferometry mode. Figure 11.17 shows the prototype sensor-measured respiration and heartbeat signals from a human participant with a heartbeat of 85 beat/min and respiration rate of 13 breath/min. Figure 11.18 presents the continuous spectrogram of radar sensed heartbeat and respiration signals. The two bright strips show clearly identifiable time evolution of the heartbeat and respiration rates. In this experiment, the human participant sat either 1.5 m in front of or with their back to the radar sensor. The participant was asked to breathe normally during the measurement period.

Additionally, an experiment was performed to differentiate a human subject from strong stationary clutter returns. In this scenario, the radar was located 0.8 m in front of a glass wall (3 m high, 10 m wide). A human subject stood behind the glass wall and a concrete wall behind the glass wall (4.2 m from the radar). A pair of 4 × 4

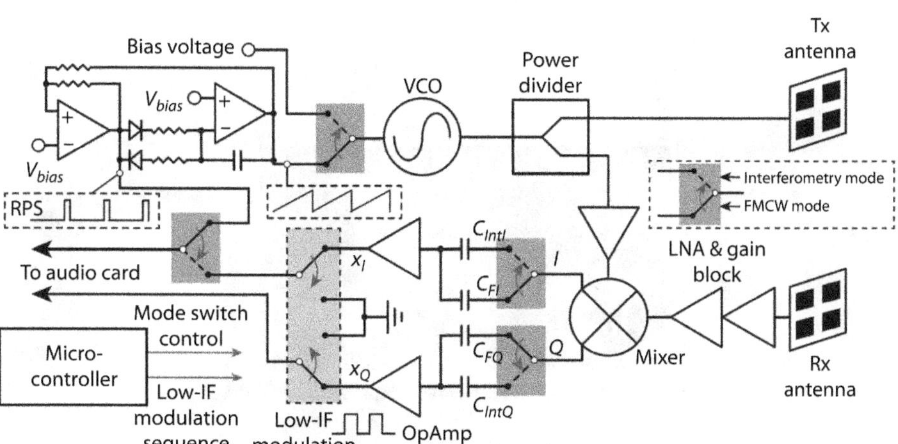


**FIGURE 11.16** Schematic diagram of an integrated frequency-modulated continuous-wave (FMCW)-interferometry radar system. (Courtesy of Changzhi Li, Texas Tech University.)

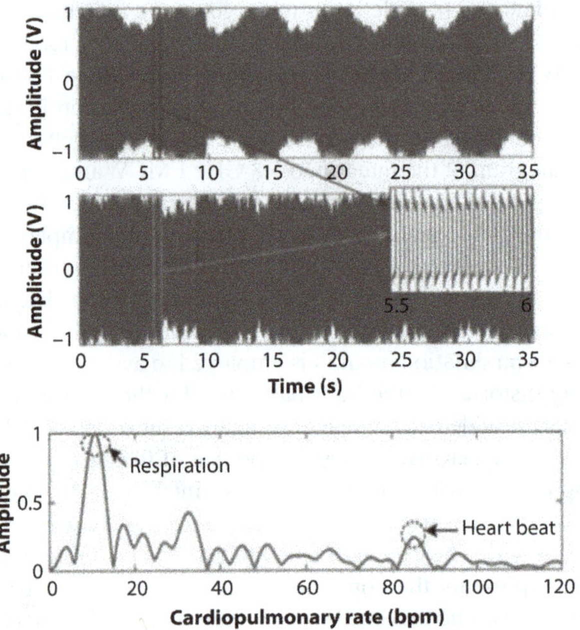


**FIGURE 11.17** Prototype sensor measured respiration and heartbeat signals of a participant: (a) Amplitude of I and Q channel output signals with detailed waveforms shown in insert and (b) normalized frequency spectrum after envelope detection.

patch antenna arrays (beamwidth of 21.6°) were used as the transmitter and receiver antennas. Figure 11.19(a) shows a range profile from measurements that clearly show reflections from the glass and the concrete walls. However, the reflected signal from a human subject displays a noticeable band of fluctuations compared with that of the glass window and concrete wall, even though the participant was instructed to keep stationary and still during the brief measurement session. However, the detected

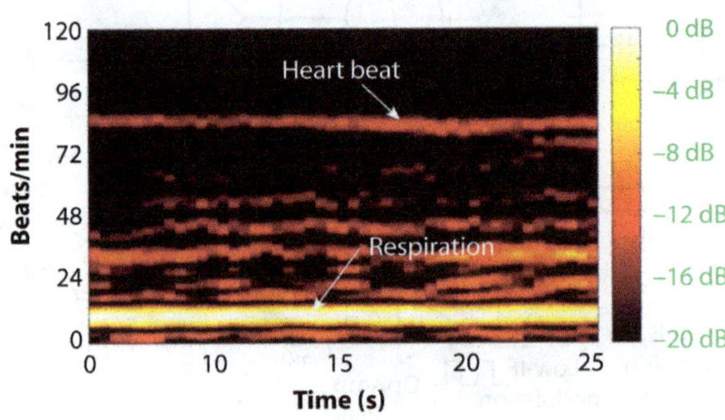


**FIGURE 11.18** Continuous spectrogram of radar-sensed heartbeat and respiration signals. (Courtesy of Changzhi Li, Texas Tech University.)

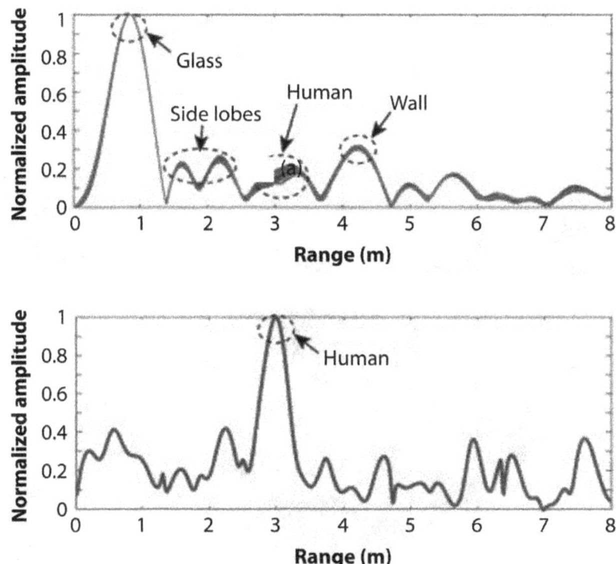


**FIGURE 11.19** Differentiation of human targets from strong stationary clutter-return scenarios: (a) Range profile corresponding to detection of human subjects behind a glass wall with various stationary targets and human-signature-associated fluctuations and (b) extraction of a human target using standard deviation enhancements.

signal from the human target reveals the Doppler effect associated with participant's cardiorespiratory movements, which introduces significant variations to the measured range profiles. By computing the standard deviation of measured data during a specific time, the human target can be separated from signatures of other stationary targets. Figure 11.19(b) depicts the normalized standard deviation for the measurements, where the human participant's range signature is enhanced while those of the stationary targets, i.e., the glass and concrete walls are suppressed.

The use of the integrated radar in identification of human subjects in a more complex environment, such as in a parking lot, was investigated with a human subject standing 1.5 m next to a parked automobile with another car parked farther away (see Figure 11.20). The 5.8 GHz radar sensor was mounted on a tripod (Figure 11.20a) and set to mechanically scan with a scan-step angle of 4° in FMCW mode. Figure 11.20(b) shows a two-dimensional (2-D) mapping of the measured range profiles. A large echo appears at 8 m, which corresponds to the location of the car and the human subject. The overlap of the two targets is the result of limited antenna directivity (21.6° beamwidth). Namely, the angular resolution is insufficient to differentiate the human subject from the automobile. The echoes on the left correspond to the radar turns from the other car in the parking lot. However, as described above, the Doppler effect associated with the subject's cardiorespiratory movements may be exploited to suppress echoes from all stationary targets, including the parked cars using the standard deviation maneuver to enhance the human subject signatures and identify the human subject in the scene. The 2-D mapping in Figure 11.20(c) was obtained

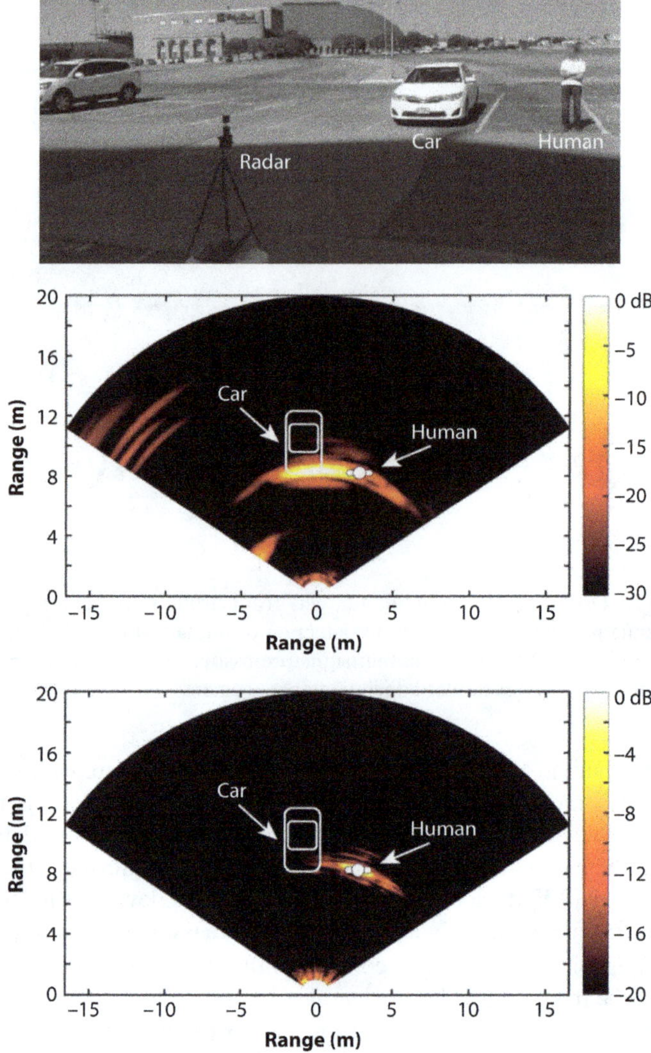


**FIGURE 11.20** Integrated radar sensor to identify human subjects in a complex environment with multiple stationary clutters: (a) Experimental scene, (b) 2-D mapping result for the scenario, and (c) human subject isolation from the 2-D mapping experiment. (Courtesy of Changzhi Li, Texas Tech University.)

after calculating the standard deviation of different measurements in each direction. The results bring out the capability of the radar sensor to isolate human subjects in a complex environment with multiple stationary clutters [Peng et al., 2017a].

Furthermore, it is often difficult to track or locate moving targets in crowded environments. The integrated FMCW interferometry radar sensor was experimentally demonstrated to enable the application of real-time inverse synthetic aperture radar (ISAR) images [Ausherman et al., 1984; Berizzi et al., 2001; Walker, 1980] to track two moving subjects in the 2-D range-Doppler domain. As mentioned earlier, a coherent FMCW radar preserves the phase history of targets during the coherent processing interval (CPI) and Doppler information can, thus, be derived, which provides two dimensions: the range and the Doppler. Hence, ISAR images, which are widely used in radar-imaging applications, can be formed for the purpose of isolating the desired moving targets from surrounding clutter.

The test scene is presented in Figure 11.21. The corridor is narrow with doors, walls, and many pillars, which produce lots of clutter-return signals. The two participants move in opposite directions in front of the radar in the corridor. The CPI for the experiment is 73 seconds. Typically, there are many strong echoes that correspond to the stationary objects. The two moving human participants are noticeable but are much weaker than the stationary clutter returns. ISAR images are obtained by performing an FFT along the slow-time direction for a given slow-time interval. A sequence of ISAR images can be combined to form a video, which can be used to evaluate the characteristics of subject movements. An image of the ISAR video when both human subjects were stopped is shown in Figure 11.22(a) (Frame 1). As a proof of the coherence of the integrated radar, the zero-Doppler echoes corresponding to the stationary objects are clearly visible. Since the two subjects were stopped at this time, both of their speeds are zero, leading to the fact that only zero-Doppler signatures are observed in this Doppler range map.

At instant 7 seconds of the acquisition time, Figure 11.22(b) (Frame 2), subject A was walking toward the radar, while subject B was walking away from the radar. In the range-Doppler image, the return associated with subject A appears above the zero-Doppler strip, while subject B produces an echo below the zero-Doppler signature. Figures 11.22(c) and 11.22(d) are two frames of the ISAR (Frames 3 and 4) relating to the 26-second and 64-second instants, respectively. In Figure 11.22(c), subject A was near the radar and prepared to turn around with a speed almost zero, while subject B was still walking away from the radar system. Concerning Figure 11.22(d), subject A was walking toward the radar and subject B was walking away from the radar. So, the ISAR images can provide the integrated radar sensor with

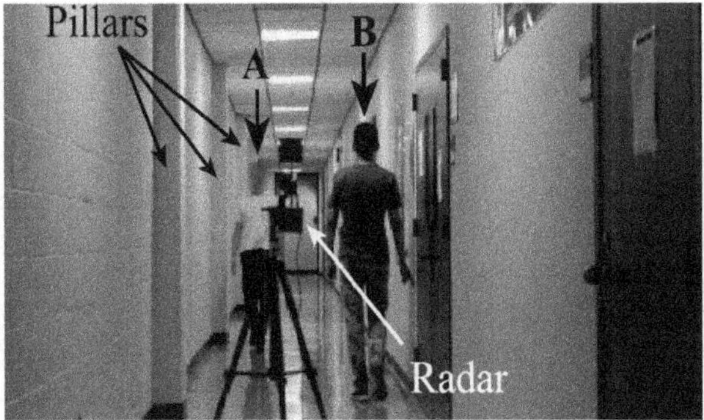


**FIGURE 11.21** Photograph of the experimental scene with two participants in an indoor corridor for demonstrating integrated frequency-modulated continuous wave interferometry radar-enabled production of inverse synthetic aperture radar (ISAR) images. (Courtesy of Changzhi Li, Texas Tech University.)

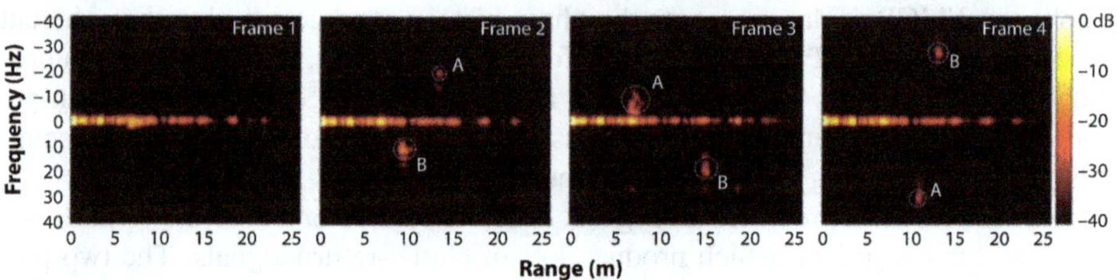


**FIGURE 11.22** A sequence of integrated frequency-modulated continuous wave interferometry radar-enabled inverse synthetic aperture radar (ISAR) images: (Frame 1) the ISAR image at the beginning of data acquisition, (Frame 2) the ISAR image at 7 seconds, (Frame 3) the ISAR image at 26 seconds, and (Frame 4) the ISAR image at 64 seconds. (Courtesy of Changzhi Li, Texas Tech University.)

2-D isolation and tracking capabilities by combining the absolute ranging and Doppler information.

The investigations described encapsulate the capability and distinct operational features of the integrated FMCW-Doppler interferometry radar sensor in several applications. They include the ability to accurately measure vital signs of human subjects, detection of human subjects behind a glass wall with various stationary objects, 2-D scanning to differentiate human subjects from other surrounding objects in complex environments, and ISAR imaging to track moving subjects in an environment with strong clutter returns.

#### 11.1.4.2 K-Band FMCW Doppler Radar with Beamforming Array

The FMCW radar system design is not frequency restricted. A printed circuit board (PCB) implementation of the FMCW radar design in K-band for short-range localization with beamforming capability was realized to take advantage of its higher resolution at the higher frequency [Peng et al., 2017b]. The PCB realization of the K-band radar system is shown in Figure 11.23, which includes both the transmitter and receiver channels. The board is 43 × 15 mm with a thickness of 0.254 mm. A photographic view of the PCB realization of K-band FMCW radar system with beamforming array is given in Figure 11.24. The size of the entire prototype radar package is 11.5 × 3.9 cm, weighs 69 g, and transmits 8 dBm of output power at a bandwidth of 500 MHz.

The transmitter channel consists of a VCO and a single patch antenna. The typical sawtooth voltage was generated by an operational amplifier-based circuit to control the VCO, which produces a frequency-modulated RF signal from 23.5 to 24 GHz centered at 23.75 GHz. The receiver channel consists of a beamforming array, a six-port circuit, and a baseband circuit. The on-board six-port is based on planar passive microwave structures and RF diodes. The distance between adjacent elements is $\lambda/2$. Each element of the four-element linear beamforming array is a series-fed microstrip patch array antenna. The beam of the array with a fixed narrow beamwidth on the E-plane can be continuously steered with a range of ± 45° on the H-plane (with low side lobes to minimize ghost images for localization) through

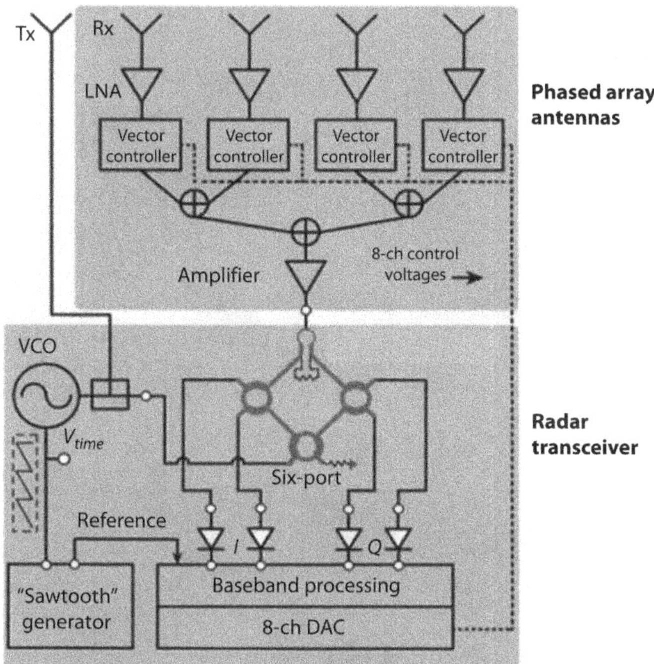


**FIGURE 11.23** Block diagram of K-band frequency-modulated continuous wave radar system with beamforming array.

an array of vector controllers. The vector controller is built on the concept of vector sum and uses microwave structures and PIN diodes. They are controlled by an eight-channel DAC, which is driven by a data acquisition device (DAQ) through a serial peripheral interface (SPI) bus and baseband signal processing. Every vector controller regulates the phase and the amplitude of the corresponding array element. The beat difference signal of the FMCW radar is detected by the six-port circuit and then sampled by a laptop.

Performance of the K-band radar sensor with beamforming array was tested in a parking lot scene (Figure 11.25), where a human participant stood roughly 4 m from the FMCW radar between the back of a passenger car and a lamppost. A 2-D mapping of the resulting range profile is shown in Figure 11.26. The radar signatures of the stationary car and lamppost, and that of the human participant, are clearly visible but blurry. However, the standard deviation of the detected range spectrum, discussed in Section 11.1.4.1, may be applied to the Doppler frequency shifts associated with the participant's cardiorespiratory movements alongside suppression of reflections from all stationary objects to isolate the signature of human participant and identify the location of human participant in the scene, as shown in Figure 11.27. Thus, the K-band radar system has the sensitivity to capture vital sign-induced motions and to discriminate human subjects from stationary targets in short-range localization applications. Moreover, FMCW radar signals can be used for their excellent range resolution in a cluttered environment. When multiple objects are present, the high

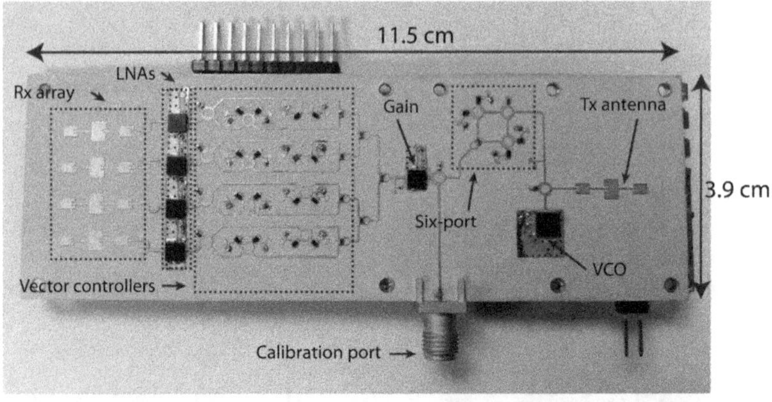


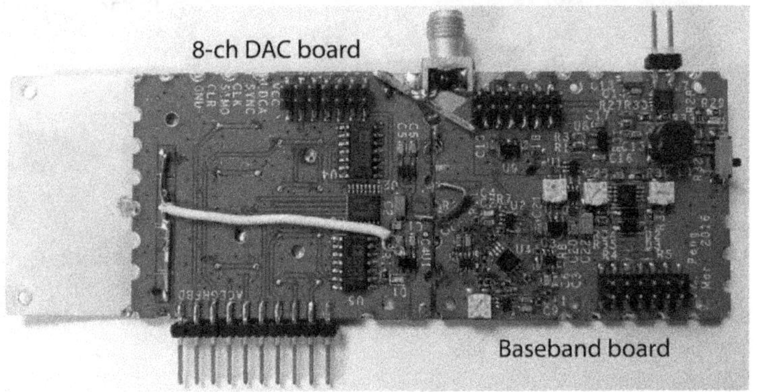


**FIGURE 11.24** Photograph of printed circuit board realization of K-band frequency-modulated continuous wave radar system with beamforming array: (a) Top view and (b) bottom view. (Courtesy of Changzhi Li, Texas Tech University.)

range resolution FMCW beamforming array radar systems with vector controllers and a six-port circuit can resolve the locations of different objects.

#### 11.1.4.3 Modulated Waveform FSK Radar for Range Tracking

Many radar range-tracking technologies are being investigated for subject localization. For example, FMCW radars can provide the absolute range of moving and stationary objects. However, a large bandwidth is required for its operation, which places high demands on system components. Furthermore, the radio spectrum is becoming an increasingly scarce commodity and resource. Recently, a spectrum-efficient, frequency-shift keying (FSK) radar technology has been investigated for both moving and stationary human subject detection and range tracking in environments with limited clutter for its operational simplicity and low-RF bandwidth requirement [Wang et al., 2019]. It specifically involves Doppler frequency-based moving target-tracking and vital-sign detection from a stationary human subject.

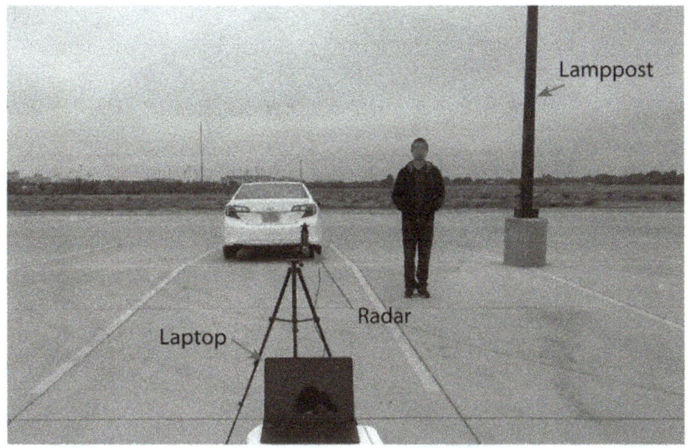


**FIGURE 11.25** Experimental scene of short-range localization with a human subject and two objects (car and lamppost). (Courtesy of Changzhi Li, Texas Tech University.)

The operation of FSK radar requires two RF frequencies. The two carrier frequencies $f_1$ and $f_2$ are transmitted in a shared RF chain at a switching rate of $f_{sqr}$ (see Figure 11.28). The frequency shift between the two carriers is usually small, i.e., in the kHz or MHz range, which is represented as $\Delta f = f_2 - f_1$, assuming $f_2 > f_1$. In a direct-conversion quadrature FSK radar system, such as that presented in Figure 11.29, two signal responses associated with the two carriers exist in I/Q channels. Note that $f_{sqr}$ should be sufficiently fast to allow proper sampling of all motion-related signals, so the target range and location can be estimated based on the phase difference associated with the motion frequency despite the square-wave modulation.

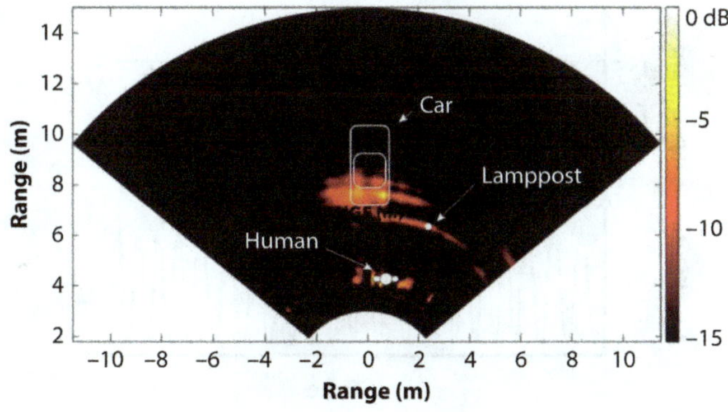


**FIGURE 11.26** Result of the short-range localization experiment with a human subject and two stationary targets using a K-band radar sensor. (Courtesy of Changzhi Li, Texas Tech University.)

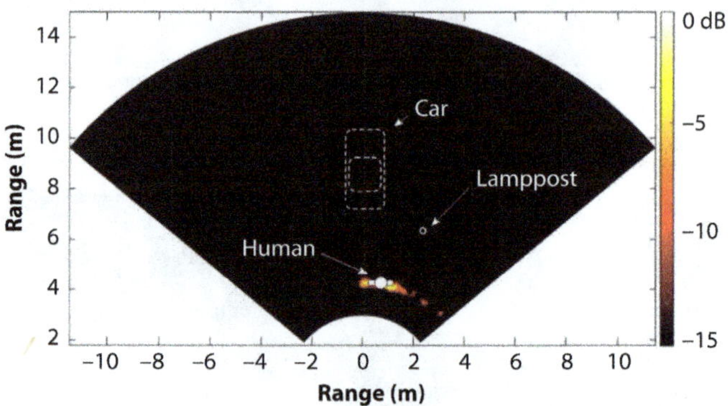


**FIGURE 11.27** Human subject extraction with a standard deviation of 10 sequencing scans. (Courtesy of Changzhi Li, Texas Tech University.)

In the reported study, range localization tracking of two subjects walking simultaneously in opposite directions was carried out in an indoor environment, as illustrated in Figure 11.30 with a 5.8 GHz FSK radar. Subject A walked from 2.5 to 11 m marks while subject B walked from 11 to 2.5 m marks. Both participants started and stopped at approximately the same time with a normal walking speed. Measurement data were recorded with a 6 kHz sampling frequency. The Doppler frequencies generated by the two subjects had opposite signs since the walking directions were opposite. After applying FFT on the baseband responses, the Doppler frequency peaks were successfully separated in the frequency domain and the phase extraction was realized separately on the associated Doppler peaks. Figure 11.31 shows the range detection results; there are three outlier points at the beginning of the measurement in the walking trajectory of subject B. Initially, subject A was much closer to the radar than subject B, thus, the signal strength of the Doppler frequencies generated by subject A was much higher than that generated by subject B. Therefore, the

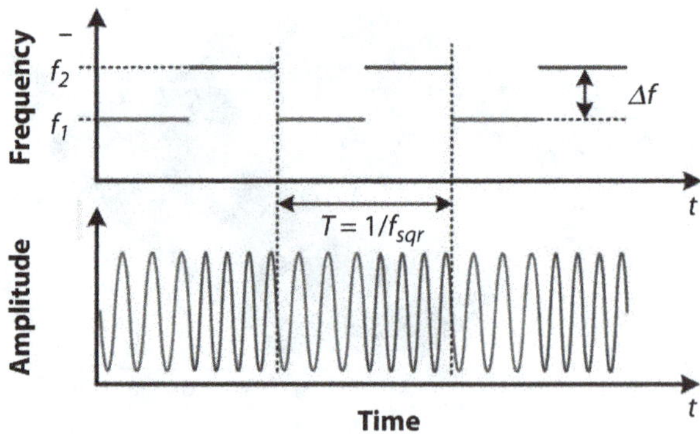


**FIGURE 11.28** The modulation scheme for a frequency-shift keying radar system: (Top) Frequency-time representation and (bottom) amplitude-time representation for square-wave modulation.

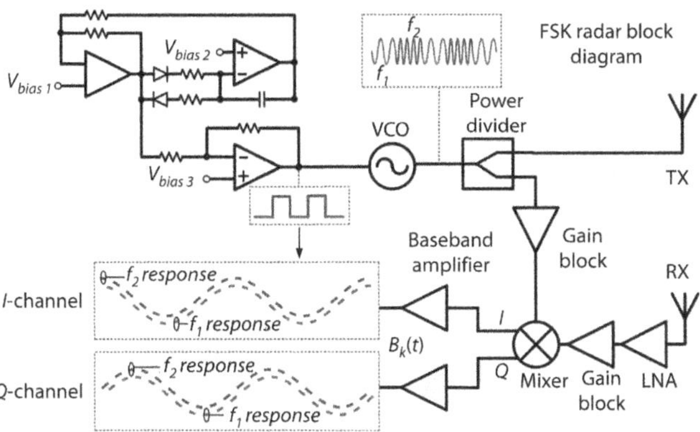


**FIGURE 11.29** Schematic diagram of a frequency-shift keying range-tracking radar system. (Courtesy of Changzhi Li, Texas Tech University.)

Doppler frequencies associated with subject B were buried under the signal leakage of the Doppler components associated with subject A. The phase information of the three outlier points was obtained from the leakage of the Doppler signals associated with subject A, which accounts for the outliers in the trajectory of subject A.

Range tracking of two human subjects walking in the same direction was performed in an outdoor open area using a 24 GHz FSK radar. Since the Doppler frequency is proportional to the carrier frequency, the higher the carrier frequencies, the more separated the Doppler peaks would be and, thus, the more accurate the range estimations. A 700 Hz square wave-control frequency was generated by an external board, which switched the transmit frequency between 23.8279 and 23.8306 GHz with a frequency shift of 2.7 MHz. The maximum unambiguous range is calculated as 55.5 m. In the experiment, both participants started the movements at approximately

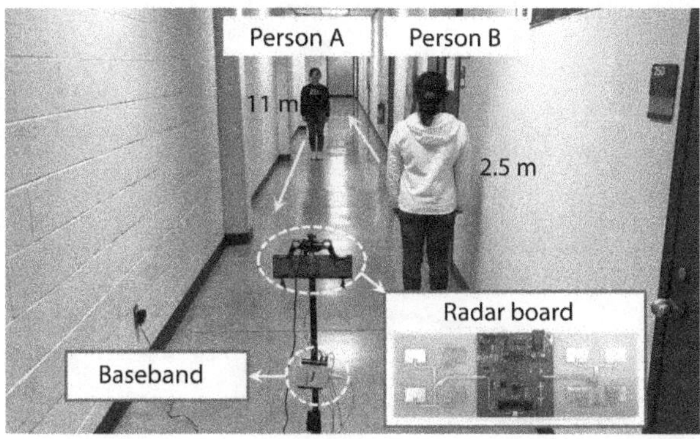


**FIGURE 11.30** Photograph of range tracking using a 5.8 GHz frequency-shift keying radar for two participants walking simultaneously in opposite directions in an interior corridor. (Courtesy of Changzhi Li, Texas Tech University.)

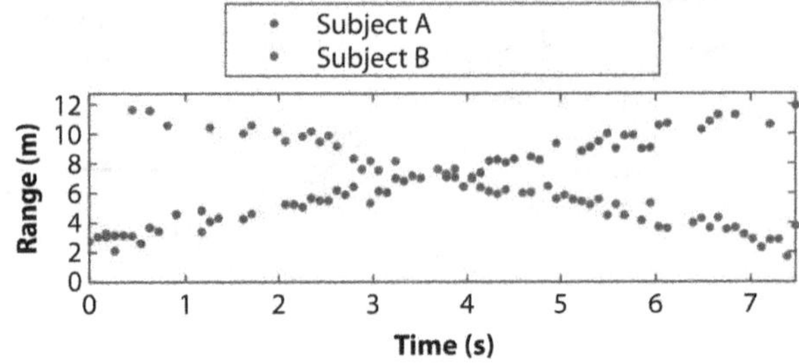


FIGURE 11.31 Measurement data for two subjects walking in opposite directions in an interior corridor using a 5.8 GHz frequency-shift keying location-tracking radar.

the same time with one walking slower than the other. The slower-moving participant walked from 2.5 to 8 m while the faster-moving participant walked from 2.5 to 12 m. Measured data were logged with a 15 kHz sampling frequency. The tracking results agreed well with the ground truth in the first 3 seconds (see Figure 11.32). The tracking performance of the faster-moving participant degraded later because of the lower received-signal strength and leakage from the slower-moving participant. Compared with the two participants walking in opposite-direction scenario, the multipath interferences are much more complex for walking in the same direction in indoor environments. Nonetheless, the 24 GHz FSK radar provided acceptable multitargets tracking performance in an outdoor open environment.

In addition, range and location tracking of single subjects were investigated using both 5.8 and 24 GHz FSK radars in environments with limited clutter. Also, range detection of a stationary human subject with different poses was demonstrated. The studies have demonstrated that the spectrum-efficient narrow-band FSK radar technology can provide absolute range and location of both moving and stationary human subjects with much less bandwidth requirement than some of the wideband counterparts. Further studies should aim toward minimizing the error contributions due to multipath, frequency drift, and I/Q channel mismatch.

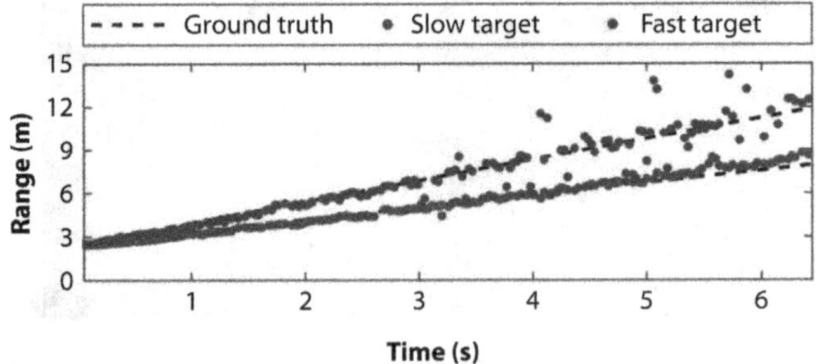


FIGURE 11.32 Results measured for two subjects walking in the same direction in an outdoor open area using a 24 GHz frequency-shift keying location-tracking radar.

### 11.1.5 Software Algorithm-Assisted 24 GHz FMCW Radar Sensing

The previous discussions on advances in microwave sensing for physiological signals from multiple subjects are driven mostly by sensor design and prototype validation. Many studies have contributed greatly to the technical development in and improvement of sensing methods for vital signs and bodily motions in environments where there is more than one subject. Section 11.1.3.2 described the effective combination of two signal processing algorithms, ICA and JADE, to offer accurate and efficient sensing of multiple subjects across a broad range of subject separation scenarios [Islam et al., 2020]. The integrated decision algorithm was shown to efficiently separate the physiological signatures of multiple subjects. Indeed, software and signal processing algorithms and methodologies for separating vital signs and localizing subjects are regarded as essential interdisciplinary research domains for continued development of extracting vital signs from multiple subjects using noncontact radar sensors.

This section describes the use of two different sets of signal processing software algorithms for improving target identification and vital-sign sensing of multiple subjects based on 24 GHz FMCW Doppler radars.

#### 11.1.5.1 Feature Extraction Algorithm for Vital-Sign Sensing of Multiple Subjects

The ability of FMCW Doppler radars to provide both range and phase information has rendered it a preferred method to determine the location of different subjects and track their vital signs. However, when two or more subjects are present within the same beamwidth, it becomes a major challenge to separate the subjects because of the resolution limited by finite bandwidth and difficulty in accurately detecting of the vital signs due to mutual interference. An algorithm in which the range information is obtained by the parametric spectral estimation method and the phase information is derived from the FFT method are combined to generate location and vital-sign information [Lee et al., 2019].

The software structure of the vital sign-sensing algorithm for multiple subjects is shown in Figure 11.33. The flow chart consists of three stages: signal acquisition, feature extraction, and vital-sign detection. In the signal acquisition stage, the beat signal is obtained from the FMCW radar system. This signal is generated by mixing the transmitted and received signals via a mixer and applies a low-pass filter to the mixer output. Range and phase information are concurrently extracted in the subsequent feature extraction stage. The role of range estimation is to determine the number of subjects and provide distance information. The role of phase formation is to determine the phase deviation caused by the Doppler effect at each location. The concurrent processing can provide more complete subject information that cannot be obtained using Doppler processing alone. In the vital sign detection stage, vital sign information is extracted from phase data at each location acquired in the feature extraction stage. Prior to extracting vital signs, the errors caused by dispersed human subjects are compensated by the range integration of the signals. Furthermore, the range integration reduces mutual interference, even in a situation where two subjects are adjacent within the radar resolution limit. The autoregressive (AR) method,

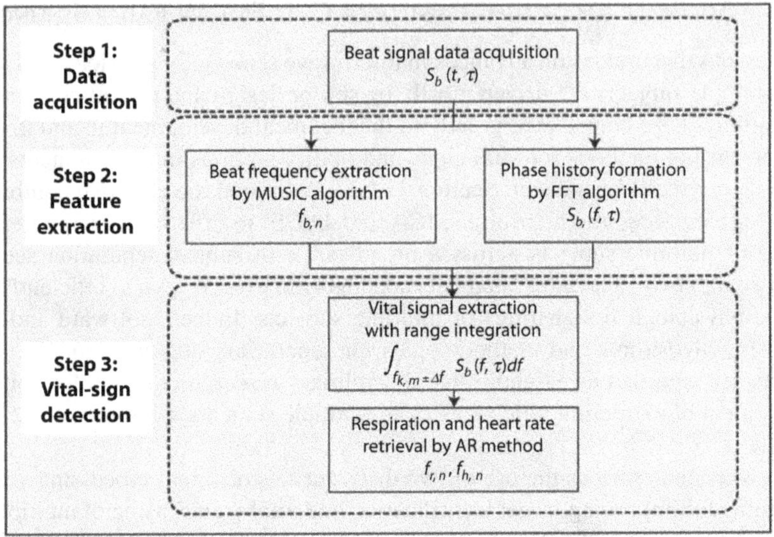


**FIGURE 11.33** Software architecture of the parametric spectral estimation feature extraction algorithm: (Step I) data acquisition from the radar system; (Step II) feature extraction for range and phase information in parallel; and (Step III) detection and tracking vital signs.

which is a parametric spectral estimation method, recovers the vital-sign data after integration.

In the feature extraction stage, the distance to each subject and the phase information necessary for the extraction of vital signs are obtained simultaneously. Respiration and heartbeat signals are very slow compared to the modulation frequency, making it appear as if the target is stationary during each modulation period. In other words, the target range may be assumed as constant for each period of the frequency modulation.

When there are two or more subjects in front of a radar, accurate extraction of the beat frequency for each subject in the frequency domain is complicated, except for the front-most subject, because of mutual interference between radar echoes. Furthermore, if subjects are within the resolution limit, the conventional FFT method cannot resolve multiple subjects due to the overlapping main lobes of the "sinc" functions in FFT. To overcome this difficulty, the multiple signal classification (MUSIC) algorithm is used to provide accurate, precise, and high-resolution outcomes in estimating the beat frequencies representing range. However, the MUSIC algorithm does not provide the necessary phase information; hence, a conventional FFT is made in conjunction with MUSIC to provide phase information for each subject. Thus, the beat frequencies $f_{b,n}$ are obtained by MUSIC, and the phase information $S_b(f,\tau)$ is simultaneously generated by FFT at each modulation period.

The range and phase information acquired are combined to recover vital-sign signals from multiple subjects. Phase information is extracted from FFT data, whose frequency is fixed at the beat frequency acquired by MUSIC. An integration is made in consideration of the property of the "sinc" function to reduce the effect of mutual interference. In a two-body model, as the two subjects approach each other, the mutual interference increases, especially in the case of two adjacent subjects within the resolution limit, and an erroneous vital sign is detected due to the mutual interference.

Despite the occurrence of some position estimation errors, the vital-sign signal of the front subject is robust against the mutual interference due to its relatively larger amplitude. In contrast, the vital sign of the back subject is susceptible to mutual interference. Thus, it is necessary to consider a method for removing the effect of mutual interference for the back subject. In this case, range integration is effective in eliminating the mutual interference for two adjacent subjects. Before the vital sign detection, the phase information is extracted from the output of the range integration at each position using arctangent demodulation.

Detecting vital signs using the FFT method is difficult because Doppler radar systems are vulnerable to small-motion artifacts and ambient noise. Thus, the AR method is advantageous under conditions where the subject to be found is clearly defined and is applied to exploit the fact that heartbeat and breathing have well-defined periodicity, given that the observation time is a few seconds.

Experimental measurements of the vital signs for two seated subjects positioned within the beamwidth of the radar are obtained using the arrangements shown in Figure 11.34. In these tests taken in an interior hallway, only the line-of-sight scenarios for each subject were considered without regard to the azimuth angle. The bandwidth of the FMCW Doppler radar is 250 MHz (24.00–24.25 GHz). The equivalent isotropic radiated power (EIRP) is 15 dBm. The horizontal 3 dB beamwidth is 45° and the vertical 3 dB beamwidth is 38°. The horizontal sidelobe suppression is 15 dB and the vertical sidelobe suppression is 20 dB. The modulation frequency is 100 Hz.

Figure 11.35 displays results obtained for two participants located at 130 and 300 cm away from the radar. The distance between participants is larger than the theoretical range resolution of 60 cm. Figure 11.35(a) shows the normalized amplitude of received signals as a function of range. The amplitude of the front subject was larger than that of the back subject. It is seen that the waveform provided by

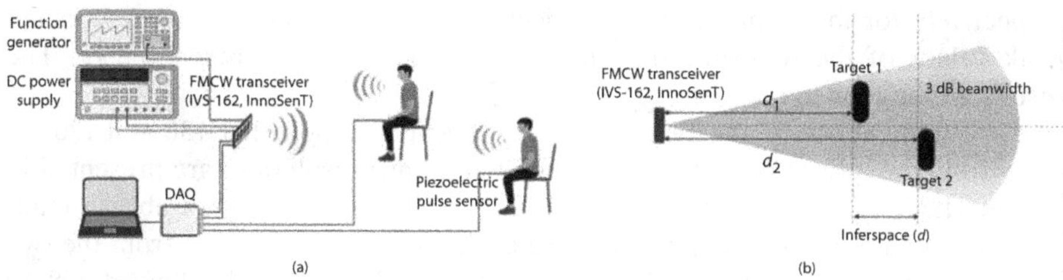


**FIGURE 11.34** Experimental setup for vial-sign measurement of two seated subjects with frequency-modulated continuous wave (FMCW) Doppler radar: (a) Block diagram showing overview of subjects with reference sensor and (b) schematic diagram giving a top view of antenna and subject spacing. (Lee et al., 2019.)

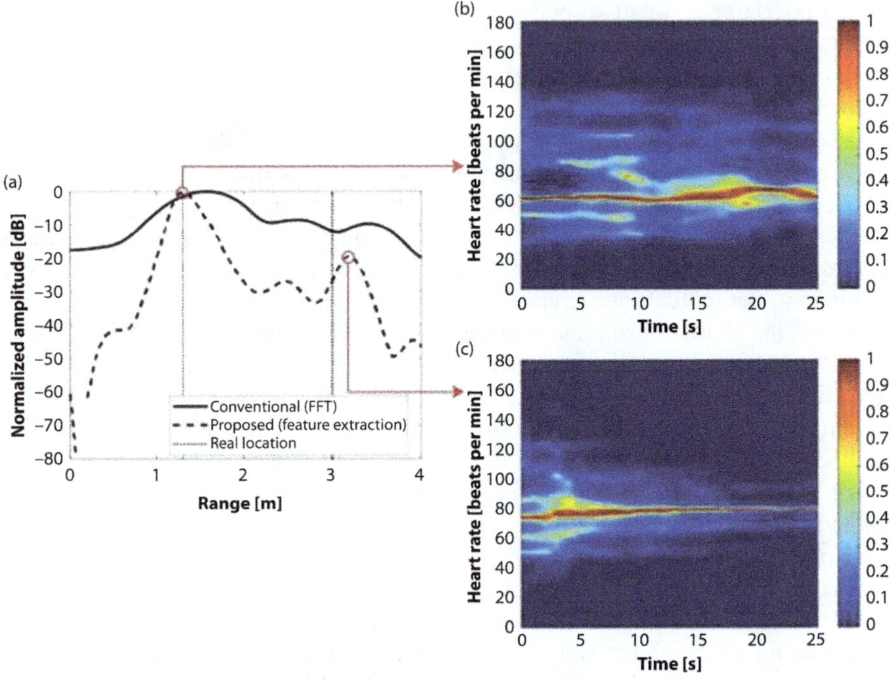


**FIGURE 11.35** Results from measurement of two subjects in the radar field: (a) Range estimation for subjects positioned at 130 and 300 cm from the radar, (b) real-time heart rate variation of the front subject at 130 cm, and (c) real-time heart rate for the back subject at 300 cm. (Lee et al., 2019.)

FFT cannot differentiate the signal from the back subject because of masking. In comparison, the result from the proposed method in the present study showed the location of the subject despite the large signal difference between the front and back subjects. For time domain data, the short-time AR method was applied at 1-second intervals with 10-second windows. Figure 11.35(b) and (c) give the time-varying heart rates extracted at each subject location (about 60 and 80 beat/min, respectively for the front and back subjects). Figure 11.36 presents the extracted peak values of the real-time data for FMCW radar and reference sensor. The results are in good agreement.

Measurement results for the case of two subjects positioned at 130 and 170 cm away from the radar (closer than the theoretical range resolution) are presented in Figure 11.37. Again, the results analyzed using FFT alone were not able to readily discriminate the two subjects because of the overlapping signals from the two adjacent subjects. In contrast, the method proposed in this study showed a clear distinction between the two positions (Figure 11.37a). However, the time-varying heart rates extracted at each subject location displayed in Figure 11.37(b) and (c) appear nearly the same (about 60 bpm) for the front and back subjects. The comparison in Figure 11.38 shows that the heart rate of the back subject did not match

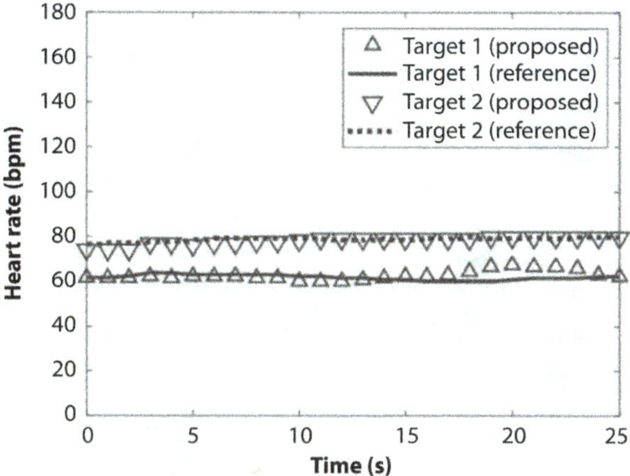


**FIGURE 11.36** Comparison of extracted peak values of the real-time heart-rate data of two subjects provided by radar and reference piezoelectric pulse sensor.

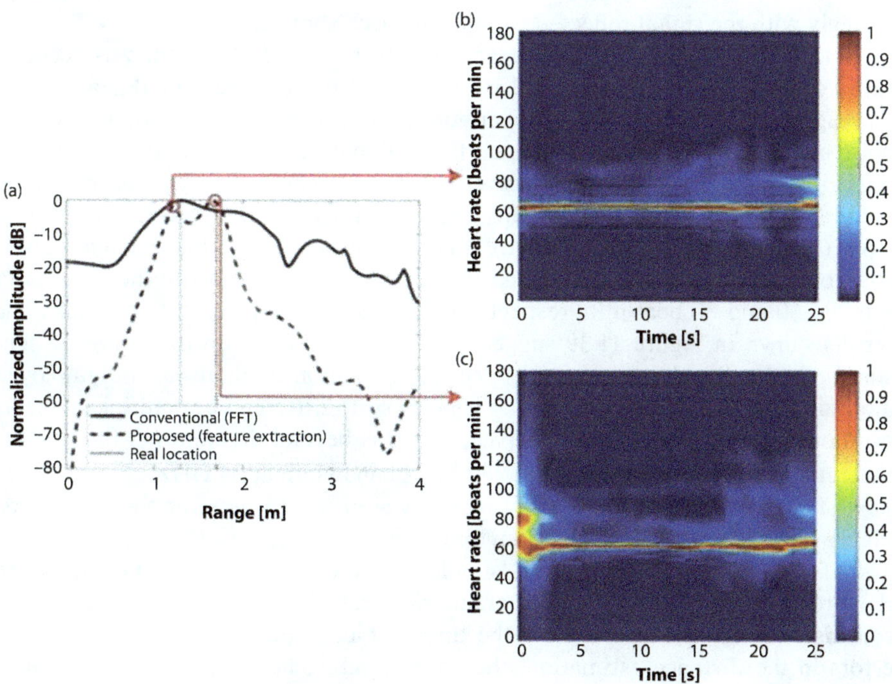


**FIGURE 11.37** Measurement results for two targets: (a) Range estimation for two targets at 130 and 170 cm, respectively, (b) heart rate for the front subject at 130 cm, and (c) heart rate for the back subject at 170 cm. (Lee et al., 2019.)

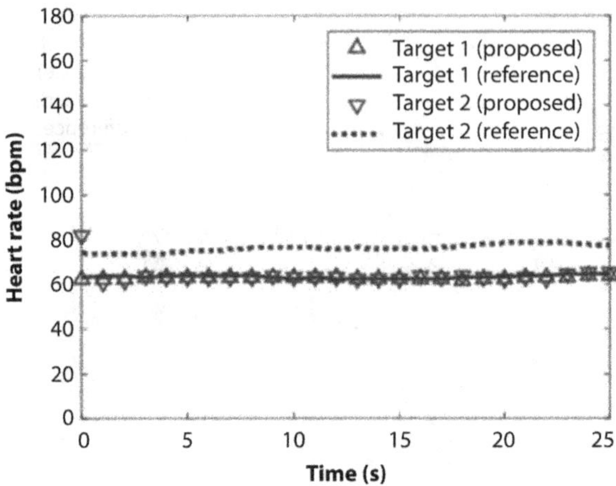


**FIGURE 11.38** Comparison between radar and reference sensor measured heart rates as functions of time.

the reference sensor data, despite their accurate localization. Instead, the FMCW radar sensed the heart signal of the subject in front, whose strength interfered strongly with the signal reflected from of the back subject.

Note that by applying range integration, the proposed algorithm was successful in compensating for the mutual interference. However, the time domain heart-rate signal exhibited considerable variations along with greater stationary clutter noise because MUSIC cannot suppress the stationary clutter, as it does not provide phase information. Figure 11.39(a) gives a comparison between the algorithm-based radar and the reference sensor-measured variations of heart rate for subjects at front (130 cm) and in back (170 cm). Figure 11.39(b) displays the frequency spectrum obtained by FMCW radar and the reference sensor showing heart rates of roughly 60 and 80 beat/min, respectively, for the subjects in front and back. The results shown in Figure 11.39 suggest general agreement with the reference sensor. Undoubtedly, the parametric spectral estimation method can be employed alongside range integration to make it possible to differentiate multiple subjects positioned approximately 40 cm apart, which is beyond the nominal limit of the theoretical range resolution for the 250 MHz bandwidth at 24 GHz.

It should be mentioned that an attempt was made to monitor three subjects. Figure 11.40 presents the results from three subjects located at 130, 180, and 300 cm away from the radar. As expected, simple FFT was not sufficient to characterize the three subjects. In contrast, the parametric spectral estimation method evidently can discriminate the locations of the three subjects. Furthermore, despite some errors in the distance estimation, the corresponding heart rates of each subject were close to those of the reference sensor measurements.

In summary, based on a 24 GHz FMCW Doppler radar, the parametric spectral estimation method was demonstrated to be capable of distinguishing between two subjects sitting 40 cm apart, overcoming the 60 cm range resolution for a

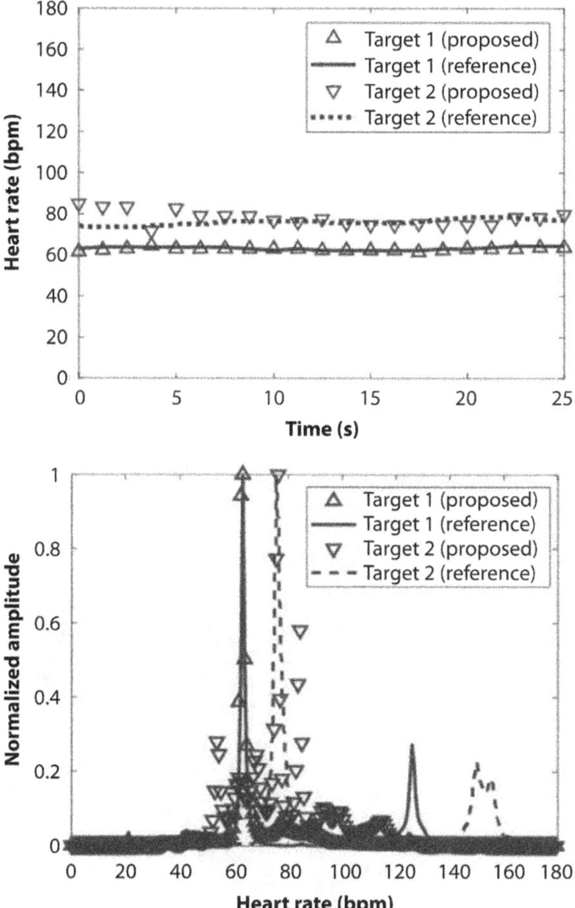


**FIGURE 11.39** Comparison between the algorithm-based radar and the reference sensor measured variations of heart rate for the subjects at front (Target1) and in back (Target2), (b) Frequency spectrum obtained by radar and reference sensor for the subjects in front (Target1) and back (Target2).

frequency bandwidth of 250 MHz. According to the Rayleigh equation for range resolution, $R$ may be either stated in terms of bandwidth or pulse width, such that

$$R = \frac{c}{2\Delta f} = \frac{c\Delta t}{2} \tag{11.1}$$

where $c$ is the speed of wave propagation, $\Delta f$ is the frequency bandwidth, and $\Delta t$ is the pulse width. This theoretical limit would, in practice, depend on the signal-processing scheme employed. The parametric spectral estimation algorithm uses signal processing techniques to overcome the ambiguity of range detection based

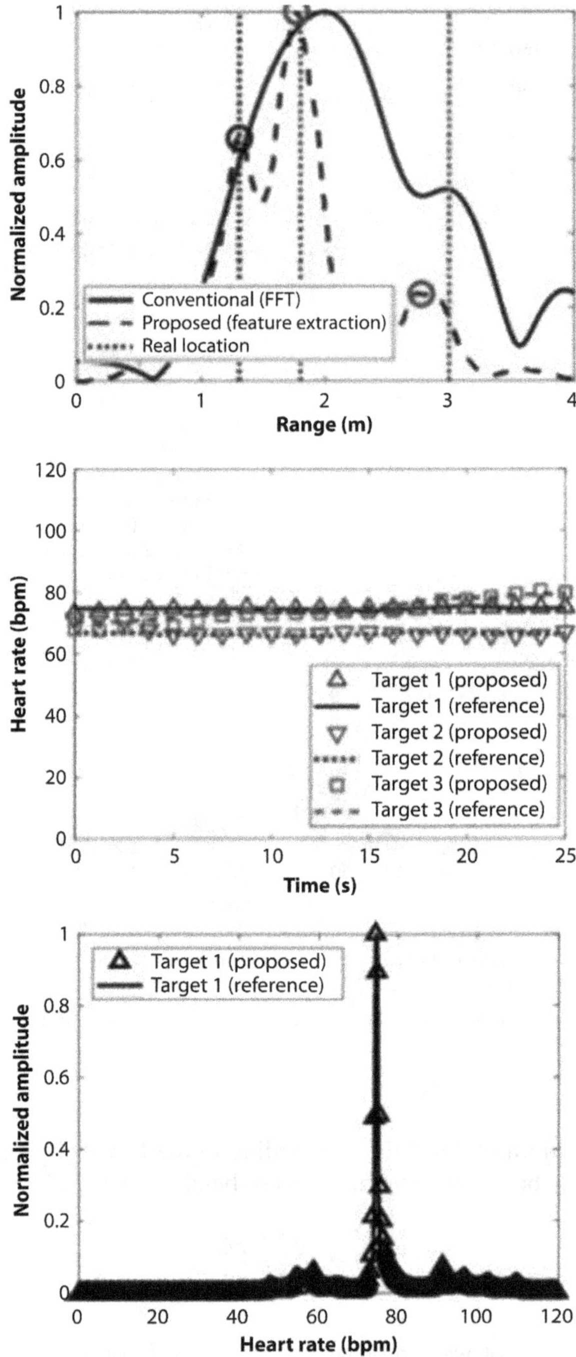


**FIGURE 11.40** Measurement results of three participants located at 130, 180, and 300 cm away from the radar: (a) Range estimation, (b) comparison of heart rates between the radar method and the reference sensor as a function of time, and amplitude distribution of heart rates (beat/min): (c) for participant 1, (d) for participant 2, and (e) for participant 3. (*Continued*)

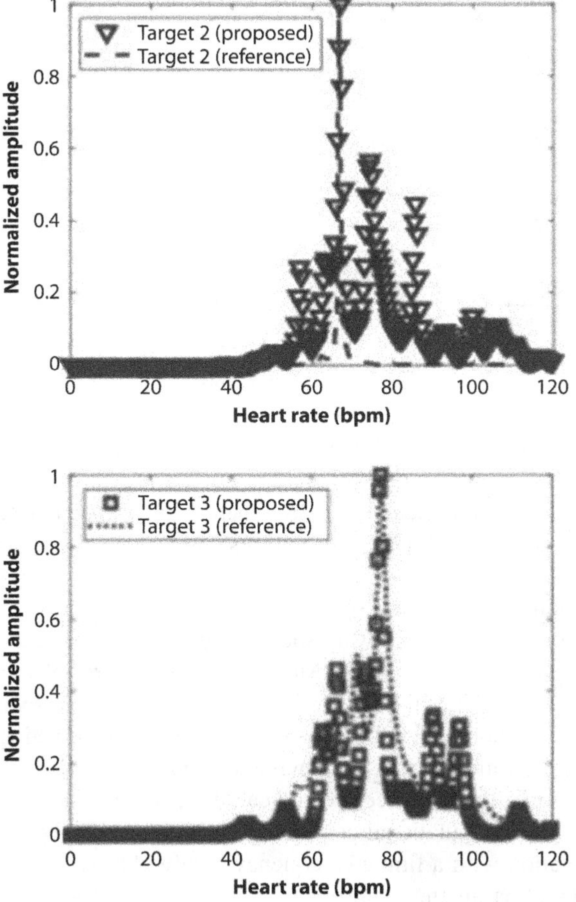


**FIGURE 11.40** (*Continued*)

on conventional FFT. Location and heart-rate information of multiple subjects is retrieved in real time by combining enhanced spatial resolution, standard deviation phase extraction, mutual interference elimination through range integration, and an AR method for detection and noninvasive sensing of vital signatures.

#### 11.1.5.2 Resolution Enhancement for Sensing Vital Sign of Multiple Subjects

The MUSIC algorithm may be employed to provide superior resolution for a given bandwidth, which can overcome the theoretical range resolution limit. However, it is difficult to suppress the effect of clutters that arise when using the MUSIC algorithm because it does not involve phase information. Moreover, real-time detection of vital signs with the MUSIC algorithm is challenging due to the high computational complexity of its eigenvalue decomposition and parametric sweep procedures. A signal-processing technique in conjunction with band-limited 24 GHz FMCW Doppler radar was reported for detecting the vital signs of two adjacent subjects with enhanced resolution, clutter mitigation, and reduced computational budget [Lee et al., 2020].

Briefly, the method exploits the fact that vital-sign signals vary slowly in comparison with the modulation frequency in FMCW radar. To enhance the resolution of the radar sensor, a mathematical manipulation was introduced to double the effective frequency bandwidth. The beat signal, $S_b\ (r,t)$ of the proposed method for two targets can be expressed as follows:

$$S_b\ (r,t) = \sum_{n=1}^{2} \phi_n\ sinc\left[\frac{4B}{c}(r - R_n)\right] + \sum_{n=1}^{2} \phi_n\ D_n\ sinc\left[\frac{2B}{c}(r - R_n)\right] \quad (11.2)$$

where $\phi_n$ is the phase information of the $n$-th target, $R_n$ is the range of the $n$-th target, and $D_n$ is a complex coupling coefficient determined by the bandwidth and range difference. The beat signal consists of a signal component which is the first term of Eq. (11.2) with a resolution of $c/4B$ and the noise component, which is the second term of Eq. (11.2), with a resolution of $c/2B$, where $c$ is the speed of microwave propagation and $B$ is the bandwidth (250 MHz in this case). Thus, the signal of interest has the resolution of a signal with twice the bandwidth, while the noise signal maintains the same resolution as the original signal. Since range estimation errors are generated by the unwanted noise signal and were shown to be roughly 10%, they do not have a significant impact on range estimation. Moreover, a range error of approximately 10% may be compensated for through the previously mentioned phase extraction using the range-integration method. Therefore, the range-estimation error does not affect the accuracy of vital-sign monitoring. Employing a standard deviation of phase information obtained via FFT, the proposed method can discriminate and extricate the stationary clutter with low computational complexity. It does not involve standard methods to improve resolution with a limited frequency bandwidth, such as MUSIC, and the estimation of signal parameters via rotational invariant techniques (ESPRIT). While MUSIC and ESPRIT are robust under noisy environments and exhibit high-resolution performance, they cannot provide phase information, have difficulty in detecting vital-sign signals in the presence of separate stationary clutter, and require parametric sweep, which imposes a large computational burden.

Furthermore, the study has demonstrated that for a stationary clutter object located 1 m from the detector and an oscillating point scatterer located 2 m away, the MUSIC algorithm detected both the stationary clutter and oscillating point scatterer. However, the proposed method can detect both targets by using only amplitude information. Moreover, by applying the standard deviation of phase information process, the proposed method can mitigate against the strong clutter and clearly detect the targeted object.

Experiments were conducted to evaluate the resolution limit of the proposed method by varying the space between two seated subjects. The position of the near (front) subject was maintained at 100 cm, while the position of the far (back) subject was changed from 180 to 140 cm in 10 cm increments. Figure 11.41 depicts results for two subjects located at 100 and 140 cm, respectively. For real-time vital-sign sensing, FFT was performed at 2-second intervals with 10-second windows. As seen

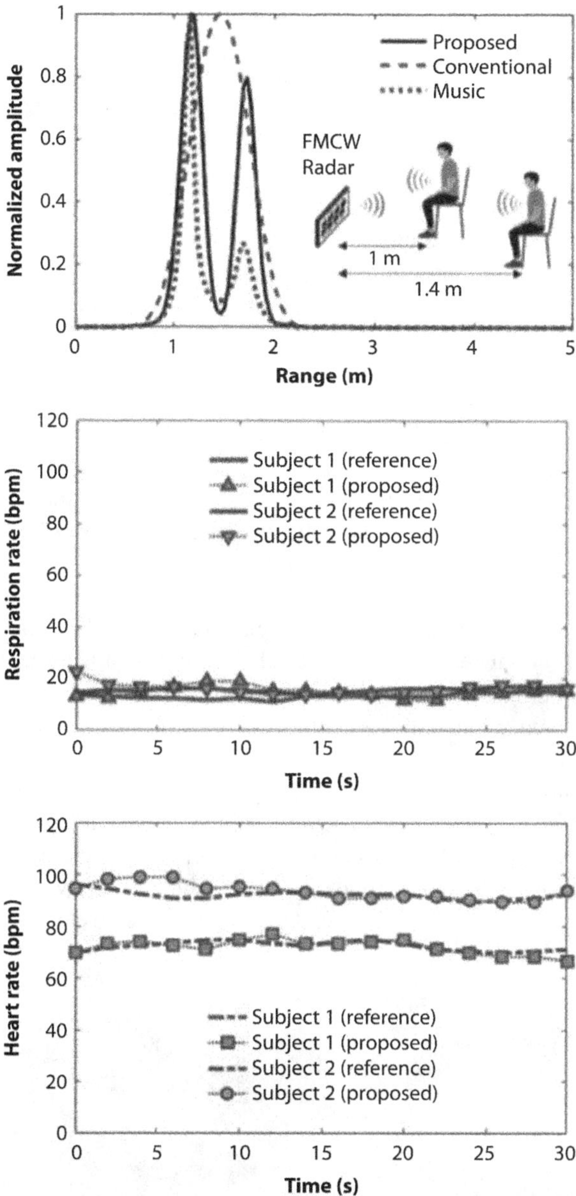


**FIGURE 11.41** Experimental results for two subjects at 100 and 140 cm: (a) Range estimation, (b) comparison of the respiration rate measured by frequency-modulated continuous wave (FMCW) radar method with that of reference sensor, and (c) comparison of the heart rate of the proposed method with that of reference sensor.

in Figure 11.41(a), with the conventional FFT method, the subjects overlapped and are undistinguishable. Both the proposed FMCW radar method and MUSIC algorithm can clearly characterize the two subjects. Figure 11.41(b) and (c) give comparisons of respiratory rate (RR) and heart rate (HR) measured by FMCW radar method with that of reference sensors. The results demonstrate that the proposed method can discriminate between subjects 40 cm apart, beyond the Rayleigh resolution of 60 cm. The vital signs are in good agreement with those obtained using commercial reference sensors in real time. The measurement errors were assessed using five different sets of data. Overall, the absolute error is roughly 4 beat/min. The relative error of the HR is about 2.5%, while the respiratory rate errors are around 9%. It appears that the respiratory rate errors are large, perhaps due to the somewhat lower frequencies of the respiratory signal.

Figure 11.42 illustrates the experimental scenario for two subjects lying side-by-side on a bed with the FMCW radar sensor mounted on the side. The total measurement time was 150 seconds. FFT was performed at 5-second intervals with 10-second windows. It can be seen from Figure 11.43(a) that the conventional FFT method failed to distinguish the two subjects. The proposed radar method showed clean detection of two subjects with successful elimination of stationary clutter such as the bed and surrounding walls. There was a false detection in the vicinity of 70 seconds for the far subject, as shown in Figure 11.43(b) and (c), due to the subject's body movement. The measured real-time HR and RR results agree well with those of commercial reference sensors.

Note that the two subjects lying side-by-side did not have visible space between them. Nevertheless, the proposed method was successful in sorting out the vital signals of two subjects despite a theoretically insufficient range resolution. FMCW radar sensing depends on the movement of the chest and abdomen. Thus, the proposed method can apparently separate the chest locations of the two subjects regardless of the positions of the human body. Since the distance between the chests of the two subjects was roughly 45 cm, the radar sensor was able to clearly differentiate the vital signs of the two adjacent subjects.

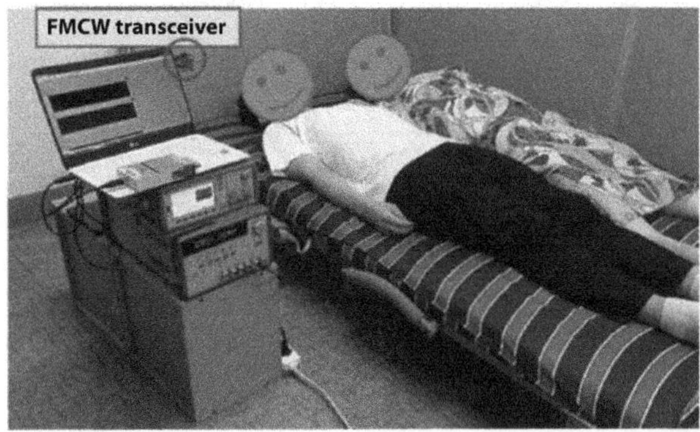


**FIGURE 11.42** Experimental scenario for two subjects lying side-by-side on a bed next to frequency-modulated continuous wave (FMCW) radar sensor. (Lee et al., 2020.)

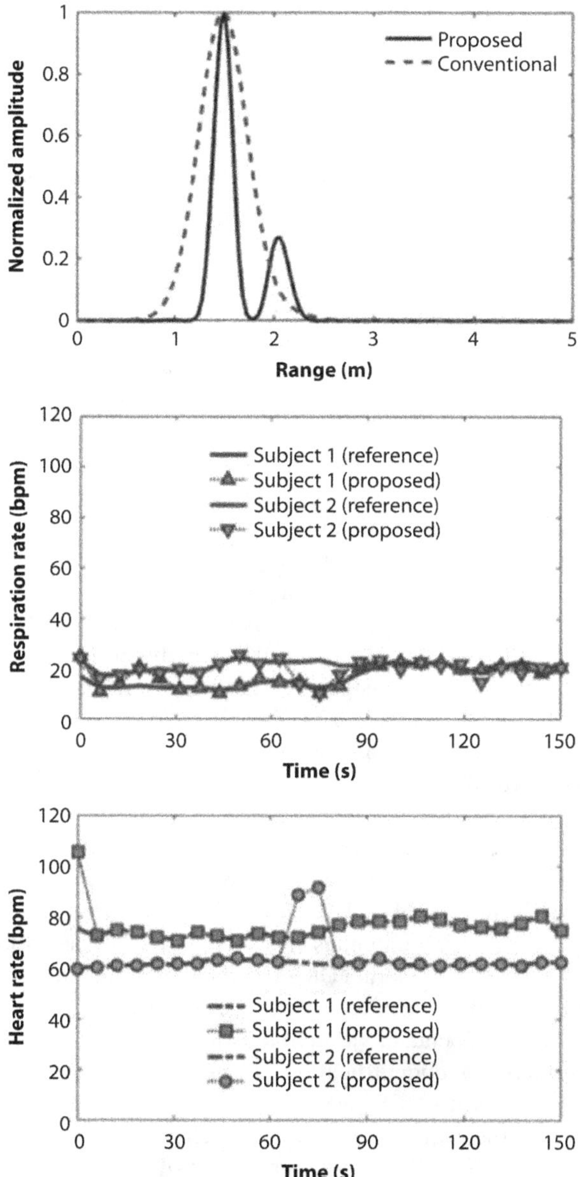


**FIGURE 11.43** Experimental results for two subjects lying side-by-side on a bed: (a) range estimation, (b) comparison of the respiratory rate (RR) obtained using the proposed radar method with commercial reference sensor, and (c) comparison of the HR obtained using the radar method with that by reference sensor.

In conclusion, the results confirmed the resolution enhancement, superior clutter mitigation performance, and reduced computational complexity. One issue that has been somewhat addressed in early discussions, but remains a challenge for practical application, is the motion artifact. A salient example is depicted in Figure 11.43. It is a common issue for remote contactless radar physiological sensors. Signals associated with body movements including hand gestures and leg motions can be much stronger than the vital signs, making it difficult to detect the vital sign when the subject is not stationary.

### 11.1.6 MM-Wave Radar Sensor for Multiple Subjects

Recently, the technological advancement and greater availability of mm-wave FMCW radars, especially at 77 GHz, are being explored for use in localizing multiple subjects and estimation of vital signs [Dai, 2022; Dai et al., 2022; Lv et al., 2021; Xu et al., 2022]. A significant attribute compared to the lower frequency FMCW radars described previously is the reduction in size of mm-wave components to support antenna arrays for vital-sign monitoring of multiple subjects. As mentioned, the ability of FMCW radars to provide both range and phase information has allowed it to become a favored radar technique to monitor locations of different subjects and track vital signs. However, the higher sensitivity afforded by the shorter mm-wave can elicit more pronounced noise sources such as body motions to degrade or interfere with remote noncontact vital-sign detection. To overcome this challenge, commercial mm-wave FMCW radars at 77 GHz were used in a MIMO architecture to improve the SNR level by taking advantage of its channel diversity [Dai, 2022; Dai et al., 2022]. The approach minimizes contributions from channels whose signals are disrupted by environmental artifacts to achieve higher accuracy estimation by using orthogonality-based channel selection.

Specifically, FMCW radars transmit mm-waves via multiple antennas (TX) in a time-division-multiplexing (TDM) scheme and the mm-wave signals are collected with multiple receiving antennas (RX). By virtue of the orthogonality of the transmitted and received signals in TDM-MIMO, the signal from each transmitting antenna can be extracted by each receiving antenna. The contributions of different TX-RX pairs present independent views of the targets, which are utilized to improve target feature estimation and identification. In one case [Dai, 2022; Dai et al., 2022], a MIMO radar system with 12 TX and 16 RX antennas was employed. In each TDM time slot, only one of the available TXs transmits. The measurements collected over 12 slots correspond to 192 TX-RX antenna pairs and are used for vital-sign monitoring of two seated subjects as illustrated in Figure 11.44. The two subjects are in different ranges — subject #1 is 0.75 m and subject #2 is 1.5 m in front of the MIMO radar — and are separated by 0.6 m between them. Figure 11.44(b) gives the range 2D-FFT profile for the experiment. The accuracy rate of heartbeat estimation for two participants showed relatively high correlation with low estimation errors (Figure 11.45). The vital-sign information was extracted by using maximal ratio combining (MRC) joined with adapted continuous wavelet transform (CWT) algorithms to enhance vital-sign estimation accuracy. Thus, the results demonstrate the successful use of a mm-wave (77 GHz) FMCW system with 192 TDM-MIMO channels to

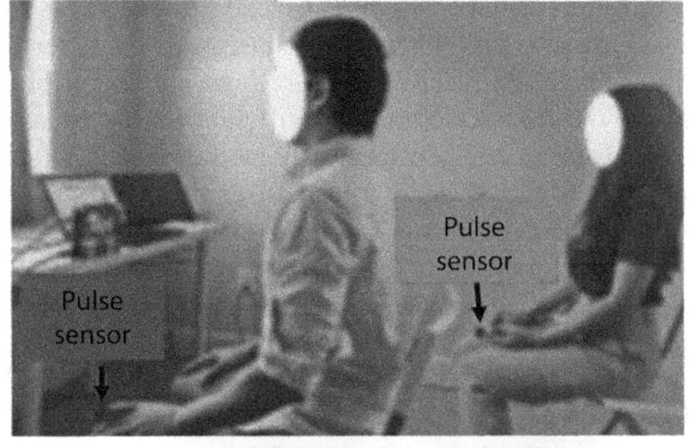


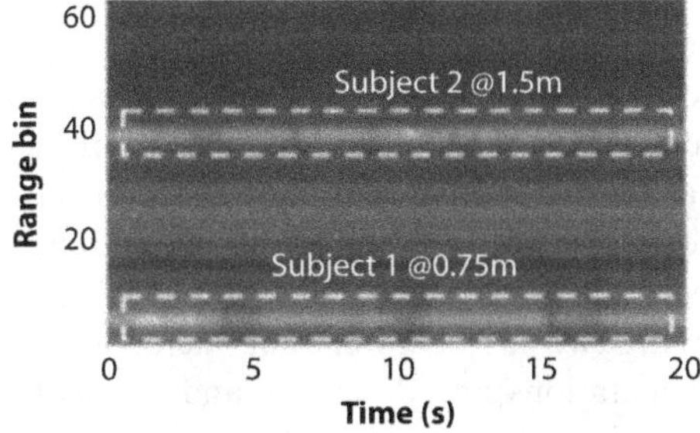


**FIGURE 11.44** The two participants at different ranges and separated side-by-side by 0.6 meters in between: (a) Experimental scenario and (b) 2-D-FFT range profile. (Dai, 2022; Courtesy of Vo Dai, Toan Khanh, University of Tennessee.)

remotely sense vital signs of multiple human subjects alongside the usage of MRC-CWT signal processing algorithms, which significantly improve the accuracy of vital-sign detection.

Another mm-wave FMCW-radar-based MIMO architecture for vital-sign monitoring of multiple subjects uses a TDM-phased-MIMO radar sensing scheme that performs beamforming to steer the radar beam toward different directions [Xu et al., 2022]. A phased-MIMO radar combines MIMO and the phased array feature, in which

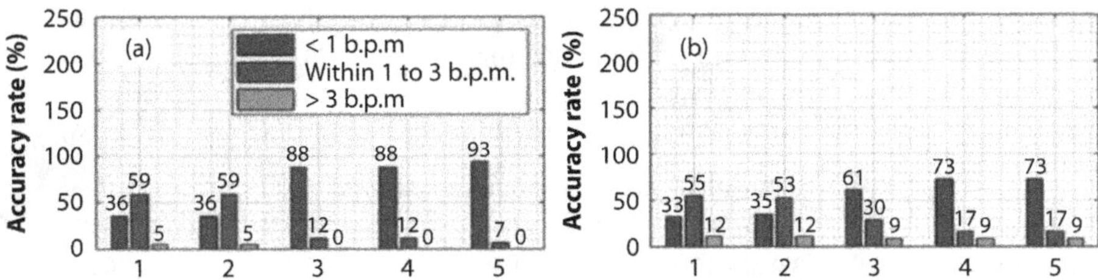


**FIGURE 11.45** Accuracy rate of heartbeat estimation for two participants (a and b). Horizontal axis shows: 1) Channel average with all channels, 2) Channel average with selected channels, 3) Channel with lowest RMS error, 4) MRC with all channels, and 5) MRC with selected channels.

an FMCW radar transmits orthogonal signals to feed a phase-array structure. The proposed TDM-phased-MIMO radar scheme combines analog beamforming and MIMO to enable both transmitter and receiver beamforming. Orthogonality is achieved by TDM transmission of the same waveform with different weights in each slot and allows the transmitted signals to be detected separately by the receiver. It effectively creates different channels that provide diversity for enhanced target estimation.

The system was implemented using a commercial 77 GHz FMCW-based MIMO radar with three TXs and four RXs. The TDM-phased-MIMO design permitted the formation of a virtual receiving array with aperture longer (eight RXs in this case) than that of the physical receiving array. Since all transmit-receive pairs corresponding to the virtual array provide independent information about the targets, combining the data collected from them boosts the receiver SNR to provide higher accuracy in the target estimation. The apparent larger aperture of the virtual array permits the receiver to better separate more closely spaced targets. Also, the receiving array focuses on scatterings coming from the desired directions and processes them through a Capon beamformer, while the power from all other directions is minimized. In this way, each beam contains the vital signs of one subject only. Since the phased-MIMO radar can steer the mm-wave beam toward different directions with a short ($\mu$s) delay, it can facilitate simultaneous monitoring of the vital signs of multiple subjects.

Experiments involving two subjects were conducted under various settings such as different subject orientations and distances and angles between the radar and subjects. Some results of single-target and two-target heartbeat and breath rate sensing are listed in Table 11.2 for different distances and angles of separation. The

**TABLE 11.2**
**Representative Result of Heartbeat and Breathing Rate Estimations for Single-Target and Two-Target Scenarios**

| Participant | Distance and Angle | Phased Array | Phased MIMO | PPG Reference |
|---|---|---|---|---|
| | | **Heart Rate Estimation (beats/min** | | |
| Participant 1 | 1.5 m, 30° | 62.89 | 84.46 | 84.07 |
| Participant 2 | 3.0 m, –10° | 61.11 | 61.33 | 61.14 |
| Participant 1 (and 3) | 1.5 m (3.0 m), 30° (–10°) | 78.22 (72.10) | 77.62 (70.81) | 78.06 (70.83) |
| Participant 3 (and 4) | 2.0 m (2.0 m), 10° (–30°) | 65.82 (65.04) | 66.02 (71.37) | 67.05 (72.06) |
| | | **Breathing Rate Estimation (breaths/min** | | |
| Participant 1 | 1.5 m, 30° | 19.03 | 20.03 | 20.01 |
| Participant 2 | 3.0 m, –10° | 18.03 | 16.03 | 16.34 |
| Participant 1 (and 3) | 1.5 m (3.0 m), 30° (–10°) | 18.05 (19.03) | 16.96 (20.00) | 17.37 (20.05) |
| Participant 3 (and 4) | 2.0 m (2.0 m), 10° (–30°) | 18.67 (17.02) | 16.56 (18.03) | 16.12 (18.14) |

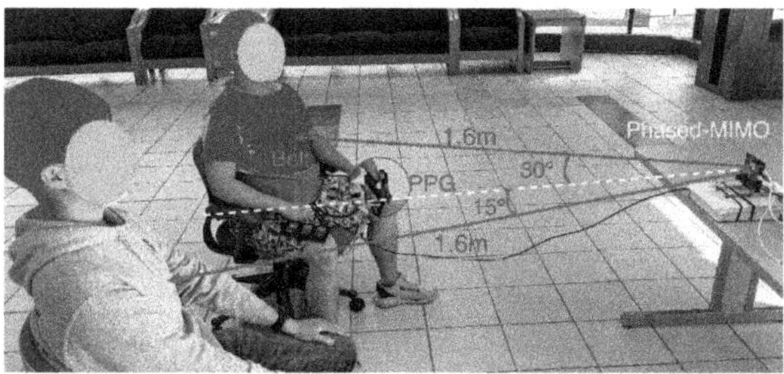


**FIGURE 11.46** TDM-phased multiple-input multiple-output sensor experimental setup for measurement of breathing and heartbeat signals of two participants. (Courtesy of Chung-Tse Michael Wu, Rutgers University.)

findings made with phased array and phase-MIMO radars sensors are compared to photoplethysmography (PPG). The accuracy rates can reach nearly 100% at distances of 1–2 m. Results shown in Figure 11.46 signify that the TDM-phased-MIMO system can achieve better than 98% accuracy for breathing rate and 83% accuracy for heartbeat estimation, at a subject-to-radar distance of 1.6 m when the targets are facing the radar. The minimal subject-to-subject angle separation was 20°, corresponding to separation of 0.3 m between two subjects (see Figure 11.47 for experimental setup). Experiments conducted with subjects not facing the radar (see Figure 11.48) indicated that when the radar sensor is used to detect vital signs from the front and back of the torso, the accuracy rates for the phased-MIMO detection are higher than when the radar sensor is located on the side of subjects.

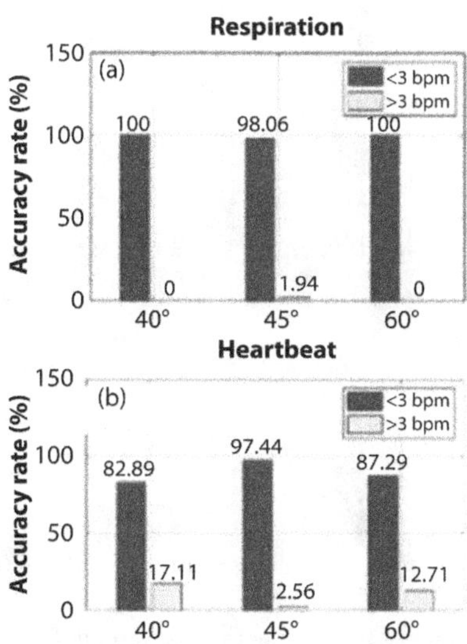


**FIGURE 11.47** Accuracy rate of two-subject measurement for different angles between two targets. The radar-to-target distance is 1.6 m: (a) Respiration and (b) heartbeat.

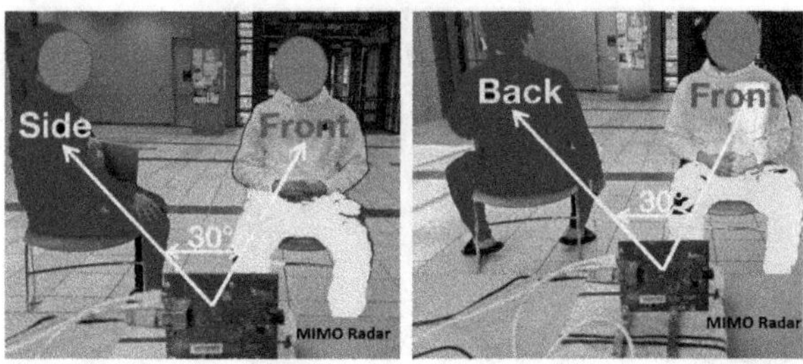


**FIGURE 11.48** Experimental setup for participants not facing the radar sensor. (Courtesy of Chung-Tse Michael Wu, Rutgers University.)

In this case, the cardiopulmonary-induced chest displacement is modest from the arm. Moreover, the chest reflections are much smaller in that orientation, thus, the breathing movement and heartbeat are more difficult to detect when the radar sensor is located on the side of human subjects.

It is noteworthy that in an experiment where two participants were at same radial distance of 1.6 m but with an angular separation of 30°, the phased-MIMO sensor was able to resolve and accurately estimate the different breathing rates of the two participants but not the heartbeat (Figure 11.49). In conclusion, by combining higher angular resolution and better accuracy target estimation, the TDM-phased-MIMO radar system is capable of providing accurate measurements of heartbeat and respiration of multiple subjects located close to each other, including when the subjects are at the same radial distance from the radar. Propagation and penetration losses

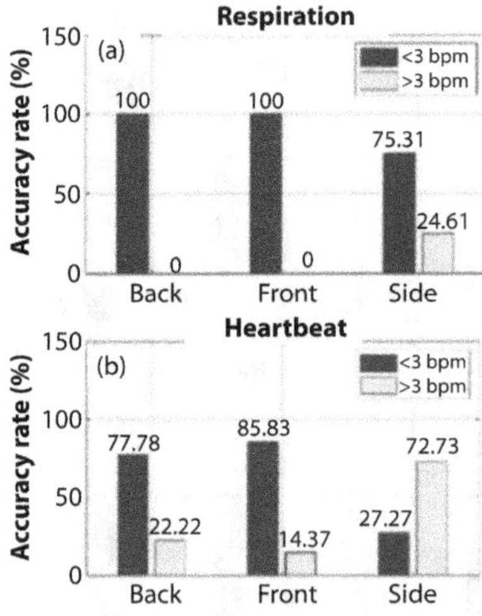


**FIGURE 11.49** Accuracy rate of two-subject measurement for different target orientations. The radar-to-target distance is 1.6 m and target angle of separation is 30°: (a) Respiration and (b) heartbeat.

are major issues for mm-wave MIMO channels. To overcome the challenges, a possible direction for extension and enhancement of the present approach could involve incorporation of active beamforming at the front end in the radar transmitters for scenarios consisting of longer subject-to-radar distances and smaller subject-to-subject separations. The tasks would obviously complicate an already complex system architecture.

## 11.2 APPLICATIONS IN MEDICINE AND HEALTHCARE

Research and technical advancement in noninvasive, unobtrusive, and contactless sensing methods for vital signs and other physiological signals can help improve diagnosis, treatment, and prevention in medical practice and healthcare. Application domains and scenarios include postsurgery recovery, respiratory syndrome, sleep medicine, intensive care, and cardiac arrhythmias as well as a variety of cardiopulmonary conditions and disorders such as diabetes, heart diseases, sleep apnea-hypopnea, and chronic obstructive pulmonary disease (COPD).

### 11.2.1 Sleep Medicine — Diagnosis of Sleep Apnea-Hypopnea Syndrome

The prevalence of sleep disorders has been increasing and the discipline of sleep medicine is growing in response. Sleep-related breathing disorders have gained the most attention among all sleep disorders [Edwards et al., 2020; Laratta et al., 2017; Penzel et al., 2018; Thompson et al., 2022; Yeghiazarians et al., 2021]. Specifically, sleep apnea-hypopnea syndrome (SAHS) is being recognized as a potential cause or significant contributor to such chronic medical conditions as hypertension, heart failure, and diabetes. As often the case, early diagnosis of the disease can positively impact treatment outcome and efficacy. The current diagnostic protocols of SAHS are based on a comprehensive evaluation of clinical symptoms and the results of a formal sleep study namely, polysomnography (PSG). However, it is difficult for a subject to maintain a normal sleep routine during the study process, with many contact monitors such as ECG, electroencephalography (EEG), electrooculography (EOG), pulse oximetry, respiratory airflow, and respiratory effort sensors. Hence, the reliability and usefulness of the PSG test are less than desired. Furthermore, the PSG test requires well-trained experts to monitor, assess, and diagnose accurately. The noninvasive contactless microwave Doppler radar respiratory measurement technique has been adopted and developed to overcome the difficulties and to provide an alternative to PSG-based formal sleep study [Kagawa et al., 2013, 2016].

The technique employs a noncontact sensing system with two microwave radars in diagnosing SAHS. The noncontact SAHS diagnostic system can provide unobtrusive detection of apneic events with minimal patient awareness of the process and is done with comfort and without any detector-induced stress in the person being monitored. Two Doppler radars are installed beneath the mattress to measure movements of the chest and abdomen (Figure 11.50). A functional block diagram of the diagnostic system for SAHS is shown in Figure 11.51.

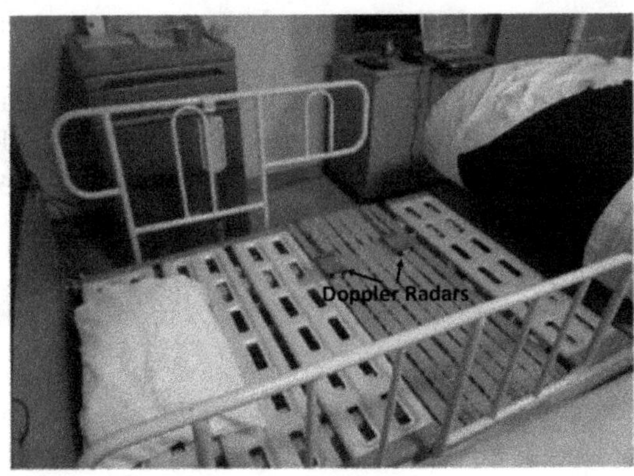


**FIGURE 11.50** Sleep apnea–hypopnea syndrome (SAHS) monitoring system showing radar location under the patient bed. (Kagawa et al., 2016.)

The hardware layer consists of two 24 GHz Doppler radars, a power amplifier (500X amplification), A/D converter (sampling frequency of 100 Hz), and a computer system for analysis. The two antennas are separated 25 cm from one another to sense chest and abdomenal movements. The output of each radar is 40 mW. The incident power density of the Doppler device is 0.15 W/m$^2$ on the body surface. The quadrature Doppler radar output signals are combined before demodulation of subject motion. The radar output signals are separated and each signal is processed through band-pass filters that correspond either to the rate of respiration (0.1–0.6 Hz) or heartbeat (pulse) (0.6–3.0 Hz). An automatic gain control technique is used to remove body-motion noise from the cardiorespiratory signals. Automatic gain control is an amplitude autoregulation method that limits signals from the heart to the maximum heart signal amplitude in the absence of body motion. This amplitude regulation processing is applied to each peak and trough as a wave fraction to reduce the effect of body motions.

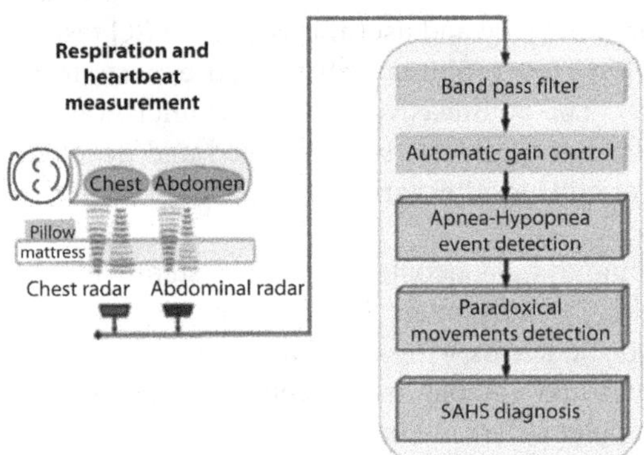


**FIGURE 11.51** Functional block diagram of sleep apnea–hypopnea syndrome (SAHS) measurement system.

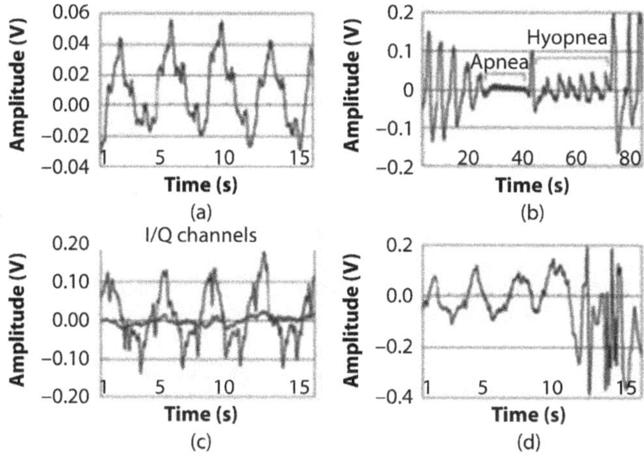


**FIGURE 11.52** Respiratory signals from radar output: (a) Heartbeat superimposed on top of respiration; (b) hypopnea signal with amplitude <50% and apnea signal with amplitude <20%; (c) I/Q channel output signals; and (d) random body movement signal starting at 11 seconds.

Apnea and hypopnea events are detected in accordance with the established SAHS diagnostic criteria based on the amplitude changes of the respiratory signals (see Figure 11.52). From the radar signals, the decrease in respiratory amplitude and the phase difference between the chest and abdominal signals are calculated. These quantities are used to detect the occurrence of apnea–hypopnea events and classify the types of apneas. Despite the subjects engagement in frequent body movements while sleeping, the Doppler radar system was very effective in the diagnosis of SAHS.

In a group of 35 test participants, the noncontact microwave SAHS diagnostic system was able to identify three types of sleep apnea: obstructive, central, and mixed. Respiratory-disturbance indices (Figure 11.53) showed a higher correlation

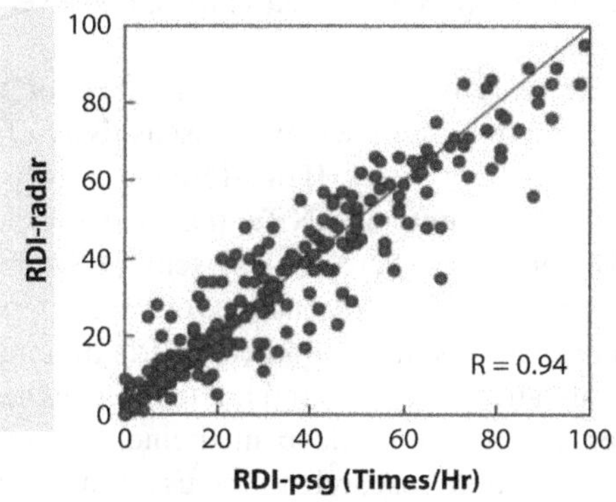


**FIGURE 11.53** Correlation of respiratory disturbance indexes between radar and PSG measurements.

**TABLE 11.3**
**Diagnostic Performance in the Test Group (35 Participants)**

| Variables | AHI Cutoff of 15/h (RDI = 12/h) | | AHI Cutoff of 30/h (RDI = 24/h) | |
|---|---|---|---|---|
| | Radar | Oximetry | Radar | Oximetry |
| Sensitivity (%) | 96.4 | 89.3 | 90.5 | 85.7 |
| Specificity (%) | 100.0 | 100.0 | 78.6 | 78.6 |
| PPV (%) | 100.0 | 100.0 | 86.4 | 85.7 |
| NPV (%) | 87.5 | 70.0 | 84.6 | 78.6 |
| AUC | 1.00 | 1.00 | 0.94 | 0.93 |

*Abbreviations:* PPV = positive predictive value, NPV = negative predictive value, AUC = area under the receiver operating characteristic curve, and RDI = respiratory disturbance index.

(r = 94%) for radar than with PSG (r = 89%). The diagnostic performances of the radar system and PSG pulse oximetry were evaluated for two different cutoffs (15 and 30 events/hour) of the apnea-hypopnea index (AHI), as shown in Table 11.3. The diagnostic ability of the radar system versus that of the PSG oximetry was assessed by comparing the sensitivity, specificity, positive predictive value (PPV), negative predictive value (NPV), and area under the receiver operating characteristic curve (AUC) between the two systems. In the group with an AHI cutoff of 15/h, the respiratory disturbance indices (RDIs) obtained from radars had a higher diagnostic performance than those of pulse oximetry, with a sensitivity of 96% and NPV of 88%. When the AHI cutoff was 30/h, the radar again had a higher sensitivity of 90% and NPV of 85%; the radar AUC was also better than that of PSG oximetry. Overall, the RDIs detected by the radar system were highly correlated with those of the PSG system, and the overall diagnostic performance of the radar system was more accurate than that of PSG oximetry. The NPV indicates the probability that subjects with a negative screening test do not have the disease; thus, it is a very important estimator when screening for a disease.

When predicting the severity of SAHS with an AHI of >15/h or >30/h using PSG as a reference, the radar system achieved a sensitivity of 96% and 90%, and a specificity of 100% and 79%, with an AHI of >15/h and >30/h, respectively. Because of the high demonstrated sensitivity and NPV, the study concluded that the Doppler radar system is suitable for use as a screening system for SAHS. The Doppler microwave radar system can be used as an alternative for apnea-hypopnea evaluation.

It is noteworthy that these results and other reports on microwave detection and monitoring for SAHS are attracting substantial attention on the application of microwave sensing in sleep research and sleep medicine. Accordingly, the promising results are helping to focus more research on the use of microwave radar techniques for remote contactless monitoring of respiratory movements during sleep [Tran et al., 2019] and to provide an important noninvasive method to observe respiratory activity of patients under general anesthesia during recovery following surgical procedures. See further discussions on these topics in sections that follow.

### 11.2.2 Real-Time Apnea-Hypopnea Event Detection

Recently, several additional noncontact microwave radar techniques were investigated to enhance their applicability, overcome practical limitations in stringent radar-subject distance requirements, and to facilitate real-time detection of apnea hypopnea (AH) events [Kang et al., 2020a, 2020b; Kim et al., 2019; Mlynczak et al., 2020; Weinreich et al., 2018]. For instance, a deep learning model for real-time AH event detection with impulse-radio ultrawide band (UWB) radar was described [Kwon et al., 2022]. UWB is a short-range wireless communication technique employing microwaves in the frequency band of 3.1–10.6 GHz. UWB radars have the advantages of superior penetrability, multipath resistance, and high spatial resolution.

In this case, a deep learning approach was adopted based on the convolutional neural network (CNN) concept in combination with a long short-term memory (LSTM) network. The CNN automatically filters out noise and extracts the valued features from the signal. Although CNN is useful in extracting patterns that appear as a local trend or appear the same in different regions of the time sequence, they are not suitable for capturing temporal dependencies. The LSTM network, which is a variant of a recurrent neural network (RNN), contains cyclical feedback designed to handle the temporal sequence. Thus, LSTM layers can encode relevant information of class-specific characteristics across time. Considering the temporal characteristics of radar signals (or images), a hybrid architecture combining CNN and LSTM was employed to detect SAHS using vital-sign sequences. Therefore, the project developed a deep learning algorithm to monitor sleep-related breath disorder using UWB radar sensors.

The performance of UWB radar with a hybrid CNN-LSTM architecture in detecting AH events was evaluated using the experimental setup shown in Figure 11.54 for UWB radar and PSG measurement. The UWB radar on a tripod set up on a bedside table was 1 m above the floor and was within a range of 0.5–2 m from a would-be human chest. The commercial UWB radar transmitter's center frequency was 7.29 GHz and had a bandwidth of 1.5 GHz. The receiver sampled the reflected signal at 23.328 GS/s and the radar signal was digitized at a speed of 20 fps. Subjects were 36 adult participants who were screened and judged as a

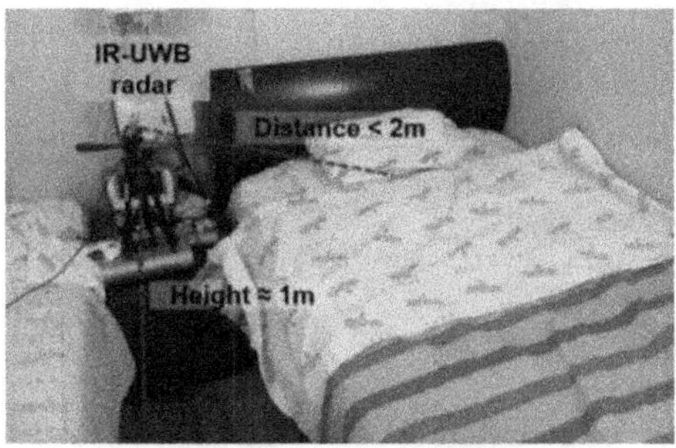


**FIGURE 11.54** Experimental setup for impulse-radio ultrawideband (IR-UWB) radar and polysomnography (PSG) measurement. IR-UWB radar on a bedside table is 1 meter above the floor and is less than 2 meters from the midline of a bed. (Kwon et al., 2022.)

high-risk group according to both the Berlin [Netzer et al., 1999,] and STOP-Bang questionnaires [Chung et al., 2016].

An important aspect of this project is to develop a diagnostic system for real-time SAHS monitoring and to detect individual AH events in real time and report the results as per segment classification performance. The system was able to determine whether an AH event occurred in the segment with only 20 seconds of radar image — a real-time performance. Moreover, a high-performance detection ability was maintained in various incidents where breathing occurs. Examples of synchronized UWB radar image, nasal airflow, and thoracic respiratory effort during a no-apnea event, central sleep apnea (CSA), obstructive sleep apnea (OSA), and hypopnea for 1 minute are shown in Figure 11.55. During a no-apnea event

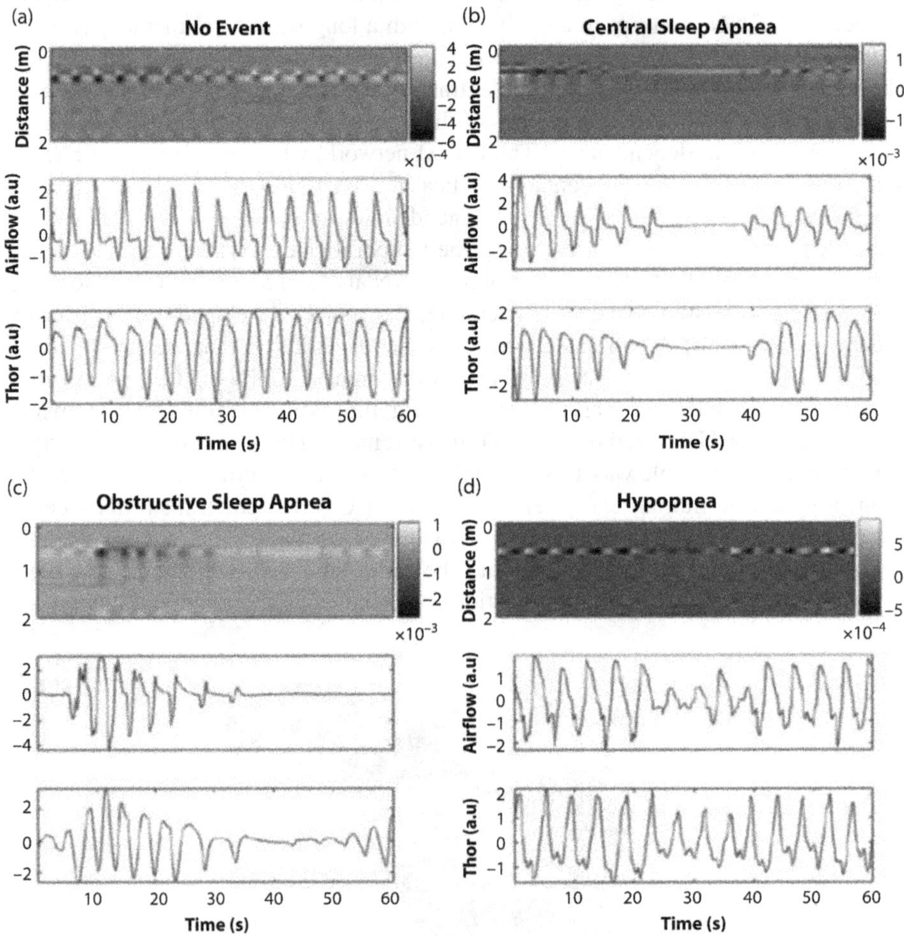


**FIGURE 11.55** Example of ultrawideband raw data and different normalized polysomnography (PSG) signals with normal breathing and three types of respiratory events: (a) normal without event, (b) central sleep apnea, (c) obstructive sleep apnea, and (d) hypopnea. The PSG signals were recorded at 500 Hz, and the UWB signals were sampled with 20 fps.

(See Figure 11.55[a]), respiratory activity that occurs at a distance of approximately 1 m in the radar image is clearly visible. In contrast, for central apnea (see Figure 11.55[b]), the airflow and thoracic waveforms disappeared, and at the same time, the breathing pattern in the radar image also disappeared. In the obstructive apnea (see Figure 11.55[c]) and hypopnea (see Figure 11.55[d]), obvious reductions are seen in the thoracic waveforms, and the contrast due to breathing in the radar image is diminished. The results clearly indicate the CNN-LSTM architecture is able to reliably detect AH events by using a single UWB radar. Figure 11.56 depicts the scatter plots of estimated AHI using UWB radar versus AHI obtained from the PSG reference for the entire sleep night. The Pearson correlation coefficient (N = 36) was 0.970 with $p < 0.001$. The Bland-Altman plot shows low mean biases (−1.983), and the limits of agreement (LoA) were −14.655 to 10.689. To verify the performance, the AHI of each hour was also computed from both the UWB radar and PSG for each participant.

Table 11.4 summarizes the SAHS severity classification and diagnostic performance for all test participants. The diagnostic performance was computed for AHI cutoffs of 5, 15, and 30 events/h. The average values for ACC, SENS, SPEC, PPV, and Kappa were 0.98, 0.97, 1.00, 1.00, and 0.96. The strong diagnostic performance and high AHI correlation of combining CNN and LSTM supports its potential use to screen for and continuously monitor SAHS severity with realistic bias toward UWB radar compared to the AHI of the PSG reference. But there are limitations, and it is incomplete for clinical apnea-hypopnea sleep study.

Appropriate assessment of each sleep stage is important for reliable AH event classification and AHI computation. The current UWB approach cannot account for sleep stages since it does not provide the essential brain electrical data. Likewise, body posture during sleep can affect sleep apnea severity and impact the occurrence of the AH events [Eiseman et al., 2012], which is not considered in the radar centered study. Nonetheless, some studies have suggested ways to provide sleep-stage classification

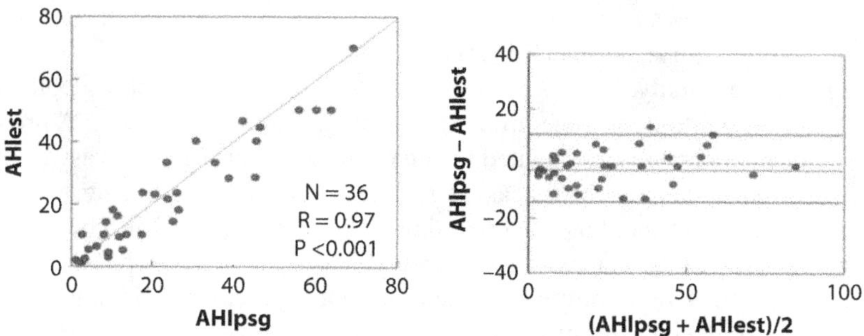


**FIGURE 11.56** Scatter plots of estimated apnea-hypopnea index (AHI) using impulse-radio ultrawideband radar versus AHI obtained from the polysomnography reference for (a) total sleep time from all subjects and (b) Bland-Altman plot for visualization of the agreement between the AHIs for total sleep time. The gray line indicates equality in (a). The gray bold line and dark lines in (b) indicate the average difference (bias) and the average ±1.96 standard deviation, respectively.

**TABLE 11.4**
**SAHS Severity Classification and Diagnostic Performance**

| UWB | | Estimated SAHS Severity | | | | AHI | | | | | |
|---|---|---|---|---|---|---|---|---|---|---|---|
| | | None | Mild | Moderate | Severe | Cutoff | ACC | SENS | SPEC | PPV | Kappa |
| | None | 0 | 0 | 0 | 0 | >5 | 1.00 | 1.00 | 1.00 | 1.00 | 1.00 |
| | Mild | 0 | 9 | 1 | 0 | >15 | 0.97 | 0.94 | 1.00 | 1.00 | 0.94 |
| | Moderate | 0 | 0 | 8 | 1 | >30 | 0.97 | 0.96 | 1.00 | 1.00 | 0.94 |
| | Severe | 0 | 0 | 0 | 11 | Ave | 0.98 | 0.97 | 1.00 | 1.00 | 0.96 |

*Abbreviations:* ACC = accuracy, SENS = sensitivity, SPEC = specificity, PPV = positive predictive value, and Kappa = Cohen's kappa coefficient.

and account for sleep posture based on UWB radar signals [Piriyajitakonkij et al., 2021; Toften et al., 2020]. Thus, combining these approaches to classify the AH events and compute the AHI could further enhance the usefulness of UWB radar with a CNN-LSTM architecture in SAHS classification and diagnosis.

### 11.2.3 Postsurgery and Anesthesia Recovery

Early and timely recognition of abnormal vital signs is a well-known marker of physiological decline. Thus, accurate continuous monitoring and early recognition of abnormal respiratory patterns can facilitate prompt intervention such as alerting the rapid response team, especially for in-hospital postsurgery and anesthesia recovery settings. Furthermore, it is noteworthy that patient comfort is an important factor in respiration monitoring as it can impact both accuracy and patient acceptance, thereby threatening the monitoring strategy under clinical settings. It may also be assistive for persons with minimized or limited body motions under caregiver situations. Respiratory movement detection based on radar appears to be the only observable body motion during coma [Kocur et al., 2017].

In a preclinical study, adult patients who underwent elective laparoscopic prostatectomy or hysterectomy were monitored after surgery during recovery. A prototype FMCW radar sensor was investigated to determine whether the noninvasive contactless radar system can reliably measure respiration in patients during mechanical ventilation (MV) and spontaneous breathing [van Loon et al., 2016]. The preclinical study involved adult patients who underwent elective laparoscopic prostatectomy or hysterectomy and were monitored after surgery during recovery. Nursing and medical staff were blinded to the study's measurement with FMCW radar.

The prototype radar sensor operated at a frequency of 9.5 GHz with a radiated power of 14 mW. The FMCW radar sensor in a small box (7.5 × 10 cm) was mounted to the ceiling above the patient's bed. Its output signals were recorded simultaneously with those from a reference standard. During MV, the reference standard was the pneumotachograph ventilator, which has an accuracy of ±1 breath/min.

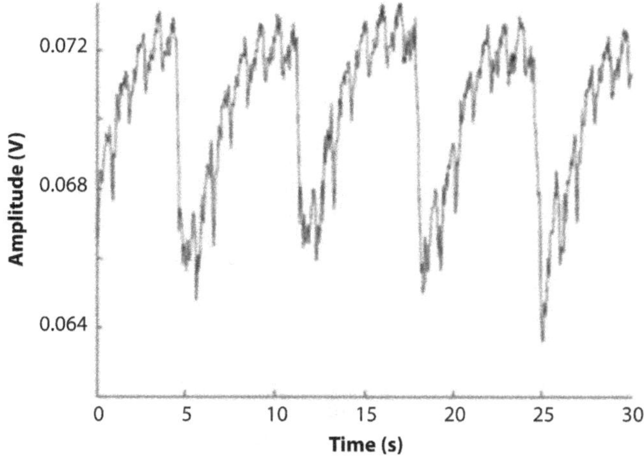


**FIGURE 11.57** Frequency-modulated continuous wave radar-detected patient breathing patterns with superimposed heartbeats during mechanical ventilation.

During spontaneous breathing, the reference standard was a capnograph, which has an accuracy of ±1 breath/min in the range 4–20 breaths/min. The capnograph measures the partial pressure of carbon dioxide ($CO_2$) in exhaled breath. A simple nonrespiratory movement artifact removal algorithm was installed to eliminate movement artifacts bias.

Figure 11.57 shows the FMCW radar detected patient breathing patterns. Although focus of this study is on detection of respiration during mechanical ventilation, as described previously, a heartbeat signal is typically superimposed on the respiration pattern, which demonstrates that the FMCW radar sensor is also capable of detecting heart rate remotely and noninvasively. An example of FMCW radar-monitored spontaneous breathing is illustrated in Figure 11.58, revealing different breathing patterns. Each inspiratory cycle is characterized by a first peak (chest-wall expansion during inhalation), followed by a curved peak (during exhalation).

A total of 796 minutes of observation time during mechanical ventilation and 521 minutes during spontaneous breathing were examined in 8 patients. The FMCW radar was able to accurately measure the respiratory rate in MV patients within the 95% LoA, but the accuracy decreased during spontaneous breathing. Considering the ability of the FMCW radar system to accurately track respiration during mechanical ventilation, it was suggested that the noninvasive contactless FMCW radar technique has the potential to support early recognition of physiological decline in spontaneously breathing patients in hospitals. However, further optimization of the signal-processing algorithms will be beneficial in tracking the respiration rate trend of spontaneously breathing postoperative patients recovering from general anesthesia on a minute-to-minute basis.

In a follow-up prospective observational study, 20 awake postoperative patients were monitored for 1203 minutes in a postanesthesia care unit with a median range of

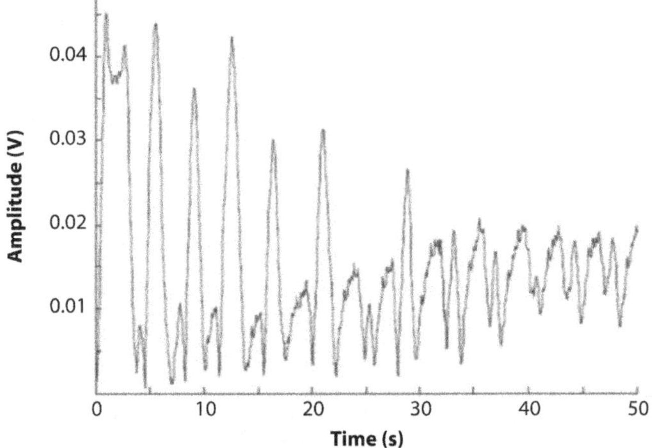


**FIGURE 11.58** Frequency-modulated continuous wave radar monitored spontaneous breathing showing different breathing patterns. Each inspiratory cycle is characterized by a first peak (chest-wall expansion during inhalation), followed by a curved peak (during exhalation).

61 minutes per patient. It was found that FMCW radar sensors adequately guided treatment decisions correctly 95% of the time [van Loon et al., 2018]. However, it deemed that the radar sensor was not sufficiently accurate to be introduced into clinical practice. The LoA did not fall within the predefined limits of ± 2 breath/min, based on clinical judgement. While the radar sensor's algorithms can provide information on patient-related movements, the study focused primarily on respiration rate determination from movement of the chest wall. Installation of software algorithms to mitigate spurious body movement-induced noise clutters such as hand gestures, leg motions, etc., could conceivably improve the precision and reliability in respiratory rate detection by better discrimination between respiratory and clutter signals. So that FMCW (and also other) radar sensors may become better suited to guide treatment decisions with enhanced accuracy and efficacy for postoperative patient monitoring.

### 11.2.4 Monitoring Diabetes-Related Physiological Signals

Diabetes is a chronic metabolic disease [Zimmet et al., 2014]. In persons with diabetes, the body either does not make enough insulin or cannot use the hormone as well as it should. It is the seventh leading cause of death in the U.S. and, in the last 20 years, the number of adults diagnosed with diabetes has more than doubled [CDC, 2022]. Records show that 422 million people suffered from diabetes worldwide, and 1.5 million deaths are directly attributed to diabetes each year [WHO, 2022]. Both the number of cases and the prevalence of diabetes have been steadily increasing over the past few decades. In persons with type 1 diabetes (T1D), their pancreas stops making insulin and would depend on daily subcutaneous administration of exogenous insulin. Common long-term complications of the disorder include cardiovascular functions and other major health problems requiring special medical attention, which increases as the patient's quality of life decreases. Monitoring of the disease is significant in preventing or minimizing complications. To date, blood glucose monitoring plays a central role in diabetes patient management. Even so, the invasive nature of current glucose meters is prone to cause pain and infections. Noninvasive blood glucose monitoring technology has become an active research topic in pursuit of a new and efficacious modality including the use of microwave technology [Bolla and Priefer, 2020; Tang et al., 2020].

Furthermore, a leading cause of mortality and morbidity in patients with diabetes is cardiovascular diseases and the pathophysiological impact is most often exhibited as coronary artery diseases. The damage can lead to abnormalities in left ventricular systolic and diastolic function and is observable through the features of heartbeat and ECG. They have important influences on heart rhythm that can occur at a relatively early stage of the disease [Bissinger, 2017; Cichosz et al., 2017; Jaiswal et al., 2014]. Thus, there is a link between these measurable physiological parameters and diabetes impaired cardiovascular anatomy and structures.

A systematic review of articles published between 2010 and 2020 evaluated evidence regarding use of contemporary wearable and mobile technology for monitoring physiological parameters that influenced the progression of diabetes, among other factors [Rodriguez-León et al., 2021]. The quality of the included studies was assessed using the Newcastle-Ottawa Scale. It was found that most of the heartbeat monitor studies applied some type of processing to the collected data, which consists of statistical analysis or machine learning for recognition and obtaining associations among health outcomes and diagnosing conditions related to diabetes. In a majority of the cases, the sensors used for physiological parameters embedded in these devices were not explicitly described. Suggestions for future work are to focus on validated clinical trials on the use of new wearable sensor technologies and the combination of mobile and clinical data in the enhancement of real-life diabetes applications with preventive or early warning strategies.

While the wearable and mobile devices are not yet extensively used in clinical settings, the technology has unique applications and capabilities in healthcare because of its capacity to gather, store, transmit, and also process the data in many cases. Both patients and physicians can pull these data for the assessment, treatment, and management of patient health conditions. Wearable heath trackers and smart watches can monitor physiological signatures such as heartbeat and ECG, which are parameters of particular interest for the monitoring of diabetes. Some of these physiological measurement capabilities can also be connected to smartphones. By processing the collected data generated by wearables, on-board or offline, it is possible to monitor the relevant parameters from patients with diabetes. The review highlighted current research achievements and limitations of noninvasive sensing systems in continuous monitoring, self-monitoring of the disease by patients, and at point-of-care and clinical settings. A salient feature of the wearables is their ability to monitor in a continuous, unobtrusive, and comfortable manner, without interfering with a person's daily life. The review on use of wearable and mobile devices for noninvasive monitoring of diabetes-related physiological parameters showed promise. Developments in the application of smart watches and health trackers can potentially benefit patients with diabetes. However, it concluded that the research is still in its early stages.

As demonstrated in this systematic review, the use of wearable and mobile devices for monitoring parameters that influence the progress of diabetes is an emerging field of study with promise, but none of the studies paid attention to common diabetes complications. Clinical trials were fairly limited or nonexistent in most of the studies. The lack of experimental details and descriptions in most studies made it difficult to judge the accuracy and precision or correlation between measurable physiological parameters and diabetes condition or the patient's health status. Some major gaps and limitations, despite its recent development, remain and include the creation or modification of existing models of wearable devices to render more reliable and robust sensors and the application of the appropriate technologies for sensing the pertinent physiological parameters. Accomplishing these challenges would require interdisciplinary teams for collaboration.

A more recent survey explored the potential of monitoring physiological parameters with wearable sensors to assist in the management of glucose levels and diagnosis and monitoring of complications in T1D [Daskalaki et al., 2022]. It explicitly inquired about whether the existing wearable, noninvasive sensors have the potential to improve how T1D is monitored and managed. It concluded that wearable sensors have the potential to augment T1D sensing with additional physiological information that can be monitored noninvasively and continuously. Moreover, in agreement with the aforementioned systematic review, despite the recent interest in wearable wireless technology for healthcare applications, the potential of wearables in T1D management has seen only limited research investigations to date. Only a few studies found in this comprehensive survey used wearable sensors and investigations of this technology in the field of T1D interventions are proceeding at a rather modest pace. Major hurdles stem from the complex relationships between the physiological signatures and glucose regulation and the data quality-related challenges such as accuracy and reliability, as they are monitored by existing wearable sensors.

For optimal T1D management, closed-loop functionality with accurate real-time sensing of essential physiological parameters could considerably improve health outcomes for persons with T1D, and it opens up new possibilities for early risk prediction and therapy. Note that current closed-loop or hybrid closed-loop (HCL) system settings only involve detailed information on the glucose, insulin, and factors affecting glucose such as food intake and exercise, without any physiological parameters. Indeed, a newly proposed single-page HCL data lists seven components including: (a) glucose metrics, (b) hypoglycemia, (c) insulin, (d) user experience, (e) hyperglycemia, (f) glucose modal-day profile, and (g) insight to help providers and patients interpret HCL data and take the necessary steps to improve glycemic outcomes [Shah and Garg, 2021].

As mentioned, features of the heartbeat and ECG are a set of physiological parameters of particular significance for the continuous monitoring of diabetes. For example, using wearable sensors and machine-learning algorithms, it was shown in a randomized cross-over study involving adult participants that the HR and blood glucose levels before exercise were predictors of exercise-induced hypoglycemia with 80–87% accuracy [Reddy et al., 2019]. Comparisons of persons who are healthy to those with T1D revealed several physiological functions or parameters are affected by T1D. Also, many studies have confirmed that T1D can impact cardiac function such as increased heart rate, reduced average heart rate variability, and modified heart rate variability features [Metwalley et al., 2018; Ribeiro et al., 2017; Silva et al., 2017; Wilson et al., 2017].

The potential of wearables and wireless technology in monitoring physiological signatures and diagnosis and management of T1D complications remains an area for further investigations, but with the aim of supporting research and development focused on enhancement of real-life T1D applications. However, there are significant challenges associated with measurement accuracy and reliability by mitigating noise clutter and artifacts. Furthermore, a prominent characteristic is the huge amount of data and extensive information generated by contemporary wearable and upcoming wireless sensors. Decision models and strategies are needed to incorporate and optimize them as inputs to achieve improved T1D interventions in the future.

Nonetheless, it is noteworthy that a recent paper described the result from a multicenter randomized controlled trial (RCT) comparing open-source automated insulin delivery (AID) system to sensor-augmented pump therapy (SAPT). Unregulated open-source AID systems are used by many T1D patients (see Figure 11.59). The patients included both children and adults. The AID system, also known as closed-loop system, consisted of a modified version of an Android algorithm paired with a preproduction insulin pump and continuous glucose monitor (CGM), which has an Android smartphone application as the user interface [Burnside et al., 2022]. AID is also known as a closed-loop system. A total of 97 patients (48 children and 49 adults) were randomly assigned (44 to open-source AID and 53 to the SAPT control group). The mean time in the target range increased from 61.2 ± 12.3% to 71.2 ± 12.1% in the AID group and decreased from 57.7 ± 14.3% to 54.5 ± 16.0% in the control group; age did not have any effect (P = 0.56). In both children and adults, the AID system was more effective for blood glucose control at 24 weeks (see Figure 11.60). The use of an open-source AID system resulted in keeping blood glucose in the target glucose range a significantly higher percentage of the time and it was efficacious and safe.

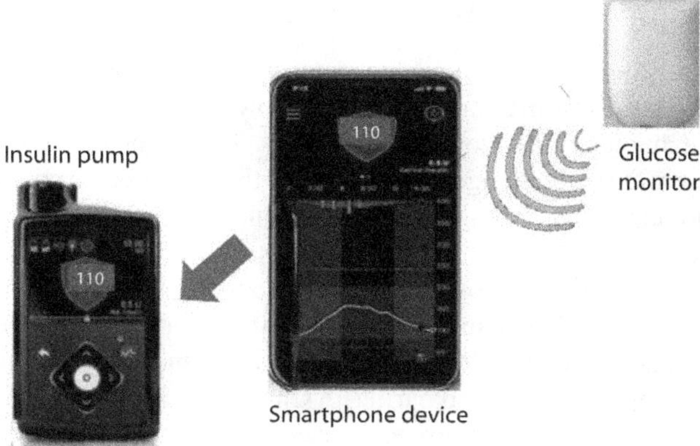


**FIGURE 11.59** Smartphone application in an automated insulin delivery (AID) system.

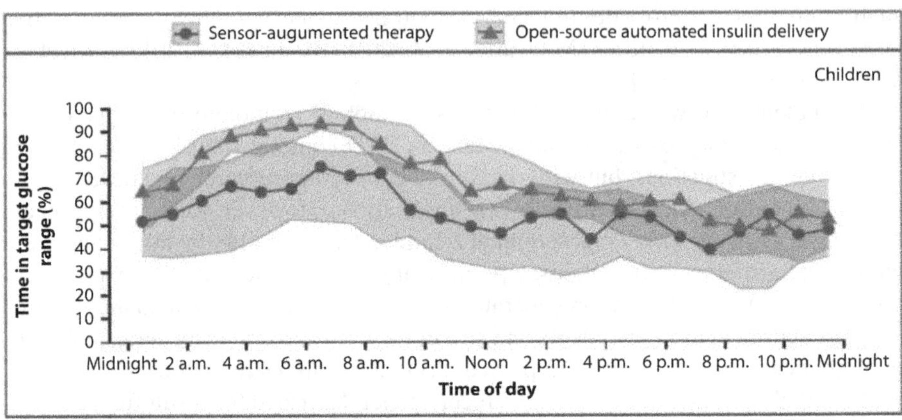


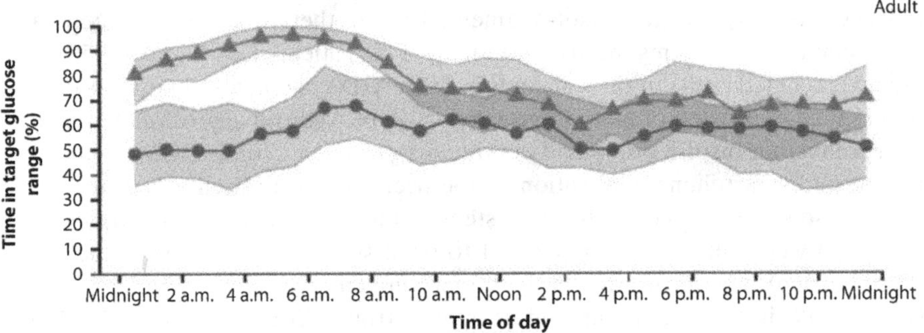


**FIGURE 11.60** The percentage of time children (a) and adults (b) in the two groups were in the target glucose range as measured by continuous glucose monitoring during week 22 and 23. Symbols represent hourly group median values, and shaded regions indicate the 25th and 75th percentiles.

### 11.2.5 Telehealth and Telemedicine for Diabetes Management

The concept of telemedicine was introduced more than 50 years ago through the use of wired telephones, facsimile machines, and slow-scan still images [Lin, 1999]. The enabling technology has grown considerably. Today, the terms telehealth and telemedicine are used interchangeably to refer to the use of electronic information and telecommunication technologies to support and provide long-distance clinical healthcare. Except in the case of telehealth, it also includes patient education and training of health promoters. A recent article advocating for prioritizing telehealth for people with diabetes [Hood and Wong, 2022] and a paper on using telehealth for diabetes self-management in underserved populations [Ju, 2020] remind the author of some related projects mentioned earlier in Chapter 2, Section 2.1. Nevertheless, it is interesting to note a 1997 systematic review of distance-medicine technology, in which clinical trials revealed significant improvements in outcomes in several disease groups including diabetes [Balas et al., 1997]. That was before the smartphone and real-time monitoring of glucose technology became generally available to connect and provide healthcare to people with diabetes remotely with better outcomes.

There are many reports documenting robust beneficial effects of telehealth for people with diabetes since then. Indeed, the effectiveness of telemedicine on diabetes management has been the subject of several meta-analyses based on RCTs. In one study involving 55 RCTs, compared to conventional in-person care, telemedicine was found to be more effective in improving treatment outcomes for diabetes patients [Su et al., 2016]. In another meta-analysis of 42 RCTs comparing the efficacy of telemedicine with typical in-person care in diabetes patients, the observed telemedicine interventions are more efficacious than conventional care in managing diabetes [Tchero et al., 2019]. Furthermore, studies have shown that telemedicine is not only instrumental in improving diabetes patient care, but also cost-effective for diabetes management and providing significant cost benefits [Lee and Lee, 2018; Tchero et al., 2019].

During the past two decades, there has been increasing interest in telehealth as a result of expanding technological capabilities and telecommunication infrastructures as well as accrued cost savings. A review of the global telehealth landscape noted that telehealth can improve both individual outcomes and the performance of health-care systems [Bhaskar et al., 2020]. Furthermore, the COVID-19 pandemic accelerated the growing trend [Choudhary et al., 2021; Danne et al., 2021; Julien et al., 2020; Scott et al., 2020; Tilden et al., 2021]. The COVID-19 pandemic may have underscored an option for the wider application of telemedicine in essential healthcare services. Available reports clearly suggest that people with diabetes view telemedicine as a viable and acceptable alternative to their healthcare. The transition to telemedicine in a pediatric diabetes care center happened easily and with high rates of patient satisfaction [Tilden et al., 2021]. Similarly, a review about telehealth based mostly in Europe also indicated high interest, and the benefits for people with diabetes included improved autonomy over the management of their condition and a substantial improvement in their quality of life [Choudhary et al., 2021]. Moreover, a survey showed a strong consensus among T1D respondents who found telemedicine consultations to be worthwhile [Scott et al., 2020].

It is noteworthy that a patient-centered telehealth program was recommended as having the potential to meet the needs of diabetes patients in underserved populations and to help to reduce healthcare and socioeconomic disparities [Agarwal et al., 2021; Ju, 2020; Hill et al., 2013]. The added value of telehealth could help achieve the missions of healthcare systems and providers in various ways. For example, by interacting with patients in their home environments, in which more than 99% of the diabetes self-management takes place, telehealth increases efficiency and efficacy. Its success is predicated on dedicated attention on health behaviors and practices of individuals in underserved populations. Therefore, the feasibility of using telehealth in underserved populations for diabetes self-management must first rely on assessed patient needs. With a clear understanding of the health behaviors and practices, telehealth programs may offer solutions to diabetes care through increased education. Nonetheless, diabetes self-management is a participatory activity and central to the well-being of patients with this chronic condition.

A few telehealth programs that offered diabetes care in rural communities have demonstrated positive patient outcomes in terms of self-reported blood glucose

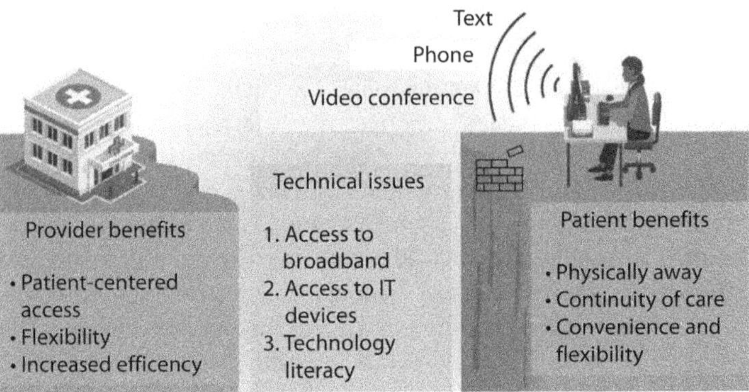


**FIGURE 11.61** The telehealth and telemedicine landscape: Access, barriers, modalities, and patient-provider benefits for successful implementation.

monitoring and have shown a positive correlation with the use of mobile technology such as effective weight management [DiFilippo et al., 2015; van Veen et al., 2019]. To improve diabetes outcomes among underserved patients, telehealth interventions and technologies need to adapt to the needs of individuals in the local communities and to develop optimal diabetes self-management behaviors to manage the lifelong disorder. An important coordinated effort needed to access telehealth diabetes self-management is the self-monitoring of blood glucose. Patients of low-income populations are aware of the importance of diabetes management but are hampered by various challenges [Cuevas et al., 2015; Hernandez et al., 2014; Onwudiwe et al., 2011]. The closed-loop functionality with accurate real-time sensing of essential physiological parameters may be assistive. In this regard, telehealth can be a platform to broaden access, increase use of diabetes-care services, and optimize health outcomes in all people suffering from diabetes. An encouraging development is that telehealth services for rural or underserved areas are offering patient access to healthcare professionals using smartphones and other devices with audiovisual capabilities. Thus, synchronous telehealth videoconferencing that helped to increase access to healthcare services are a viable strategy for improving health outcomes for patients in low-socioeconomic status populations (Figure 11.61). In addition to giving healthcare providers context to the realities of a patient's health and general condition, video calls with live messaging and content sharing including online sessions adds the capability to perform a visual medical consultation, review test results via screenshare capabilities, and perform limited physical examination. A successful telehealth and telemedicine operation requires the interactive participation of several key components: access to broadband Internet, Internet-capable devices, sufficient technology literacy, and the support of patient and healthcare providers.

## 11.3 MONITORING DRIVER VITAL SIGNS

Autonomous vehicles and driver assistance were mentioned previously as among the potential areas of application of wireless microwave sensors for short-range vital-sign tracking. Indeed, monitoring driver alertness, drowsiness, and stress has long been a subject of research interest especially for accident prevention [Béquet et al., 2020; Healey et al., 1999; Healey and Picard, 2005; Sun and Yu, 2014]. (Nearly 30 years after a failed startup attempt mentioned in Chapter 2.) Monitoring vital signs is critically important in the early detection of a patient's health or physiologic functional decline in hospital setting. Likewise, vital-sign monitoring has been explored along with opening and closing of one's eyes, head motion, and yawning among other indicators of alertness and/or drowsiness [Arakawa, 2021; Jacobé de Naurois et al., 2019; Jung et al., 2014; Murata et al., 2011; Sidikova et al., 2020].

At present, electric vehicles (EVs) are arising as a popular choice for energy-efficient and environmentally friendly forms of ground transportation compared to combustion engines. It is especially so in terms of greenhouse gas emissions over their lifetime compared to fossil fuel-powered vehicles. This trend is steering and accelerating the interest in instrumenting EVs so that they can monitor the driver's vital signs. Conceivably, the interest is facilitated by the EV's on-board capability to sense its ambient environment and road conditions, and the designs of autonomous driving systems to take over and navigate the vehicle safely while on the road.

In hospitals, a patient's vital signs are routinely monitored using wired bedside monitors for clinically significant changes in ECG, pulse rate, respiration, body core temperature, and blood pressure. In most cases, oxygen saturation ($SpO_2$) is included to assess the state of a patient, as illustrated in Figure 11.62. However, a noncontact and unobstrusive mode of operation for vital-sign monitoring is more amenable for drivers inside a vehicle's cabin.

There are several papers reviewing the unobtrusive monitoring techniques for use in the car's seat, safety belt, and steering wheel [Leonhardt et al., 2018; Sidikova et al., 2020; Wang et al., 2020]. Some potential locations may be identified for vital-sign sensing via radar sensors inside a car, including integration into the dashboard, safety belt, steering wheel, headrest, and backrest (see Figure 11.63). Reported examples involving wireless microwave sensing include the use of Doppler radar

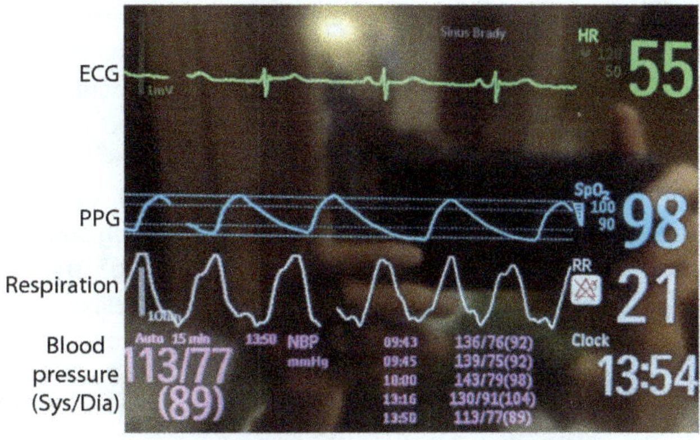


**FIGURE 11.62** Bedside monitor display of electrocardiogram (ECG, pulse or heart rate, HR), photoplethysmography (PPG), oxygen saturation ($SpO_2$), breathing (respiratory rate, RR), and blood pressure for a patient during postsurgery recovery in an actual hospital environment.

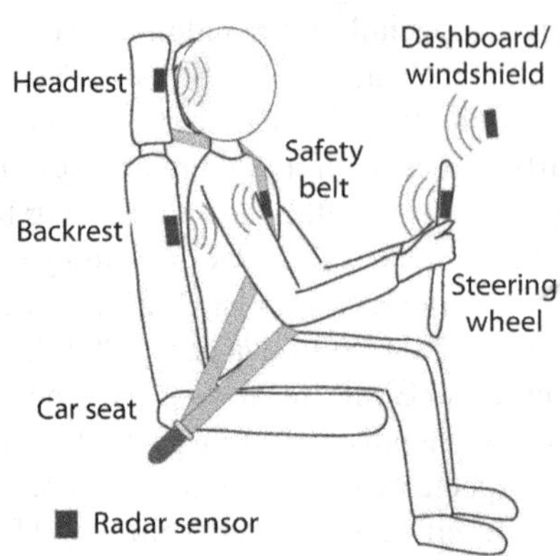


**FIGURE 11.63** Potential locations of radar vital-sign sensors inside a vehicle cabin.

sensors for monitoring vital signs while driving [Vinci et al., 2015] and a 24 GHz Doppler radar sensor installed in the backrest of the car seat [Lee et al., 2016]. The feasibility of heart and respiratory rate tracking was demonstrated using a UWB radar placed in the backrest of a car seat [Schires et al., 2018]. While those radar sensors work wirelessly, the in-car driver-monitoring systems relied on the body contact of the driver with the car seat.

For contactless unobtrusive applications, one study placed a 24 GHz radar system half a meter in front of the driver, with the antenna pointing directly at the thorax [Leonhardt et al., 2018]. Also, a novel system was proposed to monitor vital signs (HR and RR) in the presence of the driver's motion artifacts using a single-chip millimeter-wave (76–81 GHz) commercial FMCW radar sensor with two transmitting antennas and four receiving antennas configured for operation in TDM-MIMO mode [Wang et al., 2022]. The device can be mounted either on the windshield or beneath the steering wheel. The data processing system extracts from the body reflected signals which contain both the vital signals and motion artifacts. The motion artifacts are first removed by a motion compensation module, followed by the periodicity check to identify the portions with vital signals. Subsequently, the heartbeat and respiration signals are reconstructed by jointly optimizing the decomposition of all the extracted compound vital signals over different range-azimuth bins.

The system performance was evaluated in an actual driving environment. Figure 11.64 gives the reconstructed heartbeat and respiration signals, where all the bins that pass the periodicity check were used. Figure 11.65 shows the estimated vital signs and associated reference values for the 2-minute tests where it can be seen that even though there are large changes (caused by the uneven road during the driving tests), the estimation results match the reference data. The experimental results suggest that the proposed system can achieve a median error of 0.16 breath/min and 0.82 beat/min in 46 ms for RR and HR estimations. These results correspond to relative accuracies of 99.17% and 98.94%, respectively.

A recent paper described the use of noncontact in-vehicle driver vital-sign monitoring with a near-infrared (NIR) time-of-flight camera [Guo et al., 2022].

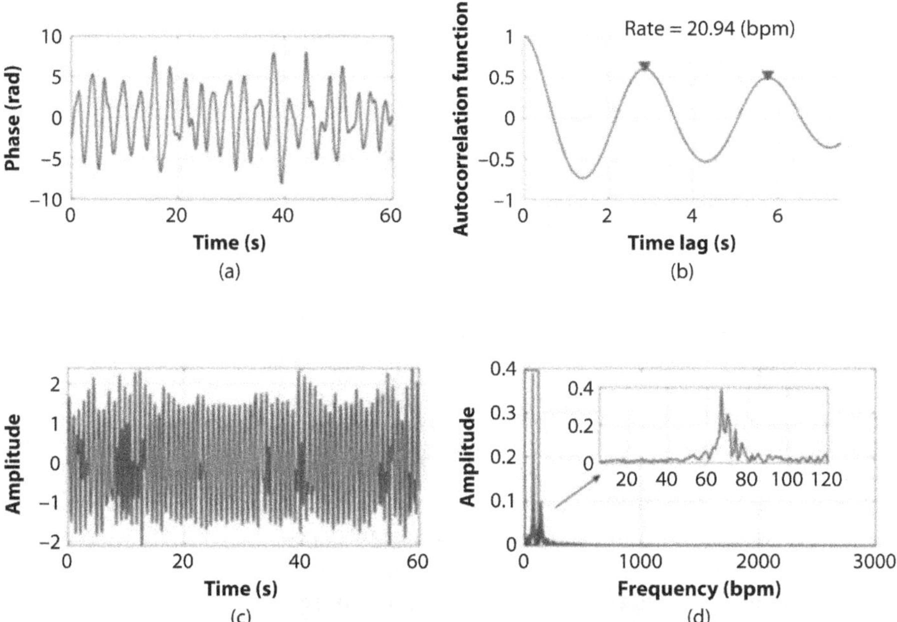


**FIGURE 11.64** Display of recovered vital-sign signals: (a) Estimated respiration signal, (b) autocorrelation function of the respiration signal, (c) estimated heartbeat signal, and (d) spectrum of heartbeat signal.

Figure 11.66 gives representative intensity and depth information obtained from the NIR camera while driving on a highway. Motions from both the driver and the road can produce artifacts that are several times greater than the HR signal. If left uncompensated, such artifacts would lead to inaccurate HR measurements (unwanted peaks in the frequency domain) (see Figure 11.66[b]). Nonetheless, the results showed reasonable rates of HR (above 70%) and RR (mean deviation of −1.4 breath/min) measurements under highway driving conditions can be extracted and the system could potentially be an enabler to drowsiness detection.

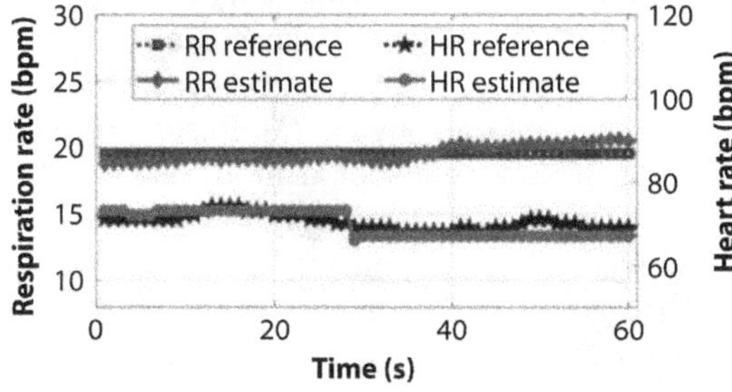


**FIGURE 11.65** Example of a single-chip millimeter-wave radar estimated result versus reference for HR and RR.

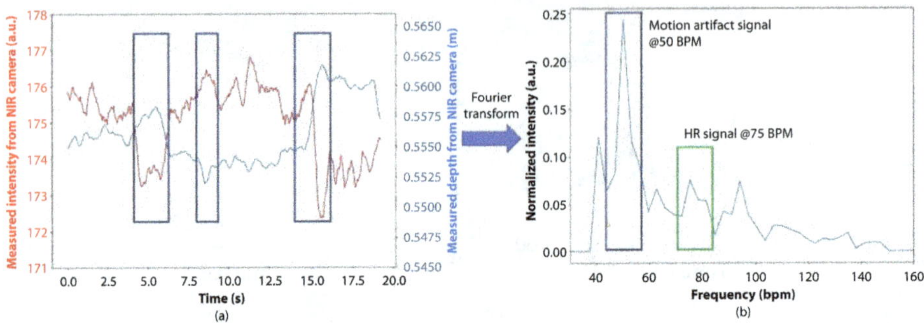


**FIGURE 11.66** Actual intensity (red) and depth (blue) obtained from NIR camera (a). Depth change induced by motion (blue rectangle) is inversely proportional to the intensity, which is a key source of errors in the HR reading. When motion clutters are present, they create noise frequency components that overwhelm the true HR signal (b). (From Guo et al., 2022.)

While some of the studies have involved participants in simulated driving and others in road tests, most of the studies are proof-of-concept investigations, albeit, in actual vehicle environments. Technologies for unobtrusive and contactless monitoring of vital signs are gaining increasing attention in recent years. However, unobtrusive and noncontact vital sign monitoring, especially using wireless microwave sensors for in-vehicle application continues as a research and development challenge. Nevertheless, to date, most research remains focused on sensor technology development for enhanced driving safety. The answers, in particular, to the questions of how wireless microwave sensors can be used for contactless unobtrusive in-vehicle health data acquisition and how the sensor-derived physiological data can be used to support driver and driving functions are still relevant and deserve greater attention in future research and development efforts.

Indeed, for autonomous driving with higher levels of automation in vehicles, the need for robust driver-monitoring systems increases. It becomes essential to ensure that the driver can intervene at any moment. Drowsiness and stress will remain the principal sources of driver distraction. Moreover, physiological state and medical condition represent significant risks for driver safety, including the ageing population. In this regard, a recent paper reported a portable cushion with multiple measurement modalities to monitor the heart and respiratory rates of a driver [Linschmann et al., 2023]. The four-sensor unit includes a capacitive ECG, reflective PPG, magnetic induction sensor for eddy current changes generated by respiratory lung-volume changes, and seismocardiography (SCG). Results of the preliminary study with 20 participants in a driving simulator demonstrated a 70% accuracy of the heart-rate estimates and a respiration rate of only 30% with errors of 2 breath/min.

Finally, it is noteworthy that the growing interest in monitoring the physiological state of drivers and driver assistance is drawing attention to the effect of mindless technologies on driving safety. The concept of "mindless" or "subtle" technology concerns the employment of technology or a strategy to perform the regulation and supervision functions that do not interfere with an ongoing task. Thus, the alertness or drowsiness management technologies and strategies on driving safety via contactless and nonintrusive monitoring may qualify or can be classified as mindless technology [Béquet et al., 2020]. It is conceivable that the effect of mindless technologies on driving safety may emerge as an important and complex topic. One question is: How much monitoring or supervision is necessary and/or appropriate? The topic could become acute as advanced driver-assistant systems (ADAS) are adopted by automobile manufacturers, aside from the growing need to monitor the physiological state of drivers to assist in the engagement of the ADAS system. Accordingly, further research are needed to better understand the effect of mindless technologies on driving safety.

## REFERENCES

Agarwal, S., Schechter, C., Gonzalez, J., Long, J. A., 2021. Racial-ethnic disparities in diabetes technology use among young adults with type 1 diabetes. Diabetes Technol. Ther., 23:306–13

Arakawa, T., 2021. Trends and future prospects of the drowsiness detection and estimation technology. Sensors (Basel), 21(23):7921. doi: 10.3390/s21237921

Ausherman, D. A., Kozma, A., Walker, J. L., Jones, H. M., Poggio, E. C., 1984. Developments in radar imaging. IEEE Trans. Aerosp. Electron. Syst., 20(4):363–400

Balas, E. A., Jaffrey, F., Kuperman, G. J., et al., 1997. Electronic communication with patients. Evaluation of distance medicine technology. JAMA, 278:152–159

Béquet, A. J., Hidalgo-Muñoz, A. R., Jallais, C., 2020. Towards mindless stress regulation in advanced driver assistance systems: A systematic review. Front Psychol., 11:609124

Berizzi, F., Mese, E. D., Diani, M., Martorella, M., 2001. High-resolution ISAR imaging of maneuvering targets by means of the range instantaneous Doppler technique: Modeling and performance analysis. IEEE Trans. Image Process., 10(12):1880–1890

Bhaskar, S., Bradley, S., Chattu, V. K., et al., 2020. Telemedicine across the globe position paper from the COVID-19 Pandemic Health System Resilience Program (REPROGRAM) international consortium (part 1). Front. Public Health, 8:556720

Bissinger, A., 2017. Cardiac autonomic neuropathy: Why should cardiologists care about that? J. Diabetes Res., 2017:537417. https://doi.org/10.1155/2017/5374176

Bolla, A. S., Priefer, R., 2020. Blood glucose monitoring- an overview of current and future non-invasive devices. Diabetes Metab. Syndr., 14(5):739–751

Burnside, M. J., Lewis, D. M., Crocket, H. R., et al., 2022. Open-source automated insulin delivery in type 1 diabetes, N. Engl. J. Med., 387:869–881

CDC, 2022. About diabetes. www.cdc.gov/diabetes/basics/diabetes.html. Accessed in October 2022

Chian, D. M., Wen, C. K., Wang, F. K., Wong, K. K., 2020. Signal separation and tracking algorithm for mulit-person vital signs by using Doppler radar. IEEE Trans. Biomed. Circuits Syst., 14(6):1346–1361

Choi, J. W., Yim, D. H., Cho, S. H., 2017. People counting based on an IR-UWB radar sensor. IEEE Sensors J., 17(17):5717–5727

Choudhary, P., Bellido, V., Graner, M., et al., 2021. The challenge of sustainable access to telemonitoring tools for people with diabetes in Europe: Lessons from COVID-19 and beyond. Diabetes Ther., 12:2311–327

Chung, F., Abdullah, H. R., Liao, P., 2016. STOP-bang questionnaire: A practical approach to screen for obstructive sleep apnea. Chest, 149(3):631–638

Cichosz, S. L., Frystyk, J., Tarnow, L., Fleischer, J., 2017. Are changes in heart rate variability during hypoglycemia confounded by the presence of cardiovascular autonomic neuropathy in patients with diabetes? Diabetes Technol. Ther., 19(2):91–95

Cuevas, H. E., Brown, S. A., García, A. A., Winter, M., Brown, A., Hanis, C. L., 2015. Blood glucose self-monitoring patterns in Mexican Americans: Further lessons from the Starr County Border Health Initiative. Diabetes Technol. Ther., 17(2):105–111

Dai, T. K. V., 2022. Remote Human Vital Sign Monitoring Using Multiple-Input Multiple-Output Radar at Millimeter-Wave Frequencies. PhD diss., University of Tennessee. https://trace.tennessee.edu/utk_graddiss/7348

Dai, T. K. V., et al., 2022. Enhancement of remote vital sign monitoring detection accuracy using multiple-input multiple-output 77 GHz FMCW radar. IEEE J. Electromagn. RF. Microw. Med. Biol., 6(1):111–122

Danne, T., Limbert, C., Puig Domingo, M., et al., 2021. Telemonitoring, telemedicine and time in range during the pandemic: Paradigm change for diabetes risk management in the post-COVID future. Diabetes Ther., 12:2289–2310

Daskalaki, E., Parkinson, A., Brew-Sam, N., Hossain, M. Z., O'Neal, D., Nolan, C. J., Suominen, H., 2022. The potential of current noninvasive wearable technology for the monitoring of physiological signals in the management of type 1 diabetes: Literature survey. J. Med. Internet Res., 24(4):e28901

DiFilippo, K. N., Huang, W. H., Andrade, J. E., Chapman-Novakofski, K. M., 2015. The use of mobile apps to improve nutrition outcomes: A systematic literature review. J. Telemed. Telecare., 21(5):243–253

Edwards, C., Almeida, O. P., Ford, A. H., 2020. Obstructive sleep apnea and depression: A systematic review and meta-analysis. Maturitas, 142:45–54

Eiseman, N. A., Westover, M. B., Ellenbogen, J. M., Bianchi, M. T., 2012. The impact of body posture and sleep stages on sleep apnea severity in adults. J. Clin. Sleep Med., 8(6):655–666

Fang, G. W., Huang, C. Y., Yang, C. L., 2020. Switch-based low intermediate frequency system of a vital sign radar for simultaneous multitarget and multidirectional detection. IEEE J. Electromagn. RF. Microw Med Biol., 4(4):265–272

Guo, K., Zhai, T., Purushothama, M. H., Dobre, A., Meah, S., Pashollari, E., Vaish, A., DeWilde, C., Islam, M. N., 2022. Contactless vital sign monitoring system for in-vehicle driver monitoring using a near-infrared time-of-flight camera. Appl. Sci., 12:4416. https://doi.org/10.3390/app12094416

Healey, J. A., Picard, R. W., 2005. Detecting stress during real-world driving tasks using physiological sensors. IEEE Trans. Intell. Transp. Syst., 6:156–166

Healey, J., Seger, J., Picard, R., 1999. Quantifying driver stress: Developing a system for collecting and processing biometric signals in natural situations. Biomed. Sci. Instrum., 35:193–198

Hernandez, R., Ruggiero, L., Riley, B. B., et al., 2014. Correlates of self-care in low-income African American and Latino patients with diabetes. Health Psychol., 33(7):597–607

Hill, J., Nielsen, M., Fox, M. H., 2013. Understanding the social factors that contribute to diabetes: A means to informing health care and social policies for the chronically ill. Perm. J., 17(2):67–72

Hood, K. K., Wong, J. J., 2022. Telehealth for people with diabetes: Poised for a new approach. Lancet Diabetes Endocrinol., 10(1):8–10

Islam, S. M. M., Boric-Lubecke, O., Lubecke, V. M., Moadi, A. K., Fathy, A. E., 2022. Contactless radar-based sensors: Recent advances in vital-signs monitoring of multiple subjects. IEEE Microw. Mag., 23(7):47–60

Islam, S. M. M., Boric-Lubecke, O., Lubekce, V. M., 2020. Concurrent respiration monitoring of multiple subjects by phase-comparison monopulse radar using independent component analysis (ICA) with JADE algorithm and direction of arrival (DOA). IEEE Access, 8(73):558–573

Jacobé de Naurois, C. J., Bourdin, C., Stratulat, A., Diaz, E., Vercher, J. L., 2019. Detection and prediction of driver drowsiness using artificial neural network models. Accid. Anal. Prev., 126:95–104

Jaiswal, M., McKeon, K., Comment, N., et al., 2014. Association between impaired cardiovascular autonomic function and hypoglycemia in patients with type 1 diabetes, Diabetes Care, 37(9):2616–2621

Ju, H. H., 2020. Using telehealth for diabetes self-management in underserved populations. Nurse Pract., 45(11):26–33

Julien, H. M., Eberly, L. A., Adusumalli, S., 2020. Telemedicine and the forgotten america. Circulation, 142(4):312–314

Jung, S. J., Shin, H. S., Chung, W. Y., 2014. Driver fatigue and drowsiness monitoring system with embedded electrocardiogram sensor on steering wheel. IET Intell. Transp. Syst., 8:43–50

Kagawa, M., Tojima, H., Matsui, T., 2016. Non-contact diagnostic system for sleep apnea-hypopnea syndrome based on amplitude and phase analysis of thoracic and abdominal Doppler radars. Med. Biol. Eng. Comput., 54(5):789–798

Kagawa, M., Ueki, K., Kurita, A., Tojima, H., Matsui, T., 2013. Non-contact screening system with two microwave radars in the diagnosis of sleep apnea-hypopnea syndrome. Stud. Health Technol. Inform., 192:263–267

Kang, S., Kim, D. K., Lee, Y., Lim, Y. H., Park, H. K., Cho, S. H., Cho, S. H., 2020b. Non-contact diagnosis of obstructive sleep apnea using impulse-radio ultra-wideband radar. Sci. Rep., 10(1):612

Kang, S., Lee, Y., Lim, Y. H., Park, H. K., Cho, S. H., Cho, S. H., 2020a. Validation of non-contact cardiorespiratory monitoring using impulse radio ultra-wideband radar against nocturnal polysomnography. Sleep Breath., 24(3):841–848

Kathuria, N., Seet, B. C., 2021. 24 GHz flexible antenna for Doppler radar-based human vital signs monitoring. Sensors, 21:3737

Kim, S. H., Geem, Z. W., Han, G. Y., 2019. A novel human respiration pattern recognition using signals of ultra-wideband radar sensor. Sensors, 19(15):3340

Kocur, D., Novák, D., Demčák, J., 2017. A joint detection, localization and respiratory rate estimation of multiple static persons using UWB radar. 18th IEEE International Radar Symposium (IRS), Prague, Czech Republic, pp. 1–11

Kwon, H. B., et al., 2022. Hybrid CNN-LSTM network for real-time apnea-hypopnea event detection based on IR-UWB radar, IEEE Access, 10:17556–17564

Laratta, C. R., Ayas, N. T., Povitz, M., Pendharkar, S. R., 2017. Diagnosis and treatment of obstructive sleep apnea in adults. CMAJ. 189(48):E1481–E1488. doi: 10.1503/cmaj.170296

Lee, H., Kim, B. H., Park, J. K., Yook, J. G., 2019. A novel vital-sign sensing algorithm for multiple subjects based on 24-GHz FMCW Doppler radar. Remote Sens., 11(10):1237

Lee, H., Kim, B. H., Park, J. K., Kim, S. W., Yook, J. G., 2020. A resolution enhancement technique for remote monitoring of the vital signs of multiple subjects using a 24 GHz bandwidth-limited FMCW radar. IEEE Access, 8:1240–1248. doi: 11.1109/ACCESS.2019.2961130

Lee, J. Y., Lee, S. W. H., 2018. Telemedicine cost-effectiveness for diabetes management: A systematic review. Diabetes Technol. Ther., 20:492–450

Lee, K. J., Park, C., Lee, B., 2016. Tracking Driver's Heart Rate by Continuous-Wave Doppler Radar. In Proceedings of the 38th Annual International Conference of the IEEE Engineering in Medicine and Biology Society (EMBC'16), Orlando, FL, USA, 16–20 August 2016

Leonhardt, S., Leicht, L., Teichmann, D., 2018. Unobtrusive vital sign monitoring in automotive environments-a review. Sensors (Basel), 18(9):3080. doi: 10.3390/s18093080. Open access

Li, C., Lubecke, V. M., Boric-Lubecke, O., Lin, J., 2021. Sensing of life activities at the human-microwave frontier. IEEE J. Microw., 1(1):66–78

Lin, J. C., 1999. Application of telecommunication technology to health-care delivery. IEEE Eng. Med. Biol. Mag., 18:28–31

Linschmann, O., Uguz, D. U., Romanski, B., Baarlink, I., Gunaratne, P., Leonhardt, S., Walter, M., Lueken, M., A portable multi-modal cushion for continuous monitoring of a driver's vital signs. Sensors (Basel), 2023 Apr 14;23(8):4002. doi: 10.3390/s23084002

Lv, W. W., Lin, X. H., Miao, J., 2021. Non-contact monitoring of human vital signs using FMCW millimeter wave radar in the 120 GHz band. Sensors, 21(8):2732. https://www.mdpi.com/1424-8220/21/8/2732

Metwalley, K., Hamed, S., Farghaly, H., 2018. Cardiac autonomic function in children with type 1 diabetes. Eur. J. Pediatr., 177(6):805–813

Mlynczak, M., Valdez, T. A., Kukwa, W., 2020. Joint apnea and body position analysis for home sleep studies using a wireless audio and motion sensor. IEEE Access, 8:170579170587

Murata, K., Fujita, E., Kojima, S., Maeda, S., Ogura, Y., Kamei, T., Tsuji, T., Kaneko, S., Yoshizumi, M., Suzuki, N., 2011. Noninvasive biological sensor system for detection of drunk driving. IEEE Trans. Inf. Technol. Biomed., 15:19–25

Netzer, N. C., Stoohs, R. A., Netzer, C. M., Clark, K., Strohl, K. P., 1999. Using the Berlin questionnaire to identify patients at risk for the sleep apnea syndrome. Ann. Internal. Med., 131(7):485491

Nosrati, M., Shahsavari, S., Lee, S., Wang, H., Tavassolian, N., 2019. A concurrent dual-beam phased-array Doppler radar using MIMO beamforming techniques for short-range vital-signs monitoring. IEEE Trans. Antennas. Propag., 67(4):2390–2404

Onwudiwe, N. C., Mullins, C. D., Winston, R. A., et al., 2011. Barriers to self-management of diabetes: A qualitative study among low-income minority diabetics. Ethn. Dis., 21(1):27–32

Peng, Z., Li, C., 2018. A short portable K-band 3-D MIMO radar with nonuniformly spaced array for short-range localization. IEEE Trans. Microw. Theory Techn., 66(11):5075–5086

Peng, Z., María Muñoz-Ferreras, J., Tang, Y., et al., 2017a. A portable FMCW interferometry raadar with programmable low-IF architecture for localization, ISAR imaging, and vital sign tracking. IEEE Trans. Microw. Theory Techn., 65(4)1334–1344

Peng, Z., Ran, L., Li, C., 2017b. A K-band portable FMCW radar with beamforming array for short-range localization and vital-Doppler targets discrimination. IEEE Trans. Microw. Theory Techn., 65(9):3443–3452

Penzel, T., Schöbel, C., Fietze, I., 2018. New technology to assess sleep apnea: Wearables, smartphones, and accessories. F1000Res., 7:413

Piotrowsky, L., Pohl, N., 2021. Spatially resolved fast-time vibrometry using ultrawideband FMCW radar systems. IEEE Trans. Microw. Theory Techn., 69(1):1082–1095

Piriyajitakonkij, M., Warin, P., Lakhan, P., Leelaarporn, P., Kumchaiseemak, N., Suwajanakorn, S., Pianpanit, T., Niparnan, N., Mukhopadhyay, S. C., Wilaiprasitporn, T., 2021. SleepPoseNet: Multi-view learning for sleep postural transition recognition using UWB. IEEE J. Biomed. Health Informat., 25(4):13051314

Reddy, R., Resalat, N., Wilson, L. M., Castle, J. R., El Youssef, J., Jacobs, P. G., 2019. Prediction of hypoglycemia during aerobic exercise in adults with type 1 diabetes. J. Diabetes Sci Technol., 13(5):919–927

Ren, L., Koo, Y. S., Wang, H., Wang, Y., Liu, Q., Fathy, A. F., 2015. Noncontact multiple heartbeats detection and subject localization using UWB impulse Doppler radar. IEEE Microw. Wirel. Compon. Lett., 25:690–692

Ribeiro, I. J., Pereira, R., Neto, P. F., Freire, I., Casotti, C., Reis, M. G., 2017. Relationship between diabetes mellitus and heart rate variability in community-dwelling elders. Medicina (Kaunas), 53(6):375–379

Rodriguez-León, C., Villalonga, C., Munoz-Torres, M., Ruiz, J. R., Banos, O., 2021. Mobile and wearable technology for the monitoring of diabetes-related parameters: systematic review. JMIR Mhealth Uhealth., 9(6):e25138

Sakamoto, T., Aubry, P. J., Okumura, S., Taki, H., Sato, T., Yarovoy, A. G., 2018. Noncontact measurement of the instantaneous heart rate in a multi-person scenario using x-band array radar and adaptive array processing. IEEE J. Emerg. Sel. Topics Circuits Syst., 8(2):280–293

Schires, E., Georgiou, P., Lande, T. S., 2018. Vital sign monitoring through the back using an UWB impulse radar with body coupled antennas. IEEE Trans. Biomed. Circuits Syst., 12:292–302.

Scott, S. N., Fontana, F. Y., Züger, T., Laimer, M., Stettler, C., 2020. Use and perception of telemedicine in people with type 1 diabetes during the COVID-19 pandemic—Results of a global survey. Endocrinol. Diabetes Metab., 4:e00180

Shah, V. N., Garg, S. K., 2021. Standardized hybrid closed-loop system reporting. Diabetes Technol. Ther., 23:323–331

Sidikova, M., Martinek, R., Kawala-Sterniuk, A., Ladrova, M., Jaros, R., Danys, L., Simonik, P., 2020. Vital sign monitoring in car seats based on electrocardiography, ballistocardiography and seismocardiography: A review. Sensors (Basel), 20(19):5699. doi: 10.3390/s20195699

Silva, A. K., Christofaro, D. G., Bernardo, A. F., Vanderlei, F. M., Vanderlei, L. C., 2017. Sensitivity, specificity and predictive value of heart rate variability indices in type 1 diabetes mellitus. Arq. Bras. Cardiol., 108(3):255–262

Su, W. C., Juan, P. H., Chian, D. M., Horng, T. S., Wen, C. K., Wang, F. K., 2021. 2-D self-injection-locked Doppler radar for locating multiple people and monitoring their vital signs. IEEE Trans. Microw. Theory Techn., 69(1):1016–1026

Su, D., Zhou, J., Kelley, M. S., Michaud, T. L., Siahpush, M., Kim, J., Wilson, F., Stimpson, J. P., Pagán, J. A., 2016. Does telemedicine improve treatment outcomes for diabetes? A meta-analysis of results from 55 randomized controlled trials. Diabetes Res. Clin. Pract., 116:136–148

Tang, L., Chang, S. J., Chen, C. J., Liu, J. T., 2020. Non-invasive blood glucose monitoring technology: A review. Sensors (Basel), 20(23):6925

Tchero, H., Kangambega, P., Briatte, C., Brunet-Houdard, S., Retali, G. R., Rusch, E., 2019. Clinical effectiveness of telemedicine in diabetes mellitus: A meta-analysis of 42 randomized controlled trials. Telemed. J. E. Health, 25(7):569–583

Thompson, C., Legault, J., Moullec, G., Baltzan, M., Cross, N., Dang-Vu, T. T., Martineau-Dussault, M., Hanly, P., Ayas, N., Lorrain, D., Einstein, G., Carrier, J., Gosselin, N., 2022. A portrait of obstructive sleep apnea risk factors in 27,210 middle-aged and older adults in the Canadian longitudinal study on aging. Sci. Rep., 12(1):5127

Tilden, D. R., Datye, K. A., Moore, D. J., French, B., Jaser, S. S., 2021. The rapid transition to telemedicine and its effect on access to care for patients with type 1 diabetes during the COVID-19 pandemic. Diabetes Care, 44:1447–1450

Toften, S., Pallesen, S., Hrozanova, M., Moen, F., Gronli, J., 2020. Validation of sleep stage classification using non-contact radar technology and machine learning. Sleep Med., 75:54–61

Tran, V. P., Al-Jumaily, A. A., Islam, S. M. S., 2019. Doppler radar-based noncontact health monitoring for obstructive sleep apnea diagnosis: A comprehensive review. Big Data Cogn. Comput., 3(1):121

van Loon, K., Breteler, M. J., van Wolfwinkel, L., et al., 2016. Wireless non-invasive continuous respiratory monitoring with FMCW radar: A clinical validation study. J. Clin. Monit. Comput. 30:797–805

van Loon, K., Peelen, L. M., van de Vlasakker, E. C., Kalkman, C. J., van Wolfswinkel, L., van Zaane, B., 2018. Accuracy of remote continuous respiratory rate monitoring technologies intended for low care clinical settings: A prospective observational study. Can. J. Anaesth., 65(12):1324–1332

van Veen, T., Binz, S., Muminovic, M., et al., 2019. Potential of mobile health technology to reduce health disparities in underserved communities. West J. Emerg. Med., 20(5):799–802

Vinci, G., Lenhard, T., Will, C., Koelpin, A., 2015. Microwave Interferometer Radar-Based Vital Sign Detection for Driver Monitoring Systems. Proceedings of the 2015 IEEE MTT-S International Conference on Microwaves for Intelligent Mobility (ICMIM), Heidelberg, Germany, 27–29 April 2015

Walker, J. L., 1980. Range-Doppler imaging of rotating objects. IEEE Trans. Aerosp. Electron. Syst., 16(1):23–52

Wang, G., Gu, C., Inoue, T., Li, C., 2014. A hybrid FMCW-interferometry radar for indoor precise positioning and versatile life activity monitoring. IEEE Trans. Microw. Theory Technol., 62(11):2812–2822

Wang, F. K., Horng, T. S., Peng, K. C., Jau, J. K., Li, J. Y., Chen, C. C., 2013. Detection of concealed individuals based on their vital signs by using a see-through-wall imaging system with a self-injection-locked radar. IEEE Trans. Microw. Theory Technol., 61(1):696–704

Wang, J., Karp, T., Munoz-Ferreras, J. M., Gomez-Garcia, R., Li, C., 2019. A spectrum-efficient FSK radar technology for range tracking of both moving and stationary human subjects. IEEE Trans. Microw. Theory Technol., 67(12):5406–5416

Wang, J., Warnecke, J. M., Haghi, M., Deserno, T. M., 2020. Unobtrusive health monitoring in private spaces: The smart vehicle. Sensors, 20;2442. https://doi.org/10.3390/s20092442

Wang, F., Zeng, X., Wu, C., Wang, B., Liu, K. J. R., 2022. Driver vital signs monitoring using millimeter wave radio. IEEE Internet Things J., (9)13, 11283–11298. doi: 10.1109/JIOT.2021.3128548

Weinreich, G., Terjung, S., Wang, Y., Werther, S., Zaffaroni, A., Teschler, H., 2018. Validation of a non-contact screening device for the combination of sleep-disordered breathing and periodic limb movements in sleep. Sleep Breath., 22(1):131138

WHO, 2022. Diabetes. World Health Organization. https://www.who.int/diabetes/action_online/basics/en/index3.html. Accessed in October 2022

Wilson, L. C., Peebles, K. C., Hoye, N. A., Manning, P., Sheat, C., Williams, M. J. A., et al., 2017. Resting heart rate variability and exercise capacity in Type 1 diabetes. Physiol. Rep., doi: 10.14814/phy2.13248

Xiong, J., Hong, H., Zhang, H., Wang, N., Chu, H., Zhu, X., 2020. Multitarget respiration detection with adaptive digital beamforming technique based on SIMO radar. IEEE Trans. Microw. Theory Technol., 68(11):4814–4824

Xu, Z., Chi, C., Zhang, T., Li, S., Yuan, Y., Wu, C. T. M., Chen, Y., Petropulu, A., 2022. Simultaneous monitoring of multiple people's vital sign leveraging a single phased-MIMO radar. IEEE J. Electromagn. RF Microw. Med. Biol., 6(3):311–320

Yavari, E., Gao, X., Boric-Lubecke, O., 2018. Subject count estimation by using Doppler radar occupancy sensor, in 40th Annual International Conference of the IEEE Engineering in Medicine and Biology Society, Honolulu, HI, 4428–4431

Yavari, E., Song, C., Lubecke, V. M., Boric-Lubecke, O., 2014. Is there anybody in there? IEEE Microw. Mag., 15(2):57–64

Yeghiazarians, Y., et al., 2021. Obstructive sleep apnea and cardiovascular disease: A scientific statement from the American heart association. Circulation, 144:e56–e67

Zakrzewski, M., Vehkaoja, A., Joutsen, A. S., Palovuori, K. T., Vanhala, J. J., 2015. Noncontact respiration monitoring during sleep with microwave Doppler radar. IEEE Sens. J., 15(10):5683–5693

Zhou, Y., Shu, D., Xu, H., Qiu, Y., Zhou, P., Ruan, W., Qin, G., Jin, J., Zhu, H., Ying, K., Zhang, W., Chen, E., 2020. Validation of novel automatic ultrawideband radar for sleep apnea detection. J. Thoracic. Disease, 12(4):1286–1295

Zimmet, P. Z., Magliano, D. J., Herman, W. H., Shaw, J. E., 2014. Diabetes: A 21st century challenge. Lancet Diabetes Endocrinol., 2(1):56–64

# Appendix

**TABLE A.1**
**Standard prefixes used with units of the international system (SI) of measurements**

| Prefix Name | Abbreviation | Magnitude |
|---|---|---|
| Atto | a | $10^{-18}$ |
| Femto | f | $10^{-15}$ |
| Pico | p | $10^{-12}$ |
| Nano | n | $10^{-9}$ |
| Micro | $\mu$ | $10^{-6}$ |
| Milli | m | $10^{-3}$ |
| Centi | c | $10^{-2}$ |
| Deci | d | $10^{-1}$ |
| Deka | da | $10^{1}$ |
| Hecto | h | $10^{2}$ |
| Kilo | k | $10^{3}$ |
| Mega | M | $10^{6}$ |
| Giga | G | $10^{9}$ |
| Tera | T | $10^{12}$ |

# Index

Note: Locators in *italics* represent figures and **bold** indicate tables in the text.

## D

## G



## H

## I



## J

## N

## O



## P

## Q



## R

## S

## T

## U



## V

## W



## X

For Product Safety Concerns and Information please contact our EU
representative GPSR@taylorandfrancis.com
Taylor & Francis Verlag GmbH, Kaufingerstraße 24, 80331 München, Germany

www.ingramcontent.com/pod-product-compliance
Lightning Source LLC
Chambersburg PA
CBHW060422220326
41598CB00021BA/2258